T0320778

Oxford Textbook of
Inpatient Psychiatry

OXFORD TEXTBOOKS IN PSYCHIATRY

Oxford Textbook of

Inpatient Psychiatry

EDITED BY

Alvaro Barrera

Consultant Psychiatrist, FRCPsych, Oxford Health NHS Foundation Trust and Honorary Senior Clinical Lecturer, University of Oxford, UK

Caroline Attard

Consultant Nurse and Head of Quality Improvement Programme, Berkshire Health Care Foundation Trust, UK

Robert Chaplin

Clinical Lead for Accreditation at the Royal College of Psychiatrists' Centre for Quality Improvement Royal College of Psychiatrists, London, UK

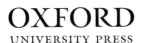

OXFORD

UNIVERSITY PRESS

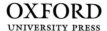

Great Clarendon Street, Oxford, OX2 6DP,
United Kingdom

Oxford University Press is a department of the University of Oxford.
It furthers the University's objective of excellence in research, scholarship,
and education by publishing worldwide. Oxford is a registered trade mark of
Oxford University Press in the UK and in certain other countries

First Edition published in 2019

Impression: 1

Published in the United States of America by Oxford University Press
198 Madison Avenue, New York, NY 10016, United States of America

British Library Cataloguing in Publication Data
Data available

Library of Congress Control Number: 2018960019

ISBN 978–0–19–879425–7

Printed in Great Britain by
Bell & Bain Ltd., Glasgow

Foreword

In nearly all health systems, hospital-based services remain an essential component of the care for people with acute and severe mental illnesses. The provision of modern, high-quality inpatient care for mentally ill patients requires a combination of clinical expertise and technical facilities plus a supportive environment and caring approach. The huge move in caring for mentally ill people in large psychiatric hospitals to community-based mental health services has probably preoccupied innovative thinkers over the last few decades. In many, but not all, countries, developments in inpatient care have somewhat lagged behind.

The editors and authors of the *Oxford Textbook of Inpatient Psychiatry* have done a wonderful job in providing a deep focus on the provision of care to the most severely ill patients. The Textbook includes an overview of the history of development hospitals for the mentally ill with Tom Burns' chapter richly highlighting some of the current thinking and challenges around the design of wards and hospitals. There is probably much to learn from countries that have really made an effort to improve patient experience. In Denmark, for example, Karlsson Architects together with Vilhelm Lauritzen Architects won the inaugural 2016 Architectural Review Healthcare Award for their design for the new psychiatric hospital in Slagelse (1). As clinicians, we should be both inspired and learn from this example, and encourage talented architects into the field, creating ever better environments for our patients.

It is hopefully obvious that the most severely ill and vulnerable patients deserve the very highest quality of clinical care, delivered by motivated, skilled, and caring teams—using the most effective and up-to-date treatments. This textbook provides a through overview of the treatments and critical processes and procedures involved in acute care. Years ago, we found that the majority of specific treatments used to treat acute illnesses on a general psychiatric ward had a reasonable evidence base (2). That was somewhat reassuring—but our aspirations should be much higher! It is clear that there is currently a great deal of innovation in this clinical area. New treatments are emerging—for example, rapid-acting antidepressants and neurostimulation—and the inpatient unit should be able to provide intensive, personalized treatments and high-quality care (3). There is also the enormous promise of remote observation using digital technologies, artificial intelligence, and machine learning which could (and should) have a transformational impact on patient care. These should allow us to move on from ancient, time-consuming, and inefficient approaches to patient observation, freeing staff time for therapeutic activity. But all these innovations will need thorough evaluation, to ensure that new approaches are evidence based. A further challenge for clinicians, architects, and funders, therefore, is how to design and resource buildings that have embedded capacity for research and are sufficiently flexible to allow the implementation of new therapies and procedures.

The *Oxford Textbook of Inpatient Psychiatry* also serves as a timely reminder that, at a time when the global burden of mental illness is increasingly recognized, we need to keep developing new treatments for the most severe illnesses as well as targeting the prevention and treatment of common mental disorders such as anxiety and depression.

Professor John Geddes
University of Oxford, Oxford, UK

REFERENCES

1. Astbury J. New psychiatric hospital in Slagelse, Denmark, by Karlsson and VLA. *Archit Rev* 2016;1435. https://www.architectural-review.com/buildings/new-psychiatric-hospital-in-slagelse-denmark-by-karlsson-and-vla/10014048.article.
2. Geddes JR, Game D, Jenkins NE, Peterson LA, Pottinger G.R, Sackett DL. What proportion of primary psychiatric interventions are based on evidence from randomised controlled trials? *Qual Health Care* 1996;5:215–217.
3. Feifel D. Transforming the psychiatric inpatient unit from short-term pseudo-asylum care to state-of-the-art treatment setting. *Psychiatry* (Edgmont) 2008;5:47–50.

Preface

This textbook has been written by practitioners for practitioners, keeping in mind the challenging work that frontline clinicians face daily. Its chapters have rather limited overlap among them, so they can be read in any order according to the demands faced by the reader. However, those readers seeking a more systematic approach can follow the order of its different sections.

The first section of the textbook provides an historical, conceptual, legal, as well as national and international context. Although a lot has been written about the big asylums now extinct in the UK, less has been said about the units built in the last few decades, with regard to their design, aspirations, and functioning; this section offers an overview of this area. The second section focuses on the crucial area of multidisciplinary team work and team leadership, including senior nursing roles such as that of the modern matron and the ward manager. Crucially related, this section also includes chapters on occupational health and the interface with community services.

The third section addresses medical aspects of inpatient care not from a traditional disorder-focused approach, but from the point of view of the dilemmas faced in clinical practice, including initial assessments, ward rounds, and the discharge process. These are covered along with highly relevant issues such as physical health care, common adverse reactions to medication, the management of substance misuse and personality disorders on inpatient wards, electroconvulsive therapy, autoimmune-related psychosis, as well as the assessment and management of violence and self-neglect. Connected with the latter, the work of rehabilitation wards is discussed here. This section closes with a chapter on clinical pharmacy, as the growing complexity of pharmacological treatments, with issues such as plasma levels, drug interactions, and non-adherence, makes it crucial for the safe running of wards.

The fourth section of the textbook covers highly relevant aspects involved in the nursing care of people in inpatient wards, including some of the daily ward processes, the all-important nursing observations, the Safewards initiative, the management of the risk of suicide, as well as the challenging topic of serious incidents and team debriefing and support. Fittingly, working with relatives and friends and the accreditation process conclude this section.

Section 5 provides an overview of the much-needed psychological work in any modern inpatient unit. The National Institute for Health and Care Excellence (NICE) has recommended several psychological interventions for severe mental health disorders so it seems unnecessary to have to argue for the importance of this section.

Section 6 returns to the daily challenges faced by teams working at the coalface, namely, those posed by the increasingly acknowledged diversity of the individuals admitted to inpatient wards, and the crucial role of advocacy on behalf of people when they are at their most vulnerable. Also, of crucial importance, this is followed by a chapter on supporting staff needs. Finally, in Section 7, the textbook comes to an end with a discussion of intensive care psychiatric units, eating disorders wards, child and adolescent units, and older adult wards, all with their specific characteristics and challenges.

This book is not organized along traditional diagnostic boundaries or written from an exclusively academic perspective. Instead, it has been developed out of the need to communicate with and be relevant to clinicians and managers who face, not uncommonly, dramatic dilemmas in their daily clinical practice.

Contents

SECTION 4
Nursing aspects

SECTION 5
Psychological aspects

SECTION 6
Diversity, advocacy, staffing issues

SECTION 7
Specialist services across the life span

Abbreviations

5-HT	5-hydroxytryptamine
ADHD	attention deficit hyperactivity disorder
AMHT	adult mental health team
AIMS	Accreditation for Inpatient Mental Health Services
AMHP	Approved Mental Health Practitioner
APA	American Psychiatric Association
ASD	autism spectrum disorder
BME	black and minority ethnic
BMI	body mass index
BPD	borderline personality disorder
C&R	control and restraint
CAMHS	child and adolescent mental health services
CBT	cognitive behavioural therapy
CBT-E	cognitive behavioural therapy for eating disorders
CCG	Clinical Commissioning Group
CI	confidence interval
CIWA-Ar	Clinical Institute Withdrawal Assessment for Alcohol, revised
CMHP	College of Mental Health Pharmacy
CPA	Care Programme Approach
CQC	Care Quality Commission
CTO	community treatment order
CVD	cardiovascular disease
DKA	diabetic ketoacidosis
DM	diabetes mellitus
DoLS	Deprivation of Liberty Safeguards
DTC	Drugs and Therapeutics Committee
ECG	electrocardiographic/electrocardiogram
ECHR	European Convention on Human Rights
ECT	electroconvulsive therapy
ECTAS	Electroconvulsive Therapy Accreditation Service
EEG	electroencephalographic/electroencephalogram
EPSE	extrapyramidal side effect
EU	European Union
FACT	flexible assertive community treatment
GABA	gamma aminobutyric acid
GP	general practitioner
HbA1c	glycated haemoglobin
IM	intramuscular
IMCA	Independent Mental Capacity Advocate
IMHA	Independent Mental Health Advocate
LGI	leucine-rich glioma-inactivated 1 protein
LPA	Lasting Power of Attorney
MAOI	monoamine oxidase inhibitor
MARSIPAN	Management of Really Sick Patients with Anorexia Nervosa
MCA	Mental Capacity Act 2005
MDMA	3,4-methylenedioxymethamphetamine
MDT	multidisciplinary team
MHA	Mental Health Act 1983 (amended 2007)
MHAA	Mental Health Act Administrator
MI	medicines information
MMT	medicines management technician
MOHO	model of human occupation
MRHA	Medicines and Healthcare products Regulatory Agency
MSO	Medication Safety Officer
NAPICU	National Association of Psychiatric Intensive Care and Low Secure Units
NC	nurse consultant
NG	nasogastric
NHS	National Health Service
NICE	National Institute for Health and Care Excellence
NJBM	*Not Just Bricks and Mortar*
NMC	Nursing and Midwifery Council
NMDAR	*N*-methyl-D-aspartate receptor
NMP	non-medical prescriber
NMS	neuroleptic malignant syndrome
NR	nearest relative
NSAb	neuronal cell surface antibody
OT	occupational therapist/therapy
PD	personality disorder
PICU	psychiatric intensive care unit
PMVA	prevention and management of violence and aggression
POM	patient's own medication
POMH-UK	Prescribing Observatory for Mental Health-UK
PRN	*pro re nata* (as required)
PTSD	post-traumatic stress disorder
RC	Responsible Clinician
RCT	randomized controlled trial
SIADH	syndrome of inappropriate antidiuretic hormone secretion
SMI	severe mental illness
SOAD	Second Opinion Appointed Doctor
SSRI	selective serotonin reuptake inhibitor
T2DM	type 2 diabetes mellitus
TSMH	Tribunal Service Mental Health
UNCRPD	United Nations Convention on the Rights of Persons with Disabilities
VGKC	voltage-gated potassium channel

Contributors

Caroline Attard Consultant Nurse and Head of Quality Improvement Programme, Berkshire Health Care Foundation Trust, UK

Agnes Ayton Consultant Psychiatrist and Medical Lead, Warneford Hospital, Oxford, UK

Tomasz Bajorek Consultant Psychiatrist, John Radcliffe Hospital, Consultant Liaison Psychiatrist, Psychological Medicine Service, Oxford University Hospitals NHS Foundation Trust, Oxford, UK

Theodoros Bargiotas Consultant Psychiatrist, MSc, Oxford Health NHS Foundation Trust, UK

Ian Barkataki Clinical Psychologist, University of Bristol, UK

Alvaro Barrera Consultant Psychiatrist, FRCPsych, Oxford Health NHS Foundation Trust and Honorary Senior Clinical Lecturer, University of Oxford, UK

Sophie Behrman Honorary Clinical Research Fellow, Oxford Health NHS Foundation Trust, UK

German E. Berrios Emeritus Professor, Department of Psychiatry, University of Cambridge, Addenbrooke's Hospital, Cambridge, UK

Sandeep Bhatti Lead Clinical Pharmacist, Oxford Health NHS Foundation Trust, UK

Gwen Bonner Clinical Director, Berkshire Health Care Foundation Trust, UK

Rachel Brown Clinical Lead Pharmacist—Medicines Information and Evidence Based Medicine, Oxford Health NHS Foundation Trust, UK

Tom Burns Emeritus Professor, Department of Psychiatry, University of Oxford, Oxford, UK

Catriona Canning Senior Quality Improvement Practitioner, Oxford Health NHS Foundation Trust, UK

Julie Chalmers Consultant Psychiatrist, The Elms Centre, Banbury, and Honorary Senior Clinical Lecturer, University of Oxford, UK

Robert Chaplin Clinical Lead for Accreditation at the Royal College of Psychiatrists' Centre for Quality Improvement, Royal College of Psychiatrists, London, UK

Gail Critchlow Consultant Psychiatrist, Oxford Health NHS Foundation Trust, UK

Dorcas Dan-Cooke Ward Manager, Oxford Health NHS Foundation Trust, UK

Karen Dauncey Consultant Psychiatrist, Oxford Health NHS Foundation Trust, UK

Lara Freeman Lead Occupational Therapist, Oxford Health NHS Foundation Trust, UK

Valeria Frighi Consultant Endocrinologist, Department of Psychiatry, University of Oxford, Oxford, UK

Jonathan Gibbons Occupational Therapist, Warneford Hospital, Oxford Health NHS Foundation Trust, UK

Georga Godwin Consultant Solicitor, UK

Jonathan Hafferty Specialty Registrar in Forensic Psychiatry, Oxford Health NHS Foundation Trust and Clinical Research Fellow, University of Edinburgh

Derek Hammond Adult Acute Operational Lead, Worcestershire Health and Care NHS Trust, UK

Jean Hammond Director of Clinical Services, Priory Hospital Woodbourne, Birmingham, UK

Anthony James Consultant Child and Adolescent Psychiatrist, Highfield Unit and Honorary Senior Lecturer, University of Oxford, Department of Psychiatry, Warneford Hospital, Oxford, UK

Claudia Kustner Clinical Psychologist, Berkshire Health Care Foundation Trust, UK

Belinda Lennox Associate Professor and Clinical Senior Lecturer, Department of Psychiatry, University of Oxford, Oxford, UK

Orla Macdonald Lead Research Pharmacist, Oxford Health NHS Foundation Trust, UK

Michelle Mbayiwa Modern Matron, Berkshire Health Care Foundation Trust, UK

Sue McLaughlin Deputy Director of Nursing, Berkshire Health Care Foundation Trust, UK

Andrew Molodynski Consultant Psychiatrist, Oxford Health NHS Foundation Trust and Honorary Senior Lecturer, Oxford University, Oxford, UK

Nicki Moone Senior Lecturer, College of Nursing Midwifery and Healthcare, University West London, UK

Christopher Morton Social Worker, Oxford Health NHS Foundation Trust, UK

Brian Murray Consultant Older Adult Psychiatry, Oxford Health NHS Foundation Trust, Aylesbury, UK

Arabella Norman-Nott Consultant Psychiatrist, Oxford Health NHS Foundation Trust, UK

Janet Patterson Consultant Psychiatrist, Oxford Health NHS Foundation Trust, UK

Steve Pearce Consultant Psychiatrist, Oxford Health NHS Foundation Trust, UK

Alyson Price Modern Matron and Senior Lecturer, Prospect Park Hospital, Reading, Berkshire, UK

David Price Department of Mental Health Social Work & Interprofessional Learning, Middlesex University, London, UK

Helen Robson Nurse Consultant, Berkshire Health Care Foundation Trust, UK

Louise Ross Clinical Psychologist, Avon and Wiltshire Mental Health Partnership NHS Trust, UK

Ashley Rule Consultant Psychiatrist, Oxford Health NHS Foundation Trust, UK

Emad Sidhom Specialty Doctor, Ashurst Ward PICU, UK

Mark Toynbee Academic Clinical Fellow, Department of Psychiatry, University of Oxford, Oxford, UK

Katalin Walsby Ward Manager, Learning Disabilities, Berkshire Health Care Foundation Trust, UK

Rose Warne Clinical Director in Patient Services, Berkshire NHS Foundation Trust, UK

David Welchew Consultant Psychiatrist, Oxford Health NHS Foundation Trust, UK

Dan White Specialist Clinical Pharmacist, BABCP accredited CBT Psychotherapist, Oxford Health NHS Foundation Trust, UK

SECTION 1
The context of acute inpatient psychiatric care

1

Historical and conceptual aspects

German E. Berrios

Introduction

'Inpatient psychiatric care' names a variety of modes of managing (caring, helping, treating, curing, etc.) persons who complain/exhibit experiences and behaviours considered by most current experts as (a) abnormal/deviant and (b) the expression of a (brain) disease (1, 2).

Writing on the history of 'inpatient psychiatric care' is difficult because of the periodic changes in meaning suffered by concepts such as 'treatment', 'experiences', 'behaviours', 'brain disease', 'madness', 'inpatient', 'recovery', etc. This variation can be dealt with by assuming that only current definitions and meanings are true. First chapters in clinical textbooks and grant applications are often based on this (anachronistic) assumption. These writings have little to contribute to historical understanding; indeed, they misrepresent the historical record.

Historiography of change

The anachronistic assumption is based on the belief that: (a) 'madness' names an object that has remained unchanged (invariant) throughout the centuries; (b) the current method of studying madness is the only one capable of uncovering its truth; and (c) past accounts of madness can be divided into those adumbrating the current truth ('pioneers') and the (erroneous) rest.

'Object invariance' was once central to Christian historiography according to which the world in toto was created by God as it is (3). The secularization of thinking in the West (4–8) led during the eighteenth century to the development of 'profane' historiographies that tried to explain the origin of man and his world without making use of 'Genesis 1:1–2:25'. Efforts to find new answers led to the gradual construction of the social and human sciences (9–11). As part of the process of re-examining traditional concepts, the old ontological (*more botanico*) view of disease (12) was replaced by a more flexible physiological view which Alienists, in turn, reinterpreted as 'psychological' by the end of the nineteenth century (13). At its widest and most productive, this view allowed for the coexistence of interacting narratives which sought to clarify not only the brain localization but also the meaning of madness.

From then on, the historiography of madness becomes fragmented according to countries. In the US, a period of interest in the meaning of madness (Freudianism) was followed by the current neurobiological fashion. European nations influenced by American psychiatry (e.g. Great Britain) followed suit; other, with strong national traditions of their own (e.g. France, Germany, and Italy) resisted for a time but eventually were forced to adopt the *Diagnostic and Statistical Manual of Mental Disorders* (*DSM*) system and its assumption that mental disorders are but 'natural kinds' (i.e. natural objects with invariant ontology) (14).

However, the fact that the neuroscientific basis of the *DSM* system must countenance Darwinian evolutionism suggests that the *DSM* system accepts that mental disorders are susceptible to biological evolution (change) over time. Its 'object invariance', therefore, is different from that of conventional 'Creationism' (15–17). Acceptance of Darwinian change, leads to two conclusions: (a) psychopathological descriptions and associated neuroscientific accounts will become blurred over the centuries and will need periodical updating, and (b) secular changes in the profile of madness will cause shifts in the content of 'inpatient' treatment. This chapter will deal with the second conclusion.

Historical background

During the nineteenth century, (a) there was an increase in the number of mental asylums (i.e. physical spaces for storage and/or care of sufferers) and (b) the process of medicalization of madness was completed (18). This made possible the formation of cohorts of patients with similar complaints, the development of descriptive psychopathology, advances in classification, and the professionalization of alienism as a medical enterprise.

Construction of alienism (psychiatry)

Each European country professionalized alienism at a different pace and with different resources. By the second half of the nineteenth century, England, Germany, France, Italy, etc. had all founded professional societies and journals and started training procedures for alienists. In spite of interruptions by wars and other conflicts, exchanges between nations continued and by the 1890s, psychiatric textbooks and classifications in the main European countries carried similar information.

To discharge their duties, alienists (or mad-doctors, as they were called) created physical, social, and legal spaces. After the 1820s, alienists participated in all national debates relating to lunacy legislation and to the housing and management of the insane (19, 20). In the asylums themselves, hierarchies became established with doctors at the top, followed by keepers (later called mental nurses), and supporting staff and the 'inmates' at the bottom (21). To facilitate patient control, functional classifications were created: public versus private, male versus female, agitated versus quiet, acute versus chronic, rational versus irrational, continent versus incontinent, epileptic versus non-epileptic, organic versus functional, criminal versus non-criminal, etc., and these categories influenced asylum architecture (22). By accumulating ever-growing cohorts of chronic patients and making possible regular postmortem examinations (23), asylums contributed to strengthening the organic (medical) theory of madness (24).

Asylum building was mostly governed by financial convenience. For example, English counties shared costs by building asylums on territorial boundaries; and regardless of the local weather, asylums in the colonies were often built on plans used in the metropolis (25). Fashion was also influential and some asylums followed the shape and ideology of Bentham's panopticon (26). Alienists worked in complex social and political contexts and skilfully used the resources available. In Roman Catholic countries, general hospitals and mental asylums were run by religious congregations (27). Frictions developed when (as happened in France) the alienist in charge was not religious and objected to practices such as regular prayer, over-modest clothing, and other religious duties. Similar frictions developed in the interface between psychiatry and the law. Insanity and dementia were traditional legal categories and lawyers used simple tests for them (28). Alienists had a less black-and-white view of such disorders and on occasions this caused major disagreement (29).

The fragmentation of madness

The nineteenth century inherited Cullen's 1785 claim (30) that from an aetiological viewpoint the Vesaniæ (insanities) were a form of neuroses, that is, 'disorders of the sense and movement of the nervous system without fever or focal lesion' (p. 182). Madness was just another bodily disease. This shaped the nineteenth-century concepts of madness and provided the criterion for the construction of neurology as the medical specialism in charge of 'neuroses' with focal brain lesions such as Parkinson's disease or multiple sclerosis (31). The original large class of 'Cullean neuroses' was gradually eroded and by the end of the nineteenth century it only included the insanities, hypochondriasis, hysteria, anxiety disorders, obsessional–compulsive disease, neurotic depressions, and Raynaud's phenomenon. In due course, the insanities themselves were reconceptualized as 'psychoses' (32) and removed from the group. From then on, the 'neuroses' were conceived as mere functional diseases, the expression of 'nervous irritation' (33, 34). Freud then suggested that the neuroses were symbolic expressions of a psychological conflict (31).

During the nineteenth century, the old concept of madness (insanity, lunacy, alienation, distraction, *vesania*, etc.) was changed into that of 'psychosis'. The word had already been in use since the early 1800s to name the subjective component of any experience. After the 1850s, it started to be used to name conditions characterized by hallucinations, delusions, mental confusion, irrationality, thought disorder, etc. (35). The new psychoses were soon classified as functional versus organic, endogenous versus exogenous, acute versus chronic, etc. If the symptoms listed previously were seen in the wake of a physical disease (such as infection, brain tumour, stroke, drug-induced state, alcoholism, neurosyphilis, etc.), the psychosis was called organic; if no organic basis could be identified (as in schizophrenia, mania, melancholia, etc.), the psychosis was called functional (35). Likewise, 'endogenous' named those psychoses whose aetiology seemed related to genes or degeneration of the seed (e.g. schizophrenia or melancholia) and exogenous those psychoses with external causes (syphilis, trauma, etc.).

Lastly, and following the introduction of time as a dimension of madness (18), acute and chronic psychosis started to be differentiated (36). The adjectives acute and chronic (as applied to disease) are old but had had a different meaning. Up to the end of the eighteenth century, 'acute' referred to a disease of rapid onset and great severity that followed a typical dichotomous path and either led to death or was followed by a period of crisis and then remission; 'chronic' meant the opposite. Thus 'acute' and 'chronic' referred to two separate groups of diseases. Madness belonged to the group of chronic diseases. The current view that an acute disease can become chronic was not available at the time. By the middle of the nineteenth century, the meaning of 'acute' and 'chronic' no longer referred to severity or type of disease but to duration.

Inpatient treatment

The current concept of 'inpatient treatment' was formed as part of the historical process described earlier in this chapter. It referred to a space of care with special characteristics. It is known that from early on in human history, places had been made available for the confinement of the madmen. Temples, gaols, bridewells, and madhouses also provided spaces of care but each symbolized a different justification for the general view that the madman and society should be kept apart. So, although the nature of, and justification for, spaces of care have changed over the centuries, their common denominator seems to have been the view that the insane need a space of their own. This chapter is about the historical epistemology of those changes. Some of the spaces provided acted as containers, others as agents of change. Since the nineteenth century, the space of care has been called 'inpatient treatment' and gradually become overregulated (37) and filled with all manner of therapeutic interventions (38).

The word 'inpatient' is relatively new in English. It seems to have appeared by 1760 in a medical report presented to the Royal Society by Mr Samuel More, an apothecary but communicated by a Fellow, Charles Morton. It concerned the case of a young man who had lost the use of his hands putatively resulting from his 'cleansing brass wire'. After attending St Thomas's Hospital in London as an 'out-patient' he showed no improvement so 'thinking, that if he was admitted as in-patient at the hospital, he should be more likely to obtain a cure, he got himself admitted …' (39, p. 938).

Changing historical views

Before the nineteenth century

In classical times, madmen could be confined in temples, asklepian sanctuaries, and other places and sometimes offered therapeutic interventions (40–42). Given the prevalent view that some forms of madness had a sacred origin (e.g. mania), it is likely that it was believed that the spaces themselves may have had curative effects (43–46).

In medieval times, 'physiological' and 'demonological' views of madness seem to have coexisted and hence confinement was justified on a different basis (47–50): 'Quite contrary to the usual impression, rather extensive and well-managed institutions for the care of the insane came into existence during the Middle Ages, and continued to fulfil a very necessary social and medical duty. For the unspeakable neglect of the insane which is a disgrace to civilization, we must look to the centuries much nearer our own' (51, p. 183).

During this period, religious institutions started to offer shelters to the insane, probably as direct expression of Christian charity. Early examples of benign and protective spaces are the Hospice de los Santos Mártires Inocentes founded in 1409 by Joan Gilabert Jofré in Valencia, Spain (52, 53) and the Bethlem Hospital in London, England, in 1247 (54). In England, the Elizabethan Poor Law of 1601 (55, chapter IV) led to the creation of bridewells which often enough were used to offer shelter to lunatics (56, 57).

This means that by the beginning of the eighteenth century, the insane could be found confined in spaces created by the poor law (21), criminal law, vagrancy law, entrepreneurial private mad houses (58, p. 9), and philanthropy such as Bedlam or St Luke's (59). Until the nineteenth century, spaces of care for the lunatic did not have a common ideological denominator. This was provided by the process of medicalization of madness.

The long nineteenth century

Before 1800, the view that madness might be a disease was already considered but not exclusively. The madman was contained in management spaces which were social and disciplinary rather than therapeutic. After 1800, all this changed as medicine sought exclusivity on all aspects of madness. As part of the philanthropic drive started by the Enlightenment and to satisfy the labour needs of the industrial revolution, governments acknowledged these new ideas and started to construct mental asylums (58). As already mentioned, these new spaces of care allowed for the accumulation of the insane, the formation of patient cohorts, and invited longitudinal observation. This led to the construction of descriptive psychopathology, the development of the concept of mental symptoms as a unit of analysis of madness and for the application of medical forms of management.

Alienists organized themselves in guilds and associations, published journals and textbooks, and created examinations, training slots, and other rites of passage. By the end of the century, 'psychiatry' had become a recognizable medical specialism in most European countries. Mental nursing, still considered as a trade during the 1850s, achieved a professional status by the 1880s (60). Since early in the nineteenth century, alienists and nursing attendants had already become the principal carers of 'inpatient treatment' (37).

Architecture

The construction of mental asylums started early in the nineteenth century and the resulting buildings expressed well the interaction between architectonical style and the ambiguous views on madness held by society at the time (61–65). Mental asylums acted as intermediaries between society and the patient (66). On the one hand, they reassured the external world that lunacy was under control; on the other, it provided the inmates with boundaries, affordances, and prohibitions. Throughout the nineteenth century, the asylums themselves became an intrinsic part of the very definition of 'treatment'. Whether mental asylums were conceived of as containers or as forms of therapy in themselves depended upon the concept of space entertained at the time. When thought of as mere containers, daily routines were filled with 'interventions' such as gyratory chairs, drugs, cold baths, physical restraint, social disciplines, moral treatment, etc. What the combined effect was of all these interventions is difficult to say but patients were discharged often enough as recovered or partially so. Although a lack of hard evidence makes it difficult to compare outcome figures then and now, what is known suggests that the differences are not very marked in favour of the present (67).

Interventions indoors

International publications, visits, and exchanges uniformized therapeutic interventions in the European asylums after the 1850s. These could be physical, psychological, and social and were rigidly inscribed into the daily asylum routine. Physical treatments were applied externally (bleeds, baths, movements, restraints) or internally (potions, drugs, alcohol, purgatives, etc.). There was a theoretical rationale for each and before overcrowding became a problem, treatments were personalized and offered with care. Massification of the inpatient population after the middle of the century rendered the same interventions mechanical. Prescriptions (usually by a superintendent) were based on clinical 'diagnosis' or more often on observed behaviour. Although duly registered in the case notes, outcomes are difficult to quantify. In general, paying patients received more personalized attention than the pauper insane but this was not necessarily the case.

The broad concept of 'moral treatment' referred to interventions that in the current language could be described as psychological and social. During the early nineteenth century, the term 'moral' meant psychological and had little ethical connotations: 'It is opposed to material, and in this sense it means mental, or that the object to which it is applied belongs to mind and not to matter. Thus we speak of moral science as distinguished from physical science' (68, p. 325, 69). Much has been written on nineteenth-century moral treatment as a sort of psychotherapy *avant la lettre* (70). This is probably not the case (71–76). Moral treatment could mean treating the insane humanly, advice, discipline, work, monetary reward, haranguing, entertainment, dinning at matron's table, removing restraints, etc. Moral treatment as practised in France, England, Germany, the US, etc. was so varied a set of activities that it is not possible to identify a psychological strategy or model of man or mind that may be common to all.

Therapeutic interventions (in England) occurred within a clear-cut legal framework until 1930, when the concept of 'voluntary patient' was enacted in law (77). In other words, until then all patients were forcibly detained. In general, the legal rights of the insane were seriously considered. Patients lost through suicide, physical disease, fights, treatments gone wrong, etc. were subject to a postmortem examination and then buried in the hospital burial ground (23).

After the nineteenth century

'Inpatient' spaces and their supporting concepts

Inpatient treatment occurs at the intersection of various conceptual dichotomies. 'Space and place' remain ever-present components in all forms of shelter for the insane. Often invisible, they have maintained a silent dialogue with the insane even when physical shelters were considered little more than containers.

Space and place

The nature of 'space' and of 'place' has been debated since classical times (78–80). The Greeks conceived of space (khôra) as either (a) a container (what was left once all objects were removed), or (b) as a boundary-property of the objects themselves because 'space' as such could not exist without occupiers. These views have vied for supremacy until the twentieth century (79): Newton conceived of space as a passive container (81); Einstein as a dynamic system intrinsically associated with time and observer (82).

The view of space predominating during a given historical period is reflected in (a) the assumptions that disciplines such as architecture, geography, physical anthropology, etc. make about their own epistemological power; and (b) the manner in which objects themselves, whether real or virtual (e.g. cities, rooms, social spaces, etc.) are conceived. Of relevance to psychiatry, concepts such as 'milieu' and 'environment' closely reflected what the nineteenth century thought of space (83) (more on this later). They also help to understand how 'inpatient' shelter was understood at the time. For example, during periods in which the 'container' definition of space predominated, the environment tended to be considered less important. Thus, during the nineteenth century, when the Newtonian view predominated, mental asylums were mostly seen as places of containment and the movement of the patient in space was rigidly structured (84). During the twentieth century, as the Einsteinian view predominated, claims began to be made as to the effects space might have on the insane. Consequently, methodologies of protection were developed to shield the patient from 'institutionalization' (see 'Institutionalization').

Over the centuries, 'space' has been metaphorized and developed into sub-concepts: geographical (85), social (86, 87), anthropological (88); and psychological (89). 'Inpatient treatment' is found at the intersection of all these types of space. Clinicians entertaining a Newtonian view of space conceive of the psychiatric ward as a mere container and insist on filling it with 'active' interventions (e.g. biological, psychological, and social). Clinicians entertaining a dynamic view of space might want to convert it into a therapeutic instrument.

The concept of place (topos, locus) has since classical times referred to the region of space when an object is located. Discussed in the work of Aristotle, 'place' was defined in terms of the boundaries of a given object within the container (90). Descartes conceived of 'place' as a point in a set of geometric coordinates (91). Definitions of place also influenced the way in which later disciplines such as social psychology and sociology were to define 'inter-subjectivity', 'group interaction', etc. These social maps are, of course, central to the conceptualization of 'inpatient treatment'.

Milieu and environment

Up to the middle of the eighteenth century, 'milieu' was being defined as 'espace matériel à travers lequel passe un corps dans son mouvement, ou en général, un espace matériel dans lequel un corps est placé, soit qu'il se meuve ou non. Ainsi on imagine l'éther comme un milieu dans lequel les corps célestes se meuvent …'. …'M. Newton conçoit de plus que les vibrations de ce même milieu, excitées dans le cerveau au gré de la volonté et portées de-là dans les muscles à-travers les filamens des nerfs …' (92, pp. 853–854).

Hartley used Newtonian ideas about the effects of the aether on the individual to explain mental disorders (93). During the nineteenth century, Comte, Taine, and Bernard transformed the concept of milieu from being a mere physical space to a dynamic notion that continuously interacted with the individual (83). Borrowing the term milieu from Blainville (94), Auguste Comte wrote: 'Cette idée suppose, en effet, non-seulement celle d'un être organisé de manière à comporter l'état vital, mais aussi celle, non moins indispensable, d'un certain ensemble d'influences extérieures propres à son accomplissement. Une telle harmonie entre l'être vivant et le milieu correspondant caractérise évidemment la condition fondamentale de la vie' (95, p. 202, lecture XL). Claude Bernard introduced the concept of 'milieu intérieur' to refer to the fluid environment of the cells (96). Hippolyte Taine (97, chapter II) listed 'milieu' (together with race and moment) as the three factors responsible for the specificity of art. It has been claimed that this choice helped to make the concept widely known (98). During the nineteenth century, Mésologie named the discipline that studied the influence of the milieu on the individual (99).

In 1828, to translate Goethe's term Umgebung, Carlyle introduced the word 'environment' (100) and soon after Spencer reused it as a synonym of 'circumstances' (101). This led to a convergence of the words 'milieu' and 'environment' whose common referent became that of (a) a surrounding, geographical space; and (b) its effects on the individual. The history of how such effects have been conceptualized goes back at least to 'Airs, Waters and Places' one of the books of the Hippocratic corpus (102). Claims that geography shaped body, mind, and culture gave rise to 'environmental determinism', a philosophical movement that remain popular well into the twentieth century (103). In the event, the *Oxford English Dictionary* (104) defined 'environment' as: 'The conditions under which any person or thing lives or is developed; the sum-total of influences which modify and determine the development of life or character'. Since then, the term has lost some of its fine grain, particularly after becoming the battle cry of the ecological movement (105, 106). 'Environment' remains the incarnation of the idea of 'dynamic' space and hence it is central to impatient treatment.

Community and society

Tönnies's (107) distinction between community and society (*Gemeinschaft* and *Gesellschaft*) is also important to inpatient treatment in psychiatry. The great German sociologist was an expert on the work of Thomas Hobbes and it has been claimed that his distinction reflects Hobbes' concepts of social 'union' and 'concord' (108, p. 6). Ideally, psychiatric wards should be open 'communities' in the sense defined by the *Oxford English Dictionary* (104): 'A body of persons living together, and practising, more or less, community of goods'. 'Open' in the sense that ordinarily there is a regular renewal of members. Thomas Main and Maxwell Jones called 'therapeutic communities' those wards in which all members (patients and staff) participated in its administration and therapeutic decision-making (109).

Institutionalization

An institution is 'An establishment, organization, or association, instituted for the promotion of some object, esp. one of public or general utility, religious, charitable, educational, etc.' (104). Institutions can thus be physical, virtual, and conceptual. Institutionalization, in turn, is defined as 'The condition or state of being or becoming institutionalized; the action of institutionalizing' (104). From being value-neutral, this definition became value-laden when, after the Second World War, it started to be applied to the 'negative' effects that the (total) 'institution' itself (space, environment of mental hospital, prison, convent, zoological garden) may have upon its inmates (patients, nuns, soldiers, etc.) (110). When applied to psychiatry, such effects included many of the 'negative symptoms' conventionally attributed to the chronic psychoses.

In Russell Barton's 1959 classical study, institutionalization is described in vivid metaphor: 'The purpose of this booklet is to present in a systematic form the dreadful mental changes that may result from institutional life and the steps that can be taken to cure them. … I have confined attention to the material readily available to me in mental hospitals where, unfortunately, there has been a tendency to assume that such mental changes are an end result of mental illness. This is not so. Institutional Neurosis is like a bedsore. It results from factors other than the illness bringing the patient into hospital. It is, so to speak, "a mental bed-sore"' (111, p. ix). Influenced by the work of Goffman (110), Barton listed loss of contact with the outside world, idleness, lack of stimulation, brutality, environmental monotony, drugs, etc., as the causes of 'mental bed sores' that would remain for as long the patient was in the hospital even if his/her psychoses had got better.

One of the consequences of this understandable concern was the rejection of the inpatient treatment offered in mental asylums (as happened in the Italy Psychiatric Reform of 1978) and the development of restricted 'inpatient' facilities in general hospitals and in the community (112). Based on scientific, social, and economic reasons, duration of stay has also been subject to some control. The fact that the ill effects of institutionalization have also been detected in patients attending day-patient facilities, sheltered homes, community placings, etc., suggests that the actual physical space of care may be less important than the way in which the intersecting social and psychological spaces are structured and managed (113).

Rehabilitation

The meaning of 'rehabilitation' in psychiatry is a metaphorical derivative. According to the *Oxford English Dictionary* (104), 'rehabilitation' means: '1. The action of re-establishing (a person) in a former standing with respect to rank and legal rights (or church privileges); the result of such action; also, a writ by which such restoration is made; or 2. The action of replacing a thing in, or restoring it to, a previous condition or status'. To rehabilitate a 'psychiatric patient' means to devolve him functions or affordances that had been taken away either by the disease, institutionalization, or the side effects of treatment. It seems clear that during the inpatient period, measures must be taken to avoid the loss of function or if that is not possible to prepare him for the period of rehabilitation.

Recovery

The Sydenham dictionary (1899) defined recovery as 'the return to the normal condition of health'. Hippocrates had called it *apotherapeia* and the Latin *medics sanatio* or *valetudinis restitutio*. Little has changed and the current definition is 'reversion of a material, object, or property to a former condition following removal of an applied stress or other influence' (104). Its medical usage is therefore metaphorical and forms part of a wider vocabulary of terms that over the centuries have been used to refer to positive (relevant) changes in someone's disease. As social context has become important in the description and evaluation of disease, recovery and suchlike have started to include the regaining of the original social, financial, and other circumstances that the patient had before he took ill. Of late, there has been a spate of works attempting to redefine 'recovery' both from the expert (114–118) and from the patient perspective (119, 120). This combination should hopefully generate a definition of recovery clinically useful for our day and age.

Extramural spaces

Therapeutic spaces can be physical or surrogate. Hospital wards are the typical purposeful space created to house/contain patients and offer them therapeutic interventions. Therapeutic spaces can also be surrogate: 'A person or (usually) a thing that acts for or takes the place of another; a substitute' (104). In addition to physical spaces (e.g. bridewells, prisons, and mental asylums), over the centuries the insane have also been housed in surrogate spaces, for example, the community itself. A well-known example of such is the Gheel colony in Belgium which managed to combine various forms of care.

In medieval times, Gheel was little more than a shrine containing relics of Saint Dyphne (the patron saint of madness) to which the insane were taken expecting a miraculous cure. Some patients were allowed to stay with local families until the next annual festivity and the tradition started. The so-called Gheel colony has survived to this day by reinventing itself and adapting its structure to successive theories of madness. When de Varigny (121) visited the place in the second half of the nineteenth century he found over 1500 patients well managed by an efficient sociomedical organization put together by central and local government and the good will of the local population. Strict rules allowed the insane and the town to live together and rates of improvement were reported to be equal to (if not higher than) the average mental asylum.

Over the years, the Gheel colony has been inspected by alienists from many countries (e.g. 122–127). Efforts to replicate the system in other countries have not been altogether successful (128). Gheel is mentioned in this chapter simply because it constitutes an exceptional example of how the role of conventional inpatient care can be diminished when effectively combined with other forms of therapeutic space.

Conclusion

Writing on the history of inpatient treatment is not easy. Secular changes in the meaning of its component concepts rob general conclusions of meaning. Madness, treatment, recovery, etc. have unstable meanings and this makes it hard to identify continuities in a historical account.

However, space and shelter seem pervading in all the systems developed by societies to deal with the madman (psychiatric patient, client, consumer of services, etc.). The current system dates to the early nineteenth century when insanity was medicalized and alienism (now psychiatry) professionalized. This chapter has dealt with the process that made these changes possible and how they survived linked to successive justificatory ideologies.

Spaces of care can be conceived as containers or as dynamic environments. After the 1810s, vast spaces of care were created that made possible the formation of patient cohorts, new observations, and classifications of madness. These new ideas fed back onto the spaces of care, justified them, and pulled them forward.

During the twentieth century, the view developed that the institutions themselves had a malignant effect upon residents. Encouraged by political and financial considerations, this led to a marked reduction of spaces of care. Smaller places were created in general hospitals and in the community but on occasions, similar negative effects seem to have appeared in the new facilities as well. Efforts have been made to render the spaces of care dynamic and therapeutic but disagreement as to which should be the leading supporting ideology (behaviourism, psychoanalysis, cognitive psychology, art-based therapy, etc.) have often enough got in the way of progress. It is also in the spirit of the times that 'inpatient treatment' has become defined by the application of neurobiological treatments.

Overly for therapeutic reasons but covertly for economic ones, the duration of stay in the spaces of care has also been reduced to the point that often enough there is no time to complete the therapeutic interventions. This celerity has in turn eroded the sheltering function of the spaces of care. 'Shelter' can of course be found elsewhere and indeed a drive towards the community has been considered as an option. However, this option is probably overdependent on voluntary contribution (by carers and others) and should not be used to release government from their social responsibility.

In summary, 'inpatient treatment' names a broad set of activities whose meaning and justification have changed throughout history. Currently, the emphasis on neurobiological treatment may give the impression to some that the spaces of care themselves are little more than short-term containers. This would be

wrong. Without having a working knowledge of the social concepts and forces that govern the hidden functioning of all inpatient facilities, the young psychiatrist may only be offering half of the help that they could otherwise do.

REFERENCES

1. Casher MI, Bess JD. *Manual of Inpatient Psychiatry*. Cambridge: Cambridge University Press; 2010.
2. Singh NN, Barber JW, Van Sant S. *Handbook of Recovery in Inpatient Psychiatry*. Berlin: Springer; 2016.
3. Breisach E. *Historiography*. Chicago, IL: University of Chicago Press; 1994.
4. Chadwick O. *The Secularization of the European Mind in the Nineteenth Century*. Cambridge: Cambridge University Press; 1975.
5. Sommerville CJ. *The Secularization of Early Modern England*. Oxford: Oxford University Press; 1992.
6. Martin D. *On Secularization: Towards a Revised General Theory*. Aldershot: Ashgate; 2005.
7. Taylor C. *A Secular Age*. Cambridge, MA: Belknap Press of Harvard University Press; 2007.
8. McKenzie G. *Interpreting Charles Taylor's Social Theory on Religion and Secularization*. Berlin: Springer; 2017.
9. McDonald L. *The Early Origins of the Social Sciences*. Montreal: McGill-Queen's University Press; 1993.
10. Heilbron J, Magnusson L, Wittrock B. *The Rise of the Social Sciences and the Formation of Modernity: Conceptual Change in Context 1750–1850*. Berlin: Springer; 1998.
11. Porter TM, Ross D. *The Modern Social Sciences*. The Cambridge History of Science, Volume 7. Cambridge: Cambridge University Press; 2008.
12. López Piñero JM. *Historical Origins of the Concept of Neurosis*. Cambridge: Cambridge University Press; 1983.
13. Berrios GE. *The History of Mental Symptoms*. Cambridge: Cambridge University Press; 1996.
14. Tsou JY. Natural kinds, psychiatric classification and the history of DSM. *Hist Psychiatry* 2016;27:406–424.
15. Scott EC. *Evolution Vs. Creationism*. Westport, CT: Greenwood Press; 2004.
16. Numbers RL. *The Creationists: The Evolution of Scientific Creationism*. Berkeley, CA: University of California Press; 1992.
17. Moore JA. *From Genesis to Genetics: The case of Evolution and Creationism*. Berkeley, CA: University of California Press; 2002.
18. Berrios GE, Marková IS. La temporalizzazione della follia nel XIX secolo [The temporalization of madness in the 19th century]. *Rivista Sperimentale di Freniatria* 2016;140:13–27.
19. Smith LD. *Cure, Comfort and Safe Custody: Public Lunatic Asylums in Early 19th Century England*. Leicester: Leicester University Press; 1999.
20. Scull AT. *Museums of Madness: Social Organization of Insanity in 19th century England*. London: Viking; 1979.
21. Bartlett P. *The Poor Law of Lunacy*. Leicester: Leicester University Press; 1999.
22. Piddock S. *A Space of Their Own: The Archaeology of 19th Century Lunatic Asylums in Britain, South Australia, and Tasmania*. Heidelberg: Springer; 2007.
23. Andrews J. Death and the dead-house in Victorian asylums: necroscopy versus mourning at the Royal Edinburgh Asylum, c. 1832–1901. *Hist Psychiatry* 2012;23:6–26.
24. Berrios GE, Freeman H. *150 Years of British Psychiatry 1841–1991*. London: Gaskell; 1991.

25. Swartz S. The regulation of British colonial lunatic asylums and the origins of colonial psychiatry, 1860–1864. *Hist Psychol* 2010;13:160–177.

26. Semple J. *Bentham's Prison: A Study of the Panopticon Penitentiary.* Oxford: Clarendon Press; 1993.

27. Walsh JJ. Asylums and care for the insane. In: *Catholic Encyclopedia*, Volume 8. New York: Robert Appleton Company; 1910. http://www.newadvent.org/cathen/08038b.htm

28. Walker N. *Crime and Insanity in England. Volume 1: Historical Perspective.* Edinburgh: Edinburgh University Press; 1968.

29. Smith R. *Trial by Medicine: Insanity and Responsibility in Victorian Trials.* Edinburgh: Edinburgh University Press; 1984.

30. Cullen W. *Synopsis Nosologiæ Methodicæ*, Volume 2, 4th edition. Edinburgh: W Creech; 1785.

31. López Piñero JM, Morales Meseguer JM. *Neurosis y Psicoterapia. Un estudio histórico.* Madrid: Espasa-Calpe; 1970.

32. Flemming CF. *Pathologie und Therapie der Psychosen.* Berlin: A Hirschwald; 1859.

33. Leven M. *La Névrose. Étude Clinique et Thérapeutique.* Paris: Masson; 1887.

34. Axenfeld A. *Traité des Névroses.* Paris: Baillière; 1883.

35. Berrios GE. Historical aspects of the psychoses: 19th century issues. *Br Med Bull* 1987;43:484–498.

36. Lanteri-Laura G. La chronicité dans la psychiatrie moderne Française. *Annales* 1972;3:548–568.

37. Pinel S. *Traité complet du régime sanitaire des aliénés.* Paris: Mauprivez; 1836.

38. Berrios GE. The history of psychiatric therapies. In: Tyrer P and Silk K (eds) *Cambridge Textbook of Effective Treatments in Psychiatry*, pp. 16–43. Cambridge: Cambridge University Press; 2008;

39. More S. An account of the case of a young man. *Philos Trans (1683–1775)* 1760;51:936–941.

40. Tzeferakos G, Douzenis A. Sacred psychiatry in ancient Greece. *Ann Gen Psychiatry* 2014;13:11–18.

41. Laín-Entralgo P. *The Therapy of the Word in Classical Antiquity.* New Haven, CT: Yale University Press; 1970.

42. Simon B. *Mind and Madness in Ancient Greece. The Classical Roots of Modern Psychiatry*, Ithaca, NY: Cornell University Press; 1978.

43. Harris WV. *Mental Disorders in the Classical World.* Leiden: Brill; 2013.

44. Dodds ER. *The Greeks and the Irrational.* Berkeley, CA: University of California Press; 1951.

45. Drabkin IE. Remarks on ancient psychopathology. *Isis* 1955;46:223–234.

46. Semelaigne R. *Études historiques sur l'aliénation mentale dans l'antiquité.* Paris: Asselin; 1869.

47. Kroll JA. A reappraisal of psychiatry in the Middle Ages. *Arch Gen Psychiatry* 1973;29:276–283.

48. Neugebauer R. Treatment of the mentally in medieval and early modern England. *J Hist Behav Sci* 1978;14:158–169.

49. Kroll JA, Bachrach B. Sin and mental illness in the Middle Ages. *Psychol Med* 1984;14:507–14.

50. Kemp S. Modern myth and medieval madness. *N Z J Psychiatry* 1985;14:1–8.

51. Walsh JJ. *Medieval Medicine.* London: Black; 1920.

52. Marco Merenciano F. Vida y obra del P. Jofré. *Archivo Iberoamericano de Historia de la Medicina* 1950;II:308–359.

53. Livianos L, Císcar C, García A et al. *El Manicomio de Valencia del siglo XV al XX.* Valencia: Ayuntamiento de Valencia; 2006.

54. Andrews J, Briggs A, Porter R, et al. *The History of Bethlem.* London: Routledge; 1997.

55. Nicholls G. *A History of the English Poor Law*, Volume 1. London: John Murray; 1854.

56. Copeland AJ. *Bridewell Royal Hospital.* London: Wells Gardner, Darton and Co.; 1888.

57. Finzsch N, Jütte R. *Institutions of Confinement: Hospitals, Asylums, and Prisons in Western Europe and North America 1500–1950.* Cambridge: Cambridge University Press; 1996.

58. Jones K. *Lunacy, Law and Conscience 1744–1845.* London: Routledge; 1955.

59. Tuke DH. *Chapters in the History of the Insane in the British Isles.* London: Kagan Paul, Trench. and Co.; 1882.

60. Tuke DH. Insane, attendants on. In Tuke DH (ed.) *A Dictionary of Psychological Medicine*, Volume 1, pp. 692–694. London: Churchill; 1892.

61. Kovess-Masféty V, Severo D, Causse D, et al. *Architecture et Psychiatrie.* Paris: Editions LeMoniteur; 2004.

62. Fussinger C, Tevaearai D. *Lieux de folie. Monuments de raison. Architecture et psychiatrie en Suisse romande 1830–1930.* Lausanne: Presses polytechniques et universitaires romandes; 1998.

63. Skålevåg SA. Constructing curative instruments: psychiatric architecture in Norway, 1820–1920. *Hist Psychiatry* 2002;13:51–68.

64. Yanni C. *The Architecture of Madness: Insane Asylums in the United States.* Minneapolis, MN: University of Minnesota Press; 2007.

65. Rutherford S. *The Landscapes of Public Lunatic Asylums in England 1808–1914.* PhD Thesis, De Montfort University, Leicester; 2003.

66. Arnold D. *The Spaces of the Hospital: Spatiality and Urban Change in London 1680–1820.* London: Routledge; 2013.

67. Healy D, Harris M, Michael P, et al. Service utilization in 1896 and 1996: morbidity and mortality data from North Wales. *Hist Psychiatry* 2005;16:27–41.

68. Fleming W. *The Vocabulary of Philosophy*, 2nd edition. London: Griffin; 1858.

69. Berrios GE. JC Prichard and the concept of moral insanity. *Hist Psychiatry* 1999;10:111–126.

70. Postel J. Le traitement moral. In: Postel J, Quétel C (eds) *Nouvelle histoire de la psychiatrie*, pp. 152–168. Paris: Privat; 1983.

71. Browne WAF. *The Moral Treatment of the Insane.* London: Adlard; 1864.

72. Charland LC. Benevolent theory: moral treatment at the York Retreat. *Hist Psychiatry* 2007;18:61–80.

73. Miller D, Blanc E. Concepts of 'moral treatment' for the mentally ill. *Soc Serv Rev* 1967;41:66–74.

74. King LS. A note on so-called 'moral treatment'. *J Hist Med Allied Sci* 1964;19:297–298.

75. Sueur L. The psychological treatment of Insanity in France in the first part of the nineteenth century. *Hist Psychiatry* 1997;8:37–53.

76. Leuret F. *Indications à suivre dans le traitement moral de la folie.* Paris: Libraire V Le Normant; 1846.

77. Jones K. *Asylums and After: A Revised History of the Mental Health Services: From the Early 18th Century to the 1990s.* London: Athlone Press; 1993.

78. Nys D. *La notion d'espace au point de vue cosmologique et psychologique.* Louvain: Institut supérieur de philosophie; 1901.

79. Jammer M. *Concepts of Space: The History of Theories of Space in Physics*, 3rd edition. New York: Dover Publications; 1993.

80. Bostock D. *Space, Time, Matter and Form: Essays on Aristotle's Physics.* Oxford: Clarendon Press; 2006.

81. Disalle R. Newton's philosophical analysis of space and time. In: Cohen IB, Smith GE (eds), *The Cambridge Companion to Newton*, pp. 33–56. Cambridge: Cambridge University Press; 2004.

82. Dorling J. Did Einstein need general relativity to solve the problem of space? Or had the problem already been solved by special relativity? *Br J Philos Sci* 1978;29:311–323.

83. Koller AH. *The Theory of Environment*. Menasha, WI: Banta; 1918.

84. Quétel C. La vie quotidienne d'un asile d'aliénés à la fin du XIXe siècle. In: Postel J and Quétel C (eds.) *Nouvelle histoire de la psychiatrie*, pp. 443–452. Paris: Privat; 1983.

85. Massey DB. *For Space*. London: Sage; 2005.

86. Lefebvre H. *The Production of Space*. Oxford: Blackwell; 1991.

87. Zieleniec A. *Space and Social Theory*. London: Sage; 2007.

88. Hirsch E, O'Hanlon M (eds). *The Anthropology of Landscape*. Oxford: Oxford University Press; 1995.

89. Dunan C. Theorie psychologique de l'espace. *Revue Philosophique de la France Et de l'Etranger* 1895;39:663–667.

90. Morison B. *On Location: Aristotle's Concept of Place*. Oxford: Clarendon Press; 2002.

91. Malpas JE. *Place and Experience: A Philosophical Topography*. Cambridge: Cambridge University Press; 2004.

92. Diderot D, D'Alambert J (eds). *Encyclopédie ou Dictionnaire Raisonné des Sciences, des Artes, et des Métiers, par una Société de Gens de Lettres*, Paris, 3rd edition, Volume 21. Geneve: Pellet; 1779.

93. Berrios GE. David Hartley's views on madness. *Hist Psychiatry* 2015;26:105–116.

94. Gouhier H. Blainville et Auguste Comte. *Rev Hist Sci* 1979;32:59–72.

95. Comte A. *Considérations philosophiques sur l'ensemble de la science biologique. Lecture XL, Cours de Philosophie Positive*, Volume 3. Paris: Baillière; 1892.

96. Holmes FL. Claude Bernard, the milieu intérieur, and regulatory physiology. *Hist Philos Life Sci* 1986;8:3–25.

97. Taine H. *Philosophie de L'Art*, 3rd edition, Volume 1. Paris: Hachette; 1909.

98. Spitzer L. Milieu and ambiance: an essay in historical semantics. *Philos Phenomenol Res* 1942;3:169–218.

99. Bertillon J. Mésologie. In: Dechambre A (ed.) *Dictionnaire Encyclopédique des Sciences Médicales*, Volume 59, pp. 211–266. Paris: Masson; 1873.

100. Jessop R. Coinage of the term environment: a word without authority and Carlyle's displacement of the mechanical metaphor. *Lit Comp* 2012;9:708–720.

101. Pearce T. From 'circumstances' to 'environment': Herbert Spencer and the origins of the idea of organism-environment interaction. *Stud Hist Philos Biol Biomed Sci* 2010;41:241–52.

102. Hippocrates. Airs, waters, places. In: Hippocrates, Volume 1 (Jones WHS, trans), pp. 65–138. Cambridge, MA: Harvard University Press; 1957.

103. Keighren IM. Environmental determinism. In: Wright JD (ed), *International Encyclopaedia of the Social and Behavioral Sciences*, 2nd edition, Volume 7, pp. 720–725. New York: Elsevier; 2015.

104. Simpson J, Weiner E (eds). *Oxford English Dictionary*, 2nd edition. Oxford: The Clarendon Press; 1989.

105. Larrère C. *Les Philosophies de l'environnment*. Paris: Presses Universitaires de France; 1997.

106. MacDonald GJ. Environment: evolution of a concept. *J Environ Dev* 2003;12:151–176.

107. Tönnies F. *Gemeinschaft und Gesellschaft*. Leipzig: Fues's Verlag; 1997.

108. Hont I. *Politics in Commercial Society: Jean-Jacques Rousseau and Adam Smith* (Kapossy B, Sonenscher M, eds). Cambridge, MA: Harvard University Press; 2015.

109. Millard DW. Maxwell Jones and the therapeutic community. In: Freeman H, Berrios GE (eds), *150 years of British Psychiatry. Volume II. The Aftermath*, pp. 581–604. London: Athlone Press; 1996.

110. Goffman E. *Asylums*. New York: Anchor Books, Doubleday; 1961.

111. Barton R. *Institutional Neurosis*, 3rd edition. Bristol: John Wright; 1976.

112. Pycha R, Giupponi G, Schwitzer J, et al. Italian Psychiatric Reform 1978: milestones for Italy and Europe in 2010? *Eur Arch Psychiatry Clin Neurosci* 2011;261:S135–S139.

113. Chow WS, Priebe S. Understanding psychiatric institutionalization: a conceptual review. *BMC Psychiatry* 2013;13:169–185.

114. Andresen R, Oades LG, Caputi P. *Psychological Recovery: Beyond Mental Illness*. Chichester: Wiley-Blackwell; 2011.

115. French P, Smith J, Shiers D, et al. *Promoting Recovery in Early Psychosis: A Practical Manual*. Chichester: Wiley-Blackwell; 2010.

116. Gumley A, Gillham A, Taylor K, Schwannauer M. *Psychosis and Emotions: The role of Emotions in Understanding Psychosis, Therapy and Recovery*. London: Routledge; 2013.

117. Rudnick A. *Recovery of People with Mental Illness*. Oxford: Oxford University Press; 2012.

118. Drake RE, Whitley R. Recovery and severe mental illness: description and analysis. *Can J Psychiatry* 2014;59:236–242.

119. Cohen BMZ. *Mental Health User Narratives: New Perspectives on Illness and Recovery*. Basingstoke: Palgrave; 2008.

120. Tucker W. *Narratives of Recovery from Serious Mental Illness*. Berlin: Springer; 2016.

121. de Varigny H. Gheel, une colonie d'aliénés. *Revue des deux Mondes* 1885;67:633–668.

122. Parigot J. *L'air libre et la vie de famille dans la commune de Gheel*. Bruxelles: Tircher; 1852.

123. Sibbald J. *The Cottage System and Gheel*. London: Adlard; 1861.

124. Duval J. *Gheel ou une colonie d'aliénés*. Paris: Hachette; 1867.

125. Byrne WMP. *Gheel: The City of the Simple*. London: Chapman and Hall; 1869.

126. Peeters JA. *Lettres Médicales sur Gheel et le patronage familial*. Bruxelles: Manceaux; 1883.

127. Lemos M. *Visite psychiatrique à la colonie de Gheel*. Porto: Typographia Occidental; 1886.

128. Bothe A. *Die Familiale Verpflegung Geisteskranken: System der Irren-Colonie Gheel*. Heidelberg: Springer; 1893.

2

Mental Health Legislation

Julie Chalmers

Introduction

This chapter will give an overview of mental health legislation as it applies to England and Wales, discuss some key concepts, and highlight the principles underpinning the law. Clinical staff need to have a working knowledge of all three elements to play their part in protecting and upholding the rights of individuals who are admitted to the inpatient unit.

People with psychiatric disorders can number among the most vulnerable in society and often experience a marked imbalance of power in their interactions with health care staff. Research has confirmed that perceived coercion is commonly experienced by people with mental disorders irrespective of whether mental health legislation has been used or not (1, p. 108).

Getting the approach right from the first point of contact and throughout the admission by applying the law through the lens of the principles underpinning the legislation may help reduce the sense of disempowerment and increase the likelihood of better outcomes (2).

Human rights

Human rights are basic rights and freedoms that protect everybody simply by virtue of being human. The British Institute of Human Rights has summarized the important rights with the easy to remember acronym FREDA: fairness, respect, equality, dignity, and autonomy (3). Everyone working on the ward has a part to play in upholding human rights, not just those in senior positions or those with statutory roles. As Eleanor Roosevelt, the first chair of the United Nations Commission on Human Rights, said: 'Where, after all, do universal human rights begin? In small places, close to home … so close and so small that they cannot be seen on any map of the world' (4).

There are several international statements and declarations outlining human rights in general or referring to the rights of those with disabilities which the UK government has agreed to be bound by but has yet to enact the relevant legislation to give the statement or declaration effect in domestic law. One exception is the European Convention on Human Rights (ECHR) as this does have legal effect. The Human Rights Act 1998 which came into force in 2000 enshrines the ECHR in English law so that it is now unlawful for a public body, such as the National Health Service, to act in a way incompatible with the Convention (Box 2.1).

Coming into hospital: an introduction

It is important that clinicians identify the appropriate legal framework governing admission to ensure the correct processes are followed and safeguards put in place. An adult admitted to an inpatient mental health unit will come into hospital under one of three legal frameworks:

1. Those with capacity, who have sufficient information and are free from the undue influence of others, can give their informed consent to admission.

2. The Mental Capacity Act 2005 (MCA) including, where necessary and relevant, consideration of the use of provisions to authorize a deprivation of liberty using the Deprivation of Liberty Safeguards (DoLS).

3. The Mental Health Act 1983 (MHA) including recall from a community treatment order (CTO).

The term informal admission simply refers to the group of patients who are not subject to detention under the MHA. Until very recently, informal patients were in the majority, although this may not have always been the case in some inner-city wards. In 2014/2015 overall, formal admissions are now just possibly exceeding informal ones (10, p. 9). This may be because of increased awareness of the need to protect Article 5 ('Right to liberty and security', ECHR) rights since the Supreme Court judgment (see 'The importance of Article 5') or reflect the severe degree of illness of the patients needing to access a reducing number of inpatient beds (11).

These legal categories are not mutually exclusive and the legal status of a patient may change over time and on occasions the legal regimes may need to run in parallel when there is a physical condition requiring treatment that is separate from the mental disorder.

The MHA does not cover treatment of a physical problem unrelated to the mental disorder so consent must be sought specifically. Depending on whether the person has capacity then the common law of consent or, if lacking capacity, the MCA will come into play for the treatment of the physical disorder.

Capacity

In deciding which framework is appropriate, it is necessary to identify if there is any evidence to rebut the presumption that a person has the capacity to make the decision in question. Capacity is a complex construct which refers to a set of functional abilities that a person needs in order to make a specific decision. UK law places considerable weight on self-determination and an adult who has capacity can refuse an intervention, however unwise that refusal might be, and this refusal must be respected and cannot be overruled even it would result in death. The exception is that when detained under the MHA, a person's decision to refuse assessment or treatment for a mental disorder can be overridden even if they have capacity. This, however, would be a very substantial step and the reasons for doing so would need to be justified. It should not be assumed that because a person suffers from a mental disorder, even one of a nature or degree requiring hospital admission, their capacity to make a particular decision for themselves will necessarily be impaired.

Capacity is time and decision specific and therefore clinicians should always remember that the standard documentation used by some hospitals to document capacity at the point of admission or when seeking consent to treatment is not fixed in stone and capacity must be regularly reassessed. The legal test of capacity is found in the MCA and will be considered later.

The importance of Article 5

Before considering the process of admission to the inpatient unit in more detail, it is essential that practitioners understand the obligations that are placed on them arising from the ECHR. The convention was drafted in the aftermath of the Second World War when millions had suffered arbitrary detention and had no recourse to appeal. The era in which it was written has shaped the language used, particularly in Article 5(1)e where people with mental disorder are referred to as 'persons of unsound mind'.

Article 5 states in part:

1. Everyone has the right to liberty and security of person. No one shall be deprived of his liberty save in the following cases and in accordance with a procedure prescribed by law:
   e. the lawful detention of persons for the prevention of the spreading of infectious diseases, of persons of unsound mind, alcoholics or drug addicts or vagrants.
4. Everyone who is deprived of his liberty by arrest or detention shall be entitled to take proceedings by which the lawfulness of his detention shall be decided speedily by a court and his release ordered if the detention is not lawful.[1]

[1] Contains public sector information licensed under the Open Government Licence v3.0 (http://www.nationalarchives.gov.uk/doc/open-government-licence/version/3/).

> **Box 2.2** Pointers to a deprivation of liberty
>
> - A request by carers for discharge is refused.
> - Restraint.
> - Sedation.
> - Staff exercise complete and effective control over the care and movement of the person.
> - Contact with family and friends is restricted by staff.
> - The person loses autonomy because they are under continuous supervision and control.
> - A decision has been taken that the person will not be allowed to live elsewhere or released into the care of others without permission.
> - Unable to maintain social contacts without restrictions.

Deprivation of liberty

Article 5 of the ECHR requires that any deprivation of liberty must be authorized by a procedure prescribed by law. In order to fulfil this legal requirement, clinicians need to be able to identify when a deprivation of liberty is potentially occurring. What constitutes a deprivation of liberty is a much broader concept than one of simple physical confinement and often includes restrictions of Article 8 rights ('Right to private and family life'). The DoLS Code of Practice at paragraph 2.5 identifies some possible pointers that a deprivation of liberty may be occurring (12) (Box 2.2).

These factors are still important but must now be read in the light of a decision of the Supreme Court in what is commonly referred to as the *Cheshire West* case although other parties were involved (13). Lady Hale identified the two questions, which she referred to as the 'acid test', and if the answer to both parts is yes then this would identify if a deprivation of liberty was occurring when the person lacked capacity to consent to the arrangements for their care or treatment (Box 2.3).

It is clear from European court judgments that the first element is not limited to those who are under continuous physical supervision (such as close observation) but is to be interpreted more broadly than that (14). Additionally, the person may not be asking to go or showing by their actions that they want to but the key issue is about how staff would react if the person did try to leave or if relatives/ friends asked to remove them.

The Supreme Court also identified factors that are no longer relevant to whether someone is deprived of their liberty. Their Lordships highlighted that whether a person objects or not to their care plan is irrelevant in determining whether there is a deprivation of liberty. As Lady Hale commented, 'a gilded cage is still a gilded cage' (15). This means that if a person is subject both to continuous supervision and control and is not free to leave they are deprived of their liberty irrespective of whether they are objecting or not. Given that patients on an inpatient unit are subject to a degree of continuous supervision

---

> **Box 2.3** The 'acid test' to identify if a deprivation of liberty is occurring
>
> Part 1: is the person subject to continuous supervision and control?
> *And*
> Part 2: is the person free to leave?

Box 2.4 Deprivation of liberty resources

- *Mental Capacity Act 2005: Deprivation of Liberty Safeguards—Code of Practice to supplement the Mental Capacity Act 2005 Code of Practice* (http://webarchive.nationalarchives.gov.uk/20130107105354/http://www.dh.gov.uk/prod_consum_dh/groups/dh_digitalassets/@dh/@en/documents/digitalasset/dh_087309.pdf) (12).
- The Law Society. *Deprivation of Liberty: A Practical Guide* (9 April 2015) (http://www.lawsociety.org.uk/support-services/advice/articles/deprivation-of-liberty/).
  - This document was commissioned by the Department of Health and is written from a legal, not clinical, perspective.
- Deprivation of Liberty Safeguards—six modules designed for doctors wanting to be authorized to undertake a specific function under DoLS (https://www.e-lfh.org.uk/programmes/deprivation-of-liberty-safeguards/). Useful introduction to deprivation of liberty including discussion of case law and also a helpful module on capacity assessment.

Box 2.5 Key information to decide whether to come into a psychiatric hospital

1 That the person will be admitted to a mental health hospital for care and treatment for a mental disorder.
2 That the doors to the ward will be locked.
3 That staff at the hospital will be entitled to carry out property and personal searches.
4 That the person will be expected to remain on the ward at least until being seen by a doctor, and most likely for at least the first 24 hours of their admission.
5 That the person will be required to inform the nursing staff whenever they want to leave the ward, providing information about where they are going and a time of return.
6 That the nursing staff may refuse to agree to the person leaving the ward (including use of the MHA) if the nursing staff believe that the person may be at risk (from themselves, or from other people) or may pose a risk to others if they leave the ward.
7 That if the person leaves the ward without informing the staff, or fails to return at the agreed time, the staff will call the police who will make attempts to find them.
8 That the person's description will be recorded by staff for the purpose of point 7.
9 In addition, it is important to include the likely consequences of the person not being admitted. This will of course vary with each individual and their personal circumstances.
10 That they will not be able to smoke (include vaping) but they will be offered nicotine replacement.

and many would not be free to leave then a number of inpatients will require protection of their Article 5 rights. This will most usually be by use of the MHA although there are currently very limited circumstances in the adult psychiatric setting where DoLS (the safeguards) could legally be used and these will be discussed later.

If a person lacks capacity and there is *no* deprivation of liberty, then a person can be treated for their mental disorder under mental capacity legislation without a need to invoke a legal procedure to protect their Article 5 rights. However, should they object to treatment then consideration of the use of the MHA would be required rather than to continue to rely on the MCA. Considerable attention needs to be given to whether someone is objecting or not as signs may be very subtle (16) (Box 2.4).

Legal frameworks: admission

Consent

A person can consent to be admitted to a psychiatric hospital if they have:

1. the capacity to make the decision and
2. sufficient information on which to base their decision, including the foreseeable consequences of not being admitted and
3. are free from undue duress or influence.

Most people will have a notion of what being on a general hospital ward for treatment of a physical illness involves through personal or family experience or even through numerous reality and fictional TV programmes. The 'rules of engagement' are broadly understood. This is not necessarily the case when considering admission to a psychiatric hospital. Practitioners do not always describe institutional restrictions of being on a psychiatric ward due to either simple omission or a reluctance to give the full facts in case these will sound unappealing and will negatively influence the decision to be admitted. However, it is not respectful of autonomy to fail to provide the necessary information in a balanced way. It has been suggested that there is key information a person must have to decide whether to come into a psychiatric hospital (17, 18) (Boxes 2.5 and 2.6). A person, who has capacity and is fully informed of the restrictions and limitations of the ward environment and makes the decision free from undue pressure, can consent to a care plan that amounts to a deprivation of liberty. Great care must be taken in how these discussions are framed as one study found that high levels of coercion were perceived by 48% of voluntarily admitted patients and a high score was associated with a poor therapeutic relationship which could negatively impact further experience of services and on the outcome (19).

The Mental Capacity Act 2005

The MCA is the legal framework for decision-making on behalf of those who are aged over 16 and lack the capacity to do so for themselves. The statute begins by laying out the principles underpinning the operation of this statute. These are summarized as follows:

1. A person must be assumed to have capacity unless it is established that he lacks capacity.
2. A person is not to be treated as unable to make a decision unless all practicable steps to help him to do so have been taken without success.

Box 2.6 Consent resources

- General Medical Council: 'Consent: patients and doctors making decisions together', 2008 (http://www.gmc-uk.org/guidance/ethical_guidance/consent_guidance_index.asp).
- General Medical Council: ten questions about consent—with useful links to various guidance including link to important legal developments (http://www.gmc-uk.org/guidance/29457.asp).

3. A person is not to be treated as unable to make a decision merely because he makes an unwise decision.
4. An act done, or decision made, under this Act for or on behalf of a person who lacks capacity must be done, or made, in his best interests.
5. Before the act is done, or the decision is made, regard must be had to whether the purpose for which it is needed can be as effectively achieved in a way that is less restrictive of the person's rights and freedom of action.[2]

The MCA does not confer any specific powers, unlike the MHA, but instead provides protection from legal liability in connection with any acts carried out on behalf of an incapacitated person if done in their best interests (Section 5, MCA). Section 6 of the MCA defines the limits of Section 5 and allows restraint to prevent harm to the persons, but not others, and does not authorize a deprivation of liberty.

The documentation of such decisions leading to acting in the absence of consent needs to outline the evidence that the person lacks capacity to make the specific decision, and what steps have been taken to help them regain capacity or to participate in decision-making, best interests decision-making including reference to their known wishes or preferences, and consideration of the least restrictive option. Care plans should not only be developed with the patient in so far that this is possible but also refer to these important aspects of the MCA if seeking to rely on the legal protection conferred by Sections 5 and 6 of the MCA.

When approaching a capacity assessment, the first three principles underpinning the MCA must be at the forefront of the clinician's mind, namely the presumption in favour of capacity, the need to support decision-making, and that unwise decisions do not necessarily indicate a lack of capacity. Of course, an extremely unwise decision or one that is out of character should prompt more careful scrutiny by the assessor to identify if there is any evidence of impairment of decision-making capacity arising directly because of mental disorder. It is not up to the patient to 'prove' they have capacity, it is up to the assessor to find evidence to overturn this starting position.

The test of capacity is contained in Sections 2 and 3 of the MCA and comprises two arms, sometimes referred to as the 'diagnostic test' and the 'functional test'. Section 2 of the MCA states:

(1) For the purposes of this Act, a person lacks capacity in relation to a matter if at the material time he is unable to make a decision for himself in relation to the matter because of an impairment of, or a disturbance in the functioning of, the mind or brain.
(2) It does not matter whether the impairment or disturbance is permanent or temporary.

Common conditions encountered in an inpatient setting such as schizophrenia, affective disorder, and, in older adult wards, organic conditions such as dementia will fulfil the diagnostic test. It is important to be aware that personality disorder and autistic spectrum disorder are also considered to be conditions that could potentially give rise to an impairment or disturbance of mind or brain.

The second arm is the 'functional' test which states that a person is unable to make a decision for himself if he is unable:

- to understand the information relevant to the decision
- to retain that information
- to use or weigh that information as part of the process of making the decision, or
- to communicate his decision (whether by talking, using sign language or any other means).

It is not sufficient that there is an impairment or disturbance of mind or brain and some evidence of functional impairment. It is essential that the assessor be satisfied that the inability to make a decision is *because* of the impairment of the mind or brain and for this direct link to be clearly documented.

What are best interests?

The MCA does not define best interests and the MCA Code of Practice states at Section 5.5:

The term 'best interests' is not actually defined in the Act. This is because so many different types of decisions and actions are covered by the Act, and so many different people and circumstances are affected by it.

Rather than define best interests, the Act outlines a process by which the decision maker acting on behalf of the person without capacity can come to a conclusion as to what is in the person's best interests. The MCA in Section 4 outlines a checklist of people to be consulted including the person's past wishes (if known) and their current preferences. This checklist is unweighted so no one point of view takes precedence over the other. It is up to the decision maker to identify what is objectively the best option taking a broad view of interests, not just medical interests. However, recent case law has placed increasingly more weight on the person's preferences both past and current and it is essential that such views be identified wherever possible and given due consideration (20).

Planning in advance

The MCA contains mechanisms to allow a person, who is over 18, to plan for future incapacity while capacity is retained. These are:

- advance decisions to refuse treatment
- Lasting Power of Attorney (LPA)
- property and affairs
- welfare.

Advance decisions to refuse treatment

A valid and applicable advance decision will be legally binding and with the exception of refusal of life-sustaining treatment need not be in writing. A person can refuse treatment for either a mental or physical disorder but not for basic care. A well-known example of an advance decision to refuse treatment is the refusal of blood and blood products by Jehovah's Witnesses who carry cards to this effect. Advance decisions to refuse treatment are a way of protecting autonomy when capacity to make a specific decision is lost, although if detained under the MHA some decisions about treatment for mental health may be overridden. Clinicians working in inpatient units need to establish whether any such instruments exist and bring these to the attention of senior clinicians, indeed this should be a routine part of the admission procedure. Decisions concerning

---

[2] Contains public sector information licensed under the Open Government Licence v3.0 (http://www.nationalarchives.gov.uk/doc/open-government-licence/version/3/).

Box 2.7 Validity and applicability of an advance decision to refuse treatment

Validity

- Capacity at the time of making an advance decision.
- Must have had sufficient information to make decision.
- Must understand the consequences of not receiving treatment—especially if refusing life-sustaining treatment.
- Freedom from duress.
- No suggestion that advance decision has been revoked.
- Evidence that this has remained fixed view.

Applicability

- Not applicable if person has capacity to make a decision at the time the decision needs to be made.
- Not applicable if the treatments proposed are not specified.
- If circumstances specified in the advance decision are absent.
- If reasonable grounds for believing current circumstances were not anticipated and, if they were, they would have affected the decision.

physical care may be particularly relevant in the care of older adults who have made advance decisions to refuse treatment prior to losing capacity. Establishing if an advance decision to refuse treatment is valid and applicable can be challenging and legal advice may need to be sought in complex cases (Box 2.7).

Advance statements

Advance statements are not legal instruments but can be a useful tool as part of the recovery model/crisis planning. They may also inform best interest decision-making by describing important values or preferences. An advance statement cannot compel a doctor to provide a specific treatment and resource considerations will also apply. In the spirit of empowerment and involvement, such statements should be followed whenever possible.

Lasting Power of Attorney

For the first time in English law, a third party, who is legally authorized to do so, may give or refuse consent on behalf of an adult who lacks the capacity to decide for themselves at the material time. One or more attorneys may be appointed when the person has capacity. There are two types of LPA, namely 'property and affairs' and 'health and welfare'.

The scope of authority may be defined and the attorney(s) must always act in the person's best interests. As with an advance decision to refuse treatment, attorneys can be appointed to make decisions about mental health treatment although they may be overridden in certain circumstances. They cannot, however, agree to a deprivation of liberty, which will need to be authorized by using the appropriate legal mechanism. The Court of Protection may appoint a deputy or deputies who, if granted authority to do so, will be able to act in a way similar to the holder of an LPA. The relationship between the MCA and mechanisms for planning in advance will be further considered under the section on treatment under the MHA.

Deprivation of Liberty Safeguards

The DoLS were introduced following the case of *HL* v *UK*, often referred to as the 'Bournewood' case when this was going through the domestic courts. This case concerned an autistic man who lacked

capacity to decide if he should be admitted to a hospital, in this instance, a psychiatric hospital. This case preceded the enactment of the MCA and he was admitted without use of any formal powers under common law on the grounds that this was in his best interests. His carers wished for him to be discharged home but this was refused and so they challenged this in the domestic courts and then in the European Court of Human Rights. The European Court of Human Rights identified that the legal framework at the time failed to provide adequate protection to individuals who lacked capacity and who were deprived of their liberty and that the State was in breach of their obligation to protect against unlawful deprivations of liberty as required to under Article 5.

DoLS were introduced in April 2009 as an amendment to the MCA. The Law Commission published proposals in 2017 for a new scheme to replace DoLS to protect Article 5 rights and a new bill, Mental Capacity (Amendment) Bill 2018, is currently being debated in parliament therefore the current safeguards will not be discussed in any further detail. The principles and reasons for the need for Article 5 protection remain, however, although the processes for doing this are likely to change.

The Mental Health Act 1983

The purpose of the MHA is for 'the reception, care and treatment of mentally disordered patients' (Section 1(1)) and the MHA provides authority to deprive someone of their liberty on the grounds of their mental health and to treat in the absence of consent provided certain criteria are fulfilled. These are substantial powers that impact individual rights and freedoms albeit with a legitimate aim of maintaining health and/or safety. The principles underpinning the MHA and a description of how they might be applied are contained in chapter 1 of the MHA Code of Practice and should be essential reading for all inpatient staff (Box 2.8). The Code was revised in consultation with expert opinion, practitioners, and most importantly involvement of users by experience and carers and was published in 2014. Although not part of the primary legislation (unlike the MCA), the Code must be followed by mental health professionals unless there are 'cogent reasons' for deviating from it (21, 22).

Formal admission under the Mental Health Act

Formal admissions to the acute inpatient unit will occur most commonly under Section 2 for assessment, which can also include treatment, and can last up to 28 days and is not renewable, or for treatment under Section 3, which can last up to 6 months in the first instance although, if certain criteria are met, this period can be extended.

Both sections require two medical recommendations, one of which must be made by a specially approved doctor, referred to as being Section 12 (2) MHA approved. Application for admission is

Box 2.8 The principles underpinning the Mental Health Act

- Least restrictive option and maximizing independence.
- Empowerment and involvement.
- Respect and dignity.
- Purpose and effectiveness.
- Efficiency and equity.

made by an Approved Mental Health Professional (AMHP) who comes from one of four qualifying professions (nursing, social work, psychology, occupational therapy) and who has had an extensive training to undertake the role. The Act also allows for an application to be made by a nearest relative but in practice this almost never occurs.

Very rarely, a patient will be admitted under Section 4, a short-term section lasting 72 hours, used on the basis of urgent necessity requiring just one medical recommendation to support the application by an AMHP or relative. Section 4 can, with a second medical recommendation made within the 72-hour period, be converted into a Section 2.

The criteria for detention are that the patient suffers from a mental disorder, defined as 'any disorder or disability of mind' that warrants detention in hospital on the grounds of:

- health and/or
- safety and/or
- with a view to the protection of other people.

For Section 3 there is an additional criterion that 'appropriate treatment be available'.

It is the right of every detained patient, other than those on short-term sections (Section 4, Section 5(4), and Section5(2)) that, as soon as practicable following admission, they must be given information both orally and in writing about how the Act applies to them. Chapter 4 of the Code of Practice (4.13–4.14) outlines the information which must be supplied.

The 2007 amendments to the MHA introduced the statutory right to advocacy for patients detained on other than the short-term sections. Section 6.3 of the Code of Practice describes the purpose of Independent Mental Health Advocates (IMHAs) as follows: 'IMHA services provide an additional safeguard to patients who are subject to the Act. IMHAs are specialist advocates who are trained specifically to work within the framework of the Act and enable patients to participate in decision making, for example, by encouraging patients to express their views and supporting them to communicate their views'. Both the provision of information and the involvement, if wanted by the patient, of an IMHA are concrete ways of bringing the principles of empowerment and involvement to life. Unfortunately, there is evidence from Care Quality Commission (CQC) inspections that this is not always followed in a minority of patients (10, p. 6).

Recall of a patient subject to a community treatment order

Inpatient staff must be aware of the differences between admission under Section 2 or Section 3 of the MHA and recall of a CTO as certain reviews and decisions must be made within the 72-hour duration of the recall.

Under the civil provisions of the Act, a patient can only be placed on a CTO having been on a Section 3 and if certain criteria are fulfilled. Once on a CTO, the underlying Section 3 goes into hibernation. The criteria for making a CTO are similar to those for detention under Section 3 (mental disorder/nature and degree/necessity criteria/appropriate treatment) but in this instance the patient no longer requires detention in hospital for treatment but could be managed in the community if the Responsible Clinician (RC) had authority to recall the patient in order that treatment could be administered. The

RC is a specially approved clinician in overall charge of the patient, most usually, but not always, a consultant psychiatrist. The Code of Practice states at paragraph 29.45: 'The recall power is intended to provide a means to respond to evidence of relapse or high-risk behaviour relating to mental disorder before the situation becomes critical and leads to the patient or other people being harmed.'

The power of recall is different from admission under the MHA in the following ways. The RC alone recalls the patient unlike detention under Sections 2 or 3 and the purpose of recall is to 'give medical treatment', not to detain in hospital. A person could be recalled, given treatment in either an outpatient setting or the ward, and then immediately return to the community. Most importantly, recall allows detention in hospital for up to 72 hours only. During this period, a decision needs to be made by the RC and an Approved Mental Health Professional as to whether further inpatient treatment is necessary or whether the patient can return to the community. If further inpatient treatment is necessary, then the CTO is revoked and the underlying Section 3 comes into play. There is also the option for the patient to consent to admission and then the CTO remains in place. Staff need to be particularly alert to the 72-hour period if the patient gets admitted over the weekend or a bank holiday and steps taken to ensure the duty consultant is informed of the recall. This is not a situation that can wait until the usual inpatient consultant is available.

Holding powers

There are two short-term holding powers. Section 5(4) can be used by a nurse from a 'prescribed class' (lasting 6 hours) when it is not possible to secure the attendance of a doctor. Section 5(2) can be used by the RC or their nominated deputy who must be a registered medical practitioner (so this excludes Foundation Year 1 doctors) lasting up to 72 hours. The purpose of Section 5(2) is to authorize the detention of the patient so that consideration can be given to making an assessment about whether an application for detention should be made. It could be argued that with careful consideration at the point of admission, the need to use such powers should diminish as the appropriate legal framework would have been identified at the point of admission. The CQC has reported that 28% of patients admitted informally were then detained under the MHA (23). Providing clear information about the nature of a stay on an inpatient ward would avoid patients agreeing to informal admission only to change their minds when they experience the reality of the ward environment. Clinicians must not write in an informal patient's notes that they should be detained on a Section 5(2) should they wish to leave. In that one sentence the second limb of the acid test described earlier is met as the patient is not free to go. As it is very likely that they will also be subject to continuous supervision and control, they are deprived of their liberty and their Article 5 rights must be protected.

Sections 135/136

Some wards may have associated areas designated as a 'place of safety' and will receive patients detained on a Section 136 (police powers to remove a person thought to be suffering from a mental disorder and in immediate need of care or control) or brought under a Section 135(1) warrant to be assessed in a place of safety. In January 2017, the duration of detention under Section 136 was reduced from

72 hours to 24 hours with the possibility of a further 12-hour extension to complete the assessment if factors such as attendance to physical health or intoxication have delayed the assessment (24). The clock is running as soon as the person is admitted to the place of safety and assessment must take place in a timely manner not only to meet the legal timeframe but to minimize the period in detention.

A complex area of law: deciding between the MHA and MCA/DoLS

All health care professionals must act to safeguard the rights of vulnerable people and they need to ensure that any deprivation of liberty of a person who lacks capacity to consent to admission to hospital for the treatment of a mental disorder is authorized in accordance with the appropriate legal regime in order to protect Article 5 rights. The most common way to protect rights, in the psychiatric setting, would be to use the MHA. However, there is one situation when DoLS could legally be used to protect the Article 5 rights of a patient admitted for assessment of a mental disorder as an alternative to using the MHA. Such a choice is only available in the following circumstances:

- The patient lacks capacity, and
- The care regime amounts to a deprivation of liberty, and
- They are not objecting to admission.

Chapter 13 of the MHA Code of Practice is particularly helpful in providing guidance on this extremely difficult area. It contains a very useful flow diagram and it also gives guidance about choosing between the two regimes in this very particular circumstance. It is important to remember that DoLS do not authorize treatment in the absence of consent. While legally available, it is likely that most, if not all clinicians, would opt to use the MHA in the setting of an acute ward.

Safeguards

Article 5 of the ECHR requires that a person who has been detained in hospital under the MHA has the right to appeal to a body able to discharge. These bodies are the hospital mangers and a First Tier Tribunal (Mental Health). A patient on a Section 2 has 14 days from the start of the period of detention to make an application to the Tribunal and those on Section 3 can apply once at any time during the first 6 months. Those who have had their CTOs revoked and are now detained on Section 3 have an automatic referral to a Tribunal.

The Tribunal comprises a judge, a tribunal doctor, and a lay member, all independent of the hospital. There is a right to be legally represented and legally aided. A medical report will be required from the RC, a social circumstances report, most often provided by the allocated care coordinator in the community, and a nursing report with a current ward care plan. The content of the report is specified in practice directions and must be followed. Section 3 reports must be available within 3 weeks of the request. These issues are discussed in the detail in the chapter on advocacy.

Following the principle of involvement and in the interests of fairness (Article 6, 'Right to a fair trial'), ECHR patients should receive the reports in good time so they can go through them with their solicitor or advocate. Zigmond (25, pp. 82–85) gives some extremely helpful tips about how to phrase the content of the report, keeping jargon to a minimum, and ways of presenting the information that is respectful of the patient's perspective.

Box 2.9 Mental Health Act resources

- Department of Health *Mental Health Act 1983: Code of Practice.* London: Department of Health; 2015 (https://assets.publishing. service.gov.uk/government/uploads/system/uploads/attachment_ data/file/435512/MHA_Code_of_Practice.PDF) (26).
- Department of Health. *Reference Guide to the Mental Health Act 1983.* London: Department of Health; 2015 (https://www.gov.uk/ government/uploads/system/uploads/attachment_data/file/417412/ Reference_Guide.pdf) (36).

Patients also have the right to appeal to the hospital managers who have the power of discharge. These 'managers' are not actually responsible for the management of the hospital but are specially appointed individuals. Patients can apply to both the hospital managers and the Tribunal.

The RC can discharge the detention at any point and the nearest relative, who is defined in section 26 MHA, can also ask for discharge but this may be barred by the RC if the patient is 'likely to act in a manner dangerous to other persons or to himself' (Section 25(1) of the MHA). Note that the criteria for barring discharge by the nearest relative are much higher than the criteria for admission (Box 2.9).

Treatment under the Mental Health Act

Treatment provisions are contained in Part 4 of the Act and Section 63 states:

> The consent of a patient shall not be required for any medical treatment given to him for the mental disorder from which he is suffering, not being treatment falling within Section 57 or 58 above, if the treatment is given by or under the direction of the approved clinician in charge of the treatment.

Medical treatment is defined in Section 145(1) of the MHA as including 'nursing, and also includes care, habilation, and rehabilitation under medical supervision'. The Act not only covers the treatment for the symptoms of mental disorder but also the physical manifestations of that disorder, for example, treatment of self-inflicted wounds. This also extends to the physical monitoring essential for safe prescription of certain drugs such as the regular blood tests needed to prescribe clozapine.

Section 63 of the MHA applies whether the patient is detained on Section 2 or Section 3 but not to the short-term sections such as Section 4, Section 5(4), nurse holding power, Section 5(2), or Sections 135(1) or 136. A patient held on one of these sections may of course, if they have capacity, consent to treatment or in an emergency be treated under the MCA if they lack the capacity to consent. Treatment must be the least restrictive, for example, oral rather than injection if possible. Any treatment must also be proportionate to the harm that treatment is seeking to address.

Having the legal power to treat is the first step. Great care must be taken to justify the decision to treat in the absence of consent as this is an infringement of the right to private and family life (Article 8 of the Humans Right Act 1998). This infringement may be justified if treatment is given in accordance with the law (in this case the MHA), deemed a medical necessity, and is proportionate to a legitimate aim, in this case, to improve health or to prevent deterioration.

It is especially important to have the principles underpinning the Act clearly in mind and be able to justify the decision to treat in the absence of consent:

- Least restrictive and maximizing independence: can medication be given orally or depots with wide administration intervals given for those who do not want injections but cannot be relied to take medication orally, or is it possible to agree and accept a treatment plan accommodating the patient's preferences even though this may not be the RC's first choice of medication?
- Empowerment and involvement: although many inpatients will be incapacitated as a result of their mental disorder, a person may still retain capacity to give or refuse treatment even if detained in hospital (26, para. 24.41). Even if a patient lacks capacity, they must be given the opportunity to be involved in the discussion if at all possible.
- Respect and dignity: compulsory treatment is capable of being inhuman treatment (or even torture) (Article 3, Human Rights Act) (26, para 24.43). Treatment must first meet a minimum level of severity if it is to fall within the scope of Article 3 and particular vigilance is required for those in 'the position of inferiority and powerlessness which is typical of patients confined in a psychiatric hospital' (27, 28). The European Court of Human Rights has concluded: 'As a general rule, a measure that is a therapeutic necessity cannot be regarded as inhuman or degrading' (29). This statement should not give rise to any sense of complacency and clinicians should always be prepared to explain their reasons to the patient for the decision to treat without consent including, where relevant, the decision to override an advance decision to refuse treatment (see 'Advance decisions to refuse treatment') or the wishes of an attorney.
- Purpose and effectiveness: the factors that need to be taken into account when considering the issue of medical necessity include the degree of certainty that the patient suffers from a treatable mental disorder, the seriousness of the disorder and the seriousness of any risk posed to others, the likelihood and extent of any alleviation of the condition, and the likelihood of any adverse consequences for the patient and the possible severity of such adverse effects (30). The RC is required to give a more detailed and carefully weighed justification for their treatment decision, or to put it colloquially, show their workings.
- Efficiency and equity: it is important that the team work together in order to deliver the treatment plan in a timely way and have clear goals.

If detained under the MHA, treatment for mental disorder, irrespective of whether a patient has capacity or not, will be governed by the MHA and the powers and duties of this Act must be followed. That is not to say that the principles of the MCA or consent should be discarded and indeed the issue of capacity and advance mechanisms to plan ahead become relevant (see 'Relationship between the power to treat in the absence of consent and mechanisms to plan in advance') when considering certain treatments. In essence, compulsion should be the last resort.

Limitations to Section 63

There are certain rules which apply to electroconvulsive therapy which limit the powers of Section 63. Electroconvulsive therapy cannot be given to a patient detained under the MHA if the patient has capacity and refuses. This is a small, albeit rather short-lived, victory for autonomy within the MHA as there is still the option for the RC to override this in an emergency. An emergency is defined in Section 62 of the MHA although, in this situation, limited to subsections (a) and (b) to:

- immediately necessary to save life, or
- prevent serious deterioration.

In the case of incapacity, electroconvulsive therapy cannot be given (unless in an emergency) unless the Second Opinion Appointed Doctor (SOAD, see below) authorizes this and:

- there is no valid and applicable advance decision refusing electroconvulsive therapy
- no authorized attorney or deputy objects
- treatment would not conflict with a decision of the Court of Protection.

Relationship between the power to treat in the absence of consent and mechanisms to plan in advance

The option to make an advance decision to refuse treatment is open to those with both physical and mental disorder. However, if detained under the MHA an advance refusal of medication for treatment for mental disorder or refusal by a welfare attorney can be overridden without any limitations although there are restrictions with respect to ECT (see above). If this occurs the RC should provide a written explanation why this decision was made.

Safeguards relating to treatment

The first 3 months of treatment with medication are at the discretion of the RC. After 3 months (calculated from the date of first administration), certain safeguards come into play. This is sometimes referred to as 'the 3-month rule'. In the first instance, the RC must consider whether the patient is 'capable of understanding the nature, purpose and likely effects of the treatment in question' (31). If the patient has capacity and consents to treatment the RC will complete a record of the discussion (trusts may have templates for this) and complete the statutory form T2.

If the patient is refusing (irrespective of capacity) or is not refusing but lacks capacity, a doctor appointed by the CQC, known as a Second Opinion Appointed Doctor (SOAD), must certify the treatment plan. As noted by a senior judge: 'Parliament devised the protective scheme of the 1983 Act as being necessary in order to guard among other things against misjudgement and lapses by the professionals involved in healthcare' (32).

The SOAD must consider if the treatment proposed would 'alleviate or prevent a deterioration of his condition' (33). The SOAD is required to consult with two other people, one a nurse and one from a discipline other than nursing or medicine, who have been professionally involved with the patient (34). If satisfied that the treatment plan fulfils the requirements of Section 58(3)(b), the SOAD then completes the relevant documentation (T3). SOADs are required, in the interests of fairness, to outline the substantive points on which they have based their decision (35) and the RC must communicate this to the patient.

Once the certificates are completed, a copy must be attached to the prescription. Care needs to be taken that any new medication is not given without it being covered by the appropriate certification.

Treatment on recall from a community treatment order

On recall to hospital, the patient is now subject to the provisions in Part 4 of the MHA including Section 63, that is, they are in a similar legal position to a patient detained on Section 2 or 3 where treatment can be given with the patient's consent or in the absence of consent under Section 63 subject to appropriate certification unless it is less than a month since the CTO was made when no certification is required. The following circumstances may apply:

1. If the community certification allows specific treatment on recall (i.e. has anticipated this eventuality) (Section 62A(4)(a)).
2. The RC can carry on with plan in the community certificate if it would cause serious suffering to delay pending a new certificate (Section 62A(5)).
3. Under provisions of Section 62 (Emergency)—in practice, this would be used to introduce a new treatment not covered by the community certification.

On revocation of a community treatment order

Revocation of a CTO means that the patient is now again detained on Section 3. The Reference Guide states at 26.60 (36): 'The Act then applies to them as if they had never been on a CTO. The only differences are that, for the purposes of expiry and renewal of the authority to detain, patients are treated as if they had first been detained on the day the CTO is revoked'. While the Section 3 period of detention starts afresh, the consent to treatment clock is still running from the original Section 3 prior to placing the patient on a CTO. This will mean that on revocation, most patients will either have to consent (documented on a T2) or will require SOAD certification.

Leaving hospital

The least restrictive principle dictates that the detention be discharged as soon as possible and the efficiency principle requires that professionals on the ward and in the community work to secure a safe, successful, and speedy discharge. It could be argued that even though still subject to the Act, a CTO offers a less restrictive option and patients may be willing to agree to the conditions in order to leave hospital. Despite unconvincing international evidence for their effectiveness and more recent evidence confirming previous findings that CTOs do not have any significant effect on hospitalization or other service use outcomes, they continue to be widely used (37–40). In the light of these concerns, patients and their representatives will rightly require professionals to justify their reasons for opting for compulsory treatment in the community. CTOs should therefore be considered on an individual basis and should never be a routine part of the discharge package for qualifying patients. A helpful starting point may be to adopt the rebuttable presumption that all patients will be discharged from compulsion as soon as possible unless there are clear reasons/individual evidence for thinking a CTO would be of benefit. A useful resource to help with this decision-making is the occasional paper published on the Royal College of Psychiatrist's website (41).

Regulation

The role of the CQC under the Health and Social Care Act 2008 is to protect and promote the health, safety, and welfare of people who use health and social care services. The CQC also has a role in monitoring the use of the MHA and DoLS and publishes yearly reports on the use of this legislation; it is also responsible for SOADs. The CQC is designated as the National Preventive Mechanism (NPM) against torture and ill treatment of people detained in health and social care establishments. The CQC describes its role in this capacity as follows:

> Establishment of an NPM is a legal requirement for states who are signatories of the Optional Protocol to the Convention against Torture and other Cruel, Inhuman or Degrading Treatment or Punishment (OPCAT), an international human rights treaty designed to strengthen the protection of people deprived of their liberty. (42)

Some challenges

There is an ethical argument to view having a separate legal regime for the assessment and treatment of mental disorder which allows the overriding of capacitated refusal as discriminatory compared to the approach to the assessment and treatment of physical illness where capacitated refusal must be respected. Despite such arguments being forcefully made by several stakeholders, the UK parliament took a different policy view when the possibility of single legislation for mental and physical disorder, so-called fusion legislation, was debated during consideration of reforms to the MHA culminating in the 2007 amendments to the MHA. Scotland, which has separate mental health law to England and Wales, has recognized the role of capacity in mental health law by requiring the presence of seriously impaired decision-making as one of the necessary criteria for detention and the Northern Ireland Assembly has passed capacity-based legislation covering both physical and mental disorder which will come into force in 2020.

The United Nations Convention on the Rights of Persons with Disabilities (UNCRPD) has taken the issue of non-discrimination even further. The UNCRPD, signed up to and ratified by the UK, takes a fundamentally different approach to previous international and domestic law having, at its heart, a social model of disability. As Bartlett and Sandland noted: 'It [the UNCRPD] directly challenges the use of state power when laws rely on the concepts of disability (including mental disability) to govern detention, involuntary treatment, and decision-making for people identified as lacking capacity' (43). Current law requires the presence of a mental disorder as necessary criteria for detention or indeed for a finding of incapacity (the 'diagnostic arm', see 'The Mental Capacity Act 2005'). While legal academics such as Peter Bartlett and others argue that current legislation is not compatible with the UNCRPD, the UK government has stated that 'After signing the Convention in 2007, the UK reviewed its existing legislation for consistency with it. Because of the approach to disability equality that has been developed over a number of years, and progress already made, it was able to ratify the Convention successfully' (44, para. 47).

Such discussions may seem rather esoteric to frontline practitioners but the ethos of equality, non-discrimination, and doing all that is possible to maximize participation in decisions as well as truly listening to the voice of the patient clearly do have a place in day-to-day work on the ward (Box 2.10).

> **Box 2.10** Fusion legislation resources
>
> - A special edition of the *Journal of Mental Health Law* considers aspects of fusion legislation and includes an account of the debates at the time of the 2007 amendments to the MHA (45).
> - Link to description of seriously impaired decision-making ability (SIDMA) as used in Scotland as criteria for detention (http://www.nes-mha.scot.nhs.uk/stdc/sigimpaired.htm).
> - Useful discussion of the ground-breaking Northern Ireland legislation (46).
> - Lively and easily readable debate about the pros and cons of fusion legislation (47).
> - Academic article about the implications of UNCRPD (48).

Concluding remarks

All staff, both clinical and non-clinical, working on the inpatient unit have an important part to play in protecting the rights of this vulnerable group of patients by adhering to the law and applying the principles that underpin the legislation. The detail and complexity of the law may seem daunting. However, genuine attention to the basics of fairness, respect, equality, dignity, and autonomy which are understandable and easily remembered and which resonate with the principles underpinning the legislation, if followed, will go a long way to improving the experience of all patients on the ward, whether detained or not.

REFERENCES

1. Sarkar S, Adshead G. Treatment over objection: minds, bodies and beneficence. *J Ment Health Law* 2002;7:105–118.
2. Nunes V, Neilson J, O'Flynn N, et al. *Clinical Guidelines and Evidence Review for Medication Adherence: Involving Patients in Decisions about Prescribed Medication and Supporting Adherence.* London: National Collaborating Centre for primary care and Royal College of General practitioners; 2009.
3. Department of Health. *Human Rights in Healthcare: A Framework for Local Action.* London: Department of Health; 2008. http://webarchive.nationalarchives.gov.uk/20130124044024/http://www.dh.gov.uk/prod_consum_dh/groups/dh_digitalassets/@dh/@en/documents/digitalasset/dh_088972.pdf
4. United Nations Foundation. 10 Inspiring Eleanor Roosevelt Quotes. 2015. http://unfoundationblog.org/10-inspiring-eleanor-roosevelt-quotes/
5. MIND. Human Rights Act 1998. 2017. http://www.mind.org.uk/information-support/legal-rights/human-rights-act-1998/about-the-human-rights-act/#.WFfBwVOLR0w
6. Kelly N. Human rights in psychiatric practice: an overview for clinicians. *BJPsych Adv* 2015;21:54–62.
7. Curtice M. Article 3 of the Human Rights Act 1998: implications for clinical practice. *BJPsych Adv* 2008;14:389–397.
8. Curtice M. The European Convention Human Rights: an update on Article 3 case law. *BJPsych Adv* 2010;16:199–206.
9. Curtice M. Article 8 of the Human Rights Act 1998: implications for clinical practice. *BJPsych Adv* 2009;15:23–31.
10. Care Quality Commission. *Monitoring the Mental Health Act in 2015/2016.* London: Care Quality Commission; 2016. http://webarchive.nationalarchives.gov.uk/20170305103418/http://www.cqc.org.uk/content/monitoring-mental-health-act-report
11. Kings Fund. Briefing: Mental Health under Pressure. 2015. https://www.kingsfund.org.uk/sites/files/kf/field/field_publication_file/mental-health-under-pressure-nov15_0.pdf
12. Ministry of Justice. *Mental Capacity Act 2005: Deprivation of Liberty Safeguards—Code of Practice to Supplement the Mental Capacity Act 2005 Code of Practice.* London: TSO; 2008.http://webarchive.nationalarchives.gov.uk/20130107105354/http://www.dh.gov.uk/prod_consum_dh/groups/dh_digitalassets/@dh/@en/documents/digitalasset/dh_087309.pdf
13. *P (by his litigation friend the Official Solicitor) (Appellant) v Cheshire West and Chester Council and another (Respondents) P and Q (by their litigation friend, the Official Solicitor) (Appellants) v Surrey County Council (Respondent)* [2014] UKSC 19.
14. *Stanev v Bulgaria* [2012] ECHR 46 (Application no. 36760/06).
15. *P (by his litigation friend the Official Solicitor) (Appellant) v Cheshire West and Chester Council and another (Respondents) P and Q (by their litigation friend, the Official Solicitor) (Appellants) v Surrey County Council (Respondent)* [2014] UKSC 19 at 46.
16. Owen GS, Szmuker G, Richardson G, et al. Mental capacity and psychiatric in-patients: implications for the new mental health law in England and Wales. *Br J Psychiatry* 2009;195:257–63.
17. List suggested by Steve Chamberlain, Social Worker and Approved Mental Health Professional as quoted in article on the implications of the Supreme Court judgement by Julie Chalmers. http://www.rcpsych.ac.uk/pdf/Steve%20Oxberry%20article%20on%20capacity%20to%20consent.pdf
18. *A PCT v LDV, CC and B Healthcare Group* [2013] EWHC 272 (Fam) 3.
19. Sheehan KA, Burns T. Perceived coercion and the therapeutic relationship: a neglected association? *Psychiatr Serv* 2011;62:471–476.
20. Ruck Keene A, Aukland C. More presumptions please? Wishes, feelings and best interests decision-making. *Elder Law J* 2015;3:293–301.
21. Legislation.gov.uk. Mental Health Act 1983, Section 118 (2D). 1983. https://www.legislation.gov.uk/ukpga/1983/20/section/118
22. *R (Munjaz) v Ashworth* [2005] UKHL 58 para. 21.
23. Care Quality Commission. Summary of findings from the 2013/14 HSCIC report. In: *Monitoring the Mental Health Act in 2013/2014,* p. 35. London: Care Quality Commission; 2014. https://www.cqc.org.uk/sites/default/files/20150204_monitoring_the_mha_2013-14_report_web.pdf
24. Legislation.gov.uk. Policing and Crime Act 2017, Section 82 (3) (b)—reducing the permitted time in a place of safety from 72 hrs to 24 hrs and Section 82 (4) allowing extension under certain circumstances. 2017. http://www.legislation.gov.uk/ukpga/2017/3/contents/enacted
25. Zigmond T. *A Clinician's Brief Guide to the Mental Health Act,* 2nd edition. London: RCPsych Publications; 2012.
26. Department of Health. *Mental Health Act 1983: Code of Practice.* London: Department of Health; 2015. https://assets.publishing.service.gov.uk/government/uploads/system/uploads/attachment_data/file/435512/MHA_Code_of_Practice.PDF
27. *T and V v UK* [2000] EHRR 30 121.
28. *Herczegflavy v Austria* (A/242B) [1992] 15 EHRR 437 at 82 and 83.
29. *Herczegflavy v Austria* (A/242B) [1992] 15 EHRR 437 at 82.
30. *R (on the application of N) v Dr M* [2002] EWHC 1911.
31. Legislation.gov.uk. Mental Health Act 1983 Section 58(2)(b). 1983. https://www.legislation.gov.uk/ukpga/1983/20/section/58
32. *R v Bournewood Community and Mental Health Trust, Ex parte L* [1999] 1 AC 458 at 492–493.
33. Legislation.gov.uk. Mental Health Act 1983, Section 58(3)(b). 1983. https://www.legislation.gov.uk/ukpga/1983/20/section/58

34. Legislation.gov.uk. Mental Health Act 1983, Section 58(4). 1983. https://www.legislation.gov.uk/ukpga/1983/20/section/58

35. *R* v *Feggetter and MHAC, ex parte JW* [2002] EWCA Civ 554 at 29.

36. Department of Health. *Reference Guide to the Mental Health Act 1983*. London: TSO; 2015. https://www.gov.uk/government/uploads/system/uploads/attachment_data/file/417412/Reference_Guide.pdf

37. Churchill R, Owen G, Singh S, Hotopf M. *International Experiences of Using Community Treatment Orders*. London: Institute of Psychiatry; 2007.

38. Maughan D, Molodynski A, Rugkåsa J, Burns T. A systematic review of the effect of community treatment orders on service use. *Soc Psychiatry Psychiatr Epidemiol* 2014;49:651–663.

39. Burns T, Rugkåsa J, Molodynski A, et al. Community treatment orders for patients with psychosis (OCTET): a randomised controlled trial. *Lancet* 2013;381:1627–1633.

40. Kisely SR, Campbell LA. Compulsory community and involuntary outpatient treatment for people with severe mental disorders. *Cochrane Database Syst Rev* 2014;12:CD004408.

41. Chalmers J. Thinking about community treatment orders: a structured clinical approach to decision-making. Royal College of Psychiatrists Occasional Paper 99. 2016. http://www.rcpsych.ac.uk/usefulresources/publications/collegereports/op/op99.aspx

42. Care Quality Commission. Monitoring the MHA. In: *Monitoring the Mental Health Act in 2013/2014*, p. 14. London: Care Quality Commission; 2014. https://www.cqc.org.uk/sites/default/files/20150204_monitoring_the_mha_2013-14_report_web.pdf

43. Bartlett P, Sandland R. *Mental Health Law: Policy and Practice*, 4th edition. Oxford: Oxford University Press; 2014.

44. Office for Disability Issues. UK Initial Report: On the UN Convention on the Rights of Persons with Disabilities. https://assets.publishing.service.gov.uk/government/uploads/system/uploads/attachment_data/file/345120/uk-initial-report.pdf

45. Gledhill K. The role of capacity in mental health laws –recent reviews and legislation. *J Ment Health Law* 2010;20;129–140.

46. Harper C, Davidson G, McClelland R. No longer 'anomalous, confusing and unjust': the Mental Capacity Act (Northern Ireland) 2016. *Int J Mental Health Capacity Law* 2016;22:57–70. http://www.northumbriajournals.co.uk/index.php/IJMHMCL/article/view/272/266

47. Smuckler G, Kelly B. We should replace conventional mental health law with capacity based law. *Br J Psychiatry* 2016;209:449–453.

48. Bartlett P. The United Nations Convention on the Rights of Persons with Disability and Mental Health Law. *Mod Law Rev* 2012;75:752–778.

3

International perspectives on inpatient mental health care

Andrew Molodynski

Introduction

Acute inpatient care is a crucial part of mental health care, and always has been. While some human rights and service user groups argue passionately that it should never be needed, most agree that there are times when an individual is so unwell that they need 'looking after', hopefully temporarily. A proportion of people with long-term mental health problems require long-term, occasionally lifelong, care. Facilities for the care and containment of the mentally ill existed long before the availability of effective interventions, as described in Chapter 1. Inpatient provision reached its height in many high-income group countries around the middle of the last century before the progressive reduction in beds began, with very significant reductions in many countries (1).

In England, bed provision has dropped from 150,000 in the 1950s to approximately 20,000 currently (2). In other countries, especially those with little or no provision, bed numbers have actually increased and provide some form of managed care for the first time. Institutions still form the mainstay of mental health care in many countries worldwide, where it can be a struggle to divert energy and resources to build a comprehensive system that includes primary and community care. In such places, inpatient units *are* care and their loss would be catastrophic in the absence of alternative provision. Conditions can be very poor, however, with relatively little treatment and overt and damaging coercion (3, 4). In countries such as the UK (and perhaps especially in the UK), progressive reductions in beds have led to a situation where there is chronic over-occupancy, high rates of detention, and increasing instances where people are admitted many miles from home as there are no beds locally. Most inpatient units in the UK are now locked, though evidence for the positive effects of this is lacking and in many countries wards remain open. These are pressing issues in contemporary British psychiatry and we will return to them later.

This chapter will first outline the investment in and relative provision of mental health services in different regions of the world and in countries with different income levels. The components of an 'ideal' mental health service will then be discussed from the point of view of the empirical evidence. This discussion necessarily concentrates on

services for adults, though it does briefly examine services for children and older people, which are considered in detail in Chapters 33 and 34 respectively.

Global mental health care investment and provision

As one would expect, there are enormous differences in levels of investment in health care globally. Such differences primarily reflect economy, but also culture and attitudes. The latter are especially important in influencing the proportion of overall health spend allocated to mental health care. For instance, in England the contribution of mental health conditions to overall disease burden is estimated at about 23% but investment is approximately 18%—a disparity no doubt unacceptable, but much better than many places. Uganda allocates approximately 1% of its overall health budget to mental health (5). As a result, services are woefully inadequate and conditions in the national hospital are reportedly poor. It is not fair though to single out a country such as Uganda, as many are in the same position and hopefully at the beginning of a journey to improve both access to care and its quality. Figure 3.1 illustrates two crucial facts:

1. The enormous disparity in mental health spend between countries (250-fold in some cases).
2. The ability of wealthier countries to invest in community care.

Figure 3.2 illustrates the number of people receiving social support in the community for mental health problems in different income groups globally. It is not surprising that many more people in high-income group countries receive social support given the wide disparities in available funds. In poorer countries, support will come from families or communities, or often not at all.

In terms of inpatient activity, there are wide variations in terms of numbers of beds available and number of admissions per head of population per year. These are illustrated in Figure 3.3.

The differences are again clear and substantial. Such statistics fail to identify any differences in the nature, quality, and outcomes of

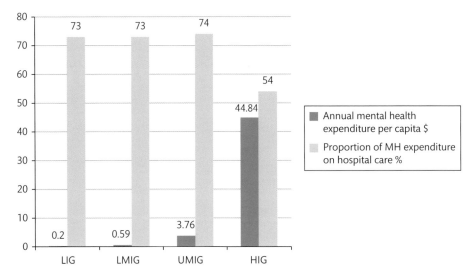

Figure 3.1 Mental health expenditure and allocation per capita in different income groups. HIG, high-income group; LIG, low-income group; LMIG, lower middle-income group; UMIG, upper middle-income group.
Reprinted from *Mental Health Atlas* 2011, World Health Organization, 2011.

care, which are difficult to measure in local areas and almost impossible on a cross-national basis. Given that the prevalence of most severe mental illnesses is relatively similar across countries, it is clear that the ability of health systems to respond will vary substantially. Informal carers shoulder much of the burden where formalized care is lacking. As a result of these differences in funding and provision, there are different issues of relevance in different places. For example, out-of-area placements—a mechanism where a patient is admitted many miles from home—cause controversy and debate in the UK but are utterly irrelevant somewhere such as Indonesia where it is the relative absence of care that matters, not where it happens. Inequalities also exist within countries, such as the well-documented fact that black British men are more likely to be subject to the mental health act than those from other communities (6) and the variable provision of beds and community services seen between

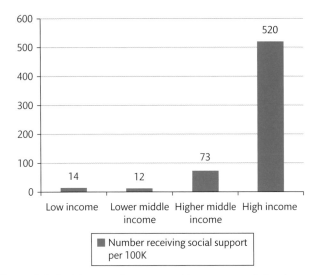

Figure 3.2 Social support for persons with severe mental disorders.
Reprinted from *Mental Health Atlas* 2014, World Health Organization, 2014.

regions in many countries. These 'within-country' differences can be about economics, but are likely to be influenced by local factors such as attitudes, existing structures, and levels of need and help-seeking behaviour.

The 'ideal' mental health service

Building blocks

Of course, the 'ideal' service does not exist, whatever some politicians (and even health managers and clinicians sometimes) might say! What is useful and acceptable in one country (or even one region of a country) may not be in a neighbouring one with different values, religious beliefs, and challenges. However, there is some evidence to guide us regarding the components needed to adequately deliver a comprehensive system of care that is *good enough* for most people in the community who might need it (7). A good starting point is an authoritative review by Thornicroft and Tansella (8). Although this was published some years ago now, changes in overall service provision are usually incremental and slow so it is still relevant and useful. Local and regional service provision can change more quickly, and we will revisit this in a UK context later in the chapter. As mentioned previously, different countries can afford very different levels of investment in mental health services. Thornicroft and Tansella argue that for the poorest countries this may mean a policy of supporting communities or primary care to identify and treat where possible the most severe mental illness. As we move up the income bands then investment in outpatient clinics, hospitals, and eventually specialized services such as employment support, crisis teams, and early intervention services (to name just a few) is possible and is justified by evidence. Table 3.1 lists suggested components to be considered at different levels of resource availability.

It is clear to anyone looking at the international literature regarding service provision and the evidence for it that much is unclear and

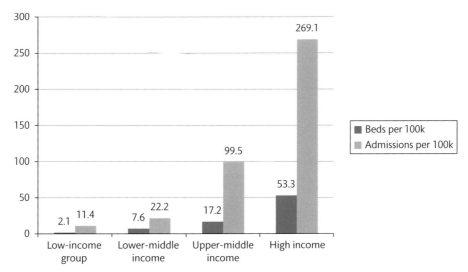

Figure 3.3 Bed numbers and admissions by country income group.
Reprinted from *Mental Health Atlas* 2014, World Health Organization, 2014.

conflicted. One key overarching issue is almost unanimously agreed upon: there is no service which is wholly community or wholly in-patient based that can adequately meet the needs of a population. A mixed approach is necessary (9). Figure 3.4 illustrates the basic building blocks necessary in a reasonably well-resourced system.

The size and exact structure of these blocks will vary significantly within and between countries but they are now widely accepted to form the bedrock of a service that can meet the needs of the majority of the population. In many places, inpatient care has been reduced and finances redirected to community care to provide a more

Table 3.1 Suggested mental health service components at different investment levels

Low level of resources	Medium level of resources	High level of resources
Step A *Step A. Primary care with specialist back-up*	**Step A + step B** *Step B. Mainstream mental health care*	**Step A + step B + step C** *Step C. Specialized/differentiated mental health services*
Screening and assessment by primary care staff	Out-patient/ambulatory clinics	Specialized clinics for specific disorders or patient groups, including: ● eating disorders ● dual diagnosis ● treatment-resistant affective disorders ● adolescent services
Talking treatments, including counselling and advice		
Pharmacological treatment		
Liaison and training with mental health specialist staff, when available	Community mental health teams	Specialized community mental health teams, including: ● early intervention teams ● assertive community treatment
Limited specialist back-up available for: ● training ● consultation for complex cases ● in-patient assessment and treatment for cases that cannot be managed in primary care, for example in general hospitals	Acute inpatient care	Alternatives to acute hospital admission, including: ● home treatment/crisis resolution teams ● crisis/respite houses ● acute day hospital
	Long-term community-based residential care	Alternative types of long-stay community residential care, including: ● intensive 24h staffed residential provision ● less intensively staffed accommodation ● independent accommodation
	Employment and occupation	Alternative forms of occupation and vocational rehabilitation: ● sheltered workshops ● supervised work placements ● cooperative work schemes ● self-help and user groups ● club houses/transitional employment programmes ● vocational rehabilitation ● individual placement and support service

Reproduced from Thornicroft, G. and Tansella, M., 2004. Components of a modern mental health service: a pragmatic balance of community and hospital care. *The British Journal of Psychiatry*, 185(4), pp. 283–290.

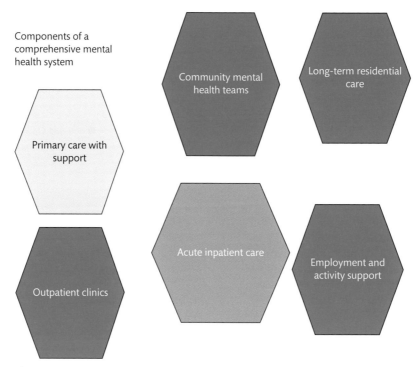

Components of a comprehensive mental health system

Primary care with support

Community mental health teams

Long-term residential care

Outpatient clinics

Acute inpatient care

Employment and activity support

Figure 3.4 Suggested basic components of mental health care systems.

balanced system. In other countries, this is simply not possible as inpatient care is limited already. The different services will be briefly described in the following subsections, with reference to their evidence base.

Community mental health teams

Generic community mental health teams are the bedrock of most community services and closely allied to inpatient and crisis care teams (10). They first began to develop in the latter half of the twentieth century in the UK as a response to several factors, including the new welfare state, the availability of psychotropic medications, and deinstitutionalization. The new Mental Health Act 1959 and its principle of 'reciprocity' was crucial as it introduced a responsibility to provide aftercare following discharge. Also important was the 'water tower' speech by then Health Minister Enoch Powell in 1961 in which he called for strategic change in the whole nature of mental health care:

> There they stand, isolated, majestic, imperious, brooded over by the gigantic water-tower and chimney combined, rising unmistakable and daunting out of the countryside—the asylums which our forefathers built with such immense solidity to express the notions of their day. Do not for a moment underestimate their powers of resistance to our assault … the transformation of the mental hospitals is not only a matter of buildings, the change of a physical pattern, it is also the transformation of a whole branch of the profession of medicine, of nursing, of hospital administration. Politics apart, let us admit that we all have a great deal of the conservative in our make-up, and find it easier to envisage things going on much as at present, or with small or gradual modifications, than deliberately to choose and favour the unaccustomed, the drastic and voluntarily to bring about a pattern of organisation in which new tasks will be performed in a new and wider setting … it is the duty of a Minister of Health and the duty of the National Association for Mental Health, to lean with all their

might … to choose and to favour the course of more drastic and fundamental change.

These powerful forces came together to allow the creation of the first fledgling services outside institutions. Since that time, community mental health teams have increased in scope and complexity and are now common in many countries around the world. They generally cover a discrete geographical area (that varies in size depending on resources) and are multidisciplinary in nature, with doctors, nurses, social workers, occupational therapists, and (hopefully) psychologists working together to be able to meet the needs of most people with mental illnesses in the local area. The overall model predates the era of mental health services research but has been durable and robust for several decades now, unlike many other services (11).

Day hospitals

Day hospitals form part of most mental health services, including in low-income group countries, as they can be relatively easily provided from traditional institutional bases such as inpatient units. Like community mental health teams, they were introduced prior to the era of collecting systematic evidence but have formed part of services nevertheless for many decades now. They vary significantly in size and approach, but can be crudely subdivided into acute day hospitals and longer-term day centres. In the former, there will characteristically be trained professionals and the ethos is to work acutely with people with severe mental illness or high levels of acute distress and risk to prevent them being admitted to hospital. In the latter, people may attend for years for social contact, structured activities, and monitoring. The reader will not be surprised that there is considerable overlap and blurring and it is often the case that even those who pay for and run services are not clear what they have.

Early intervention in psychosis services

Early intervention in psychosis services are now commonplace as part of well-resourced systems and have a particular remit to reduce the duration of untreated psychosis, as this is known to be associated with a worse long-term outcome (12). Early intervention in psychosis services vary significantly but a core role is the early identification and treatment of psychosis using a broad biopsychosocial model, while preserving as much function and community engagement as possible (13). There is evidence of effectiveness in the short term but accumulating concerns that gains may be lost over time (14). Nevertheless, the concept is attractive to clinicians, politicians, and those who use services and their carers. As a result, these services look more likely to survive than other specialist teams.

Assertive outreach teams

Assertive outreach teams originated from North America following a truly ground-breaking study in Wisconsin in 1980, in which it was proven that highly disabled psychotic patients could be successfully cared for outside institutions with an active and practical approach called the 'training in community living program' (15). Patients received active, practical support focusing on day-to-day life. Crucially, this support assertively reached out to people and did not wait for them to attend appointments themselves. As with early intervention in psychosis services, this model has enormous intuitive appeal and early research findings were very positive. However, later studies in more developed and supportive general services failed to find a significant advantage in terms of readmission, costs of care, or symptom and functioning levels (16, 17).

Crisis resolution and home treatment teams

The early research on crisis resolution and home treatment teams was conducted by Hoult and colleagues in Sydney, Australia, with profound results that ushered in a wave of teams across the world over the following years (18). Early pioneering results haven't generally been replicated, though an innovative study in England and Wales by Glover and colleagues (19) looked at rates of admissions over a period of several years and mapped them onto availability and type of crisis service. The study demonstrated a positive effect in well-managed services.

Liaison psychiatry

These services are at the interface of physical and mental health care and are generally multidisciplinary teams with more medical input and less input from other disciplines due to their nature and remit (20). Again, they have been enthusiastically adopted as part of health care systems in many high-income group countries, following positive research findings (21). They are not widely available in low- and middle-income group countries, though presumably the need is the same, or perhaps greater when one considers the relative paucity of mental health services.

Eating disorder services and personality disorder services

Separate services now exist in many systems as recognition that the presentation and needs of people with eating and/or personality disorders can be quite different from those of people with psychosis or severe affective disorders. It goes without saying that, as with all specialized services, this sophistication comes at a financial cost and also creates a more complex system for the patient to navigate and for managers to administer.

Employment services

There is considerable variation in the nature and extent of these services, more so than the services mentioned above. This may be partly because work and meaningful activity are often very culture bound and lack of activity (whatever the cause) is generally highly stigmatized by societies. The intervention with the strongest evidence base is undoubtedly 'Individual Placement and Support'. Again, this originated in North America (22) and studies in Europe have replicated the positive results of the early US studies (23). Again, however, it has been little tested outside a small group of similar countries with high gross domestic product. Other models exist, everything from long-term 'sheltered work' with support staff and limited expectations to small business start-up grants for individuals to 'make a go' of things. The later increasingly form part of the overall model in low-income group countries, with profoundly positive effects in some cases.

Alternative solutions

The previous paragraphs follow the traditional pattern of suggesting that low- and middle-income group countries should follow the example of wealthier countries. The latter are predominantly 'westernized' countries with a set of values that favours the rights of the individual over wider community values. Interventions commonly used in such societies may not be appropriate or helpful where families play a greater role in care, such as in many parts of Africa, Asia, and South America. It is difficult to be clear, however, as the enhanced family role is often a result of necessity due to the absence of statutory services (4). One example of a different approach is a project in Uganda that prioritizes making loans and support available to those with mental health problems to work and help support their families (24). They cite numerous examples where this has led to significantly improved quality of life and productivity from the allocation of really trifling levels of resource. Examples include buying seeds or granting a loan for someone to buy a small solar panel and become a living, cycling mobile phone charger—an indispensable resource and a sustainable living in rural areas. While these interventions may not form part of a 'standard set' applicable in countries like the US or many European countries, they may improve or save lives elsewhere and should not be underestimated. They may be more cost-effective and more palatable than the large-scale importation of approaches tested elsewhere, and thus do more good overall. Perhaps the traditional approach in the largely westernized literature of encouraging poorer countries to adopt 'as much as possible' of approaches that have evidence bases formed in this relatively small group of countries with similar legal systems, social structures, and prevailing attitudes should be lessened and an acceptance or encouragement of different models be developed. For example in countries with severe economic challenges, high levels of stigma, and high levels of unemployment it may be less stigmatizing to focus on opportunities to work and contribute, as in the example from Uganda. The components might then look more like the following (in order of capacity, not cost):

- Educational and work schemes.
- Stigma reduction.
- Community support and outreach to distribute medications.
- Some provision for supported accommodation in each region.
- Hospital beds for treatment-resistant patients or those for whom community tenure is not safe.

In such a system, though the basic building blocks will be similar, the relative weight given to each one and the capacity of it may be very different from the generally accepted model in wealthier countries. The difficulty in making decisions regarding provision in lower-income group countries (where full overhaul may be needed) is the stark lack of evidence or even statistics on the need to inform change.

Key international challenges for inpatient care

It is clear that inpatient care will form part of any mental health service internationally, and as far as can be ascertained all countries have inpatient beds, though as shown earlier, the number of these varies significantly. Key recurrent themes in the international literature regarding inpatient care are briefly outlined in the following subsections with examples from different countries and systems.

Amount of provision and access

We have already looked at global figures for investment in services, as well as the wide disparity in psychiatric bed numbers between countries in different income groups. These overarching statistics (25) hide some illuminating differences, however. A study by Priebe compared bed numbers in different European countries, all of whom have comparatively well-resourced mental health and social care systems (26). Despite having adequate resources and broadly similar societal attitudes (compared to countries outside Western Europe), bed provision varied enormously. Reported bed numbers varied between 5.3 per 100,000 inhabitants in Italy to 135.5 in the Netherlands. England was approximately midway with a reported 62.8 beds per 100,000 population. This strongly suggests that mental health systems and responses to crises differ substantially between countries due to factors apart from wealth or significant differences in culture—Italy is a little different to England and the Netherlands but not that different! These differences in bed provision reflect differences in practice. For example, admission to hospital in Germany for people with anxiety disorders is common and cognitive behavioural therapy and medication are used early and in conjunction. This would seem unthinkable in the UK where inpatient care is generally reserved for those with psychosis or very severe affective disorders and people with anxiety may wait months or even years (sadly) for appropriate intervention. The reasoning behind the German model (crucially an insurance-based set-up) is that although early intervention and hospitalization is expensive, it is cost effective if welfare use is less and the individual can return to work faster. This is perhaps food for thought for those who practise in the UK, and it

was certainly part of the thinking in setting up 'Improving Access to Psychological Therapies' services.

Having recently visited excellent inpatient services in Geneva, a city with substantial inpatient care and little in the community, I can bear witness to the fact that the atmosphere and approach of hospitals is very different, with open doors, less distress, and a more collaborative atmosphere than our busy, locked, and cramped units in the UK. The price that is paid, however, is clear on the streets, with manifestly unwell individuals lacking care and treatment that they would likely receive in the UK.

Outside of Europe, variations in bed provision are even more marked. Overall statistics for the Americas disguise an enormous difference between North America and Canada and 'the rest' with the US being calculated to have 910 admissions per 100,000 population for adult acute psychiatric care in 2004 (27). This relatively high rate in a large country skews the continental data significantly; many countries, for example Chile, have services that do not provide adequate beds or community care for their population (28). Even in the US, it is widely reported that there are more mentally ill people in prison than hospital following the latest rounds of deinstitutionalization—a shocking reflection on a society (29). Across South America too, prison numbers have risen while psychiatric beds have reduced (30), seemingly confirming the inverse relationship between the two forms of custody—the so-called Penrose principle (31). However, a recent systematic review of the international evidence over recent years (32) casts doubt on such a clear relationship and rightly highlights the number of wider factors that influence whether an individual is admitted to prison or not. Many of these are not related to changes in service provision, but some have used recent research like this to argue against deinstitutionalization in South America. It is more likely that a mixed approach of investing adequately in community services and support alongside rationalizing hospital estates and improving conditions would do more for those with severe mental illnesses in countries such as Chile.

Asia is undoubtedly the most diverse continent, both in terms of number of different countries and in societal and economic variation. China is the most populous country and an interesting example in terms of mental health care. Information can be difficult to come by regarding Chinese health care (I recently co-wrote a book and several leading psychiatrists in the region were fearful of taking part in case of repercussions). This is changing though and we increasingly know more. Over recent years, a massive programme of reform called the '686 Project' has been ongoing. It principally aims to make available community care to as many of the population as possible, but crucially also has a huge mental hospital building programme to create 550 new modern psychiatric hospitals. From a global perspective, this increase in bed provision is highly unusual, but records appear to show that China previously had very low bed numbers overall, as little as 1 per 100,000 population. There is also enormous variation between urban and rural areas (33). Also unusual by international standards is the fact that a high proportion of beds were (and still are) in institutions with over 500 beds. India, the other giant that is awakening in terms of mental health care provision and reform, also has great shortages of both hospital beds and community care facilities and is seeking to address these.

Moving to Africa, there is a more uniform picture of inadequate services, with some exceptions. Many countries in sub-Saharan Africa, for example Uganda, have very low levels of relative and absolute investment and as a result, inpatient services are centrally located and inadequate. Access for much of the population is thus very limited (34, 35). In South Africa, progress has been made with de-institutionalization and decentralization. There has been an increase in community services and a reduction in bed numbers over the years since the introduction of more modern mental health legislation in the form of the Mental Health Care Act 2002, which focused more on holistic care and individual rights (36).

Quality of provision

The quality of inpatient care varies as much as the amount internationally. Quality is a hard notion to define but must encompass such things as relative comfort, freedom from fear, adequate nutrition and general health care, and an acceptable level of mental health interventions. At one end of the scale, there are highly staffed and resourced units in many high-income group countries with input from psychologists, psychiatrists, nurses, occupational therapists, and others. There is ready access to all available medications and other interventions needed and patients generally have individual rooms, often with en-suite facilities. At the other end of the scale are units such as those described below in Indonesia, where an influential human rights charity report contained the following:

> In Panti Laras 2, approximately 90 women live in a room that can reasonably accommodate no more than 30 … to enter one had to literally tiptoe over hands and feet … as a consequence of sleeping close together on the floor or sharing wooden slats, many people have lice. Instead of providing anti-lice shampoo, staff forcibly shave their heads.[1]

These differences are principally related to economy, but also reflect prevailing social attitudes to those affected by mental illness and their families. Where mental illness is still seen as a curse or affliction of some kind, and where there is a strong collectivist culture (and expectation on the family to care for their relative), it can be understood why adequate facilities are not felt to be a priority among competing demands for very limited resources. It is easy to find numerous similar reports, particularly relating to low-income group countries in Africa, Asia, and South America. There are worrying reports from North Korea of poor conditions and the ongoing use of insulin coma therapy (37). However, poor conditions are not confined to poor countries. There have been widespread concerns regarding conditions in many former Soviet bloc and central European countries (38, 39), as well as some in the southern Mediterranean regions of Europe. Major international newspapers reported food shortages at a large Greek asylum only in 2012, reportedly a result of ongoing austerity following the global financial crisis.

Coercion and human rights abuses

Psychiatry, particularly that within institutions, has a long and inglorious history of human rights abuses, most notably in Fascist Germany, Soviet Russia, and Communist China. These, however,

were only the most extreme and large-scale abuses. What one sees as an abuse of human rights or the use of excessive coercion is very contextual. An example from my practice a few years ago in urban Southern England comes to mind:

> I had to detain a young Bangladeshi woman who was suffering with a severe manic episode and not responding to treatment. Her very supportive family offered to tie her up and bring her the 20 miles to hospital that afternoon to help out. I was initially horrified and we of course arranged for the police to come instead; they handcuffed her and bound her legs before putting her in a van and transporting her to the same place. Undoubtedly this was safer, but was it less traumatic—perhaps not?

It would not be appropriate in this chapter to attempt to explore issues of coercion and human rights in any detail. Accounts can easily be found (34, 40, 41) and this section is simply a very brief introduction to some of the issues. Very crudely put, issues of coercion in wealthy countries tend to relate to the increasing scope and use of legislation such as community treatment orders in the absence of evidence for effectiveness (42), the use of physical/mechanical/chemical restraint, and the increasing phenomenon of locked units. In lower-income group countries, coercion includes these things as well but often results from a relative or total absence of available treatment. This leaves a vacuum in which many mentally ill people are simply contained by desperate families or within institutions with no legislative safeguards or external scrutiny (4).

Prominent human rights concerns relating to inpatient care in the UK at present relate primarily to increasing rates of detention in hospital and an associated increased proportion of detained patients, locked environments, seclusion, and the use of physical restraint, particularly so-called face-down restraint. It has been argued by some that the increasing use of out-of-area placements far from where a person lives breaches their right to a family life as enshrined in the United Nations Universal Declaration of Human Rights. Though significant noises have been made by senior members of the profession and especially politicians regarding this practice, and despite the fact that it is undeniably counterproductive and unhelpful, it persists and if anything is increasing. It does not appear to be a prominent feature of mental health systems in other countries, except in very impoverished systems where the nearest unit may be 200–300 miles away and there is no alternative. Practices of restraint in the UK have been changing over recent years, with an increased focus on de-escalation, amending rigid routines, and generally trying to make the environment and interventions fit the patient, rather than vice versa. There are encouraging reports from units that have adopted this approach, such as in Cambridge, but much work remains to be done and rigorous evaluation will be needed.

While mechanical restraints are not used in acute inpatient care in the UK, they are fairly commonly used in North America, Scandinavia, and other European countries. Cage beds, structures where a standard single bed has bars up to the ceiling and the patient remains in there, often including defecating, remain in use in some central European countries such as the Czech Republic, though numbers are declining (43).

Outside Europe, and especially in low-income group countries across Asia and Africa, human rights issues tend to relate to very impoverished and poor conditions such as those described earlier in Indonesia and in Uganda. Chaining, shackling, and tying are common as is the use of painful physical treatments, such as excoriating the skin and beating to remove the symptoms experienced by the sufferer, often ascribed to evil spirits. That these practices continue to occur in open view in many countries around the world brings shame on our professions and societies. Change is slow, but is occurring. Many countries have now developed legislation, but it is frequently outdated and not really used in practice, leading to little if any oversight and scrutiny of detention and treatment.

Conclusion

Variations in the amount and quality of inpatient care vary enormously internationally, from literally nothing to 1500-bedded asylums in some parts of Russia and China. This variation is clearly associated with economics, as the graphs early in the chapter illustrate vividly. If a country only allocates $0.20 to health care it will not be able to afford what a country allocating $44 can: a 220-fold disparity. These economic differences relate both to the overall wealth of countries and the political and strategic decisions that are made regarding how much to invest in health care overall and subsequently what proportion of that should be invested in mental health care. Several earlier examples show that in many low-income group countries the proportion of an already tiny health budget allocated to mental health is small, a double whammy causing widespread absence and insufficiency of care. These decisions to allocate disproportionately small budgets are likely to be influenced by stigma and the ongoing widespread opinion that many with mental health problems cannot be helped.

Acute inpatient care must be seen within the systems it is part of, increasingly so as more people receive community care and the systems to provide it in many countries are increasingly well resourced, specialized, and complicated. These systems also vary significantly between countries, and even within them, and influence the need for and conditions within institutions. There is no 'perfect model' for any country, and in this chapter I have elaborated on some key components and variations in different circumstances.

The very brief overview given here serves only to highlight the variation in provision, conditions, and current issues that exist globally. Issues that are currently of great concern in wealthy countries are utterly irrelevant in many countries that have very different and undoubtedly more fundamental difficulties to overcome. Many factors hamper efforts to develop effective overall systems and solid, respectful models for inpatient care—economy, political conditions, stigma, and geography. Many of these are outside our control, but not all. By developing a better understanding of systems and models of care around the world, and crucially by gathering high-quality evidence from developing systems outside traditionally research active countries, we can undoubtedly learn lessons to improve and refine acute inpatient care everywhere.

REFERENCES

1. Fakhoury W, Priebe S. The process of deinstitutionalization: an international overview. *Curr Opin Psychiatry* 2002;15:187–192.
2. House of Commons. *NHS Indicators: England, December 2016.* Briefing Paper Number 7821. London: House of Commons; 2016.
3. Hammond R. Condemned. Mental health in African countries in crisis. Fotoevidence; 2015. http://www.robinhammond.co.uk/condemned-mental-health-in-african-countries-in-crisis/
4. Human Rights Watch. Living in hell; abuses against people with psychosocial disabilities in Indonesia. 2016. https://www.hrw.org/report/2016/03/21/living-hell/abuses-against-people-psychosocial-disabilities-indonesia
5. World Health Organization. Country overview, Uganda. 2016 http://www.who.int/countries/uga/en/
6. Health and Social Care Information Centre (England and Wales). Mental Health Bulletin 2014–2015. 2015. http://content.digital.nhs.uk/catalogue/PUB18808/mhb-1415-ann-rep.pdf
7. Thornicroft G. *Oxford Textbook of Community Mental Health.* Oxford: Oxford University Press; 2011.
8. Thornicroft G, Tansella M. Components of a modern mental health service: a pragmatic balance of community and hospital care. *Br J Psychiatry* 2004;185:283–290.
9. Jacob KS, Sharan P, Mirza I, et al. Mental health systems in countries: where are we now? *Lancet* 2007;370:1061–1077.
10. Burns T. *Community Mental Health Teams.* Oxford: Oxford University Press; 2004.
11. Cowen P, Harrison P, Burns T (eds). *Shorter Oxford Textbook of Psychiatry.* Oxford: Oxford University Press; 2012.
12. Marshall M, Lewis S, Lockwood A, Drake R, Jones P, Croudace T. Association between duration of untreated psychosis and outcome in cohorts of first-episode patients: a systematic review. *Arch Gen Psychiatry* 2005;62:975–983.
13. Birchwood M, Todd P, Jackson C. Early intervention in psychosis: the critical-period hypothesis. *Int Clin Psychopharmacol* 1998;13:S31–S40.
14. Gafoor R, Nitsch D, McCrone P, et al. Effect of early intervention on 5-year outcome in non-affective psychosis. *Br J Psychiatry* 2010;196:372–376.
15. Stein LI, Test MA. Alternative to mental hospital treatment: I. Conceptual model, treatment program, and clinical evaluation. *Arch Gen Psychiatry* 1980;37:392–397.
16. Molodynski A, Burns T. What does research tell us about assertive outreach? In Williams et al. *Assertive Outreach in Mental Healthcare: Current Perspectives*, pp. 1–14. Oxford: Blackwell; 2011.
17. Burns T, Creed F, Fahy T, Thompson S, Tyrer P, White I. Intensive versus standard case management for severe psychotic illness: a randomised trial. UK 700 Group. *Lancet* 1999;353:2185–2189.
18. Hoult J, Rosen A, Reynolds I. Community orientated treatment compared to psychiatric hospital orientated treatment. *Soc Sci Med* 1984;18:1005–1010.
19. Glover G, Arts G, Babu KS. Crisis resolution/home treatment teams and psychiatric admission rates in England. *Br J Psychiatry* 2006;189:441–445.
20. Leentjens AF, Rundell JR, Wolcott DL, Guthrie E, Kathol R, Diefenbacher A. Reprint of: Psychosomatic medicine and consultation-liaison psychiatry: Scope of practice, processes, and competencies for psychiatrists working in the field of CL psychiatry or psychosomatics. A consensus statement of the European Association of Consultation-Liaison Psychiatry and Psychosomatics (EACLPP) and the Academy of Psychosomatic Medicine (APM). *J Psychosom Res* 2011;70:486–491.
21. Tadros G, Salama RA, Kingston P, et al. Impact of an integrated rapid response psychiatric liaison team on quality improvement and cost savings: the Birmingham RAID model. *Psychiatrist* 2013;37:4–10.

22. Drake RE, McHugo GJ, Bebout RR, et al. A randomized clinical trial of supported employment for inner-city patients with severe mental disorders. *Arch Gen Psychiatry* 1999;56:627–633.

23. Burns T, Catty J, Becker T, et al. The effectiveness of supported employment for people with severe mental illness: a randomised controlled trial. *Lancet* 2007;370:1146–1152.

24. BasicNeeds. Our approach. 2015. http://www.basicneeds.org/our-approach/

25. Saxena S, Thornicroft G, Knapp M, Whiteford H. Resources for mental health: scarcity, inequity, and inefficiency. *Lancet* 2007;370:878–889.

26. Priebe S, Badesconyi A, Fioritti A, et al. Reinstitutionalisation in mental health care: comparison of data on service provision from six European countries. *BMJ* 2005;330:123–126.

27. Blader JC. Acute inpatient care for psychiatric disorders in the United States, 1996 through 2007. *Arch Gen Psychiatry* 2011;68:1276–1283.

28. Saldivia S, Vicente B, Kohn R, Rioseco, P, Torres S. Use of mental health services in Chile. *Psychiatr Serv* 2004;55:71–76.

29. Lamb HR, Weinberger LE. The shift of psychiatric inpatient care from hospitals to jails and prisons. *J Am Acad Psychiatry Law* 2005;33:529–534.

30. Mundt AP, Chow WS, Arduino M, et al. Psychiatric hospital beds and prison populations in South America since 1990: does the Penrose hypothesis apply? *JAMA Psychiatry* 2015;72:112–118.

31. Penrose LS. Mental disease and crime: outline of a comparative study of European statistics. *Br J Med Psychol* 1939;18:1–15.

32. Winkler P, Barrett B, McCrone P, Csémy L, Janoušková M, Höschl C. Deinstitutionalised patients, homelessness and imprisonment: systematic review. *Br J Psychiatry* 2016;208:421–428.

33. Liu J, Ma H, He YL, et al. Mental health system in China: history, recent service reform and future challenges. *World Psychiatry* 2011;10:210–216.

34. Molodynski A, Rugkåsa J, Burns T. *Coercion in Community Mental Health Care: International Perspectives*. Oxford: Oxford University Press; 2016.

35. Mental Disability Advocacy Centre. Psychiatric hospitals in Uganda: a human rights investigation. 2015. http://www.mdac.org/sites/mdac.info/files/psyciatric_hospitals_in_uganda_human_rights_investigation.pdf

36. Petersen I, Lund C. Mental health service delivery in South Africa from 2000 to 2010: one step forward, one step back. *S Afr Med J* 2011;101:751–757.

37. Kim SJ, Park YS, Lee HW, Park SM. Current situation of psychiatry in North Korea: from the viewpoint of North Korean medical doctors. *Korean J Psychosom Med* 2012;20:32–39.

38. Ougrin D, Gluzman S, Dratcu L. Psychiatry in post-communist Ukraine: dismantling the past, paving the way for the future. *Psychiatrist* 2006;30:456–459.

39. Krasnov VN. Psychiatry in Russia. *Die Psychiatrie* 2014;11:51–55.

40. Dudley M, Silove D, Gale F. *Mental Health and Human Rights; Vision, Praxis, and Courage*. Oxford: Oxford University Press; 2012.

41. Molodynski A, Turnpenny L, Rugkåsa J, Burns T, Moussaoui D. Coercion and compulsion in mental healthcare—an international perspective. *Asian J Psychiatr* 2014;8:2–6.

42. Kisely S, Hall K. An updated meta-analysis of randomized controlled evidence for the effectiveness of community treatment orders. *Can J Psychiatry* 2014;59:561–564.

43. Mental Disability Advocacy Centre. Cage beds and coercion in Czech psychiatric institutions. 2014. http://www.mdac.org/en/content/cage-beds-and-coercion-czech-psychiatric-institutions

4

The design and function of inpatient wards

Tom Burns

Introduction

The origins of modern psychiatry are usually dated to Pinel's 'striking off the lunatics' chains in Paris in 1793 and the establishment of the York Retreat by the Tuke family in 1796 (1). Mental hospitals (or asylums as they were called until the 1930s) differed significantly from the madhouses that preceded them. An inpatient stay aimed to actively encourage a return to reason, rather than simply isolate and control disturbed behaviour. The Tukes called their approach 'moral treatment', what we would now probably call 'social therapy' or 'occupational therapy'. It consisted of a calm, predictable routine, an emphasis on care and encouragement, and an absence of punishment. The original Retreat was small and domestic, housing just 30 patients, but already had separate wards for the more disturbed and recovering patients. The physical environment was considered to be critical to recovery right from the start.

For much of psychiatry's history, the inpatient ward was the centre of treatment and thinking. It was the only care available, as it still is in several parts of the world. Because they were taken so much for granted, little active attention was paid to their purpose and design. This was to change, like so much else in psychiatry, with the advent of evidence-based medicine in the 1980s. Prior to that, developments consisted of local improvements in the level of comfort and facilities for activities and association.

Configuration of wards and hospitals up to 1980

The shift from madhouse to asylum placed a focus on the environment in which patients lived. The cells and squalid public areas that characterized the former were abandoned for more domestic settings with normal furniture and level of cleanliness. Privacy was not common in early asylums any more than it was in patients' homes and so sleeping and leisure rooms were shared. As the asylum building programme took off in the early nineteenth century, wards were modelled essentially on those in general hospitals. In the UK, these were large dormitories, usually with two rows of beds stretching down their entire length. These are referred to as 'Nightingale wards' after Florence Nightingale's influence (2). Intended originally for severely ill, bed-bound patients, Nightingale wards provided ease of oversight and monitoring but they afforded no privacy and only

minimal space for personal belongings or recreation. The sexes were rigidly segregated from the beginning in asylum buildings, not only by ward, but by whole wings and villas. Dormitory wards characterized most asylum accommodation but individual rooms were not that uncommon in parts of continental Europe and the US.

Psychiatric patients are, of course, not bedbound so Nightingale wards became more spacious and better furnished over time. They provided lockers for patients' possessions and also areas for eating and daytime activities as shown in some rather idealized pictures from the Bethlem Royal Hospital in 1860 (Figures 4.1 and 4.2). As overcrowding overwhelmed mental hospitals, the distance between beds was reduced and extra rows placed down the middle as locker and association spaces were squeezed out.

Patients were expected to be off the ward during the daytime, either in day rooms, attending activities, or in the airing courts. Overcrowded, dingy dormitory wards with their impersonal and dehumanizing regimes came to symbolize all that was wrong with mental hospitals. They were portrayed in an influential Hollywood film as the 'snakepit' and contributed impetus to early deinstitutionalization. Public opinion was outraged in the US by shocking revelations of neglect and abuse in a *Life Magazine* May 1946 article containing photographs from State Hospitals in Philadelphia and Ohio. These were smuggled out by the conscientious objectors sent to work there (3). Reports of abusive care such as the Ely enquiry had the same effect in the UK (4).

The first 30 years of deinstitutionalization (1950–1980) saw a substantial reduction in bed numbers. This was mainly achieved by discharge and provision for long-stay and elderly patients. Deinstitutionalization started early in the UK, somewhat later but more precipitously in the US, and with a dramatic flourish in Italy in 1978. This early period of bed reduction was not accompanied by any significant reduction in staffing nor in the closure of hospitals or buildings. As a result, wards became better staffed and less crowded. By 1980, few wards contained over 25 patients. Long-stay provision in most of Europe and the US was now restricted to highly disturbed and offender patients.

Rehabilitation and mixed-sex wards

A return to wards as mainly sleeping areas developed after the Second World War as structured rehabilitation became a clinical goal in mental hospitals. Previously, less disabled patients had been

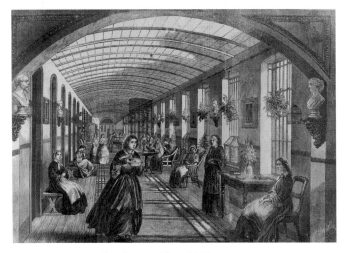

Figure 4.1 Women's gallery, Bethlem, 1860.
The Royal Hospital of Bethlehem, the Gallery for Women (engraving), Vizetelly, Frank (1830–83)/Private Collection/© Look and Learn/Illustrated Papers Collection.

active in running much of the hospital, working in hospital farms and kitchens. However, a recognition that much of their apparent disability arose from habit and social impoverishment (institutionalization) (5, 6) prompted the development of workshops and occupational therapy departments to address deficits and disabilities (7). Getting off the ward and spending time in these training settings (and often eating in a central dining room) were themselves important parts of rehabilitation.

This generally positive development had some unanticipated consequences. One was a change in the nurse's role. Rehabilitation became increasingly the remit of specialist occupational therapists and psychologists so nurses became less involved in shared activities with patients. In addition, as admission wards reduced their length of stay, an increasing number of more disturbed patients were unable to leave the ward for these activities. They stayed behind, often inadequately supervised in their bed spaces in a deserted, unstimulating environment, and often with reduced staffing.

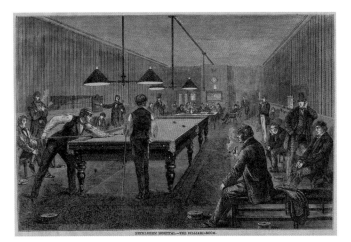

Figure 4.2 The billiard room, Bethlem, 1860.
The Hospital of Bethlem [Bedlam], St. George's Fields, Lambeth: the billiard room. Wood engraving by F. Vizetelly, 1860. by Frederick Vizetelly. Credit: Wellcome Collection. Used under the Creative Commons Attribution 4.0 International Public License (https://creativecommons.org/licenses/by/4.0/).

The therapeutic community

The 'therapeutic community' was a post-war development that had a powerful impact on ward structure and functioning. The psychoanalyst Tom Main coined the term in 1946 (8) to mean that the ward, and how it was run, had a therapeutic effect in itself; it was not just a space in which treatments could be delivered. Maxwell Jones, who had been working with disabled soldiers, was responsible for the spread of the therapeutic community concept. He emphasized the role of the ward as a 'living-learning' situation where all the relationships and activities were open to active scrutiny (9). Maxwell Jones relaxed the then very formal hierarchy on the ward, with the abandonment of uniforms, the use of first names, and the introduction of various ward groups. He emphasized an active striving after more normal relationships and healthy behaviour as a vehicle for recovery. He believed single-sex wards inhibited such rehabilitation and often promoted inappropriate behaviour. Between the 1950s and 1970s, most wards became mixed sex (as did their staff). Reconfiguring wards to accommodate both sexes became possible as discharges freed up sufficient space for day rooms and separate dormitories. In some of the older hospitals, ensuring separate bathrooms and day spaces proved difficult and some inadequate solutions exposed women to compromised privacy (10).

Ward developments since 1980

The year 1980 serves as a useful, if somewhat arbitrary, turning point in the development of inpatient wards for a number of reasons. The publication of Stein and Test's landmark study on assertive community treatment (11) was the first mental health service trial to have a global impact, generating a wave of replications both of the service and its evaluation (12). It can be seen as marking the start of evidence-based mental health care rather than the theoretically driven developments that had been the practice before. Now, when considering new treatments or developments, the expectation was that experience and evidence would be sought internationally. In addition, deinstitutionalization moved up a gear with the first closures of admission wards and soon of whole hospitals. As acute capacity was dramatically reduced, what was left had to be used with maximum efficiency. Lastly, the controversial but hugely influential Italian reforms of 1978 explicitly legislated for a maximum of 15 beds in admission wards. This figure was based on local consensus—there was no empirical or theoretical basis for it. It was pitched as low as it was thought possible to staff and manage. Despite its arbitrary nature, having a definite number served as a focus for consideration; was it about right, or was it too low or too high? Future planning would be tested against it.

While the advent of evidence-based medicine has failed to provide experimental tests of different ward sizes, it has tested their necessity for acute care. Two early randomized controlled trials demonstrated that admissions for a significant proportion of patients could be avoided using an acute day hospital (13). However, replicating this in a less research-intensive setting proved difficult (14) and the approach has failed to generalize. A recent revival in interest in this approach, usually as part of a crisis resolution home treatment service, also demonstrates some successful diversion from admission (15). However, no resultant closure of wards or fundamental change in practice has followed.

Not Just Bricks and Mortar

The absence of rigorous research evidence on the characteristics of admission wards does not mean that it is all guesswork. As new wards are being built, or older units reconfigured, decisions about their structure and size need now to be based on some consistent principles that can be explained and understood. The Royal College of Psychiatrists Council Report *Not Just Bricks and Mortar* (*NJBM*) (16, 17) was an attempt to address this issue comprehensively. Its remit was to examine the size, staffing, and security of acute admission wards. It was tasked to gather whatever consensus was available on these issues, to visit a range of differing inpatient units, and to produce recommendations for a model for a psychiatric unit that could 'stand alone' as a self-contained clinical facility.

The authors of *NJBM* found that there was no coherent, focused body of literature to guide them. There was, on the other hand, a rich architectural literature on the aesthetics of hospital building and on the practical engineering problems of their construction. Similarly, there was a vast sociological literature on the impact of group size on human behaviour and also on the nature of therapeutic relationships and the impact of ward atmosphere on patient behaviour. Not surprisingly, what evidence existed was observational; this is not an undertaking that lends itself easily to experimental testing.

NJBM made recommendations about the establishment of a broad and representative working group to plan for new or redesigned wards. It pointed out the need for careful consideration of the local context plus an inventory of local needs, assets, and collaborations. The document addressed the issues in specific chapters focused on size, staffing, security and structure, and siting. Siting was about the location of new-build units (whether alongside general hospitals, isolated, or in larger mental health campuses) and is not relevant here. What follows is a review of the four broad areas plus the recent considerations of functional versus integrated clinical responsibility and current approaches to the assessment of ward functioning.

Ward size

The Italian reforms in 1978 stipulated that their 'diagnostic and curative' wards should be limited to 15 beds (18). Before this, there was little published material recommending optimal ward size. Presumably this reflected a general consensus that the wards that most services had inherited were too large and simply needed to be slimmed down. How small they should be was most often determined by the availability and configuration of buildings. In the UK and much of Europe, the aim of 15-bed wards has been generally accepted but is often compromised in practice. Many new wards are still being built with up to 20 beds, and occasionally a few more. However, there is rarely a rationale, other than staffing and cost contingencies, advanced for this larger size.

There are, of course, smaller inpatient wards to cope with specific clinical needs and many of these accommodate only eight to ten patients. Examples are psychiatric intensive care units (PICUs), forensic wards, and mother and baby units where patients require enhanced security and monitoring. There was a movement in the 1980s and 1990s to provide 24-hour routine acute admission care in less formal, more domestic settings. These small units were designed to distance themselves from the 'institutional' feel of more standard wards and were sometimes referred to as crisis houses or 'acute alternatives to admission' facilities. They were often restricted to first-onset psychosis patients or vulnerable women (19). Many services continue to provide such alternatives but as *additions* to admission wards rather than *alternatives*.

The hope that these ultra-small wards would replace standard wards (20) has not been fulfilled as their ability to contain disturbed or compulsory patients proved very limited. The *NJBM* team visited a number of these and found that the rate of transfer to PICUs was strikingly higher than that from comparable local admission wards, despite them admitting fewer compulsory patients. Units of under ten also make it difficult for patients to form healthy 'subgroups' and to choose their own friends, so they can become over-intense. The TAPS group compared the success of different sizes of hostels in reprovision for discharged long-stay patients (21). They concluded that residents in slightly larger hostels with 10–15 places settled in better, at least in part because they could choose their own company.

Structure and siting

This chapter in *NJBM* (16, 17) is concerned with the ward as a single entity; however, wards are not stand-alone facilities but are part of a hospital or larger mental health unit. *NJBM* considered the optimal number of wards needed in any setup to ensure safe staffing and care. It concluded that anything less than three wards on a given site was unlikely to be able to provide adequate back-up staff for emergencies or enough flexibility to cover sickness and leave. It also concluded that having more than about five wards in one building starts to introduce an excessively institutional feel because of long corridors and the associated anonymous and impersonal office spaces.

Single en-suite bedrooms

Despite concerns about supervision, there is now broad agreement that all new-build psychiatric wards should aim to provide each patient with their own bedroom. In addition, the bedroom should have its own toilet and showering facilities. Where established wards are being refurbished and reconfigured, single rooms should be the goal with, at the very most, some shared bedrooms of two to four patients.

The judgement of virtually all staff with experience of both older and new wards is that the availability of single rooms markedly reduces tension and disturbance. By being able to retire to their own rooms, patients are able to get relief from others they may find stressful such as overactive manic patients. Simply being able to choose what they watch on television avoids a potent and ever-present source of conflict. Admission wards can be frightening places for patients and having their own space and some privacy can be very reassuring. Individual accommodation also permits greater flexibility for fluctuations in the demand for male and female admissions (see 'Single-sex wards'). Having their own private room reflects what people now expect and are used to in modern homes. Most hospitals are still struggling with the principles of providing the other common necessities of modern life such as Wi-Fi and constant access to smartphones. The latter are particularly challenging as their cameras present real issues about confidentiality for other patients. The provision of such levels of comfort is not simply a matter of acceptability but also raises important ethical dilemmas. With over half of inpatients being there against their will for some of the time, this becomes an issue of 'reciprocity' (22). Depriving patients of some of their normal expected comforts needs to be justified carefully—it is not enough to simply say that money is tight.

The costs of en-suite facilities in new-build wards are not excessively more than providing separate facilities. They also remove a potentially risky shared space that is difficult to monitor. The design of single en-suite rooms to ensure their safety is discussed in 'Security'.

When considering the design or renovation of inpatient wards it is easy to overlook the vital importance of the external environment. Not only does there need to be somewhere to go outside but thoughtful landscaping of the areas around the ward has a direct influence on the experience inside. Decent views from the windows have a major impact on the atmosphere, as we all know from our own homes. Given that psychiatric patients are up and about, it is essential for all wards to have direct access to gardens or courts. Consequently, the practice of placing wards several floors up in a tower would be impossible to justify. *NJBM* concluded that inpatient wards should not be more than one floor up.

Staffing

It goes without saying that the most important factor in a ward is the staffing. Wards have to be run as multiprofessional units. Sensitivity is required to ensure that medical authority over patient management is maintained while allowing space for the full range of professional judgements and for legitimate nursing authority to be respected. The UK is remarkable in the degree of informality between staff and the way lines of authority tend to be downplayed. In other countries, they are generally much more rigid and explicit. The advantage of flexible, mutually respectful relationships is obvious in engaging all opinions and in the message of individual worth it conveys to patients. It does, however, carry risks for misunderstanding (and even conflict) and requires regular attention from all involved. In our increasingly litigious times, it is essential that all are aware of their individual professional responsibilities and those of their colleagues. Professional distinctions and hierarchy tend to be reasserted temporarily in times of increased stress and tension on the ward, subsequently to be relaxed.

Most services establish minimum staffing levels and skill mixes for wards. These are constantly changing—both the range and ratio of trained to untrained staff and the ratio of staff to patient. Staff mix is surprisingly culture specific and not all countries have specific training for mental health nurses. In the US and several European countries, for instance, the nurses in charge of the ward have general training. There are relatively few of them and aids and attendants make up the bulk of the staff. The level of training required to be a nurse also varies in different countries. Minimum staffing levels have to reflect these local differences. *NJBM*, for instance, recommends three (mental health) trained nurses during the day and two at night per ward. Staffing levels should not fall below agreed minimum levels but in many circumstances they may be higher if patient

need requires it. Too much striving for cost efficiency (e.g. minimum staffing levels and 100% bed occupancy) is a false economy. Wards that are overcrowded with very high occupancy levels are more difficult to manage and are poor environments for patients (23). An early study from New Zealand (24) reports occupancy levels at around 70% which would be considered utopian currently in much of Europe and the UK where occupancy is often at 100% and 85% is considered the goal (25).

The presence or absence of dedicated occupational therapists, psychologists, and doctors on wards also varies enormously. As the length of admission has reduced and the acuity of patients has increased, occupational therapists and psychologists have often found inpatients too disturbed to engage with. By the time they are well enough they are discharged. In most European countries there are dedicated junior doctors who work only on the ward and the numbers can seem surprising to UK observers. In Switzerland or Germany, a mixed admission ward of 20 patients may have two full-time junior doctors and a full-time consultant all with no duties off the ward. Such international variations mean there is little to be gained by exploring the range of staffing combinations in this chapter. Suffice it to say that the more staff, and the more experienced and better trained those staff members are, the better the ward tends to function.

In the UK, we have experienced a dramatic increase in the bureaucratic burden placed on inpatient nurses. This has resulted in less face-to-face interaction with patients and more time writing notes in the nursing office.

Wards vary in whether they title their lead nurse 'ward manager' or 'charge nurse/sister'. This is not just a semantic issue but may reflect a fundamental difference in philosophy. Ward managers emphasize management by regular, comprehensive, and structured supervision of their nurses in formal sessions and tend to have less of a presence out on the ward with the patients. Charge nurses, while they also supervise staff, emphasize more an 'apprenticeship' training model which has traditionally characterized medicine and nursing (26, 27). In visiting wards, I have been struck by the differences of these two different styles of working. Where the charge nurse is out there dealing directly with difficult problems, working alongside more junior staff and teaching flexibly by example, the ward has almost invariably seemed to me more harmonious and settled for both staff and patients.

Security

Staffing is clearly crucial for security and safety in wards. Overcrowded and understaffed wards are invariably less secure. There are well-established building standards for psychiatric wards that cover everything from the strength of window frames to the choice of fireproof materials, and furniture that is durable and safe. Most of these standards are common to general and psychiatric wards but there are some that are specific to psychiatric settings. These include spindle-locking, outward-opening bedroom doors that allow for privacy but cannot be barricaded and can be opened from the outside. Similarly, there are restrictions on the extent of window opening and the design of bedrooms with en-suite facilities to avoid blind spots when they are being viewed from the outside (17, 28).

The use of CCTV for public areas in wards has become increasingly common in new-build units and seems to be well accepted by patients. The risk of nurses retreating to 'monitoring stations' rather than being out on the ward with patients is, of course, a concern. Most experienced practitioners believe that active engagement with patients is the most effective protection against disturbance and risk, rather than a range of specified 'security measures'.

Locked doors

A generation ago, admission wards were not locked and those involuntary patients who could not be nursed without such measures were transferred to a 'locked ward', now referred to as a PICU. In the UK, it is not legal to nurse a voluntary patient on a PICU although this is accepted in several European countries. Increasingly, wards keep their doors locked much or most of the time although it is made clear that voluntary patients can leave by asking a nurse or member of staff to open the door. This is a more significant change than many staff who have only experienced this current state of affairs may realize.

Many hospitals used to manage completely without locked wards (29); Dingleton Hospital in Scotland was the first general catchment area hospital in the UK to operate entirely without any locked doors. It did so from 1948 (long before the introduction of antipsychotics) and never closed them before the hospital itself was closed in 1981 (30). The 'open-door' movement was a talisman for an increasing liberalization of psychiatry throughout the 1960s and 1970s. Some recent research from Germany suggests that locked doors may have little or no effect on absconding, self-harm, or suicide (31).

Several factors contribute to the increasingly routine use of locked doors and the international rise of compulsion in psychiatry (32). The first is our increasingly risk-averse society with its blame culture and unrealistic expectations of medicine and psychiatry. This is manifest in a failure to accept that while we can reduce risk, we cannot eliminate it. It leads to a fading confidence in professional judgement and a demand for external, increasingly bureaucratic, assessments of quality of care. What can be measured and documented (locked doors, frequency of observation, and absence of ligature points) takes precedence over more nebulous factors such as ward atmosphere and nurse engagement. The ostensible purpose is to reduce absconding, self-harm, and suicide, although the German research gives pause for thought about this. Undoubtedly it is also driven by the reduction in bed numbers (33) with the consequent high level of disturbances on wards. In the UK, half of all patients are involuntary for at least part of their admission. Levels of disturbance are not helped by the wide availability of street drugs, and 'keeping undesirables out' is certainly a part of the motivation for locking doors in inner-city units (29).

Habit and expectation, however, may be the main reason. The use of 'mechanical' restriction in psychiatry is enormously variable between different countries and cultures, with no obvious rationale or difference in outcome. In Scandinavia, Northern Europe, and the US, mechanical restraints (leather straps to bind patients to their beds) are common and considered humane and essential, just as caged beds were until very recently in parts of central and eastern Europe. Yet in the UK such techniques would be considered outrageous. Here they were abandoned in the 1840s in the 'non-restraint movement' spearheaded by John Connolly (34). In the Netherlands,

seclusion is widespread and considered humane while rapid tranquilization is considered abusive and hardly used—the reverse of the situation in the UK. Once established as a routine in care, clinicians quickly come to believe such restrictions were essential and that effective care would be impossible without them, even though, as with community treatment orders, the evidence is that they make no difference (35, 36). The current widespread locking of doors may be just such an unhelpful habit.

Single-sex wards

Moving from the rigid separation of the sexes in the old asylums to mixed-sex wards was considered enlightened progress in the 1960s and 1970s. Psychiatrists were concerned about the risk of institutionalization, with patients becoming demotivated by a regimented and depersonalized environment (5, 6). Along with the abandonment of staff uniforms, mixed-sex wards were seen as a move based on earlier therapeutic community thinking (9) to 'normalize' as much as possible the inpatient environment. This was to protect the patient's fragile self-esteem and promote recovery.

The last decade has seen a reversal of this policy with a move back to single-sex wards. This has been driven by concerns about sexual exploitation and assault of female patients by male patients in increasingly disturbed wards with high levels of compulsory admissions (37). The recommendation in *NJBM* was not for single-sex wards but for mixed wards with shared day rooms and facilities but with clearly separated sleeping and bathroom facilities. In fieldwork for that report, we visited a number of pioneering units that had introduced strict single-sex provisions and found mixed responses from both female patients and staff.

Staff were concerned about inflexibility and the possibility of beds being oversubscribed on one ward and empty on another. They also recognized the challenge that single-sex wards posed for conducting ward rounds and providing continuity of care (see 'The functional split'). All staff we interviewed recognized the need to protect young, disinhibited female patients, particularly those who were manic. Many female patients and several staff disliked the segregation and experienced the atmosphere as less relaxed. However, these visits were early on in the process and attitudes may have changed with familiarity. Unfortunately, as with many service changes which are imposed centrally, it has not proved possible to evaluate the impacts. There are suggestions, however, that the separation is not necessarily enough in itself to remove all risk (38).

The functional split

Internationally, most mental health services have dedicated inpatient staff. The degree of outpatient development varies from almost none in some countries to well-established multidisciplinary teams providing both outpatient care and extensive outreach to patients in their homes and neighbourhoods (39). The UK led the way in sectorized community mental health care in part because the Mental Health Act 1959 required hospitals that admitted involuntary patients to provide aftercare themselves. The model in the UK was thus one where the same consultant-led multidisciplinary team managed their patients both in and out of the hospital (although there was, of course, a dedicated inpatient nursing team). Italy has gone one step further in some of its most progressive sites with inpatient nurses following discharged patients and visiting them at home but this is not widespread.

During the last decade, the UK has unpicked this continuity of care and introduced separate inpatient and outpatient consultants. The implied rationale for this is to address acknowledged failings in the leadership and management of busy and overcrowded wards but also clearly with the hope that it will reduce pressures on beds (40, 41). It has also been driven by the pressure experienced by ward staff in serving an increasing number of ward rounds. Instead of one or two teams admitting all their patients to one ward there is now a range of admitting teams (crisis teams, early intervention teams, and recovery teams) and the whole structure has been doubled up by the impact of single-sex provision. European experience suggests that this split responsibility is unlikely to streamline bed usage and there are, rather late in the day, reservations being expressed about the functional split (42).

Assessing the quality of inpatient wards

In insurance-funded health systems, there are invariably processes for accrediting wards. In the UK, inspections by the Care Quality Commission assess the quality of wards as part of their overall service assessments. They ask five key questions: are they safe? Are they effective? Are they caring? Are they responsive? Are they well-led? A specific matrix for self-assessment of mental health wards has been produced by the Royal College of Psychiatrists (Accreditation for Inpatient Mental Health Services (AIMS)) (28). The standards are derived from government policy documents and consultations and aim to ensure compliance with guidelines from the National Institute for Health and Care Excellence. The standards are aspirational and very detailed indeed and they suffer from not having a summary. They are intended to be assessed annually and cover five areas:

1. General.
2. Timely and purposeful admission.
3. Safety.
4. Environment and facilities.
5. Therapies and activities.

Standards are classified into three types:

Type 1: failure to meet these standards would result in a significant threat to patient safety, rights, or dignity and/or would breach the law.

Type 2: standards that an accredited ward would be expected to meet.

Type 3: standards that an excellent ward should meet or standards that are not the direct responsibility of the ward.

Fortunately, the Royal College of Psychiatrists produced an occasional paper in 2011 with a shorter, more manageable, and useful checklist: 'Do the right thing: how to judge a good ward' (43). This has ten standards that all of us can quickly ascertain and understand (Box 4.1).

Box 4.1 Do the right thing: ten key standards checklist

1 Bed occupancy of 85% or less.
2 Ward size: 18 maximum.
3 Environment offers gender-specific bedrooms and toilet facilities, and direct access to external space and a quiet room.
4 Daily therapeutic activities.
5 Positive risk management policy.
6 Information sharing on diagnosis and treatment to inform the care pathway.
7 Linking with external community for housing, faith communities, employment, voluntary services, etc.
8 Access to at least one psychological intervention a week.
9 Daily one-on-one contact.
10 Cultural sensitivity: staff trained in cultural awareness with access to interpreters.

Royal College of Psychiatrists, OP79: *Do the right thing: how to judge a good ward* (2011).

Current controversies

Mental health wards and mental health inpatient care are inevitably controversial. It is not surprising they attract critical attention and usually receive the lowest ratings in patient satisfaction returns. This is because they are, by definition, where patients do not want to be. Many patients are legally compelled to be there and few would voluntarily seek inpatient care if they could manage with an alternative such as a day hospital or home care. Inpatient stays are also when patients are feeling at their worst. They are the setting, par excellence, where starkly conflicting assessments are played out: 'I want to be at home and don't need any medicine', 'No, I'm afraid you have to stay here for now and take this medicine'.

So understandably there is a constant search for how to improve the patient and staff experience. None of the current models can truly claim to be 'evidence based', rather they reflect constant shifts in ideological and ethical preoccupations in our professions and in society more widely. Consequently, they remain controversial and open to further change, or even reversal. The most obvious controversy currently is the degree of security that is now so pervasive. Locked doors, TV screens behind Perspex sheets, and institutionally designed furniture convey an oppressive emphasis of avoiding risk rather than fostering a welcoming, domestic, therapeutic atmosphere. We need to find ways of asking and answering the questions of whether such practices achieve real benefits or not. The comparison of locked and unlocked wards in German hospitals was one lucky opportunity afforded by a natural experiment.

Similar questions surround the move to single-sex wards. It can be endlessly argued whether this reflects a long-overdue recognition of the risks to women or a damaging overreaction to isolated events. Such strict segregation of the sexes is not routine in countries where these decisions are made more locally by clinicians. As with locked doors, the onus should surely be on those who introduce these restrictions to show that they bring real benefits.

How 'luxurious' should an inpatient ward be? In *NJBM*, we proposed that design and décor should convey a strong message that patients are valued and respected. Pleasing design, imaginative lighting, and a choice of materials that do not simply indicate 'durable and cheap' all seem to make sense. In our original draft, we proposed that the wards should match the standard of a three-star hotel but the phrasing was considered too provocative. The point being made was that standards and expectations will inevitably rise and it will be patient and family expectations, not professional judgements, that will matter. Provision needs to keep up with them or patients and families will reject it. Linking these standards to what we take for granted in our own lives would drive this steady improvement. It would also avoid having to produce voluminous, detailed policy documents itemizing every trivial detail. It also reminds us that these wards are for people like us—not some strange 'other'.

Many staff we talked to also worried that increased expenditure on wards and décor would be wasted as patients would inevitably damage them. Early experience in therapeutic communities demonstrated the failure of this logic—promptly repairing windows broken by patients reduced the rate of breakages. The evidence more generally is overwhelming that neglected or shabby properties get vandalized more. The tasteful décor and level of furnishing in Northern European wards is in striking contrast to that in the UK and does not seem to lead to more damage—flower pots and advent lights were not thrown around by angry patients when I worked on Swedish admission wards. Whether the standard of the rehabilitation ward in Denmark shown in Figures 4.3 and 4.4 is necessary may be debated, but it undoubtedly conveys a sense of personal worth to patients and staff. Staff taking pride in the ward environment, keeping it clean and homely, certainly seemed to pay off when I worked in Scandinavia.

All of these concerns about the physical environment (important though they undoubtedly are) can distract us from what all researchers into inpatient care consistently eventually identify as *the* most important factor. This is the quality of interaction with staff. The establishment of trusting relationships and time spent together make it clear to patients that they are understood, sympathized with, and valued. Whether it is in studies of rates of seclusion, aggression, or satisfaction levels it is these relationships that invariably feature in the conclusions.

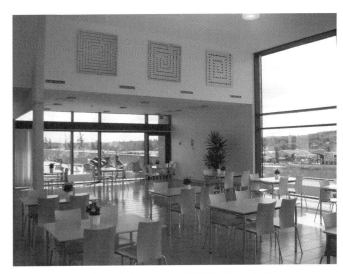

Figure 4.4 Danish rehabilitation ward (2006): dining hall.

Some final thoughts

I will finish this chapter by hazarding my own thoughts, based on working in such settings over 40 years of major change. Ward atmosphere and practice have been changed by the drastic shortening of admissions and the focus on admitting only the most ill. However, a more pervasive change has accompanied this that warrants some reflection. This period has witnessed a marked retreat from close engagement with patients. This is undoubtedly imposed in part by a risk-averse culture with its burden of bureaucracy and a clinical governance regime that is based on looking back over your shoulder rather than focusing on the patient in front of you. It is at its most obvious in the sight of staff trapped in nursing stations dealing with a plethora of detailed policies. These policies have been developed to deal with problems, many of which would never arise if those nurses servicing them were freed up and encouraged to 'be with' patients rather than endlessly providing evidence of 'doing evidence-based things to them'.

There is nothing, of course, fundamentally incompatible between humane and person-centred practice and evidence-based medicine. However, there is a recognizable temperamental difference between those who naturally wish to intervene and those who wish more to understand and support. Good care needs both, and both require time and personal investment. The issue is whether our current system of managing and monitoring wards gives both adequate scope and importance.

Why this shift in emphasis has become so is open to speculation. Much of it reflects the societal pressures on us such as burdensome bureaucracy and risk management. However, much of it may be due to changes in how we view our jobs and what core skills we value most highly.

I have been regularly struck by the differences in ward atmosphere in mental health cultures which stress relationships and understanding, and which place a premium on warmth and engagement rather than efficiency. This understanding and engagement is often understood in narrative terms (attention to the patient's personal story) and it is often expressed in language that originates from the

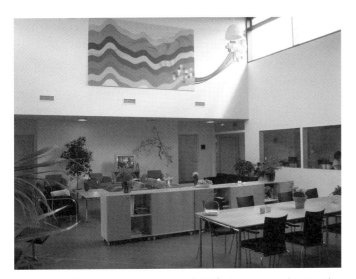

Figure 4.3 Danish rehabilitation ward (2006): day space and patients' kitchen.

now unfashionable traditions of psychodynamic therapy and counselling. Shifting that balance back somewhat towards this joint exploration of personal meaning might resolve many of the current seemingly intractable problems faced by inpatient wards.

REFERENCES

1. Burns T. *Our Necessary Shadow: The Nature and Meaning of Psychiatry.* London: Penguin; 2013.
2. Nightingale F. *Notes on Hospitals.* London: Longman, Green, Longman, Roberts and Green; 1863.
3. Taylor SJ. *Acts of Conscience: WWII, Mental Institutions and Religious Objectors.* New York: Syracuse University Press; 2009.
4. Committee of Inquiry. *Report of the Committee of Inquiry into Allegations of Ill-Treatment of Patients and Other Irregularities at the Ely Hospital, Cardiff, Presented to Parliament by the Secretary of State of the Department of Health and Social Security.* London: Department of Health; 1969.
5. Barton R. *Institutional Neurosis.* Bristol: John Wright; 1959.
6. Goffman I. *Asylums: Essays on the Social Situation of Mental Patients and Other Inmates.* Harmondsworth: Penguin Books; 1960.
7. Anthony WA. *The Principles of Psychiatric Rehabilitation.* Baltimore, MD: Human Resource Development Press; 1979.
8. Main TF. The hospital as a therapeutic institution. *Bull Menninger Clin* 1946;10:66–70.
9. Jones M. *Social Psychiatry: A Study of Therapeutic Communities.* London: Tavistock; 1952.
10. Barlow F, Wolfson P. Safety and security: a survey of female psychiatric in-patients. *Psychiatric Bull* 1997;21:270–272.
11. Stein LI, Test MA. Alternative to mental hospital treatment. I. Conceptual model, treatment program, and clinical evaluation. *Arch Gen Psychiatry* 1980;37:392–397.
12. Catty J, Burns T, Knapp M, et al. Home treatment for mental health problems: a systematic review. *Psychol Med* 2002;32:383–401.
13. Creed F, Black D, Anthony P, Osborn M, Thomas P, Tomenson B. Randomised controlled trial of day patient versus inpatient psychiatric treatment. *BMJ* 1990;300:1033–1037.
14. Creed F, Black D, Anthony P, et al. Randomised controlled trial of day and in-patient psychiatric treatment. 2: comparison of two hospitals. *Br J Psychiatry* 1991;158:183–189.
15. Johnson S, Nolan F, Pilling S, et al. Randomised controlled trial of acute mental health care by a crisis resolution team: the north Islington crisis study. *BMJ* 2005;331:599.
16. Royal College of Psychiatrists. *Not Just Bricks and Mortar.* Council Report CR62. London: Royal College of Psychiatrists; 1998.
17. Burns T. Not just bricks and mortar: Report of the Royal College of Psychiatrists Working Party on the size, staffing, structure, sitting, and security of new acute adult psychiatric in-patient units. *Psychiatric Bull* 1998;22:465–466.
18. Jones K, Poletti A. Understanding the Italian experience. *Br J Psychiatry* 1985;146:341–347.
19. Johnson S, Gilburt H, Lloyd-Evans B, et al. In-patient and residential alternatives to standard acute psychiatric wards in England. *Br J Psychiatry* 2009;194:456–463.
20. Haycox A, Unsworth L, Allen K, Hodgson R, Lewis M, Boardman AP. North Staffordshire Community Beds Study: longitudinal evaluation of psychiatric in-patient units attached to community mental health centres. 2: impact upon costs and resource use. *Br J Psychiatry* 1999;175:79–86.
21. Dayson D. The TAPS project 15: the social networks of two group settings: a pilot study. *J Ment Health* 1992;1:99–106.
22. Eastman N. Mental health law: civil liberties and the principle of reciprocity. *BMJ* 1994;308:43–45.
23. Bowers L. Association between staff factors and levels of conflict and containment on acute psychiatric wards in England. *Psychiatr Serv* 2009;60:231–239.
24. Bradley N, Kumar S, Ranclaud M, Robinson E. Ward crowding and incidents of violence on an acute psychiatric inpatient unit. *Psychiatr Serv* 2001;52:521–525.
25. Gilburt H. *Mental Health under Pressure.* London: The King's Fund; 2015.
26. Sennett R. *The Craftsman.* London: Penguin Books (Allen Lane); 2008.
27. Sinclair S. *Making Doctors: An Institutional Apprenticeship.* London: Bloomsbury; 1997.
28. Royal College of Psychiatrists. *Accreditation for Inpatient Mental Health Services (AIMS): Standards for Inpatient Wards – Working-Age Adults,* 4th ed. London: Royal College of Psychiatrists Centre for Quality Improvement; 2010.
29. Burns T. Locked doors or therapeutic relationships? *Lancet Psychiatry* 2016;3:795–796.
30. Jones D. The Borders Mental Health Service. *Br J Clin Soc Psychiatry* 1982;2:8–12.
31. Huber CG, Schneeberger AR, Kowalinski E, et al. Suicide risk and absconding in psychiatric hospitals with and without open door policies: a 15 year, observational study. *Lancet Psychiatry* 2016;3:842–849.
32. Priebe S, Badesconyi A, Fioritti A, et al. Reinstitutionalisation in mental health care: comparison of data on service provision from six European countries. *BMJ* 2005;330:123–126.
33. Keown P, Weich S, Bhui KS, Scott J. Association between provision of mental illness beds and rate of involuntary admissions in the NHS in England 1988–2008: ecological study. *BMJ* 2011;343:d3736.
34. Haw C, Yorston G. Thomas Prichard and the non-restraint movement at the Northampton Asylum. *Psychiatric Bull* 2004; 28:140–142.
35. Maughan D, Molodynski A, Rugkåsa J, Burns T. A systematic review of the effect of community treatment orders on service use. *Soc Psychiatry Psychiatr Epidemiol* 2014;49:651–663.
36. Rugkåsa J, Dawson J, Burns T. CTOs: what is the state of the evidence? *Soc Psychiatry Psychiatr Epidemiol* 2014;49:1861–1871.
37. Henderson C, Reveley A. Is there a case for single sex wards? *Psychiatr Bull* 1996;20:513–515.
38. Mezey G, Hassell Y, Bartlett A. Safety of women in mixed-sex and single-sex medium secure units: staff and patient perceptions. *Br J Psychiatry* 2005;187:579–582.
39. Medeiros H, McDaid D, Knapp M, MHEEN Group. *Shifting Care from Hospital to the Community in Europe: Economic Challenges and Opportunities.* MHEEN II Policy Briefing. London: MHEEN Group; 2008.
40. Burns T. The dog that failed to bark. *Psychiatrist* 2010;34:361–363.
41. Burns T. Splitting in-patient and out-patient responsibility does not improve patient care. *Br J Psychiatry* 2017;210:6–9.
42. Laugharne R, Pant M. Sector and functional models of consultant care: in-patient satisfaction with psychiatrists. *Psychiatrist* 2012;36:254–256.
43. Royal College of Psychiatrists. *Do the Right Thing: How to Judge a Good Ward. Ten Standards for Adult In-Patient Mental Healthcare.* London: Royal College of Psychiatrists; 2011.

5

The context of inpatient mental health care in England

Robert Chaplin

Introduction

This chapter, which is of special interest to mental health professionals who are unfamiliar with the UK health care system, reviews the practice of inpatient care in relation to the provision of overall psychiatric care in England. The structure of mental health care in the UK National Health Service (NHS) is outlined and in particular the various subspecialties of inpatient care. Recent trends in the provision of inpatient psychiatric care in the UK are considered in comparison to those in Europe and North America. There follows a review of the role of public sector care under the NHS and a debate about the effectiveness of inpatient care and whether it should be a separate psychiatric subspecialty. Finally, local service developments are discussed as a type of case study to illustrate how services are currently undergoing rapid changes.

Psychiatric care in England

The UK NHS is free at the point of delivery, is paid for by general taxation, and is designed to provide a comprehensive service. This includes primary care where all people are registered with a local general practitioner. General practitioners treat the majority of people with mental disorders but can refer to secondary mental health services to receive opinions on patients with more severe, enduring, or complex mental disorders or those who are assessed as being at higher risk. Patients stay registered at the same general practice surgery for years and are often seen by the same doctor who may know other family members as well.

The NHS currently runs on an 'Internal Market'. Services are commissioned by Clinical Commissioning Groups (CCGs) which were established in April 2013 and are overseen by NHS England (1). They are responsible for two-thirds of all NHS spending and have general practitioners as their members. There are currently 209 CCGs in England with a mean health population of 250,000 people. Following changes in 2013, the majority of NHS care is provided by NHS foundation trusts which were first introduced in 2004. They are independent legal entities and have unique governance arrangements.

They are also accountable to local people, who can become members and governors. They are free from central government control and are self-standing, self-governing organizations. They have financial freedom and can raise capital from both the public and private sectors. Mental health care and social care for people with mental disorders who require secondary care is provided by mental health trusts of which there are currently 60 in England. For example, locally Oxford Health NHS Foundation Trust provides secondary mental health care to people in the counties of Oxfordshire and Buckinghamshire as well as physical and social care for people of all ages across the areas of Oxfordshire, Buckinghamshire, Swindon, Wiltshire, Bath, and North East Somerset. It is responsible for the inpatient care described in this chapter.

Individuals who meet the threshold of needing secondary care are allocated a mental health professional called a 'care coordinator' (usually a community psychiatric nurse or social worker) and are reviewed regularly by psychiatrists. There is a statutory framework called the Care Programme Approach (2) which underpins the delivery of care and ensures the person has a care coordinator (who is usually the first point of contact), a care plan, and a review date. Prescribing is often initiated in secondary care but the majority of prescribing is handed over to general practice and patients would expect to be in touch with their general practitioner throughout their period of secondary mental health care. The basic unit of community care has traditionally been the community mental health team consisting of psychiatrists, community psychiatric nurses, and social workers and this may also include clinical psychologists and occupational therapists. The team is usually aligned with specified general practices and will serve a dedicated geographical area (around 30,000–40,000 people). The consultant psychiatrist in the team used to assume responsibility for the care of the team's patients when admitted to hospital; however, decreasing bed numbers has made this a difficult type of service to run and people will now generally be cared for by a different consultant psychiatrist when they are admitted to hospital. There have been more recent initiatives to streamline community mental health care and this has been achieved locally using a care pathway approach. This essentially provides functional teams to provide assessment, community treatment, early intervention for people with psychosis, and inpatient teams. The interface with community mental health care is discussed in more detail in Chapter 9.

When a person is in relapse or needs a higher level of support, this can be provided in the community through the secondary mental health team either by a crisis resolution and home treatment team or equivalent 'step-up' service where a person can be seen up to twice daily at home. Alternatively, they may attend a day hospital on a short-term basis for up to 5 days a week for participation in a structured programme of activities and therapy, often in a group setting. Their care coordinator and mental health team would remain working with the individual throughout this period. On recovery, their care would usually be 'stepped down' back to their usual care plan and care coordinator.

People may be admitted to psychiatric hospital when their illness and/or risk is at a level of severity that cannot be managed safely in the community, even with stepped-up care usually following a referral from the community mental health services. Inpatient care is provided locally with separate admission units for different ages of people: services for adults of working age (usually aged 18–64), older adults (usually aged 65 or over), and child and adolescent mental health units (aged under 18) which are the subjects of further chapters in this book. Additionally, there are inpatient units that have special functions which include psychiatric intensive care units (short-term admission for people with more severe illness who need extra care), forensic units for people with mental illness and offending behaviour and high risk referred by the criminal justice system, and inpatient units that specialize in the treatment of people with severe and enduring mental illness (psychiatric rehabilitation), eating disorders, and those with alcohol and drug dependency, and mother and baby units. Not all localities provide the full range of services (e.g. the local services in Oxford and Buckinghamshire do not have a mother and baby unit or inpatient care for those with a primary drug or alcohol behaviour). Where such care is not available it can be purchased elsewhere either within the private sector or at other NHS trusts. Care coordinators from in-reach services work alongside the individual patients on the inpatient unit and are involved in discharge decisions leading to the goal of 'seamless' care.

About 50% of people are admitted under compulsory powers of the Mental Health Act 2007 although voluntary admission (usually referred to as informal admission) is common. People may be regraded to informal status prior to discharge if they have sufficiently recovered or be discharged still subject to compulsion. To accept a voluntary admission, capacity to consent to admission and treatment is generally necessary although there are safeguards under the Mental Capacity Act 2005 for those who lack capacity. People admitted under the Mental Health Act 2007 have the right of appeal to the Mental Health Review Tribunal and the Hospital Managers (these are discussed in detail in Chapter 31). Treatment in hospital is underpinned by the National Institute for Health and Care Excellence who have produced a series of authoritative evidence-based practice guidelines for the majority of mental health conditions. The Care Quality Commission is the statutory regulator and each inpatient unit is thoroughly inspected on a regular basis and must pass rigorous standards in five domains of care (safety, caring, responsiveness, effectiveness, and good leadership). Additionally, individual wards are encouraged to achieve accreditation with the Royal College of Psychiatrists Accreditation of Inpatient Mental Health Services (AIMS) (this topic is the subject of other chapters).

There is a responsibility to investigate serious untoward events (e.g. suicides and serious violence) which usually takes the form of a Root Cause Analysis and may be either internal to the organization or external in more severe cases.

Currently, there is a staffing crisis nationally with regard to inpatient staff around retention and recruiting which every trust is facing. It is now a serious problem and is getting worse. The Royal College of Nursing in London have published a review of staffing levels for registered nursing in London in 2015 (3). The data published in this report shows more than 10,000 nursing vacancies, a rate of around 17%—an increase from 14% in 2014 and 11% the year before. At some London trusts, 30% of nursing posts are now vacant. Locally, the situation is not dissimilar, possibly due to the nursing bursary being discontinued. This could have a major impact on the ability of inpatient mental health services to deliver a high quality of care.

The international context of inpatient care

In many European countries, the number of psychiatric hospital beds has decreased, accompanied by an increase in forensic psychiatric beds (4). A good, recent overview of the context of inpatient admissions in the UK relative to the international situation of provision of inpatient care has been provided by Craig (2016) (5). There has been a reduction in public sector inpatient capacity in the UK which is not reflected in all European countries with Germany, Croatia, Lithuania, and Latvia all increasing capacity while Belgium and the Netherlands have proportionally much higher provision of inpatient beds. The US has seen a reduction in the total number of psychiatric beds including provision of private psychiatric beds and private hospitals (6), while the UK has seen a rise in admissions to private sector beds and a rise in compulsory admissions (7). Cohen et al. (8) highlight the lack of an international priority given to psychiatric institutional care despite ongoing media reports of human rights abuses. They call for the establishment of a global commission on mental health institutions which would in particular outline poor conditions and disseminate strategies that have been successfully applied to improve quality in some notable international sites. Although many high-income countries are have been reproviding psychiatric services in the community from the closure of large institutions (9), high-income countries still have a greater number of inpatient beds and inpatient admissions than low-income countries (10). Most people who are admitted to hospital globally are discharged within a year and are followed up within a month of discharge (5).

Research and evidence into inpatient care

Research into novel interventions in psychiatric care in the UK has focused on community services: for example, day hospitals, crisis intervention, and assertive outreach as alternatives to hospital admission. Inpatient care has been used as a measure of the negative outcome of the intervention under trial. An authoritative review of hospitalization as a negative outcome of schizophrenia is provided by Burns (11). He argues that hospitalization is the most frequently reported outcome measure for studies evaluating mental health services as it has been used as a proxy for relapse of severe mental illness as it is clearly understandable to clinicians (face validity), has utility for service planning, and represents the majority of costs. However, disadvantages of this approach assume that it is a negative therapeutic goal and may not be seen as relevant to patients and carers. The following studies have used hospitalization as a negative outcome and are reviewed for the perspective of whether hospital admission is necessary or effective.

There have been a series of service innovations in community mental health with a primary aim of reducing the need for inpatient admissions. Increased community support, evaluated by the UK700 controlled trial of intensive case management, for people with psychosis resulted in 'no significant decline in overall hospital use' for the intervention over the control group over the 2-year study period (12). This was the converse of the original finding from Stein and Test (13) in the US that assertive community treatment reduced the need for inpatient admission. A study of compulsory community treatment (14) found there was no difference in readmission rates over a 12-month follow-up period for people randomized on hospital discharge to receive a community treatment order. Conversely, joint crisis planning for people with psychosis afforded no reduction in the need for compulsory inpatient admission (15). A review of studies evaluating the use of the acute psychiatric day hospital (16) found weak evidence in support of it avoiding the need for inpatient admission. Likewise, a review of crisis intervention studies (17) found low- to moderate-quality evidence for the reduction of inpatient admissions. The provision of alternative residential accommodation instead of acute admission did not reduce the mean number or length of hospital admissions over a 12-month period (18). Finally, a study from rural Buckinghamshire, a relatively affluent area of the UK with a stable population with low psychiatric morbidity, showed that even with the development of enhanced community mental health services this did not prevent the need for hospital admission for two individuals over a 2-year period (19).

A separate speciality for inpatient psychiatry?

Debate about whether acute inpatient psychiatry should become a new psychiatric speciality began as long ago as 2006. With a reduction in inpatient beds, increasing proportions of patients admitted to hospital being detained, increasing amounts of substance misuse, comorbidity, and complexity among inpatients, Dratcu (20) argued that the local response in Guy's Hospital, inner London, has been to create a speciality of acute hospital psychiatry which has rolled out to other services. Holloway (21) argues against the development of a separate speciality, citing that the skills that consultants need for the management of inpatients are eclectic and develop over a career working in all aspects of general adult psychiatry and the patients admitted to hospital do not generally differ from those cared for in mental health services. He does accept that more consultant time needs to be devoted to inpatient care. Finally, Middleton (22) has argued for the patient's 'journey' through the service to guide service design and advocates that individual organizations are free to make their own decisions according to the skills of individual staff working within them. Currently, the Royal College of Psychiatrists does not have a separate subspecialty for general adult inpatient psychiatry among its 14 subspecialty groups of psychiatry. Experience of inpatient psychiatric care is provided to trainees in their core and specialist training years with an overall qualification in general adult psychiatry.

Current challenges to the delivery of inpatient care in England

Inpatient psychiatric care in England is currently facing high levels of demand. Numbers of beds fell by 62% between 1987/1988 and 2009/2010 with figures from NHS Benchmarking indicating a 3.7% reduction in beds in the year to March 2015 while the number of admissions has not changed over a 10-year period (23). These reductions have mirrored the increased provision of services providing alternatives to admission. Admissions have often been unnecessarily prolonged due to the shortage of supported specialized accommodation provision for people with severe and enduring mental health problems and complex needs. The Commission on Acute Adult Psychiatric Care in England reported in February 2016 that there was inadequate access to acute psychiatric inpatient care with a monthly average of 500 people with acute mental illness needing to travel more than 50 km away from their home to receive inpatient psychiatric treatment, mainly as a result of not finding local inpatient beds or services. The Commission has introduced two substantial recommendations to improve access to inpatient care by October 2017: a maximum 4-hour wait for admission to an acute psychiatric ward for adults and the end of sending adults out of area for non-specialized admission. The practice of out-of-area admissions and their outcome is currently subject to an ongoing research project.

It has long been the case that inpatient beds have been unavailable to people needing acute admission due to difficulties in discharging people who have been successfully treated because of the lack of appropriate supported accommodation or services to provide care in the community. One potential solution to the problem has been to develop acute or 'triage' admission wards where people are admitted for a maximum of 10 days to have a thorough and rapid assessment in order to try to prevent longer hospitalizations. They would either be discharged at the end of this stay or transferred to another less acute ward to continue their treatment. Williams et al. (24) compared such a service in London with a neighbouring service where people were admitted to the same ward for the whole length of their admission. The results were that the triage system did not reduce the overall length of stay, but was similar in costs and readmission rates and the authors could not conclude that the triage system was superior to standard acute admissions. Furthermore, the same authors (25) reported on patient and staff experiences of inpatient care in the two systems. Although they found no difference between the triage and control wards, a deteriorating picture of patients' experiences was noted over the 18-month follow-up period in both systems. This coincided with local and national reductions in budgets, increased pressure on beds and shorter admission length, and a reduction in time that staff spent with patients. Finally, as mentioned earlier, there are serious problems in recruiting nursing staff to work on acute inpatient wards in London and elsewhere in England.

Changes in the management of local inpatient care

Following the development of community mental health teams, the focus on mental health care has been primarily community orientated with consultants aligned to a defined area of the population often around boroughs or counties and general practice populations rather than discrete inpatient wards. The effect of such a system was that the consultant psychiatrist follows the patient on their pathway through the service, working alongside them at initial assessment, in the community, outpatients, as a day patient and as an inpatient, as well as organizing their follow-up after discharge. The benefits appeared obvious in enabling the patient to be treated by a consultant who is familiar with them with good knowledge of their treatment, history, and risks. Continuity of care was assured and reassessment and repetition of information gathering from unfamiliar doctors is avoided. Consultant psychiatrists generally enjoyed working in this system where they were able to develop trust and therapeutic alliances with patients and their carers which are used to the patient's advantage. Conversely, the system can appear inflexible to the patient and carers with little choice in their consultant unless they specifically ask to change, and people with complex needs generally do not receive a specialist second opinion unless this is requested formally. Generally, one or two consultants admitted patients to one mixed-sex ward and managed their patients when inpatients.

As numbers of acute adult inpatient beds have declined over the past 20 years and consultant psychiatrist numbers have expanded, there has been an inevitable increase in the number of consultants and community mental health teams admitting to single inpatient wards. This has resulted in a number of problems. Firstly, there has not been a medical input into the prioritization of patients who are ready for admission or discharge. With each consultant visiting the ward usually for a minimum frequency of weekly, patient reviews have not been timely and patients may have needed to stay longer in order to be discharged at the next ward round. This has had the effects of delaying patient discharge and not managing the beds efficiently to admit acutely unwell individuals. Moreover, if there is a high demand for inpatient admissions from different admitting consultants and teams, consultants have not been in a position to prioritize or triage patients referred to the unit for admission. Secondly, it has become increasingly difficult to accommodate an expansion of different admitting teams to have time and space to review patients on a regular basis. It has been difficult for the inpatient nursing staff to allocate time when the individual psychiatrists and their teams visit on a weekly basis in order to conduct ward rounds. There have been problems in identifying which particular consultant or their junior doctor the nursing staff should contact at times of clinical emergency and at times there have been no regular medical staff covering the wards. Thirdly, doctors have not been involved in the leadership of the wards they admit patients to although this was partially addressed locally by the development of clinical lead psychiatrists for each ward. There has been the potential for disagreement about priorities for admission and discharge between medical and nursing staff and there is less potential to develop close working relationships between the professions. This has been compounded as consultants have often had their patients admitted to more than one inpatient unit.

Single-sex inpatient accommodation was adopted locally following a Department of Health requirement in 2010 (26) in response to the need to protect the safety, privacy, and dignity of individuals at times of increased vulnerability. Admitting an adult to a mixed-sex mental health unit was deemed as 'never' acceptable. This has compounded the situation with consultant alignment to inpatient units further, effectively doubling the number of consultants and junior doctors the wards aligned with. This was clearly a situation which could not continue to operate locally, resulting in a very complex network of medical input to individual wards. The response to the situation locally was that community mental health teams aggregated to include three consultant-led teams and one consultant from each team worked with the inpatients of the combined team and the other two with patients in the community. The advantage was that each inpatient consultant retained direct links with their community mental health team and shared office space, enabling efficient handover of care. They still did not, however, align with one particular ward and often still had patients in many different wards, although the inpatient units had a reduction by over 50% in the number of medical teams they related to.

Since 2013 in Oxford, there have been major improvements in the staffing of the inpatient units and in the development of the identity of the inpatient psychiatric medical group within the local organization. Individual consultants have been appointed to each of the six general adult acute admission wards who work in partnership with newly appointed modern matrons and the ward managers. Each inpatient unit has leadership meetings on a regular basis to review quality and activity data, staffing, staff development, and development of the ward environment. Psychologists have been appointed to cover wards for 1 day per week, increasing the access of psychological therapies to inpatients which were previously not available (see Chapter 28 for a discussion). There has been a development of the medical group with 3-monthly clinical medical meetings involving psychiatric trainees where the cases of difficult-to-treat patients are presented and reviewed. Monthly supervision groups also take place involving just the inpatient consultants where clinical, audit, and quality topics are discussed.

Conclusion

The delivery of inpatient psychiatric care has undergone many changes in the last 10 years. There have been changes in the mix of patients admitted and increased staffing levels. Although inpatient psychiatry has not gained recognition as a separate psychiatric subspecialty, wards increasingly have had their own dedicated psychiatrist who plays an active role in ward leadership. Inpatient admission has been seen in research as an undesirable outcome measure in novel community initiatives but remains an essential short-term component in a care pathway for people with severe mental illness and who are at high risk. Despite this, numbers of acute adult beds continue to decline. Quality of care is underpinned by the Care Quality Commission and the Royal College of Psychiatrists' Quality Improvement Service and services are regularly audited against their standards. Currently we are awaiting further research findings to inform existing service organization and practices.

REFERENCES

1. NHS Clinical Commissioners. About CCGs. 2016. http://www.nhscc.org/ccgs
2. NHS. Care programme approach: your guide to care and support. 2015. https://www.nhs.uk/conditions/social-care-and-support-guide/help-from-social-services-and-charities/care-for-people-with-mental-health-problems-care-programme-approach/

3. Royal College of Nursing. *London Safe Staffing Review.* London: Royal College of Nursing; 2015. http://www.rcn.org.uk/news-and-events/news/london/safe-staffing-report-2015

4. Priebe S, Badesconyi A, Fioritti A, et al. Reinstitutionalisation in mental health care: comparison of data on service provision from six European countries. *BMJ* 2005;330:123–126.

5. Craig T. Shorter hospitalizations at the expense of quality? Experiences of inpatient psychiatry in the post-institutional era. *World Psychiatry* 2016;15:90–91.

6. Russakoff M. Private inpatient psychiatry in the USA. *Psychiatr Bull* 2014;38:230–235.

7. Keown P. Retrospective analysis of hospital episode statistics, involuntary admissions under the Mental Health Act 1983, and number of psychiatric beds in England 1996–2006. *BMJ* 2008;337:a1837.

8. Cohen A, Chatterjee S, Minas H. Time for a global commission on mental health institutions. *World Psychiatry* 2016;15:116–117.

9. Fakhoury W, Priebe S. The process of deinstitutionalization: an international overview. *Curr Opin Psychiatry* 2002;15:187–192.

10. World Health Organization. *World Mental Health Atlas 2014.* Geneva: World Health Organization; 2015. http://www.who.int/mental_health/evidence/atlas/mental_health_atlas_2014/en/

11. Burns T. Hospitalisation as an outcome in schizophrenia. *Br J Psychiatry* 2007;191(Suppl 50):s37–s41.

12. Burns T, Creed F, Fahy T, et al. Intensive versus standard case management for severe psychotic illness: a randomised trial. UK700 Group. *Lancet* 1999;353:2185–2189.

13. Stein LI, Test MA. Alternative to mental hospital treatment. 1. Conceptual model, treatment program and clinical evaluation. *Arch Gen Psychiatry* 1980;37:392–397.

14. Burns T, Rugsaka J, Molodynski A, et al. Community treatment orders for patients with psychosis (OCTET): a randomised controlled trial. *Lancet* 2013;381:1627–1633.

15. Thornicroft G, Farrelly S, Szmukler G, et al. Clinical outcomes of joint crisis plans to reduce compulsory treatment for people with psychosis: a randomised controlled trial. *Lancet* 2013;381:1634–1641.

16. Shek E, Stein AT, Shansis FM, Marshall M, Crowther R, Tyrer P. Day hospital versus outpatient care for people with schizophrenia. *Cochrane Database Syst Rev* 2009;4:CD003240.

17. Murphy SM, Irving CB, Adams CE, Waqar M. Crisis intervention for people with severe mental illness. *Cochrane Database Syst Rev* 2015;12:CD001087.

18. Byford S, Sharac J, Lloyd-Jones B, et al. Alternatives to acute inpatient care in England: readmissions, service use and cost after discharge. *Br J Psychiatry Suppl* 2010;53:s20–s25.

19. Wilkinson G, Piccinelli M, Falloon I, Krekorian H, McLees S. An evaluation of community based psychiatric care for people with treated long term mental illness. *Br J Psychiatry* 1995;167:26–37.

20. Dratcu L. Acute in-patient psychiatry: the right time for a new speciality. *Psychiatr Bull* 2006;30:401–402

21. Holloway F. Acute in-patient psychiatry: dedicated consultants if we must but not a speciality. *Psychiatr Bull* 2006;30:402–403

22. Middleton H. A new speciality of acute in-patient psychiatry. *Psychiatr Bull* 2006;30:404–405.

23. Crisp N, Smith G, Nicholson K (eds). *Old Problems: New Solutions. Improving Psychiatric Care for Adults in England.* London: The Commission on Acute Adult Psychiatric Care.

24. Williams P, Csipke E, Rose D, et al. Efficacy of a triage system to reduce length of inpatient hospital stay. *Br J Psychiatry* 2014;204:480–485.

25. Csipke E, Williams P, Rose D, et al. Following the Francis Report: investigating patient experience of mental health inpatient care. *Br J Psychiatry* 2016;209:35–39.

26. Department of Health. *Eliminating Mixed Sex Accommodation in Hospitals.* London: Department of Health; 2010.

SECTION 2

Team leadership and multidisciplinary work

6

Multidisciplinary work, multidisciplinary team

Jean Hammond and Derek Hammond

Introduction

It is generally accepted that patients admitted to today's acute mental health wards are more severely ill than they were in the past (1). Previous changes to models of care provision and the changes to patient expectations have changed the role of inpatient wards. The poorly understood interactions between biological and psychosocial influences (2) create a complex level of need among patients with severe and enduring mental illnesses, requiring multiprofessional and often multiagency involvement in planning and delivering care. Team work is a strategy (3) which clinicians long ago (4) adopted to meet the challenge of delivering care where there are complex treatment decisions to be made (5).

As health care teams developed, they have used a variety of terms to describe themselves (4), such as multiprofessional, interdisciplinary, and multidisciplinary. Identifying an agreed definition for any of these terms proves challenging. In a review of terms used to describe health care teams from a range of clinical specialities, 17 varying definitions of these terms with ten definitions of 'multidisciplinary team' alone were identified (4). There is some commonality of theme within the definitions, for example, they each provide a description of individuals from different disciplines working together as a team and how these care teams collaborate together to meet the patient's needs.

The lack of a consistency in describing health care teams has led to these terms often being used interchangeably (6) within the literature. This chapter will use the descriptor multidisciplinary team (MDT); this is not an attempt to enter the debate over definitions but merely to simplify the complex idea of the 'team' using a descriptor term which most nursing staff will have experience of working with (6).

The patient journey and changing expectations

The MDT approach has long been recognized as being effective in providing individualized care to patients (7) and effective team working is vital for the provision of high-quality care (8) though as Oynet tells us: 'teamwork means nothing if the patient is not central to the process ... and where possible coproduces a care plan that supports the patient direct their own care' (9). Out of the 17 definitions found by Chamberlain-Salaun et al., only one included patient participation as part of the definition of the health care team (4).

Patient participation in the decision-making process is considered to be a significant contributor to the overall patient experience (10); similarly, professional listening to the patient is positively associated with patient satisfaction. Several studies have demonstrated a link between positive patient experiences and clinical safety and effectiveness and Doyle et al.' s systematic review concludes that taking steps to improve patient experiences will increase the chance of improvements within clinical safety and effectiveness outcomes (11).

The relationship between patients and mental health professionals has not always been viewed as positively as that between patients and other clinical specialities. A recent study found that mental health patients' experiences contrasted with those of physical health patients regarding the care provided by their MDT. Mental health patients identified involvement in the decision-making as an area of particular dissatisfaction, expressing a desire to be more involved in the process (12).

To understand some of the tensions that need to be navigated to include the patient in the decision-making process, it is necessary to consider the social journey the concept of the mental health patient has undertaken.

From asylum inmate through passive patient to mental illness survivor, then service user, and now consumer, the role of the patient has changed as dramatically as the services they use. Mental health patients and service user groups have a long history of activity within the UK existing long before there was any supportive legislation to mandate their involvement in service provision. During the 1970s and 1980s, the service user movement campaigned for changes to the institutional care model that was prevalent and improved living conditions for those suffering from mental illness (13). This activism was supported latterly by the publication of the National Health Service and Community Care Act 1990 which laid a duty on local authorities to consult the users of services on the planning, delivery, and purchasing of services (11), arguably causing the closure of the asylums. It also, crucially, changed the internal structures of health and local authorities, creating the separation of the purchasers and providers of health and social care. This, in effect, introduced an element of competition for the providers of these services and gave the first hint of the patient as a consumer of services.

As the asylums closed, service user and patient groups began to identify themselves as 'survivors' of mental illness and of mental health services and started to organize themselves into groups, possibly influenced by the antipsychiatry movement of the 1960s (14), and created what has been described as a new social movement reacting against, among other things, the disempowerment created by psychiatric practice at the time (13). National and international user groups developed which provided different narratives of mental illness from that of the professionals and looked towards different solutions (15). In recent times, service user groups appear to have reduced in number and size, being replaced by larger mental health charities which have proved effective for pulling smaller groups together to advocate change (16).

Though dwindling in number, user-led groups have been at the forefront of promoting a new approach in mental health care. This approach focuses on recovery as an end point of the patient's engagement with services and is a growing concept in health services nationally and internationally (17). There is no one definition of recovery though it can be argued that it is a social model of illness which focuses on a number of elements which include instilling hope, empowerment, and inclusion; supportive social relationships, and coping strategies (18). The focus on these elements of recovery helps cement the concept that the patient should be front and centre in making decisions about their care as an active partner and not a passive recipient (19).

Supporting policy

The 'Care Programme Approach' provided a framework for care planning for those with serious mental illnesses and introduced the role of the care coordinator as a clinician specifically responsible for coordinating the care provided from multiple agencies to individual service users (20). This was further augmented by the publication of *Building Bridges* (21) which directed that service users should have involvement in drawing up their care plans. Successive governments have since built on this foundation and have promoted patient involvement as an essential part of their health care reform (19).

Additionally, there is now a greater awareness of the deep understanding patients have of living with their illness and navigating mental health services. Patients are now recognized as being experts in their own care and service providers are beginning to recognize the benefits of harnessing this expertise by developing peer support worker roles (22), again reflecting wider developments.

The introduction of 'personal budgets' has further developed the patient role to one of consumer (23). There is now an opportunity for patients to demand to be involved with their care, identifying outcomes which are meaningful to them supported by clinicians who help to realize these or they can purchase their care elsewhere. As patient expectations have developed, government policy has also changed to promote service user involvement at all levels.

Meeting the complex needs and expectations of acutely ill patients and meeting the policy obligations presents significant challenges to acute mental health inpatient ward staff. Providing care where the patient is the key decision maker, particularly where there is the necessity of managing a risk of harm to the patient and others or where there are concerns about a patient's capacity to consent to any element of the treatment plan, complicates things further. In practice, an element of compulsion may be used in these circumstance utilizing provisions laid out in the Mental Health Act 1983 as amended by the Mental Health Act 2007, to ensure that the appropriate level of care is given and that patients' rights and best interests are safeguarded. Regulation 9 of the Health and Social Care Act 2014 outlines that providers are required to ensure the patient's ability to consent, and where this is compromised, an individual who is lawfully acting on behalf of the patient is involved in the planning and review of their care (24). The Mental Capacity Act 2005 also places a duty on care teams to consult the patients, carers, families, or advocate where possible to ensure their views are considered (25).

Thus, the MDT is recognized as the appropriate approach to do this while placing the patient at the centre of the decision-making process. In fact, MDT working is now core to several standards contained within the Royal College of Psychiatrists Accreditation for Inpatient Mental Health Services (AIMS) (26).

The multidisciplinary team

Multidisciplinary and multiagency working is defined as a process 'involving the appropriate use of knowledge, skills and best practice from multiple disciplines and across service boundaries to reach solutions based on improved collective understanding of complex patient needs' (27). It has been argued that MDT working is the 'main mechanism to ensure truly holistic care' (28). Currently, there is growing demand within the wider National Health Service that team-based approaches and in particular the MDT approach are adopted to optimize the care of patients with complex needs (29). The MDT is currently recommended as the approach of choice in the delivery of cancer care (30) and a range of other complex conditions (31).

The adoption of a MDT approach to providing care is assumed by professionals to have several benefits for both the patient and the clinicians of the team (30). There is a perception held by professionals that patients and their carers find reassurance in the fact they are being supported by highly specialized teams with the appropriate skills and abilities (32), improved care planning, increased clinical effectiveness, and an increased focus on patient needs (6). It has also been argued that the patient receives a more holistic and seamless service and there is a higher level of user satisfaction with this model compared to more traditional models of planning health care (33). Other benefits include peer support, recognizing the high degree of resilience needed to deal with complex and often distressing clinical situations. The delivery of high-quality care through the process of peer review and the cross fertilization of skills between different professions can improve clinicians' sense of job satisfaction (33). Additionally, improved clinical decision-making, provision of evidence-based interventions, and better coordinated care were also identified as benefits in a survey of breast cancer MDT clinicians (34).

On the other hand, while it has been argued that there is little evidence to support these perceptions (35), a recent study suggested that some MDT members held a degree of scepticism about the MDT concept, describing it as idealistic (6), and it may be argued that the practice and function of the MDT is idiosyncratic to individual teams and can change frequently within a team depending on which professionals are involved (36).

Within the field of acute inpatient mental health care there is surprisingly little published about the use, effectiveness, or perceived benefits of the MDT approach. To gain some clarity on the key characteristics of the MDT, it is perhaps useful to look at the teams working in different health care contexts, such as cancer care, where there is a long tradition of using the MDT approach for service provision (31) and where performance and clinical outcomes are audited against national guidelines (30).

The National Cancer Action Team identified several characteristics which MDTs should have; they suggest that the MDT members should possess the right knowledge, skills, and experience to provide diagnosis and treatment of high quality and consider the MDT meeting as a forum to consider the patient as a whole and not just to consider disease management (37). To do this they identify the following five key characteristics that MDTs require to be effective, namely the team, the meeting infrastructure, meeting organization, making person-centred decisions, and team governance.

The team

There are numerous models which attempt to describe 'the team' but in general it is accepted that teams consist of a group of individuals, with varying skills coming together, with a shared purpose and high task interdependence (38). The nested model of mental health team relationships used by the Mental Health Commission of Ireland (33) places the patient, their carers, and their families in the centre of a number of concentric circles with their community resources and with primary care services surrounding them in the second layer. The next layer surrounding the latter is the core MDT, in this case the community mental health team who then link on to other mental health services.

While putting the patient at the centre of the approach, the nested model does not illustrate the patient as part of the MDT. As an entity, the MDT continues to function and develop prior to, and following, the involvement of any particular patient. Furthermore, the MDT provides a function to a number of patients at any given time. This and other cultural elements such as team dynamics, understanding of each role within the MDT, and team objectives mean that patients and their carers will need support to engage with the MDT process (39). It has been proposed that patients should be considered extraordinary or as 'VIP' members of the MDT (39), recognizing their unique contribution but also acknowledging their position as a consumer of the services provided by the MDT and wider health care system.

In the nested model, the acute inpatient team sits in the circle surrounding the MDT core team, demonstrating that the inpatient teams are extended members of the core MDT and only become active when the patient enters their sphere of responsibility. At this point, the inpatient team become responsible for managing the acute illness and meeting the patient's day-to-day needs. Links are maintained with the community team through the engagement of the care coordinator who should also be considered a core member of the inpatient MDT, as information regarding the admission, and tasks to support the patient's discharge pathway, need to be completed and coordinated with the wider MDT. The care coordinator role is recognized as providing a 'continuous point of contact' for the patient, their carers, and a range of professionals and agencies involved in providing care to the patient (27).

Core members of the inpatient multidisciplinary team

Consultant psychiatrist

This is the senior medical doctor on the team and is the team's specialist in the diagnosis, treatment, and management of the full range of mental health disorders; they are responsible for the biological aspects of the treatment, for diagnosing mental disorders, and prescribing treatment (39). Within the MDT they act as a consultant to the team, promoting distributed responsibility and leadership. In the past, the consultant was regarded as the person who had the overall say in planning care and who would direct other professionals. While this model has experienced challenges in community mental health teams, within the inpatient environment it is often perceived as still dominant (6). Within acute inpatient wards, the consultant is the clinician who most often holds 'Responsible Clinician' status under the Mental Health Act 1983 (amended 2007), a role that is pivotal to the decision-making process in this context.

Social worker

The social worker is a vital component of the MDT, providing the necessary link with the wider social care arena, as well as providing the support and care that the patient requires to promote discharge from inpatient services. The social worker will assess how aspects of the social environment may affect the patient's mental state and may impede recovery, and in consultation with the MDT addresses these issues as appropriate. Using theories of human behaviour and social systems, social workers bring a cultural and community perspective to the deliberations of the MDT (40). Depending on the service provision model, social workers may be employed by the local authority or by the local health service and are often the patient's care coordinator.

Inpatient nurse

The inpatient nurse is the only member of the MDT who is responsible for meeting the patient's needs 24 hours a day. As a discipline they have the most engagement with the patient and are therefore in an excellent position to be able to work closely with the patient and assess how they interact, look for the effect of any medication, and observe for any changes in behaviour. Nurses aim to achieve their outcomes by providing individual nursing care, by ensuring the care is safe and effective, and by promoting a culture where safe and effective care can be sustained by all members of the MDT (41). The nurse has responsibility for coordinating inpatient care as well as implementing treatment decisions (6) and managing clinical risk within the ward context (42).

Occupational therapist

Promoting the individual's capacity to maximize their independence in the context of their social, physical, and occupational environments is a key contribution provided by the team's occupational therapist (39). This focus on occupational performance means there has to be close collaboration with the patient to identify what activities are meaningful to them and what prevents the patient from engaging with these activities. By promoting independence, they reduce the need for external support and also ensure that any additional support is appropriately targeted (see Chapter 8).

Psychologist

The unique contribution of this discipline is considerable. Through assessment and the process of formulation, the psychologist brings a reflective psychological perspective to the team decision-making. The psychologist also considers team development and peer supervision as key contributions to the MDT. Unfortunately, team make-up and local commissioning arrangements often have the result that psychologists are not always included in the core MDT.

Pharmacist

In all care settings the pharmacist is considered the expert in medicines and processes; this is particularly relevant when we consider the potential side effects of a number of the medicines used within psychiatry and the impact this may have on concordance. Pharmacists support medication management (43), act as educators to the team (44), and can provide second opinions regarding medication (45). Though not always recognized as part of the MDT, a systematic review showed that where they were included in the MDT there were improved clinical outcomes, better prescribing practices, and improved patient satisfaction (44).

Dietician

Similarly as with pharmacists, dieticians are not always available to the MDT within an acute mental health care context. However, there is an increasing recognition of the physical health care needs of mental health patients and the current drive to improve their physical health outcomes suggests that there will be a greater involvement of dieticians in the mental health acute care pathway in the future. Dieticians are able to contribute an interpretation of current research findings on food and health, translating this into practical guidance that supports the patient making informed choices regarding their nutrition, hydration, and lifestyle. They provide assessment of nutritional problems and provide advice and training to the MDT in their area of expertise (39).

While the core MDT provides the skills, knowledge, and expertise to support the patient, there is also a degree of flexibility regarding additional members of the MDT depending on the needs of the patient. For example, the role of the advocate, police and probation services, and community services such as housing should be involved in planning and implementing MDT decisions where appropriate.

Key roles within the multidisciplinary team

The main vehicle for delivering an MDT approach is the MDT meeting (46) at which all core and necessary extended team members are present to discuss the patient's care and treatment and agree with the patient a treatment pathway (37). For the MDT meeting to function effectively, a number of key responsibilities need to be considered. These roles are allocated to individual members of the MDT and should be considered distinct from their clinical or other roles.

The leadership functions within the MDT can be categorized into three distinct roles (33). The clinical lead role focuses on ensuring that there is a set of clear and agreed objectives for the team to achieve as well as promoting team cohesion. The clinical leader

should consider issues related to team effectiveness and governance while providing a vision for team development. This role is often considered the role of the ward manager. The team coordinator role is concerned with providing a central point of communication within the team. This role has responsibility for informing members of the MDT of relevant clinical issues and auditing the team's activity. The team administrator role is concerned with ensuring the smooth running of the MDT meeting, making sure the right clinicians are in attendance, and that all equipment is available. This role ensures the supportive systems that the MDT requires to function are in place. In practice, on busy acute wards these roles may often be completed by one individual or several individuals depending on who is on duty at the time (6), but on the whole are assumed by the ward manager or senior nurse currently on duty. Senior doctors also assume the leadership role though some researchers have found that senior doctors tend to focus their attention on the medical management of the patient and risk management while ward managers and team leaders had a more holistic focus considering work and organizational factors (47).

The meeting infrastructure

The MDT meeting is the key decision-making forum and communication route for the clinical team (31, 46) and requires a high degree of organization and infrastructure to enable it to function effectively (48). An appropriate meeting environment needs to be provided, and not only should the size of the meeting room and the privacy it affords (30) be considered but also the processes and technology to record and communicate MDT discussions (39).

The meeting organization

To be effective, MDT meetings need to be highly organized but there is a lack of guidance for mental health MDTs to refer to so MDT meeting objectives and structure are generally locally developed (31). A number of areas to consider are outlined by the National Cancer Action Team (30) though not all those identified will be relevant to the acute mental health care context. Meeting organization includes not only the scheduling and attendance of meetings but should consider managing the agenda and ensuring sufficient time to discuss all the patients. The preparation clinicians should undertake for the meetings, such as ensuring adherence to a minimum dataset when completing case presentations, should be made clear to all core members of the team. Access to relevant clinical information, to support clinical decision-making, is essential to the MDT making appropriate decisions and processes need to be in place to ensure all MDT recommendations are discussed with the patient and other members of the MDT if they are not present at the meeting. A process to monitor the implementation of MDT decisions is recognized as being an important element of the meeting structure and to inform the MDT where treatment decisions are not completed (30). A process for establishing the patient's views prior to the meeting must also be established as often patients can find MDT meetings an anxiety-provoking experience (49).

Person-centred/shared decision-making

The main objective of the MDT is to support the patient and the care team to make evidence-based decisions on care and treatment. The clinical decisions made by the team should result in unambiguous recommendations for the treatment plan. The recommendations should be evidence based and in line with National Institute for Health and Care Excellence guidelines and standard treatment protocols. The MDT should support the patient to be involved in making any clinical decision-making. Although there has been little research into the impact of shared decision-making (50), we know that a number of features of the discussion must be present (51). Involving the patient in the discussion and listening to what the patient is aware of and being clear on what the patient understands their problem to be are essential. Allowing the patient adequate time to express their concerns and expectations as well as outlining treatment options, and providing the relevant information in a format that is accessible to the patient supports the process of shared decision-making. Other significant features of the process are that the MDT spends time clarifying if the patient is comfortable with the decision made as well as setting an review date (50).

Team governance

There is a considerable amount of debate concerning the effectiveness of MDT working with very little high-quality evidence to support the effectiveness of the approach (6, 31, 35), though other authors argue that this situation is changing in some clinical specialities (5).

To monitor the effectiveness of the clinical decisions made by the MDT it is important to ensure the objectives of the MDT and the expected clinical outcomes are agreed locally and that there are policies and protocols in place that support the team achieving these. Policies and protocols for the team should cover aspects of who the team are and what their roles are. They should also outline how the team should work together including communication routes outside the meeting and when the policies and protocols will be reviewed (30).

The collection of and review of data are also key characteristics of the MDT; this data may be related to national datasets but should also focus on clinical outcomes and, importantly, patients' experiences of their engagement with the MDT.

Barriers to effective multidisciplinary team working

Much has been written about the obstacles that prevent effective MDT function. Issues of leadership (47), professional relationships and perceived power differences between disciplines (6, 52), staff morale (53), the lack of a clear model or guidelines for MDT working (31), and differing conceptual models of mental illness (40) have been highlighted as impacting team function and effectiveness. Role ambiguity, staff shortages, and a lack of confidence and assertiveness in nursing staff have also been cited in the literature (6). While it is clear that MDT working has its own limitations and many authors have written extensively on models or features that impact team working within the health care context, there are very few systematic reviews of the interventions aimed at improving it. One such review into improving effectiveness in acute hospital teams (54) suggested that much of the literature reviewed had significant limitations with very little high-quality research. The conclusion of the review was that issues in MDT functioning should be clearly understood before identifying an intervention to improve functioning (54).

The acute inpatient ward context

The necessity of having an effective team approach is emphasized when the issue of why patients are admitted to acute mental health inpatient services is considered. Bowers et al. (55) found the main reason for admission was to manage risk during a crisis episode. The risk was often categorized as risk to self, such as suicidal ideation, self-harm, vulnerability, and neglect, while risk to others was categorized as including violent behaviour, homicidal ideas, and threats to kill (55). Need for respite, carer breakdown, and acuity of symptoms were also identified as significant drivers of inpatient admissions.

The purpose of admission leads directly to what the function is of an acute mental health inpatient ward. Bowers et al. (55) identify five themes, including assessment of the patient's needs and response to treatment, providing treatment, supporting the patient meet their self-care needs, the management of physical health needs, and perhaps most significantly, managing risk and keeping the patient safe. Achieving these functions requires effective team working. Governments are beginning to understand that mental health services need support on how to put the idea of the MDT into practice. The Welsh government has published *Multidisciplinary Working: A Framework for Practice in Wales* (39) which attempts to clarify issues related to MDT working and offers a number of useful exercises and actions for team leaders to help develop their teams. The Mental Health Commission of Ireland has published a discussion paper on multidisciplinary working which debates some of the issues discussed here in greater depth (33). NHS England published a handbook on MDT development which provides a number of models of effective MDTs taken from clinical practice (27).

Acute inpatient mental health wards have to overcome a number of challenges if they are to keep pace with the growing demands of their patients. From passive recipient to consumer and now expert, the patient is now more invested in their care than in previous times. They are more articulate and through successive governmental changes there are better structures to make their voices heard. Though there appears to be a lack of consensus around the terminology to describe a MDT and define its functions, there is broad agreement that having a range of experts and skills has a beneficial effect on clinical outcomes and patient experience. Other key elements include providing patients with choices that are evidence based as well as involving patients in the decision-making process, ensuring, where this is not possible, that the patient's views are taken into account. Finally, clear aims and objectives, identifying individuals to assume key functions, and having clear processes in place to plan, deliver, and monitor the effectiveness of the inpatient MDT's interventions will help to meet the challenge faced by inpatient teams.

REFERENCES

1. Rethink. *The Lie of the Land In: Behind Closed Doors: Acute Mental Health Care in the UK*. London: Rethink; 2007. http://www.rethink.org

2. Orovwuje P. Contemporary challenges in forensic mental health: the ingenuity of the multidisciplinary team. *Ment Health Rev J* 2008;13:24–34.

3. Salas E, Cooke J, Rosen M. On teams, teamwork, and team performance: discoveries and developments. *Hum Factors* 2008;50:540–547.

4. Chamberlain-Salaun J, Mills J, Usher K. Terminology used to describe health care teams: an integrative review of the literature. *J Multidisc Healthc* 2013;6:65–74.

5. Taylor C, Shewbridge A, Green JS. Benefits of multidisciplinary teamwork in the management of breast cancer. *Breast Cancer (Dove Med Press)* 2013;5:79–85.

6. Atwal A, Caldwell K. Nurses perceptions of multidisciplinary team work in acute health care. *Int J Nurs Pract* 2006;12: 359–365.

7. Dorahy M, Hamilton G. The 'narcissistic' we model: a conceptual framework for multidisciplinary team working, researching and decision-making with traumatised individuals. *Couns Psychother Res* 2009;9:57–64.

8. Royal College of Nursing. *Developing Effective teams: Delivering Effective Services. Executive Summary*. London: Royal College of Nursing; 2006.

9. Onyett S. Connecting the parts of the whole: achieving effective teamwork in complex systems. In: Stickley T, Basset T (eds), *Learning About Mental Health Practice*, pp. 311–328. Chichester: John Wiley & Sons Ltd; 2008.

10. Doyle C, Lennox L, Bell D. A systematic review of evidence on the links between patient experience and clinical safety and effectiveness. *BMJ Open* 2013;3:e001570.

11. Legislation.gov.uk. National Health Service and Community Care Act 1990. 1990. https://www.legislation.gov.uk/ukpga/1990/19/contents

12. O'Driscoll W, Livingston G, Lanceley A, et al. Patient experience of MDT care and decision-making. *Ment Health Rev J* 2014;19:265–278.

13. Rose D, Barnes M, Crawford M, Omeni E, Macdonald D, Wilson A. How do managers and leaders in the National Health Service and social care respond to service user involvement in mental health services in both its traditional and emergent forms? The ENSUE study. *HS&DR* 2014;2:10. https://www.ncbi.nlm.nih.gov/books/NBK259692/ doi: 10.3310/hsdr02100

14. Crossley N. *Contesting Psychiatry: Social Movements in Mental Health*. London: Routledge; 2005.

15. The Survivors History Group. The Survivors History Group takes a critical look at historians. In: Barnes M, Cotterell M (eds), *Critical Perspectives on User Involvement*, pp. 7–18. Bristol: Policy Press; 2012.

16. Gilburt H, Peck E. *Service Transformation: Lessons from Mental Health. The Kings Fund Ideas that Change Health Care*. London: The King's Fund; 2014.

17. National Institute for Mental Health in England. *NIMHE Guiding Statement on Recovery*. London: Department of Health; 2005.

18. Terry L, Cardwell V. *Understanding The Whole Person: What are the Common Concepts for Recovery and Desistance Across Fields of Mental Health, Substance Misuse and Criminology?* London: Revolving Door Agency; 2016.

19. Corrie C, Finch A. *Expert Patients*. London: Reform; 2015.

20. Department of Health. *Effective Care Co-Ordination in Mental Health Services: Modernising the Care Programme Approach; A Policy Booklet*. London: Department of Health; 1990.

21. Department of Health. *Building Bridges: A Guide to Arrangements for Interagency Working for the Care and Protection of Severely Mentally Ill People*. London: Department of Health; 1995.

22. Gillard S, Holley J. Peer workers in mental health services: literature overview. *Adv Psychiatr Treat* 2014;20:286–292.

23. NHS England Patient Participation Team. *Guidance on the "Right to Have" in Adult Continuing Health Care and Children and Young Peoples Continuing Care*. London: Department of Health; 2014.

24. Care Quality Commission. *Health and Social Care Act 2008 (Regulated Activities) Regulations 2014*. London: Care Quality Commission; 2014.

25. Department for Constitutional Affairs. *The Mental Capacity Act 2005: Code of Practice*. London: TSO; 2007.

26. Cresswell J, Beavon M. *Accreditation for Inpatient Mental Health Services (AIMS); Standards for Inpatient Wards—Working Age Adults*, 4th edition. London: Royal College of Psychiatrists; 2010. http://www.rcpsych.ac.uk/AIMS

27. NHS England/Nursing/LTC. NHS England: multi-disciplinary team handbook. 2014. https://www.england.nhs.uk/wp-content/uploads/2015/01/mdt-dev-guid-flat-fin.pdf

28. Jeffries N, Chan K. Multidisciplinary team working: is it both hostile and effective? *Int J Gynaecol Cancer* 2004;14:210–211.

29. Care Services Improvement Partnership, National Institute for Mental Health in England. *New Ways of Working for Everyone: A Best Practice Implementation Guide*. London: Department of Health; 2007.

30. National Cancer Action Team. *National Cancer Peer Review Programme Manual for Cancer Services: Haemato-oncology Cancer Measures*. London: National Cancer Action Team; 2013.

31. Raine R, a' Bháird CN, Xanthopoulou P, et al. Use of a formal consensus development technique to produce recommendations for improving effectiveness of adult mental health multidisciplinary team meetings. *BMCV Psychiatry* 2015;15:143.

32. Carter S, Garside P, Black A. Multidisciplinary team working, clinical networks, and chambers; opportunities to work differently in the NHS. *Qual Saf Health Care* 2003;12:i25–i28.

33. Mental Health Commission. *Multidisciplinary Team Working: From Theory to Practice*. Discussion Paper. Dublin: Mental Health Commission; 2006.

34. Saini KS, Taylor C, Ramirez AJ, et al. Role of the multidisciplinary team in breast cancer management: results from a large international survey involving 39 countries. *Ann Oncol* 2012;23:853–859.

35. Lemieux-Charles L, McGuire WL. What do we know about health care team effectiveness? A review of the literature. *Med Care Res Rev* 2006;63:263–300.

36. Deady R. Studying multidisciplinary teams in the Irish Republic: the conceptual wrangle. *Perspect Psychiatr Care* 2012;48:176–182.

37. National Cancer Action Team. *Multidisciplinary Team Member's Views about MDT Working: Results from a Survey Commissioned by the National Cancer Action Team*. London: National Cancer Action Team; 2009.

38. Dyer JL. Team research and team training: a state of the art review. In: Muckler FA (ed), *Human Factors Review*, pp. 285–323. Santa Monica, CA: Human Factors Society; 1984.

39. Continuing NHS Healthcare National Programme. *Multidisciplinary Working: A Framework for Wales*. Cardiff: Welsh Government; 2011.

40. Giles R. Social workers perceptions of multi-disciplinary team work: a case study of health and social workers at a major regional hospital in New Zealand. *Aotearoa N Z Soc Work* 2016;28:25–33.

41. Royal College of Nursing. *Measuring for Quality in Health and Social Care*. RCN Position statement. London: Royal College of Nursing; 2009.

42. Royal College of Nursing. *Principles of Nursing Practice*. London: Royal College of Nursing; 2010.

43. Wheeler A, Crump K, Lee M, et al. Collaborative prescribing: a qualitative exploration of a role for pharmacists in mental health. *Res Social Adm Pharm* 2011;8:179–192.

44. Finley P, Crimson ML, Rush AJ. Evaluating the impact of pharmacists in mental health: a systematic review. *Pharmacotherapy* 2003;3:1634–1644.

45. National Institute for Mental Health England. *Medicines Management: Everybody's Business.* London: Department of Health; 2008.

46. Rushtaller T, Roe H, Thurlimann B, Nicoll J. The multidisciplinary meeting: an indispensable aid to communication between different specialities. *Eur J Cancer* 2006;42:2459–2462.

47. West M, Alimo-Metcalfe B, Dawson J, et al. *Effectiveness of Multi-Professional Team Working (MPTW) in Mental Health. National Institute for Health Research Service Delivery and Organisation Programme.* London: HMSO; 2012.

48. Ke M, Blazeby J, Strong S, Carroll F, Ness A, Hollingworth W. Are multidisciplinary teams in secondary care cost-effective? A systematic review of the literature. *Cost Eff Resour Alloc* 2013;11:7.

49. White R, Karim B. Patients' views of the ward round: a survey. *BJPsych Bull* 2005;9:207–209.

50. Duncan E, Best C, Hagen S. Shared decision making interventions for people with mental health conditions (Protocol). *Cochrane Database Syst Rev* 2008;3:CD007297.

51. Charles C, Gafni A, Whelan T. Shared decision making in the medical encounter: what does it mean? (Or, it takes at least two to tango). *Soc Sci Med* 1997;44:651–661.

52. Vetere A. Bio/psycho/social models and multidisciplinary team working—can systemic thinking help? *Clin Child Psychol Psychiatry* 2007;12:5–12.

53. Totman J, Lewando Hunt G, Wearn E, Moli P, Johnson S. Factors affecting staff morale on inpatient mental health wards in England: a qualitative investigation *BMC Psychiatry* 2011;11:68.

54. Buljac-Samardzic M, Dekker van Doorn C, van wijngaarden J, van Wijk K. Interventions to improve team effectiveness: a systematic review. *Health Policy* 2010;94:183–195.

55. Bowers L, Simpson A, Alexander J, Hackney D, Grange A, Warren J. The nature and purpose of acute psychiatric wards: the Tompkin Acute Ward Study. *J Ment Health* 2005;14:625–635.

7

Modern matron, ward manager, consultant nurse

Caroline Attard, Catriona Canning, and Rose Warne

Introduction

In the late 1980s and 1990s, the ward sister and matron were seen as key to nursing and nursing leadership and were essential to the delivery of patient care and the development of nursing staff. The ward sister was responsible for both nurses and patients on a ward and was expected to supervise all nursing practice and ensure the clinical standards of the ward were met.

In 1966, the Ministry of Health (1) reviewed the senior staff structure in hospitals and a new management structure for nursing was proposed for the UK National Health Service (NHS) with lines of senior management, middle management, and first-line management. This was a significant difference to the way in which hospitals had been run previously; many felt that this undermined the ward sister and matron roles and as a result, many nurses left healthcare (2, 3).

Over 30 years later in 2000, the Department of Health published *The NHS Plan* (4) which admitted the need to strengthen the ward sister role within hospital settings. *The NHS Plan* was created as a reform with far-reaching changes across the NHS. The intention was to provide a health service designed around the needs of the patient. Clinical leadership was seen as an important part of this change and this included the introduction of the modern matron role. The revisiting of the matron role had the aim of providing strong clinical leadership on the wards, utilizing this authority to get the basics right. The Secretary of State acknowledged in 2007 that there was a need to look further at the ward sister and matron roles and to give them more power so that they could fulfil their function without the bureaucracy that the roles often entailed (5).

These developments in nursing leadership were further strengthened when the Department of Health (6) announced the introduction of the nurse consultant (NC) role in response to a lack of clinical career pathways for senior nurses in England and the need to ensure expertise was kept at the bedside (7). The NHS set out guidance for NHS trusts in the recruitment and appointment of NCs. This was followed by the Department of Health (6), and then the Scottish Executive, Wales, and Northern Ireland respectively. NCs were then introduced into the NHS in the UK as part of the modernizing strategy outlined in *The NHS Plan* (4). Nurses practising at higher levels were seen as key to reforming the health service, with particular emphasis on their working across professional and organizational boundaries, as outlined in the Chief Nursing Officer's report (8). Key roles for nurses were discussed by the Department of Health (9). Also, the Bristol Royal Infirmary Inquiry (10) highlighted a need for change in practice and team culture to develop a health service that was well led through programmes of training and support for clinicians. The role of a specialized NC was born which along with the ward manager and modern matron roles would provide a strong nursing leadership structure where quality and improvement are central.

The ward manager

The ward manager role in mental health services is responsible for ensuring high-quality, safe, and effective care in the inpatient setting. The Royal College of Nursing (RCN) (11) identified that ward managers are responsible for overseeing the day-to-day running of the ward or unit and nurses in this role typically will:

- ensure the assessment, planning, and evaluation of evidence-based care is carried out in line with best practice
- provide professional leadership for a team of multiprofessional registered and unregistered staff
- provide the line management for a team of multiprofessional registered and unregistered staff
- provide expert evidence-based clinical advice
- have continuous responsibility for their ward, ensuring systems are in place for the safe delegation, monitoring, and supervision of care
- be responsible for the ward budgets and the safe and efficient delegation of resources
- be responsible for the safety of the ward and the clinical environment
- build the capacity and competency of the ward team through the effective planning, facilitation, and delivery of education and training opportunities.[1]

[1] Adapted from Royal College of Nursing (2009) *Breaking Down Barriers, Drive Up Standards: the Role of the Ward Sister and Charge Nurse.* London: RCN. Tinyurl.com/barriers-standards

This is in no way an exhaustive list; however, it is clear that this is not an easy role to undertake. It may feel a relentless task to the newly appointed ward manager at times, with competing demands and limited training available at the start, although local authorities may well provide some leadership training, once a person is in post. The ward manager role is seen as the interface between health care management and clinical delivery and links to the standards of patient care. *The NHS Plan* (4) states that the 'NHS organizations should be led by the brightest and the best of public sector management'. It is important therefore to ensure the right person is in the right position and that they have the best possible training and guidance.

The role of ward manager is fundamental to the smooth running of the ward as they provide a central point of contact, stability, and consistency to the ward team. Management is a sensitive function, as staff spend a great deal of their time at work and may need varying degrees of support at times during their employment. It is helpful therefore if the ward manager spends time getting to know their staff and to some extent their personal lives and/or circumstances to help promote trust within the team. If staff have a sense of trust and security from the ward manager and within the team, they are more likely to share information and seek support or advice when they need it. This can then be reflected in the safe delivery of care for patients.

Taking up a ward manager position for the first time may be challenging as there can be a lot to learn in a short space of time. The ward manager can significantly influence the successful functioning or failure of a ward. Tasks such as managing the budget, the rota, the e-procurement orders, and the wages are straightforward with the appropriate training. However, what can often be the most challenging and something rarely touched on in nurse training is ensuring that all staff are fully supported while also ensuring each staff member fulfils their required role and responsibility. This is an important balance to achieve as staff may present at work with an assortment of problems such as challenges within their roles, sickness and absence, and/or performance-related problems. It is therefore important for the ward manager to get to know their team, how they learn, what motivates them, and indeed what does not. Staff work harder when they are developed and feel appreciated for doing a good job. Staff should feel valued for the work that they do and the ward manager is in a prime position to develop a culture of positive recognition for work well done and can act as a role model giving praise and saying thank you. This can help staff and teams to maintain motivation and moral. It is apparent that to achieve a successful ward the ward manager needs to adapt their leadership style to the staff that they manage and the situation that they are in (12).

The Hay Group (13) argue that high-performing ward managers consistently use a broader range of leadership styles with their teams, varying their approach in line with the needs of the situation and the people that they are managing. This supports the idea that without having the ability to change the style of working or engaging with people, it is very difficult to lead a team/service in the direction the ward manager wishes to lead them. Little can be achieved if the leader fails to take people with them.

Another significant challenge for the ward manager is the need to balance clinical and administrative tasks. Different ward managers may approach this differently depending on their view of the role; however, Bonner and McLaughlin (14) found that administration was one aspect of the role for which ward managers felt unprepared

for and was a source of frustration when these tasks took them away from frontline clinical work. This in turn reduced opportunities for role modelling good clinical practice to the team.

Given the varied tasks and aspects of the ward manager role, time management is vital but can be difficult to achieve at times. Managing time has of course many benefits, not only in planning the day-to-day running of the ward but also for the health and well-being of the ward manager. Learning how to organize time can help most people cope better and reduce their level of stress (15). Pedler et al. (16) suggest that after considering what you do with time it is important to make decisions about what could be delegated. There is an expectation that ward managers can successfully manage the ward budget, the ward risk assessments, and many more tasks. Francis (17) advised that nurse managers should operate in a supervisory capacity and that they should not be bound to an office. He also suggested that they should work alongside staff as a role model to develop clinical skills and competencies, know all there is to know about patient care plans, ensure that there is a caring culture, be a leader of the ward, and educate those that work there. The RCN (11) found that it is often very difficult to achieve all of this, as managers lack the time, resources, and sometimes the authority to lead effectively.

As well as challenges, there are opportunities to make a difference as a ward manager. The role is central to care delivery. It is a well-rounded role as there is the room to act as the catalyst between senior management and front-line staff. This is a powerful position, as managers have access to a wide variety of disciplines and professionals creating opportunities for networking and developing relationships. This can have a significant impact on accessing support, involvement of others in developments, and improvements and so influence the delivery of high-quality care. Further to this, the ward manager is often the messenger between senior management and frontline staff but they can also be the cushion when changes are imminent and potentially anxiety provoking for staff.

With all these competing demands, challenges, and opportunities it is particularly important for a ward manager, indeed any leader, to understand the importance of self-development and self-awareness as this helps support growth for the individual as well as for their team. Without self-awareness, it is difficult to see how a person can lead a team successfully. The self-aware ward manager takes time to understand their own responses and emotions as well as their teams, to ensure an understanding of how best to react and respond to the team and so learn what works well for them, what does not, and how to help the team grow.

It is clear therefore that the role of a ward manager is a complex one, balancing the differing demands of the job. Thus, the ward manager needs to be a skilled clinician, a manager, and be able to support and educate staff to do their job effectively. The RCN (11) carried out some research into the demands of this role and they found that many managers struggle to balance the complexity of the role and the competing demands. It takes a very good manager to effectively set priorities and ensure that they can achieve all that the ward and service requires of them.

Modern matrons

The need for modern matron posts to be developed was proposed by *The NHS Plan* (4) in response to the perceived need following a public consultation for stronger clinical leadership with sufficient authority that could be easily identified by patients and was accountable for a group of wards. Thus, modern matrons were to be highly visible and accessible to patients and their loved ones and were to be present on the wards to lead by example in driving up standards of clinical care and empowering nurses to do the same.

The role of the modern matron therefore focuses on the provision of high-quality, visible, and professional leadership. Modern matrons have a clear role in setting and maintaining standards of clinical excellence, improving outcomes and the experience of patients, families, and carers. The Department of Health (18) identified key responsibilities for the modern matron role:

- Making sure patients get quality care.
- Ensuring staffing is appropriate to patients' needs.
- Empowering nurses to take on a wider range of clinical tasks.
- Improving hospital cleanliness.
- Ensuring patients' nutritional needs are met.
- Improving wards for patients.
- Making sure patients are treated with respect.
- Preventing hospital-acquired infections.
- Resolving problems for patients and their relatives by building closer relationships.

However, the role of the modern matron often becomes much more than the above especially when the ward environment is busy and many of the patients are acutely unwell. Modern matrons may have responsibility for managing beds across the wards and in supporting the day-to-day management of the ward as well as involvement in senior management issues and meetings. It can then be difficult to balance the different aspects of the role, particularly if the demand for beds for acutely unwell patients falls at the door of the modern matron, as it can then often overtake other priorities such as quality and service improvement.

The modern matron is in a position to lead change in a team despite challenges to time and resources. Part of being an effective leader is facilitating the development of employees' skills and abilities by delegating challenging duties that push them to go beyond their current level of functioning (19). The modern matron role offers ward-dedicated time to focus on the team and their development while the ward manager deals with the day-to-day management. The modern matron is a clinical role model who can work with a variety of other practitioners to ensure that the clinical aspects of the ward are of a high standard. The modern matron can lead on a variety of quality targets and audits that are required to measure, quantify, and make visible the impact of nursing on care quality outcomes. The modern matron must have excellent clinical skills and therefore can add more to the monitoring of standards and in turn ensure that the delivery of the service is improved while relieving the ward manager of this time-consuming but important task.

The Hay Group (13) explained that the ward manager's job is to provide day-to-day line management of nursing staff and arrange the available resources to best meet the needs of the ward. However, roles such as the modern matron are also picking up issues that are closely aligned to managing ward staff such as training, development, setting standards, and monitoring quality. Consequently, the responsibility of the ward manager may now be less clear because they are only partly responsible for the resources on their ward. It

is clear from this that the ward manager and modern matron roles interface very closely and to get the best out of both they need to work effectively together. The main challenge is the potential for a lack of clarity in understanding the two roles and how they differ, which can be a source of conflict between them (20), which can be exacerbated if other wards divide their roles and responsibilities differently. Furthermore, the Hay Group (13) looked at the morale of ward managers and adds that the overlap can lead to a job that is less satisfying to do, and therefore it may not attract high-quality clinicians. It can also be hard for ward managers to stand back from a role they had been doing for some time and allow modern matrons to take over some of the work they had previously been responsible for. It can help the process if a trust's senior management teams support ward managers, modern matrons, and ward consultants to invest time into developing their own senior ward leadership team, which can then help to effectively address any issues related to lack of clarity and areas of responsibility.

It is important for modern matrons to work with the ward managers to support them to maintain some of the control and tasks they previously had but also to help relieve some of the pressure from them. It will undoubtedly be difficult for ward managers to let go of the clinical leadership and to focus solely on the day-to-day management; therefore, it is essential to make sure that ward managers retain some clinical responsibilities. The more clarity there is in the understanding of each other's roles, the better they will be able to work together as a leadership team providing consistency and a clear vision for the ward staff. The senior clinical leadership team is crucial, as it shows the ward manager, the modern matron, and the consultant psychiatrist providing positive role models for the ethos that working together improves clinical standards and are seen by the staff as a joint force for advice and support on difficult clinical issues.

The RCN (20) summarizes the modern matron role as one that can strengthen nursing leadership particularly in relation to responding quickly to problems raised by patients and their families, improving the ward environment, developing and improving nursing practice as well as staff morale, and ensuring quality of care. They indicate that the role is complex and its success will depend on the authority given to it, the resources available, and the relationship they built with ward staff and other clinicians and managers.

Nurse consultants

NCS are advanced nurses who have a higher level of comprehensive skills, experience, and knowledge in nursing care and practice (21). Each NC specializes in an area of expertise. Advanced roles have evolved over time to broaden the scope of nursing practice (22–24) in the domains outlined in the following summary:

- The practice of nursing for a specific client group.
- Developing a learning culture.
- Practice-based research approaches and evaluation.
- Providing consultancy from clinical to organizational levels.
- Transformational leadership.
- Facilitating individual, team, and organizational learning.
- Cultural change.
- Practice and service development.

Furthermore, the Department of Health (6) helpfully structures the role around main functions:

- Expert practice.
- Professional leadership and consultancy.
- Practice and service development, research, and evaluation.

Being an expert in an area of practice means delivering high-quality care to patients and carers. It also means enabling other practitioners to maintain professional expertise, and exercising a high degree of personal autonomy within their role. A NC is expected to spend at least half the time available in direct contact with patients and families. A NC also has a direct role in education, training, and contributing to the development of others. They establish formal links with local education providers such as universities and contribute to the development of qualified staff in their specialist fields, extending to the education of other professionals, particularly if their expertise is core to the day-to-day business, such as risk assessment and management on inpatient wards. NCs are also professional leaders and have a direct consultancy role within their area of expertise. Their leadership skills support and motivate others to continuously improve quality of care and standards of practice. The NC can support teams in service development, research, and evaluation as well as contribute to the development of professional practice, through the promotion of evidence-based practice, the audit of standards of care, and evaluation of practice within their specialist fields (6).

Evaluations of the NC role during the first decade of their introduction noted a wide variety of job descriptions and qualifications being required (24) and in more recent years, the NHS funding cuts have fallen disproportionately on nurses in specialist and consultant roles with evidence of recruitment freezes and 'down banding' of posts, as employers attempt to make savings (25). Many trusts and organizations decided not to employ NCs and so very few trusts have active NC roles that fall within the remit set by the government. As a result, some NCs in the UK have had to change and adapt their role and their professional identity. However, in determining what was regarded as central to their role, NCs were faced with a dilemma. On the one hand, their promotion to a consultant post had inevitably taken them away from day-to-day clinical nursing work, yet on the other hand, this clinical nursing work, and their expertise in it, was the very basis of their professional identity.

Nurse consultant role

The NC role in the UK healthcare system is firmly established in clinical practice while the literature on the consultancy role of the nurse developed from the US (26–31), where the role is one of providing expert and professional advice. The consulting role as an explicit area of expert nursing practice was identified by Fenton (32), in addition to seven domains of nursing practice identified by Benner (33) which include the helping role, coaching function, diagnostic and patient-monitoring function, effective management of rapidly changing situations, administering and monitoring therapeutic interventions, monitoring and ensuring the quality of practices, and organizational and work-role competencies

The NC role emerged out of the many examples from nurses studying for masters and PhDs. These nurses seemed to be consistently providing expertise and guidance, both formally and informally, to other health care providers (33). The role was then created to provide a career pathway for experienced nurses who wished to maintain a clinical role, rather than moving into administration or education which historically were the pathways available for further progression (34).

Inpatient mental health nurse consultant role

The NC's knowledge, skills, expertise, personal qualities, and attributes as well as being patient centred, available, visible, and flexible are vital to the role. An inpatient NC needs to be enthusiastic and provide a role model for the nursing profession. Being self-aware and having emotional intelligence is essential and using the role as a catalyst for excellent practice and service improvement is central to success. An inpatient NC must have a vision of how nursing should be and work strategically and politically within the organization to make this vision a reality. An inpatient NC is also heavily involved in processes on the wards and needs to demonstrate transformational leadership to develop and share the vision for improvement and inspire nurses in their roles.

The clinical leadership role of the NC is an under-researched area and so lacks the literature to provide tangible evidence of the impact this aspect of the role has made, particularly in relation to how NCs spend their clinical time and work with colleagues. Organizations will therefore need to provide support and commitment if they are to maximize the benefits of the NC role. Strategic positioning of where the NCs sit within the organization is also vital (22, 23) and Woodward et al. (35) suggest that this is achieved by reporting directly to the director of nursing rather than being part of the management tier within the organization; this then ensures the clinical focus is in line with the organizational structure. McIntosh and Tolson (36) recognized the challenges that a lack of authority creates for NCs as a result of having this clinical focus and no or limited operational responsibility. They identified the need for the NC to have influencing skills in order to manage upwards and the courage to defend such a position. Organizations where the NC role has been successful have promoted and endorsed the role as the pinnacle of the clinical career ladder in nursing and one that bridges practice, education, and research.

Nursing leadership

The development of these three roles in nursing (ward manager, modern matron, and NC) provides an opportunity for strengthening nursing leadership and creating a culture where quality and improvement is the focus as well as providing strong role models and the potential for nurses to develop further in their career pathway. However, leadership is not just a role and requires individuals to be able to manage themselves as well as others. Goleman (37) found that while the qualities traditionally associated with leadership such as intellect, strength, determination, and vision are required for success, they are insufficient. Effective leaders are also well known as having a great amount of emotional intelligence. Goleman (37) adds that this would include skills in self-awareness, self-regulation, motivation, empathy, and social skills. Leaders and managers who perform at a higher standard often have greater self-awareness than those who do not perform so well (38). Those leaders with emotional intelligence are more able to effectively manage not only their own emotions but the emotions of those that they lead (39). It is often the case that leaders who are more in tune with their own emotions can also have an impact on not only increasing the positive emotion in others but also alleviating negative feelings too. This is so often needed in stressful environments such as inpatients wards. It is also a skill that can be used by nurse leaders to coach and support staff to develop when managing patients on the ward. Nursing leaders that are self-aware often have the desire and need to learn which in turn promotes excellence.

Supporting staff to have opportunities for reflection is also an important part of the nursing leadership role, ensuring that staff recognize the commitment to reflection and so improving individual and team practice. Reflection is considered a process of reviewing an experience of practice to describe, analyse, and evaluate it and so to inform learning about practice (40). Reflection is paramount to both personal and team development. Nursing leaders should actively encourage the use of reflection in the inpatient setting as it encourages teams to learn and provides them with additional support. The Practice Education Group (41) explains that critical analysis varies between each professional and finding a preferred style is a personal choice. There are many tools available for teams to use, including the reflective cycle designed by Gibbs (42). This is often seen as a useful tool in nursing and in leadership. This reflective tool goes beyond explaining what has happened and looks closely at making sense of the situation which can be of great benefit to the ward environment. It looks at the positive and negative aspects of the situation, and can therefore aid improvements in future practice.

The Kings Fund (43) suggests that compassionate leadership creates cultures where people can deliver sustainable improvements quickly. NHS Improvement has identified compassionate leadership as one of the five conditions it is seeking to create in its new national framework ('Developing People – Improving Care') (44). While empathy is described as understanding how someone feels, and trying to imagine how that might feel, compassion is described as feeling what that person is feeling, holding it, accepting it, and taking some action. Compassionate leaders look after themselves and model this self-care to others. They realize it is acceptable to make mistakes and to learn from them and they give themselves and others around them permission to do the same without blame. Working on busy inpatient wards with constant competing priorities can be difficult and compassion can therefore sometimes be forgotten. Compassionate leaders have the courage to work against the norms and challenge the wider systems that can restrict teams. Teams need to know that their nurse leaders are with them and are supporting them in times of difficulty. Compassionate leaders portray this. Among the many traits and skills that good leaders possess, such as trust, communication skills, respect, knowledge, and experience, trust is one that staff must have in their leader and leaders must have in their teams. It is well known that trust takes a long time to build yet can take a very short time to lose. As a leader, it is important to be proactive in developing an environment where trust is apparent to all.

Conclusion

Effective leadership is central to the delivery of quality care. It is particularly important in the current financial climate where there are increasing demands on ward teams with the constant need for beds and fast turnover of patients. Nursing leadership is key to the safe delivery of care and to the quality of care delivered. Having nurses at the heart of this leadership will only strengthen the ward teams. It is hard to define what nursing leadership is, especially when roles are becoming increasingly complex. Lord Darzi explained the importance of effective leadership, emphasizing the need for greater involvement of clinicians in leadership (13). Compassionate leadership can develop a positive culture for change, improvement, and development which in turn will increase morale in teams and will have a more positive impact on staff retention and recruitment. Good leadership leads to patient satisfaction and is a requirement for care to be effective. The roles of ward manager, modern matron, and NC play an important part in developing this culture within the inpatient setting, transforming the care provided as well as the image of inpatient nursing.

REFERENCES

1. Ministry of Health Scottish Home and Health Department (Salmon report). *Report of the Committee on Senior Nursing Staff*. B. Salmon (Chairman). London: HMSO; 1966.
2. Paulley J. Is it too late to scrap Salmon—a charter for incompetents? *Nurs Times* 1971;67:212–213.
3. Calne R. The ward sister. *Br Med J* 1971;3:45.
4. Department of Health. *The NHS Plan: A Plan for Investment, A Plan for Reform*. London: HMSO; 2000.
5. Johnson A. United Kingdom Parliament. Hansard column 566. Response: 15 October. 2007. https://publications.parliament.uk/pa/cm200607/cmhansrd/cm071015/debtext/71015-0005.htm
6. Department of Health. *Nurse, Midwife and Health Visitor Consultants: Establishing Posts and Making Appointments*. Health Service Circular 1999/217. London: Department of Health; 1999.
7. Department of Health. *Making a Difference: Strengthening the Nursing, Midwifery and Health Visiting Contribution to Health and Healthcare*. London: Department of Health; 1999.
8. Chief Nursing Officer Report. *From Values to Action: The Chief Nursing Officer's Review of Mental Health Nursing*. London: Department of Health, 2006.
9. Department of Health. *Implementing the NHS Plan—Ten Key Roles for Nurses*. London: Department of Health; 2002.
10. Department of Health. *Bristol Royal Infirmary Inquiry. The Report of the Public Inquiry into Children's Heart Surgery at the Bristol Royal Infirmary 1984–1995: Learning from Bristol*. London: Department of Health; 2001.
11. Royal College of Nursing. *Breaking Down Barriers, Drive Up Standards: The Role of the Ward Sister and Charge Nurse*. London: Royal College of Nursing; 2009. Tinyurl.com/barriers-standards
12. Darzi A. *High Quality Care for All: NHS Next Stage Review Final Report*. London: Department of Health; 2008.
13. Hay Group. *Nurse Leadership: Being Nice is Not Enough*. London: Hay Group; 2006.
14. Bonner G, Mclaughlin S. Leadership support for ward managers in acute mental health inpatient settings. *Nurs Manag* 2014;21:2.
15. Brown G, Esdaile S, Ryan S. *Becoming an Advanced Practitioner*. Edinburgh: Butterworth-Heinemann; 2003.
16. Pedler M, Burgoyne J, Boydell T. *A Manager's Guide to Self-Development*, 5th edition. Maidenhead: McGraw Hill Professional; 2007.
17. Francis R. *Report of the Mid Staffordshire NHS Foundation Trust Public Inquiry*. London: Stationery Office; 2013. Tinyurl.com/HMSO-Francis2

18. Department of Health. *Modern Matrons—Improving the Patient Experience*. London: Department of Health; 2003.

19. Quinn RE, Faerman SR, Thomson MP, McGrath MR. *Becoming a Master Manager: A Competency Framework*. Hoboken, NJ: John Wiley & Sons; 2003.

20. Royal College of Nursing Institute, The University of Sheffield School of Nursing and Midwifery. *Evaluation of the Modern Matron Role in a Sample of NHS Trusts*. Sheffield: The University of Sheffield; 2004.

21. Barton TD, Bevan L, Moone G. Advanced nursing. Part 1: The development of advanced nursing roles. *Nurs Times* 2012;108:18–20.

22. Manley K. A conceptual framework for advanced practice: an action research project operationalizing an advanced practitioner/nurse consultant role. *J Clin Nurs* 1997;6:179–190.

23. Manley K. *Nurse Consultant: Concept, Processes, Outcome*. Unpublished PhD thesis, London: Manchester University/Royal College of Nursing Institute; 2001.

24. Manley K. Refining the nurse consultant framework: commentary on critique of nurse consultant framework. *Nurs Crit Care* 2002;7:84–87.

25. Buchan J, Calman L. Skill-Mix and Policy Change in the Health Workforce: Nurses in Advanced Roles. OECD Health Working Papers No. 17. https://www.oecd.org/els/health-systems/33857785.pdf

26. Oda D. Specialized role development: a three-phase process. *Nurs Outlook* 1977;25:374–377.

27. Blake P. The clinical nurse specialist as a consultant. *J Nurs Adm* 1977;7:33–36.

28. Stevens BJ. The use of consultants in nursing service. *J Nurs Adm* 1978;8:7–15.

29. Kohnke MF. *The Case for Consultation in Nursing: Designs for Professional Practice*. New York: John Wiley; 1978.

30. Lareau SC. The nurse as clinical consultant. *Top Clin Nurs* 1980;2:79–84.

31. Norton D. The nursing process in action—1. The quiet revolution: introduction of the nursing process in a region. *Nurs Times* 1981;77:1067–1069.

32. Fenton MV. Identification of the skilled performance of masters prepared nurses as a method of curriculum planning and evaluation. In: Benner P (ed), *From Novice to Expert: Excellence and Power in Clinical Nursing Practice*, pp. 262–274. Menlo Park, CA: Addison-Wesley; 1984.

33. Benner P. *From Novice to Expert: Excellence and Power in Clinical Nursing Practice*. Menlo Park, CA: Addison-Wesley; 1984.

34. Abbott S. Leadership across boundaries: a qualitative study of the nurse consultant role in English primary care. *J Nurs Manag* 2007;15:703–710.

35. Woodward VA, Webb C, Prowse M. Nurse consultants: organizational influences on role achievement. *J Clin Nurs* 2006;15:272–280.

36. McIntosh J, Tolsen D. Leadership as part of the nurse consultant's role: banging the drum for patient care. *J Clin Nurs* 2008;18:219–227.

37. Goleman D. What makes a leader? *Harv Bus Rev* 2004;82:82–91.

38. Bruno L, Lay E. Personal values and leadership effectiveness. *J Bus Res* 2008;61:678–683.

39. Peterson S, Luthans F. The positive impact and development of hopeful leaders. *Leader Organ Dev J* 2003;24:26–31.

40. Reid B. But we're doing it already! Exploring a response to the concept of reflective practise in order to improve its facilitation. *Nurse Educ Today* 1993;13:305–309.

41. The Practise Education Group. *Mentoring: A Resource for those who Facilitate Placement Learning*. Oxford: Oxford Brookes University; 2006.

42. Gibbs G. *Learning by Doing: A Guide to Teaching and Learning Methods*. Oxford: Further Education Unit, Oxford Brookes University; 1988.

43. Nursing and Midwifery Council. Preceptorship Guidelines. 2006. tinyurl.com/NMC-preceptorship

44. National Improvement and Leadership Development Board. Developing People – Improving Care. A national framework for action on improvement and leadership development in NHS-funded services. 2016. https://improvement.nhs.uk/documents/542/Developing_People-Improving_Care-010216.pdf

8

Occupational therapy: values, evidence, and interventions

Jonathan Gibbons and Lara Freeman

Introduction

Occupational therapists are unique in their approach to promoting the physical and mental well-being of their clients, in that they are primarily guided by a fundamental belief in the positive relationship between meaningful activity and good health: 'The philosophy of occupational therapy is founded on the concept that occupation is essential to human existence' (1). An occupational therapist is concerned more with the consequences of an illness in terms of its effect on an individual's ability to function than with the illness in itself, and the primary aims of intervention are to help the individual to function at their optimal level in the occupations that they themselves choose to engage in. The role of the occupational therapist in an inpatient psychiatric multi-disciplinary team (MDT) is to explore with the individual what is most meaningful and important to them in their lives, and to support them in identifying and achieving their goals in these areas. By doing so, we can not only play a vital role in improving a patient's experience of their admission, but also in helping that individual to restore foundations on which they can build and sustain a life which has quality and meaning outside of the hospital environment (2).

Despite being valued members of inpatient psychiatric MDTs, there is limited empirical evidence about the impact of occupational therapy on recovery in acute mental health settings. Wimpenny et al. (3) describe the challenge in reporting therapeutic effectiveness as being 'not only to find ways to demonstrate clear links between the intervention used and its effect on functioning but also how to capture the impact of these interventions on improving an individual's quality of life and ability to overcome obstacles to participation' (p. 277).

In this chapter, we outline instead the philosophy and values of occupational therapy and discuss how this complements the medical model to support individuals' recovery from an acute mental health crisis and their development of the skills required to maintain health and well-being on discharge.

Philosophy and aims of occupational therapy within the inpatient setting

The occupational therapy profession was founded on the belief in the therapeutic value of meaningful occupation and the importance of satisfying interpersonal relationships, alongside a routine which supports a balance of self-care, work/education, and leisure activities (4) in order for individuals to maintain their mental and physical well-being.

The occupational therapy process is a holistic one, and aims to help people to lead lives that are as fulfilling as possible by focusing on their occupation in self-care, work/education, and leisure, and how this can be supported or inhibited by their physical and psychological health, and the social, economic, environmental, and spiritual context of a person's life. Fundamental to this process is an emphasis on improving the competence of the individual rather than focusing on the disability or dysfunction which may influence their performance (2). Occupational therapists routinely work in a person-centred manner, firmly holding that an individual's unique values and beliefs should be at the centre of all intervention planning and treatment.

Models of practice

Models of practice provide a philosophical basis for a service, define key concepts, and guide clinicians in selecting interventions. There are multiple occupational therapy models of practice in use around the world, however the model of practice that is often chosen to use in acute adult psychiatric services is the model of human occupation (MOHO). This is the model selected to guide practice in the inpatient occupational therapy service where the authors work and is explored here to give an insight into the ways that occupational therapists conceptualize individuals, and also into the guiding philosophy that governs our work to support them towards living meaningful lives.

Model of human occupation and the inpatient setting

There are several advantages of using MOHO in the acute psychiatric setting. Firstly it has a strong evidence base, with a large number of accompanying standardized assessments which allow therapists to design a wide range of interventions which are tailored to an individual's very specific needs. In this way, it facilitates person-centred practice, and encourages a holistic view of patients, which in turn can help to support the building of strong therapeutic relationships (5).

Kielhofner (6), who developed this model of practice, asserts that: 'humans possess a complex nervous system that gives them an intense and pervasive need to act' (p. 12), and that human occupation can be summed up by talking about three broad areas of activity. These areas are activities of daily living, productivity, and leisure, or play:

- Activities of daily living are the routine tasks that we need to regularly carry out in order to maintain our personal hygiene and nutritional needs, and these would often include washing, dressing, eating, drinking, shopping, and preparing meals.
- Productivity pertains to activities that 'provide services or commodities to society' (p. 5), so this includes any kind of work-related activity, whether they be paid or unpaid. Education also falls into this category, because studying can improve our ability to provide those services in the future. Additionally, productivity also encompasses our family and social roles.
- Leisure, or play, refers to the activities that we take part in simply for the enjoyment of doing so, and encompasses anything that we may refer to as a hobby. These might include playing sports or games, playing a musical instrument, or socializing with friends.[1]

Although these categories are relevant to all of us they are still very broad descriptions and in terms of the specific activities that we choose to do we are all unique. We are also unique in terms of the way in which we organize these activities into routines or patterns of behaviour, and also in terms of the level of skill with which we carry out these activities. In order to understand these differences, we need to look at a further three components which influence our individual occupational behaviour:

- Volition.
- Habituation.
- Performance capacity.

An advantage of using MOHO in a psychiatric setting is that it places an emphasis on the person's volition, or motivation for engagement in occupation, and explains that it is the complex interplay between a person's values, interests, and level of self-efficacy which partly determine their occupational choices. Individuals' motivation to engage in meaningful activity is often adversely affected by mental ill health and one of the occupational therapist's primary aims is to gradually engender in their patients a renewed enthusiasm for activities that they have previously found valuable and enjoyable. It is this idea of volition which dictates whether a particular activity is meaningful or not to somebody, and it is vital for the occupational

therapist to remember when planning and carrying out interventions with their patients that what might be meaningful and important to one person might not be to another. It is also crucial that the occupational therapist seeks to understand what specific activities are important to the individual, and why, in order to formulate appropriate occupation-focused intervention plans with them which are most likely to promote their recovery.

There are two main challenges which occupational therapists face in their aim to stimulate their patients' motivation to engage in meaningful occupation. The first is the often inherent aspect of poor mental health: a reduced interest in activity. In order to address this, the occupational therapist may use a process which aims to build the individual's self-efficacy to engage in activity, and also to explore with the individual future options to engage in meaningful occupation (7). The second challenge is that an admission to the ward often limits opportunities for engagement in meaningful occupation, especially for those patients who are particularly unwell and who may be unable to access resources outside of the hospital. Enabling patients to meet their occupational needs on the ward, while also managing risks and maintaining patients' safety, is a challenging yet crucial aspect of the occupational therapist's role. This is managed through the provision of a carefully risk-assessed 7-day therapeutic activity programme which aims to provide patients with the opportunity to engage in a wide range of occupations from each of the three areas of occupation outlined previously: self-care, productivity, and leisure. Because of the constantly changing patient group, this programme should be reviewed and updated regularly by the occupational therapist and activity coordinator in close collaboration with the patients on the ward at that time in order to ensure that it continues to align with the group's needs.

The concept of 'habituation' pertains to the process through which occupation is often organized into patterns or routines (6). Much of our daily occupation is guided by habits, and these habits are formed through repetition of the same tasks, often at the same times of the day, until they become automatic and no longer require concentration. Having a routine helps us to carry out the basic fundamental tasks that we need to do to manage our activities of daily living, and to fulfil our roles and responsibilities as workers, students, and family members. Frequently, the routines of individuals with severe mental illnesses break down and without the solid foundations that routine can provide, their lives can become chaotic and their ability to look after themselves and others, as well as being able to engage in more complex activities, can become very compromised. It is the role of the occupational therapist to support individuals to re-establish routines through engagement in meaningful occupation, with a view to supporting their wider recovery through this process.

Again, in the interest of patient and staff safety, the ward environment is a necessarily restrictive one, and this can pose challenges to this process. In the absence of opportunities to work and engage in other meaningful activities in their own community which might normally provide routine to patients, the occupational therapist must take the lead on promoting structure and routine on the ward to address this need during an individual's admission. With the necessary support of the whole MDT, routine can be promoted via both the 7-day therapeutic activity programme, and also the facilitation of regular daily/weekly patient planning and community meetings.

Finally, it is also important to explore an individual's 'performance capacity' in order to fully understand their occupational behaviour.

[1] Adapted from Kielhofner G. *Model of human occupation: theory and application.* 4th ed. Baltimore: Lippincott Williams & Wilkins; 2002.

Severe mental illness can have a massive impact on people's day-to-day functioning because it can affect not only their motivation to engage in previously meaningful activities, and disrupt the routines through which they organize them, but also their mental and sometimes physical capacity to do them successfully. So, for example, someone who is affected by the negative symptoms of schizophrenia is likely to be affected from a cognitive perspective and may have a reduced ability to concentrate for long periods of time, or have difficulty planning the stages necessary to carry out tasks. When the resulting reduced capacity to successfully manage tasks combines with lack of motivation and disrupted routines, it can often result in severe self-neglect and, if the person doesn't receive the necessary treatment in a timely fashion, in a gradual process of deterioration in which the skills that are necessary for them to function independently become lost.

So in summary, as guided by MOHO, the occupational therapist's role on an acute psychiatric ward is to promote their patients' engagement in occupations which are meaningful to them, to help them to establish routines which support them to be able to do them, and to promote an optimum level of independence in these activities in light of any cognitive or physical difficulties that they may have.

Ensuring the best and most effective use of occupational therapy resources in meeting the occupational needs of the inpatient population: pathways, prioritization, and outcome measures

The nature of acute inpatient services providing short-term admissions and the ratio of patients to therapists means that occupational therapists need to be able to identify how best and most effectively to use their finite resources. Service pathways and prioritization criteria are useful in ensuring that this is standardized and based on patient need and agreed local priorities rather than the individual preferences of the therapist (8). Each of these is discussed in the following subsections.

Service pathways

Service pathways provide a clear structure to the input provided by inpatient occupational therapists. These help to guide clinicians in providing a standard against which individual clinical care and service provision can be measured, and in ensuring that a standardized approach is adopted across the service. Pathways should be based on the occupational therapy process (discussed in detail in 'Stages of the inpatient occupational therapy process'); however, they will need to be tailored to reflect the inpatient population, the model of care adopted in the locality, and resources available. By resources we mean the amount of clinical input available, the skills mix of the occupational therapy team, and the availability of activity support workers and wider MDT to input into recovery-orientated care plans alongside the environmental and financial resources. They need to be regularly reviewed (annually or in response to significant change in local health economy) and refined in response to feedback from clinicians, changes in local service priorities and demands, and feedback from service users and carers to ensure a responsive provision.

Service pathways also provide a valuable means of communicating to MDT colleagues, service users, and carers how occupational therapy input is structured and delivered within the inpatient service. This ensures that clear expectations are established about how and when occupational therapists will be in contact with individual service users and how decisions relating to levels of interventions are made.

Figure 8.1 provides an example of an acute inpatient occupational therapy service pathway (created for the service within which the authors practice).

Prioritization criteria

Inpatient mental health wards provide short, focused periods of treatment for individuals during mental health crises. It is widely agreed that individuals' recovery is best supported in their own homes, social networks, and local communities and therefore admissions are kept as short as possible. This leads to a rapidly changing population on the ward. In order to respond effectively to this and the needs of the population at any given time, inpatient occupational therapists need to be able to quickly identify and prioritize individuals' needs. Although most individuals admitted to an inpatient ward have some form of occupational need, the ratio of occupational therapists to patients means that they have finite resources and therefore need to identify how best to allocate their input to meet the needs of the population at any given time. Prioritization criteria support clinicians in this decision-making, guiding their allocation of clinical input based on best practice and need, and ensuring equity of provision.

Figure 8.2 provides an example of an acute inpatient occupational therapy prioritization decision tree adapted from a template created by Heasman and Morley (8). As with the service pathway, prioritization decision trees need to reflect the local population, service provision, and priorities.

Outcome measures

The use of standardized outcome measures provides a number of benefits to inpatient occupational therapy service provision, and quality of care. Firstly, and importantly, these enable the individual clinician and service user to measure the impact of interventions adopted (discussed further in 'Stages of the inpatient occupational therapy process'). Secondly, the information gathered can be used more widely to measure effectiveness and efficiency of the local service being provided, offering a quality measure to ensure that patients' needs are being met and that resources are used effectively and efficiently (8, 9). And finally, the data collected across multiple services can contribute to meaningful evidence about the impact and value of occupational therapy within inpatient settings, which as we outlined in the introduction is currently lacking.

Stages of the inpatient occupational therapy process

Occupational therapy intervention is largely governed by a process in which the clinician and individual (with corroborative input from carers, family members, and other clinicians involved in the individual's care) identify an individual's occupational needs and then work to address these (10).

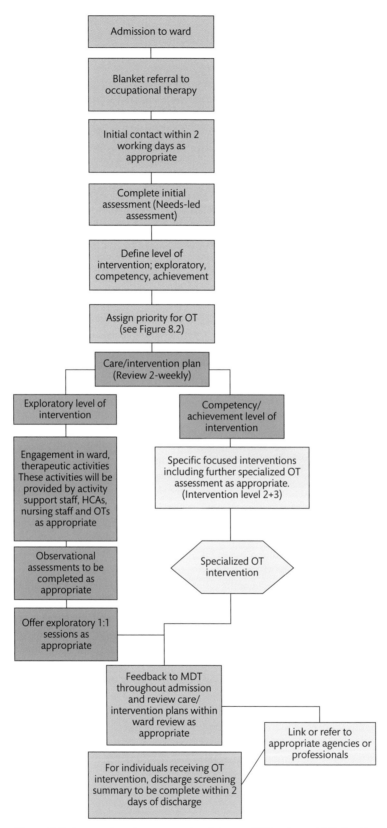

Figure 8.1 An acute inpatient occupational therapy (OT) pathway. HCA, health care assistant; MDT, multidisciplinary team.

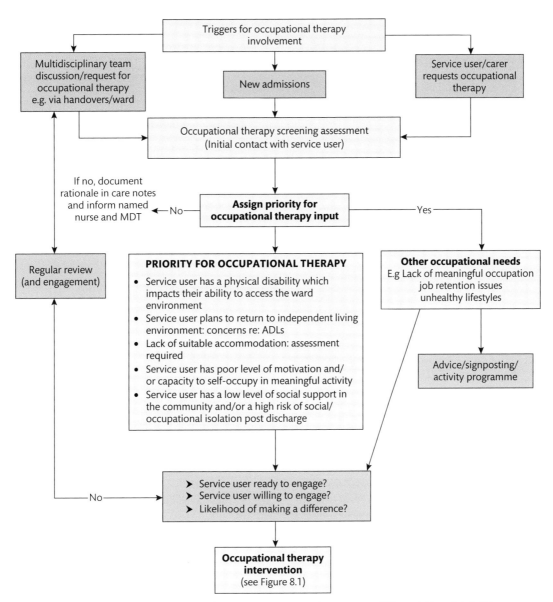

Figure 8.2 An acute inpatient occupational therapy prioritization decision tree. ADLs, activities of daily living.
Adapted from Heasman D, Morley M (2012) Introducing prioritisation protocols to promote efficient and effective allocation of mental health occupational therapy resources. *British Journal of occupational Therapy*, 75(11), 522–526.

This section provides an overview of the inpatient occupational therapy process which underpins occupational therapy practice. Two key areas of this process—interventions and discharge planning—have been selected to provide a practical exploration of how occupational therapists work with individuals and contribute to MDT care within the inpatient setting and are discussed in more detail later in this chapter.

Initial screening

This forms the initial information gathering and is based on review of clinical notes, reasons for admission, and discussions with the patient (and their carers where appropriate). This should be guided by set screening questions informed by the occupational therapy model adopted within the service.

Assigning priority

This is completed through the application of locally agreed prioritization criteria on the information gathered during the initial

screening process (as discussed earlier). Priority for intervention will be determined by individual need and the patient's readiness/willingness to engage.

Assessment

The primary role of the occupational therapist during assessment is to determine 'the relationship between health, illness and occupational functioning' (11). Occupational therapists use the selected activities to assess the individual's occupational performance (12). This will be completed through clinical observation and use of standardized assessment tools linked to the model used by the service. Occupational therapists assess occupational performance skills and participation in activities of daily living and make an assessment of psychopathology which forms a vital part of the clinical assessment of the individual's needs (12). The information gathered informs MDT treatment planning, person-centred occupational goals, and decisions relating to placement and housing.

Goal setting and intervention

The primary factor influencing goal setting and intervention should be what is meaningful to the individual involved (13). Occupational therapists use a wide range of interventions and treatment modalities which are selected based on the needs of the individuals, their goals, preferences, and occupational performance. Some of these are discussed in more detail in 'Occupational therapy interventions in the inpatient setting'. Not all interventions will be delivered by occupational therapists but might form part of a wider MDT plan. For example, if the individual's needs or goals focus on establishing participation in specific activities of interest, this might be facilitated by the activity coordinator or occupational therapy assistant. If an individual has goals relating to self-care, these may be supported by health care assistants with guidance and monitoring from the occupational therapist.

Outcome evaluation

On an individual level, outcome measures provide a means of monitoring an individual's progress and attainment of their personal goals as well as changes in their skills and occupational performance. This supports occupational therapists and individuals to reflect on their progress, building the individual's understanding of their abilities and competences. This can provide a basis for review of treatment and intervention plans, inform discharge planning and support discussion with individuals, carers, and MDT members about the level of support that will be needed in the community.

Discharge planning and links to community resources

Inpatient occupational therapists work with individuals to identify their personal goals and begin making changes to achieve these; however, the establishment and embedding of these will take place after discharge within their own homes, communities, and social networks. Cohesive links between inpatient occupational therapists and community resources are essential in ensuring that the individual's recovery continues. A key part of discharge planning is to support the individual to re-establish the roles and routines they had participated in prior to admission alongside identifying opportunities to build on these (14).

Occupational therapy interventions in the inpatient setting

As we have discussed, occupational therapy input within the inpatient setting has a key role in developing the skills and/or compensating for skill deficits required for safe discharge. This naturally leads to interventions which are focused on occupational performance in activities of daily living being prioritized. It is important, however, even in this environment which requires short, focused interventions, to retain the holistic, person-centred approach that governs occupational therapy practice and ensure that all domains of an individual's occupational life are considered. Individuals' recovery from mental health crisis is rooted in their ability to retain, sustain, and develop their ability to live meaningful lives (15) and it is therefore important that occupational therapy input does not overlook the importance of interventions that support an individual's aspirations relating to productivity and leisure.

Personal activities of daily living

It is not uncommon for individuals admitted to acute inpatient wards to have issues relating to the maintenance of their personal care. This can be related to active symptoms of their mental health condition or secondary triggers such as poor volition or low self-worth. The role of the occupational therapist is to establish the contributory factors to an individual's self-neglect. Working collaboratively with the individual and MDT, the occupational therapist will devise goals and intervention plans to address these. By focusing on the individual's values and on the occupations that are meaningful to them, occupational therapists can encourage the motivation to attend to personal activities of daily living. Often the individual does not place inherent value in the act of maintaining personal activities of daily living; however, this can be promoted by identifying activities of meaning which require them to attend to these, for example, cooking or social activities.

Domestic activities of daily living

Self-neglect can also extend to individuals' management of their domestic activities of daily living, with extended periods of self-neglect sometimes resulting in a gradual loss of the necessary skills to be able to manage these post discharge. As with other areas of occupation, their performance in this area may also be inhibited by cognitive and/or physical deficits. One of the roles of the inpatient occupational therapist, in tandem with practical input from activity coordinators, is to ensure that patients who require support with domestic tasks are given the opportunity to build their skills in this area, for example, with regular one-to-one shopping and cooking sessions to support the development of budgeting and meal planning skills, and a greater awareness of different cooking techniques and healthy nutrition. Individuals are also encouraged to engage in regular cooking groups on the ward in order to support them to maintain the domestic activities of daily living skills that they may already possess partly in order to reduce the risk of a loss of these skills as a result of what in some cases can be lengthy admissions.

Productivity

Being able to engage meaningfully in our chosen roles, contribute to our community, and be meaningfully employed provides individuals with a sense of purpose and value. It allows us to feel connected to others and see ourselves as a contributing member of society. While it is unlikely that an inpatient occupational therapist will be working with the individual to create new opportunities, it is essential that individuals are supported to maintain their skills and ability to participate in their valued roles during their admission. The identification of an individual's roles, particularly relating to employment, is a key area for discussion during initial contact between the occupational therapist and the individual. Interventions may include: ensuring that individuals have sick notes to cover periods of absence from work, and liaison with employers; assessing readiness and coordinating visits from children and families (to maintain a role as parent); and ensuring spiritual support from relevant faith communities, supporting visits to a normal place of worship where appropriate.

Leisure

Leisure activities are those that bring joy, enjoyment, and relaxation. They contribute to an individual's quality of life and, given the unique nature of the activities that people enjoy, their identity. These activities provide opportunities to create social bonds, supporting individuals to develop social networks. Due to the combination of the impact of mental health symptoms such as anhedonia and avolition, and a lack of opportunities or resources, individuals admitted to acute inpatient settings often have reduced participation in their leisure activities of choice. For some individuals, where their mental health condition has impacted significantly on their functioning, it may have been an extended period of time since they actively participated in leisure activities. In this instance, occupational therapists play a key role in supporting individuals to explore their interests and identifying opportunities to participate in these in the community. Access to a ward-based therapeutic activity programme is a key part of interventions to support individuals in identifying, reconnecting to, or sustaining their interests. Occupational therapists will work closely with the individual and the activity coordinator to identify key activities of interest and ensure they are encouraged to participate. In this way, occupational therapists may take a consultative role in overseeing an individual's participation, with the activity coordinator leading on the delivery of the session. The occupational therapist, activity coordinator, and individual will work closely together to monitor participation and identify any key occupational performance issues that may be significant.

Functional mobility

The social model of disability, in contrast to the medical model, explains that disability is caused by the way that society is organized rather than by the person's physical or cognitive impairment itself. This may be as a result of an inaccessible physical environment, or of negative attitudes and a lack of understanding from others in society (16).

In line with this person-centred model, an important role of the occupational therapist on an acute inpatient ward is to ensure that the ward environment is accessible to patients in light of their impairments. Although patients are admitted primarily for the mental health needs, it is not uncommon for individuals to also be affected by concurrent physical health and mobility problems which might affect their ability to access the ward environment, and by extension, its facilities and resources which would normally enable engagement in meaningful occupation (Box 8.1).

This would normally involve an assessment of their ability to safely and independently mobilize around the ward and access its

---

Box 8.1 Clinical vignette

Beatrix is a 42-year-old woman with a diagnosis of schizophrenia who has lived with her parents for most of her adult life. She was admitted to the ward as a result of a relapse of psychotic symptoms, including a re-emergence of derogatory voices and paranoid thoughts. Although she had had several previous psychotic episodes and hospital admissions since the age of 19, the episode which led to this admission was particularly acute. This high level of acuity caused Beatrix and her parents significant distress in the weeks prior to admission, and resulted in her parents' decision to request that alternative housing be identified for Beatrix post discharge as they found it increasingly difficult to cope with her chaotic and sometimes hostile behaviour when she is unwell.

In the early stages of Beatrix' admission, she had difficulty understanding the reasons for her admission and did not recognize that she was unwell. Despite this, in her first few days on the ward she was able to discuss her interests and hobbies with the occupational therapist, who used an 'interest checklist' to facilitate this, and she identified that she very much enjoyed gardening and listening to music—her main role at home was to grow vegetables for family meals in their garden and she greatly valued this responsibility. With encouragement from the occupational therapist and activity coordinator she began regularly attending the activity groups being run, especially gardening and music-related groups, and appeared to be significantly less distressed during these times. She later reported that these particular activities lessened the frequency and volume of the voices that she heard and, as a result, the level of distress that they caused her. Additionally, as Beatrix is a practising Christian, the occupational therapist helped to ensure that her spiritual needs were addressed throughout her admission by linking her in with the hospital chaplain for regular one-to-one meetings, and accompanying her to weekly chapel services.

Although she had a very active and valuable role at her parents' home growing and providing vegetables for the family, Beatrix had not had the opportunity to develop other domestic skills such as meal planning, budgeting, and cooking as these were the responsibilities of her parents. As a result of this, and because she was not going to return to her parents' home post discharge, Beatrix and the ward team had concerns about how she might manage her domestic tasks in the community. The occupational therapist therefore carried out a functional assessment of Beatrix's meal planning, shopping, and cooking skills, using the MOHOST (model of human occupation screening tool), and was able to identify areas of strength and need. Although Beatrix found the tasks challenging, it was clear that she had the cognitive potential to manage them with practice, and she was also very motivated to do so. Therefore, alongside encouragement to join group cooking sessions on the ward, a programme of regular weekly one-to-one meal planning and cooking sessions was also formulated in collaboration with Beatrix, and over the course of her remaining 6 weeks on the ward her confidence and performance improved greatly, as evidenced by a follow-up MOHOST assessment.

As her treatment progressed, Beatrix began to recognize that she had been unwell, and she became more motivated to understand her illness and learn about ways of managing her mental health. With some encouragement from the occupational therapist, she began attending their twice-weekly psychoeducation and discussion 'recovery' groups whose main aim was to empower patients to manage their mental health more independently. The sessions which Beatrix reported finding particularly valuable were those which focused on coping with voices, and managing anxiety. She reported that as a result of her participation in these sessions, and the use of the practical strategies that were shared by other patients and the occupational therapist during them, her sleep greatly improved, and this in turn helped to enhance her mood and her ongoing ability to successfully manage her symptoms.

Beatrix was anxious about her discharge, especially because she had never lived without the daily support of her parents before. It was agreed by Beatrix, the MDT, and her community care coordinator that because of her ongoing mental health needs and lack of experience of living independently, the most suitable discharge destination would be to a supported accommodation placement. In order to make this transition more manageable for her, the occupational therapist liaised with staff at the placement in order to advise them of Beatrix's level of function, and recommend the level of input that she would require in order to allow her to continue developing her domestic skills. Prior to her discharge, the occupational therapist also referred Beatrix to a community mental health service which offered a range of daily activities, including gardening, to meet her ongoing occupational and social needs. Beatrix began attending these groups twice per week in the final weeks of her admission, serving as a very valuable bridge between the ward and the community, and this continuity helped her to manage her anxiety about the transition more successfully.

facilities (e.g. toilet, shower, kitchen, therapeutic activity room, and medical treatment room). This would also include an assessment of their transfers to ensure that ward furniture and toilets enable safe usage in light of any impairment. Following this assessment, if any physical barriers have been identified (e.g. the toilet is too low to allow for safe transfers), the occupational therapist would then consider provision of daily living equipment to remove this barrier.

Due to the risks inherent on a ward such as this, any temporary or permanent alteration to the physical environment must be thoroughly risk assessed and a risk management plan be formulated. For example, if a patient who has poor standing endurance requires a shower seat to allow for independent self-care, the risks of providing this equipment must be considered and managed prior to its provision, both for the individual's safety but also for the safety of other patients and staff.

Following a mobility assessment and potential daily living equipment provision, if any concerns remain regarding an individual's safety when mobilizing, a falls risk assessment should be completed which may subsequently indicate referral to the physiotherapy team for their input. This may involve the provision of walking aids (which would also need a risk management plan) and/or musculo-skeletal exercises/stretches to improve functional mobility or reduce associated discomfort, or both.

Where equipment has been provided and/or an individual's physical functioning has changed during admission, inpatient occupational therapists have a role in ensuring that they are able to safely navigate their home and community setting. In order to support safe discharge, occupational therapists may be required to complete an assessment of the individual in their own home and ensure equipment is provided where required. If the individual has required support from health care staff to manage their self-care, mobilize, or complete transfers, occupational therapists will work with families and carers to ensure they are able to safely support the individual. Where the individual's physical functioning has changed and/or they do not have support at home, occupational therapists' assessments contribute to applications for care packages to be funded and implemented in the community setting.

Managing mental health/psychosocial interventions

One of the most significant barriers to our patients' engagement in meaningful occupation relates to their ongoing experiences of their mental health. One of the key roles for occupational therapists is supporting individuals' understanding of their experiences and development of strategies to minimize the impact of these on their participation and inclusion in activities of meaning. Interventions to address this area can be delivered in group or one-to-one settings. Through the delivery of psychosocial groups, occupational therapists provide an opportunity for education, discussion, and peer support. Through participation in these sessions, individuals come to understand their experiences, are supported to share these in a safe environment, and learn strategies to use in managing these. Focused one-to-one interventions may explore the practical application of these strategies to increasing or maintaining participation in important roles and occupations. An example of a particularly relevant recovery-focused group for this patient group might be a relapse prevention planning group. In this, the occupational therapist explores the meaning of 'relapse' with group participants, and then explains that evidence shows that individuals can reduce their

risk of relapse through the identification and ongoing monitoring of their own unique triggers and early warning signs of relapse, and crucially the identification and implementation of a daily maintenance plan, again which is tailored to the experience and needs of that individual. As with all psychosocial intervention-focused groups offered on the ward, individuals are then given the opportunity to continue this work on a one-to-one basis with the occupational therapist if they wish to do so.

Discharge planning

One of the key contributions occupational therapists make to MDT care planning relates to the assessment of individuals' level of independence in their activities of daily living. This informs key decision-making relating to their ability to manage these safely within their home environment and is used to guide the identification of appropriate housing and support packages. As occupational therapists adopt a strengths-focused approach, their assessments of function support the team and individual in positive risk-taking by providing the evidence to promote individuals' opportunities to maintain their independence.

This strengths-focused approach can play a valuable role in supporting the discharge planning process. Without taking positive risks it would be difficult to accurately assess patients' suitability for discharge. Occupational therapists work with and assess individuals in different environments where risk can be graded to provide evidence for an individual's ability to manage and tolerate this. For example, within the hospital setting this might involve completion of unfamiliar tasks, demanding social situations (groups), and environments which contain risk (therapeutic kitchens). Or, outside the hospital setting this might include graded exposure to settings which provide high stimulus for the individual.

As already referenced earlier, discharge planning should not only include a focus on the physical environment required by an individual to live safely to their maximum level of independence but also on continuing the learning made by the individual about how to embed recovery and live a meaningful life. It is important to ensuring continuity of the recovery process that opportunities are identified for individuals to work towards their personal goals in relation to meaningful activity. Occupational therapists must therefore establish an understanding of the resources available in their locality and develop strong working relationships with these organizations. This enables recovery pathways to develop from the inpatient setting into the community.

Conclusion

Occupational therapists in acute inpatient settings have to be skilled in building strong therapeutic relationships, identifying a shared understanding of the individual's occupational identity, and establishing treatment goals. Occupational therapists help individuals to think about what it was that was really valuable and enjoyable for them, and how they can build on that as they start to think about their life outside the hospital. The inpatient setting provides many restrictions on an individual's patterns of occupation (17); however, this environment can also provide opportunities by providing structure and routine, safe settings to explore interests, and social situations to develop skills and confidence (3). As Lloyd and Williams (17) put it: 'in such situations occupational therapists are required to engage in a full range of services from assessment to active treatment, with a focus on assisting service users to engage in meaningful occupational roles both during and after their admission' (p. 437).

The value of occupational therapy in the inpatient setting is not solely drawn from their therapeutic interventions with individuals and their recovery but also in the role they play within the MDT. Occupational therapists' underpinning philosophy and values bring an alternative view to the traditional medical model. Their assessments and strengths-focused perspective support the team in making complex decisions relating to an individual's skills and their support needs. This enables the identification of post-discharge care that both supports individuals to maintain their independence, and also to manage safely in the community. By establishing an individual's occupational goals and supporting the development of the skills required to meet these, occupational therapists provide individuals with tools to support their ongoing personal recovery in the community.

REFERENCES

1. The College of Occupational Therapists. *Mental Health (Scotland) Bill*. MHB003. London: The College of Occupational Therapists; 2014.
2. Blair SEE, Hume CA, Creek J. Occupational perspectives on mental well-being. In: Creek J, Lougher L (eds), *Occupational Therapy and Mental Health*, 2nd edition, pp. 17–30. Philadelphia, PA: Churchill Livingstone Elsevier; 2008.
3. Wimpenny K, Savin-Baden M, Cook C. A qualitative research synthesis examining the effectiveness of interventions used by occupational therapists in mental health. *Br J Occup Ther* 2014; 77:276–288.
4. Paterson CF. A short history of occupational therapy in psychiatry. In: Creek J, Lougher L (eds) *Occupational Therapy and Mental Health*, 2nd edition, pp. 2–13. Philadelphia, PA: Churchill Livingstone Elsevier; 2008.
5. Wook Lee S, Kielhofner G, Morley M, et al. Impact of using the model of human occupation: a survey of occupational therapy mental health practitioners; perceptions. *Scand J Occup Ther* 2012;19:450–456.
6. Kielhofner G. *Model of Human Occupation: Theory and Application*, 4th edition. Baltimore, MD: Lippincott Williams & Wilkins; 2002.
7. De las Heras CG, Llerena L, Kielhofner G. *A User's Manual for Remotivation Process: Progressive Intervention for Individuals with Severe Volitional Challenges (Version 1.0)*. Chicago, IL: The Model of Human Occupation Clearinghouse, Department of Occupational Therapy, College of Applied Health Sciences, University of Illinois at Chicago; 2003.
8. Heasman D, Morley M. Introducing prioritisation protocols to promote efficient and effective allocation of mental health occupational therapy resources. *Br J Occup Ther* 2012;75:522–526.
9. Rajkumar RS, Loughran MF, Secker J. Evaluating outcomes of therapies offered by occupational therapists in adult mental health. *J Mental Health* 2012;21:6:531–538.
10. Creek J. *Occupational Therapy Defined as a Complex Intervention*. London: College of Occupational Therapists; 2003.
11. Hawkes R, Johnstone V, Yarwood R. Acute psychiatry. In: Creek J, Lougher L (eds), *Occupational Therapy and Mental Health*, 4th edition, pp. 393–408. Philadelphia, PA: Churchill Livingstone Elsevier; 2008.
12. Shorten C, Crouch R. Acute psychiatry and the dynamic short-term intervention of the occupational therapist. In: Crouch R, Alers V (eds), *Occupational Therapy in Psychiatry and Mental Health*, 5th edition, pp. 115–125. Oxford: John Wiley & Sons, Ltd; 2014.
13. Lesunyane A. Psychiatry and mental health in Africa: The vital role of occupational therapy. In: Alers V, Crouch R (eds), *Occupational Therapy: An African Perspective*, pp. 286–304. Johannesburg: Sarah Shorten Publishers; 2010.
14. Synovec CE. Implementing recovery model principles as part of occupational therapy in inpatient psychiatric settings. *Occup Ther Ment Health* 2015;31:50–61.
15. World Health Organization. *Towards a Common Language for Functioning, Disability, and Health*. Geneva: World Health Organization; 2002.
16. Harrison M, Angola R, Forsyth K, Irvine L. Defining the environment to support occupational therapy intervention in mental health practice. *Br J Occup Ther* 2016;79:57–59.
17. Lloyd C, Williams PL. Occupational therapy in the modern adult acute mental health setting: a review of current practice. *Int J Ther Rehab* 2010;17:483–493.

9

The interface with community services

Christopher Morton and Arabella Norman-Nott

Adult community mental health teams and partnership agencies

Adult mental health teams (AMHTs) provide health and social care to people aged 18 to 65 who suffer mental health problems, whose needs cannot be met at primary care level. Each AMHT provides mental health services to the population of a geographical catchment area. This population is usually defined by a cluster of general practitioner (GP) services. *The Spectrum of Care* guidance (1) made explicit their role as the cornerstone of specialist mental health service provision. Studies have shown that community teams help engagement, reduce suicides, reduce length of hospital admissions, reduce costs, and lead to increased patient satisfaction among people with severe mental illness (2). Community teams vary in their structure depending on the country and within Britain each county, reflecting different local commissioning as well as historical differences in population and needs.

AMHTs aim at providing an evidence-based, biopsychosocial approach to care, working closely with families and carers, primary care, general hospital, as well as the voluntary sector. AMHT services generally include outpatient clinics, day services, in-reach teams, and work in partnership with housing services such as supported accommodation with full or part time levels of supervision. The professional make-up of the AMHT teams are multidisciplinary with social workers, support workers, psychiatric nurses, occupational therapists, psychiatrists, voluntary sector workers, and psychologists all undertaking key roles in helping to ensure holistic care. In Oxford, as a university-linked trust, we also have research assistants embedded in teams to link patients to relevant research studies. The teams also have a dedicated pharmacy technician ensuring efficient and safe oversight of the medication management processes.

Through any journey of care there is a beginning, and in Oxford, the AMHT provides a single point of access for patients with mental health needs. The aim of the single point of access is to avoid unnecessary delays and prevent multiple barriers into care. This single point of access to the service is provided by an assessment function, which will provide a comprehensive first assessment and depending on the outcome of this assessment, either discharge the patient back to primary care, provide a short-term intervention, admit the patient to the inpatient ward, or transfer the patient to one of the longer-term treatment teams with the allocation of a care coordinator or lead professional.

Increasingly, mental health trusts have developed partnerships with the third sector to provide more seamless and comprehensive interventions with a focus on both enhancing recovery as well as preventing crises (3, 4). In Oxfordshire, such a partnership has been established between the mental health trust and five charitable organizations (5), with a principle of a shared responsibility in supporting patients and reducing barriers to accessing health and social care. This approach can both relieve the burden on the National Health Service (NHS) as well as provide innovative support for patients both during their hospital stay and upon discharge. For example, housing providers with well-established criteria for offering differing levels of support can work across inpatient services ensuring timely review of patients' needs and start the processes necessary for accessing appropriate accommodation.

The Care Programme Approach

The Care Programme Approach (CPA) was introduced in England in 1991 and revised and updated in 1999 and 2008. It is a form of case management to improve the community care of people with severe mental illness. Changes in policy have emphasized the need for incorporating crisis and contingency planning and risk assessments, detailing employment, accommodation, and financial concerns of patients, into care plans. Generally, within the team the patients with the highest needs and greatest risks are managed under the CPA.

The principles of the CPA are that:

- patients in contact with secondary services under the CPA have a care coordinator, who can be a social worker, a community psychiatric nurse, or an occupational therapist
- the patient will have a full, holistic assessment of their needs
- the care coordinator will work with the patient to write a care plan, which will set out how services will support the patient in addition to what strategies they will use to promote their self-care
- where applicable, it is recognized that carers play a pivotal role in a person's recovery and their needs should be incorporated into the care plan

- there are regular review meetings to discuss how the care plan is working and to agree changes that may be needed.

Some have criticized the CPA for being too bureaucratic and over-structured and taking clinicians away from face-to-face work with patients (6). Recent reviews of care have suggested that some trusts are using the CPA flexibly or abandoning it altogether (7). An example of a care plan can be seen in Figure 9.1.

The CPA process serves clinical and administrative functions. The clinical duties involve assessing patients' needs, their risks, their recovery status, and to consider referral for appropriate interventions or to offer interventions themselves if they have the required skills (e.g. administering a depot antipsychotic). The administrative duties include coordinating meetings and making appropriate referrals and documenting regular updates on care plans, risk assessments,

diagnosis, physical health reviews, and clustering the patient's presentation and level of need (used as a tariff band payment system) (8). CPA meetings take place at least once every 6 months, although national guidance indicates once a year (9), and should include all those involved in the patient's care, such as family members and carers or primary care and third-sector agencies. At the CPA meeting, progress is reviewed and care is planned.

Importantly, care plans are 'living documents' and should be kept up to date, reflecting the current circumstances of the patient and reflecting patient and carer wishes. Care coordinators provide continuity for patients throughout their journey through care, both in the community and on inpatient wards, keeping links with patients' networks, facilitating transitions, and making sure that the care provided is patient centred and recovery focused.

NEEDS AND GOALS	INTERVENTIONS WITH ANTICIPATED OUTCOMES	BY WHOM OR PERSONS RESPONSIBLE
1		
2		
3		
Current Medication		
Patient's thoughts and level of involvement in the care plan		Comments from others on the care plan
Triggers and early warning signs		
Crisis and contingency plan		
1.		
2.		
3.		
Is the patient a parent, carer or being cared for?		Information sharing statement
Copy of the care plan shared with the patient		
Date		

Figure 9.1 Care Programme Approach document.

In ensuring that care planning is patient centred, there are many nuances to consider ranging from cultural needs to legal status. Patients who are under the Mental Health Act 1983 (amended 2007) on leave from the ward present unique challenges for professionals when it comes to ensuring that care planning is focused on recovery and is self-determined. Inevitably, the need to maintain a legal framework around a person's care reduces a patient's autonomy and so great care is needed in describing the aspects of care planning that are enforced and those that are voluntary. The care plan should also detail how the recall or revocation functions can be used. The clinician should always aim to do this as collaboratively as possible and to be mindful of documenting advanced directives and explore opportunities for patients or carers to contribute to decisions.

Numerous factors are likely to impact the effectiveness of teams providing CPA-led community care. These factors include caseload size, availability of therapeutic interventions (10), quality of the therapeutic relationships (11), complex interrelationships between social, personal, and psychiatric factors (12), and inpatient bed availability (13). Unfortunately, recruitment and retention problems cause high levels of vacancies with an increasing use of agency staff. This can lead to patients experiencing discontinuity of care and a reduction in the standard of care they experience. Care coordinators are increasingly experiencing high caseload sizes and have insufficient time to carry out the tasks they are asked to complete. This can inevitably have an impact on mental health staff's ability to treat patients with sensitivity, patience, and empathy (14). This may well have an impact on the ability of community staff to prevent patient deterioration or consequent admission.

Interface between the adult mental health team and inpatient wards

Admission options should be discussed in care planning for patients if appropriate. This applies to those who have needed admissions as part of care planning before or for those who are likely to in the future due to their perceived risks. Particularly for patients who have never been admitted, there needs to be a clear account of what the experience and the environment will be like and an agreement about expectations of staff and patients in terms of their care. Exceptional care should be taken with patients who will find transitions challenging, for example, those on the autistic spectrum or with learning disabilities. Here, efforts should be made to visit inpatient services or to give details of how wards work to prepare in case an admission becomes necessary.

Vigilance should be paid to patients who care for others, be it children, elderly relatives, or pets. Liaison with primary care services will help identify potential risks for others in the family. Children's services, health visitors, and school nurses should be included in any CPA process for parents with children. Similarly, older adult teams should be included when patients care for elderly relatives. On occasions, teams only become aware of situations involving dependants, pets, or issues such as severe hoarding when a crisis has taken place and access to the property is allowed for the first time or it is forced during a Mental Health Act assessment. This clearly poses immediate challenges in terms of reassessing risks and making appropriate arrangements if patients are admitted.

Admissions from community teams usually happen in the context of a patient suffering a mental health crisis but can occasionally be part of a planned process. Mental health crisis care is commissioned 24 hours a day, 7 days a week with local core services offering care between 07:00 and 21:00. Crisis care during these times is delivered using the flexible assertive community treatment (FACT) model within the AMHT. This provides continuity of care and ensures that clinicians with established relationships with the patient are there to provide the intensive support needed. Outside of these hours, there are a small number of care coordinators on shift to provide additional crisis support if needed. While this may not always provide continuity for patients, it is assessed as a necessary additional level of support for some patients. Efforts are made by staff to give good handovers of care to prevent unnecessary repetition of assessments or lack of knowledge of care planning. Although aimed at improving the availability of care, the increased hours of working with a lack of resources to support it have left teams with staff more thinly spread and more vulnerable when demands increase.

Community mental health teams work closely with emergency statutory organizations such as the police, emergency departments, and street triage teams to provide timely and appropriate care for patients who are suffering from an acute mental health crisis and arrange admissions when necessary. Similarly, our local psychiatric emergency department service and psychiatric liaison team in the general hospital refer to our services when crisis care is needed. Patients in crisis can be diverse in nature and include those well known to the service with multiple problems to those who have not experienced mental ill health before. The people who have chronic disabling illness are more likely to be characterized by having a dual diagnosis, complicated physical health problems, homelessness, and forensic histories. In Oxfordshire, there is a clear homeless person care pathway with a homeless person's GP practice, which helps coordinate care and identify needs for this group. When admission is warranted for the homeless and disengaged, this can be an opportunity to tackle some of these complex issues but the challenge is often in how to safely discharge these patients and how to continue their care in the community.

It is necessary for mental health services to work closely with police, the courts, and ambulance services to coordinate some care planning actions involving mental health act assessments, recalls to hospital under the Mental Health Act, and welfare checks. It is often a challenging process to find an available and suitable inpatient bed, obtain a section 135(2) warrant when needed and then organize police, ambulance services, an approved mental health professional, and doctors to allow these assessments and processes to go ahead. In addition, the patient may not always be available or be difficult to locate when an assessment is needed. Often the process falls to the patient's care coordinator in liaison with their community consultant psychiatrist and can require repeated efforts over protracted periods of time as priorities change for all involved. Careful risk management and utilization of crisis support is done in parallel with this process and close contact is kept with the patient's social network.

Models of community care

The evolution of community mental health services has been somewhat cyclical in nature. Changes in services over the years have been driven by numerous factors including an improved evidence base, financial implications, political directives, and patient as well as carer views. In the 2000s, the UK saw a significant drive to 'functionalize' care with services broken up into teams with specific functions, for example, some teams specialized in crisis and home treatment while other provided assertive outreach care. More recently, the amalgamation of these functional teams has become the norm, primarily due to the financial pressures faced by health services. Early intervention for psychosis teams remain as independent teams running alongside the AMHT.

The flexible assertive community treatment model

In Oxford, the assertive outreach team and the crisis resolution and home treatment team were dismantled and replaced by a flexible assertive community treatment (FACT) model, adapted from the FACT model developed in the Netherlands in 2000s and updated in 2008 (15). A key component of the FACT model is enabling people to seamlessly move to a high-intensity team approach at times of increased need. The FACT teams work in a group of 11 or 12 staff members, managing a caseload of around 200 patients from a total population patch of around 40,000–50,000. Patients can access intensive support in the community using a team caseload and assertive outreach team principles, as and when they require it. In this model, care coordinators manage individual caseloads, but also work together to provide shared care for people at times of increased need, enabling seamless transition between high- and low-intensity care (16).

If a patient is at risk of relapse, neglect, or readmission to hospital, they receive intensive assertive outreach care. Supportive interventions can include frequent contacts within or out of hours by care coordinators or partner agencies, home visits, supervision of medication, day hospital attendance, medical reviews, as well as carer assessments and respite. Also, interventions such as liaising with the police or other agencies can be crucial in reducing stress and risks. Emphasis is given to managing people at home, with an increased focus on the social milieu, engagement with social networks, and identifying social triggers and perpetuating factors. FACT teams are in a good position to be the gatekeepers for hospital admission as well as retaining contact with patients during hospital admissions and facilitating timely and safe discharge from the inpatient wards.

The FACT team meet daily during the working week to discuss staff availability and allocation of tasks for those patients who are being team-worked, sharing responsibility for those patients with high needs and complex presentations, offering a consistent approach to care to avoid deterioration and need for hospital admission. FACT team boards are used to highlight patients who are in crisis in the community as well as those who are working towards discharge from hospital. Tasks related to patients in crisis in the community are prioritized over those offered to the rest of the team's caseload. A rotated team member coordinates activities for the day, chairing the meeting and delegating tasks or offering interventions themselves.

Importantly, some patients cared for under the Mental Health Act have conditions to adhere to while in the community, which if broken require recall to hospital. These conditions usually include compliance with medication, residing at a certain address, and making themselves available for assessment by the mental health team. If recall becomes necessary it often requires a warrant, police attendance, and ambulance escort to hospital, a process often described by patients and carers as challenging and stressful. Patients in this situation are offered advocacy where appropriate while their support networks, carers, and family are closely involved in planning their care and sharing information regarding the hospital admission.

Daily teleconference call

An outcome of the daily AMHT meeting is identifying those individuals who may need hospital admission, either voluntarily or under the Mental Health Act. This information is then fed into the twice-daily telephone conference held by senior clinicians from the AMHTs and the inpatient wards. Available inpatient beds are identified, community patients in need of admission are prioritized, and barriers to discharge from hospital are addressed (e.g. accommodation). Also, patients who had been placed in out-of-area hospitals are discussed and plans made for repatriation are put in place. Importantly, any patients needing hospital admission should have a clear plan of the aims of the admission and a rough estimate of its length. Community networks are involved and informed of the team's decision, with care coordinators maintaining the links with all those involved in the patient's care. Recent guidance from the National Institute for Health and Care Excellence (NICE) has emphasized the need for patients to be kept informed and educated about what to expect when admitted to an inpatient ward to ease the transition (17).

Risk management and contingency planning

A focused, succinct, and critically considered risk assessment with clear crisis and contingency plans offers invaluable guidance to a clinician assessing a service user in crisis. Without such plans, the risk of poor therapeutic outcomes and reinforcing maladaptive behaviours such as self-harm will become more likely (18); similarly, a crisis and contingency plan has been found to reduce the occurrence of compulsory admissions to hospital and reduce admission overall (19). The key to developing such plans is the collaboration between patient and clinician with an emphasis on a person-centred recovery with positive risk-taking approach (20). Patient and clinicians will identify indicators of relapse and will agree a plan of intervention if those relapse indicators occur. Such plans can contain advance statements outlining specific requests regarding treatment if the patient were to lose their capacity or were unable to make decisions. Care coordinators in collaboration with patients, carers, and other key people will consider the steps to avoid further deterioration or relapse, including actions such as the patient moving back home to live with their parents, taking time off from work, stopping driving, avoiding substances, improving sleep pattern, utilizing relaxation techniques, complying with medications, etc. The crisis plan may indicate when risks are too high for a patient to remain in the community (e.g. carers are unavailable, there are concrete suicidal plans, or disengagement from services).

Clinical vignette

- It is Monday morning and Steve (a community psychiatric nurse) uses the planning meeting to talk about the fourth police alert that has been received this month about Darren, a 38-year-old white British male with a dual diagnosis of paranoid schizophrenia and substance misuse. He has been seen in the local area shouting out at members of the public, talking to himself, and appearing dishevelled. He has a history of intermittent engagement with services and frequent admissions to hospital under the Mental Health Act. He is currently under threat of eviction due to neglect and damage to his property, unpaid utility bills, and long-term concerns about antisocial behaviour.

- It is agreed that a more assertive intervention is needed. The team discuss the need for crisis management and possible admission. The psychiatrist suggests that Steve contacts the GP and pharmacist to establish if Darren has been collecting his medication. Another colleague suggests contacting Darren's father as he usually tries to contact Darren once a week and may have more information. Darren's name is added to the team working list and it is agreed that there will be daily visits to try and review him. Each of the visits are to try and locate Darren, who is known to spend time either in his flat, a local homeless drop in, or an area off the local main street. The whole team will report back with any updates.

- It was subsequently established that Darren has not collected his medication for over a month and his father reports that his last contact with him was 2 weeks earlier, when he appeared guarded and paranoid. His father is concerned about Darren as he has been receiving frequent texts messages from him that are muddled and paranoid in content, and Darren has been sleeping on the streets, and has been asking for more money, all indicators of Darren's relapse. After 5 days, the team discuss their efforts in trying to contact Darren. One of the social workers in the team, Julie, managed to see him off the local main street with another male known to use substances. Julie explains that she managed to speak with him for 5 minutes but that he was mainly questioning why she was looking for him; he also told her that he wanted to be left alone and that he did not want to see the team. He also stated that he could not stay in his flat at night as people were coming in and moving things around and trying to poison him.

- After reviewing his risk assessment and crisis contingency plan, the team concluded that admission to hospital was needed as he appeared unwell, he had disengaged from services, and his risk of vulnerability and self-neglect were high. A referral was made to the Approved Mental Health Professionals (AMHP) service for an assessment under the Mental Health Act 1983. It was agreed with the AMHP service that a Section 135(1) warrant would be needed to gain access to his flat, and that the assessment should be attempted in the morning as Darren was reported to return home for a few hours most days. Steve and the AMHP agreed that Steve would contact the police to advise them about the concerns about Darren's mental health and safety; it was suggested that if they had any contact with him they should consider using their detaining powers under Section 136 of the Mental Health Act 1983.

- After 4 days, an inpatient bed was found for Darren. Unfortunately, the AMHP, the psychiatrist, and an independent Section 12 approved doctor did not find Darren at his flat. Two days later, Darren was detained by the police on Section 136 after he had become verbally threatening to a member of the public. After an assessment at the 'place of safety', Darren was admitted to hospital under Section 2 of the Mental Health Act.

Inpatient admissions

Most mental health patients are cared for in the community with only around 6% a year, spending time as inpatients (21). For the small number of patients who do require admission, it can be needed for many reasons, for example, suicidal or homicidal ideation or behaviour, serious self-neglect or risk of physical harm, severe mental illness, acute drug intoxication, adjustment of medication where supervision is needed, or due to serious physical health comorbidity (22, 23). Bowers (24) and others have detailed historically how some admissions in the past have been offered in a planned way for patients to give respite for carers and respite for the patient themselves. As care in the community has been increasingly promoted, perhaps the view that inpatient admission is a failure of care or should be a last resort has become the prevailing view. This, along with the reduction in total number of beds available, has led to less pre-planned or respite admissions and more admissions for patients in crisis who are too high risk to manage safely in the community.

Often, the decision-making about whether to admit a patient lies with the community team's judgement, on whether community care can be safely sustained or not. Thresholds for admission are changeable and affected by local and national factors. Local factors include availability of beds, adequate community service provision, and professional judgement of risks. Increasingly, inpatient beds are being used for patients detained under the Mental Health Act (25). Informal or voluntary patients usually have capacity to make decisions about their care and having deteriorated, cannot keep themselves safe in the community.

When patients require admission and beds cannot be locally found and alternatives to admission are not available, then patients are considered for 'out-of-area treatment', which is unsatisfactory for all involved as continuity of care is often lost, geographical separation from family and carers occurs, and care planning quality reduces, leading to longer admissions as well as having cost implications for trusts. Recent recommendations from the Commission on Acute Adult Psychiatric Care (14) have set targets to first reduce and then stop all non-specialist out-of-area treatments in 2017. The commission reviewed practice in England and found that although some trusts had many out-of-area treatments, others had had none, which could be related to variations in the strength of community services (e.g. homelessness pathways, social housing, crisis accommodation, day centres, and community team crisis management).

Community team involvement for patients in hospital

If a patient did not have a care coordinator prior to admission, they will be allocated one by the community team within 24 hours of admission. Care coordinators will usually make planned visits to the ward and try and attend ward rounds where their patients' care is discussed. They will then share this information with the community team who will update the FACT boards with their progress and care needs. Discharge planning is a process that starts at admission and involves goal setting and careful consideration for what needs to be achieved before discharge can happen.

The care coordinator is often the team member who works closest with the patient and has the most frequent contact with them. The care coordinator can usually have the most influence on maintaining continuity for patients and allowing the sharing of relevant information between care settings. They will liaise with specific staff on the wards, who will in turn help to deliver certain aspects of the patient's health and social care needs; for example, an inpatient social worker will assist in looking at accommodation or benefits issues and the ward's occupational therapist will assess the patient's daily living skills. Patients who were in employment or education will require help in keeping links with those areas of their life, which in turn will facilitate their engagement when recovered. This is particularly the case with young people, who may suffer significant and long-term setbacks if not given appropriate help and support with regard to employment or education. Another important role for the care coordinator will be communicating with the patient's family, carers, and friends.

While the average length of stay on admission is in the range of weeks, longer stays of a year or even more may occur when patients have complex social and health needs that prevent any easy solutions being found to facilitate transfer into a community setting. These patients often have challenging behaviours, multiple physical and mental health needs, difficult relationships with services, care networks that have broken down, and a perceived continuing risk of dangerousness. Some of these patients would have previously been considered as suitable for rehabilitation units, but with significant reductions in rehabilitation beds they are increasingly managed on adult wards (26). It is recognized for more complex patients, where care planning is challenging and discharge delayed or admission seen as counterproductive, that additional support may be required for clinical teams. Oxford has a specialist risk panel made up of senior managers and clinicians who convene to help review and support care planning for this group of patients.

The discharge planning process

Discharge planning should start early in the admission and continue as an active process throughout the patient's time on the ward. Unmet needs such as finding new accommodation, arranging benefits, house cleaning, or setting up care packages must be addressed early, to avoid delays in discharge. In fact, a recent systematic review supported the implementation of discharge planning, stating that it was effective in reducing readmission to hospital and improving adherence to aftercare among people with mental health disorders (27).

During the discharge planning process, the patient, ward staff, and the care coordinator should work in partnership to update the care plan, review the crisis contingency plan, review early warning signs, do a piece of work with the patient and carers regarding psychoeducation, and try and encourage the patient's support network to support their transition to the community. Sadly, the Commission on Acute Adult Psychiatric Care (14) found that 30% of delayed discharges were associated with the absence of good

quality, well-resourced community teams, and patients and carers reported inadequate support and planning for and after discharge.

At the point of discharge from inpatient settings, there needs to be a clear summary of progress on the ward and clear planning for how any improvements are going to be sustained or improved upon in the community. For a successful transition into the community, a timely, collaborative engagement with the patient and their support network is needed. Current risks need to be identified and crisis and contingency planning thought about. This planning then needs to be formalized into the care plan document with specific reference to the inpatient interventions that need to be continued and how the community network is going to affect or contribute to the care plan. Where delays in communication occur, critical lapses in support may result, leading to ineffective follow-up or errors in medication management. Documents such as discharges summaries should be provided by wards to community teams in a timely manner.

The period following discharge from hospital is associated with increased rates of completed suicide. The 'National Confidential Inquiry into Suicide and Homicide by People with Mental Illness' (28) found that between 2003 and 2013 in England, 2368 mental health patients died by suicide in the first 3 months after discharge compared to 1295 inpatient deaths in the same period, with a peak in the first 2 weeks. Community teams need to be aware of the change in circumstances affecting patients leaving the ward, such as job loss, homelessness, relationship breakdowns, and loss of income. This in addition to coping with active mental illness while living in the community can be destabilizing and increase risks. The time immediately following discharge is also the period of highest risk of readmission, with 20–40% of patients being readmitted within the first 6 months (29, 30), but is the highest in the first month (31). The lesson is clear that careful consideration must be given to the level of support patients will need after discharge. This support may include daily home visits, supported living arrangements, attending day hospital, having daily contacts with services such as drop ins or rehabilitation facilities, and using social networks for additional support.

Well-organized follow-up during the period post discharge is crucial. Thus, a follow-up within 7 days of discharge must be carried out. Indeed, NICE recommends that patients with a clear risk of suicide should be followed up within 48 hours of discharge, that there is a 2-week follow-up by a psychiatrist for patients with bipolar disorder, and that an appointment with their GP within 2 weeks of discharge should be considered for all patients. NICE also recommends that peer support is provided by patients who have previously been in hospital (17).

Accommodation issues such as homelessness, either recent or long standing, need to be considered at early stages of admission, and often need reassessment after the patients have received treatment on the ward. At discharge, some patients will return to a homelessness situation, being signposted for the homeless pathway in the community, while other patients will be appropriate for various levels of supported or social care housing. Of course, some patients may be offered housing by their social networks once contact is reestablished and risks have lessened. Section 117 aftercare planning should be available for all patients who have previously or currently been detained in hospital under Section 3 of the Mental Health Act (25). Social workers working within the NHS as part of the Section 75 partnership agreement with local authorities are pivotal in ensuring that social care needs of patients in mental health services are given appropriate support and housing (32). In fact, a lack of suitable housing has been identified as a major factor, affecting 49% of delayed discharges from hospital (14). Unfortunately, there is an identified lack of social workers in mental health services as well as general cuts in local budgets (33) which limits local expertise and connections in getting social care issues addressed in a timely way.

When planning the care of patients detained under the Mental Health Act, the ward and the community team need to consider whether an application for a community treatment order or for guardianship is required for 'revolving door' patients or where the episode of care has not improved the patient's risks sufficiently that they can be managed safely as a voluntary patient in the community. The Mental Health Act 'Code of Practice' (34) provides invaluable guidance in addressing these issues.

Discharge planning should fulfil several characteristics. It should be collaborative, person centred, and suitably paced according to NICE guidance (17). One aspect of this process is offering patients a trial of leave from the ward. Unfortunately, with the high demand for beds, overnight leave is not usually available. In these circumstances, ward teams try and facilitate increasing levels of leave during the day to try to make the transition smoother.

Conclusion

High-quality care planning is central to achieving transitions between community and inpatient services that are safe, well organized, and perceived by patients and carers as supportive. Navigation of the interface between services can be complex, involve multiple agencies, and require careful negotiation between service areas that have competing demands. Services and teams are increasingly trying to develop a culture that encourages responsiveness to patients' and carers' needs as well as focusing on recovery. Under-resourced services can find it difficult to provide the high-quality care they strive to offer.

Care coordinators working with the principles of the CPA provide the continuity and information sharing which is crucial for patients' care planning across the transition. The adapted FACT team model of care in collaboration with our partnership organizations' support can offer a more integrated and thoughtful approach to meeting patients' needs. This in turn helps keep patients stable in the community and allows any crisis or deterioration to be managed in a timely way, utilizing all necessary resources in the third sector and NHS services. Admissions, we hope, are then used in a more measured way, for care that cannot be delivered in the community.

REFERENCES

1. Department of Health. *The Spectrum of Care: A Summary of Comprehensive Local Services for People with Mental Health Problems*. London: Department of Health; 1996.
2. Simmonds S, Coid J, Joseph P, Marriott, S, Tyrer P. Community mental health team management in severe mental illness: a systematic review. *Br J Psychiatry* 2001;178:497–502.
3. Ham C, Imison C, Jennings M. *Avoiding Hospital Admissions: Lessons from Evidence and Experience*. London: King's Fund; 2010.
4. Tait L, Shah S. Partnership working: a policy with promise for mental healthcare. *Adv Psychiatr Treat* 2007;13:261–271.
5. Oxfordshire Mental Health Partnership. We Are The Oxfordshire Mental Health Partnership. 2018. http://omhp.org.uk/#about
6. Simpson A. Community psychiatric nurses and the care co-ordinator role: squeezed to provide 'limited nursing'. *J Adv Nurs* 2005;52:689–699.
7. Gilburt H. *Mental Health under Pressure: A Briefing*. London: King's Fund; 2015.
8. NHS England. Mental health clustering booklet (version 5). 2016. https://www.gov.uk/government/uploads/system/uploads/attachment_data/file/499475/Annex_B4_Mental_health_clustering_booklet.pdf
9. Department of Health. *Refocusing the Care Programme Approach. Policy and Positive Practice Guidance*. London: Department of Health; 2008.
10. Burns T, Perkins R. The future of case management. *Int Rev Psychiatry* 2000;12:212–218.
11. McCabe R, Priebe S. The therapeutic relationship in the treatment of severe mental illness: a review of methods and findings. *Int J Soc Psychiatry* 2004;50:115–128.
12. Wakefield P, Read S, Firth W, Lindesay J. Clients' perceptions of outcome following contact with a community mental health team. *J Ment Health* 1998;7:375–384.
13. Tyrer P, Evans K, Gandhi N, Lamont A, Harrison-Read P, Johnson T. A randomised controlled trial of two models of care for discharged psychiatric patients. *Br Med J* 1998;316:106–109.
14. Crisp N, Smith G, Nicholson K (eds). *Old Problems, New Solutions – Improving Acute Psychiatric Care for Adults in England*. London: The Commission on Acute Adult Psychiatric Care. 2016)
15. van Veldhuizen JR. FACT: a Dutch Version of ACT. *Community Ment Health J* 2007;43:421–433.
16. Sood L, Owen A, Onyon R, et al. Flexible assertive community treatment (FACT) model in specialist psychosis teams: an evaluation. *BrJPsych Bull* 2017;41:1–5.
17. National Institute for Health and Care Excellence. *Transition Between Inpatient Mental Health Settings and Community or Care Home Settings*. NICE guideline [NG53]. London: National Institute for Health and Care Excellence; 2016.
18. Dawes RM, Faust D, Meehl PE. Clinical versus actuarial judgment. *Science* 1989;243:1668–1674.
19. Henderson C, Flood C, Leese M, Thornicroft G, Sutherby K, Szmuckler G. Effect of joint crisis plans on use of compulsory treatment in psychiatry: single blind randomised controlled trial. *BMJ* 2004;329:136.
20. Neill M, Allen J, Woodhead N, Sanderson H, Reid S, Erwin L. A positive approach to risk requires person-centred thinking. *Tizard Learn Disabil Rev* 2009;14:17–24.
21. Community and Mental Health Team, Health and Social Care Information Centre. Mental Health Bulletin, Annual Report from MHMDS Returns (2013–14). 2014. https://digital.nhs.uk/data-and-information/publications/statistical/mental-health-bulletin/mental-health-bulletin-annual-report-from-mhmds-returns-2013-14
22. Allness D, Knoedler W. *Recommended PACT Standards for New Teams. Programs of Assertive Community Treatment, Inc. Madison, Wisconsin*. Washington, DC: Center For Mental Health Services, Substance Abuse and Mental Health Services Administration; 1998.
23. Allness D, Knoedler W. *The PACT Model: A Manual for PACT Start-Up*. Arlington, VA: NAMI Campaign to End Discrimination; 1998.

24. Bowers L. Reasons for admission and their implications for the nature of acute inpatient psychiatric nursing. *J Psychiatr Ment Health Nurs* 2005;12:231–236.

25. Department of Health. Code of Practice: Mental Health Act 1983. 2008. http://webarchive.nationalarchives.gov.uk/20130107105354/http:/www.dh.gov.uk/en/Publicationsandstatistics/Publications/PublicationsPolicyAndGuidance/DH_084597

26. Holloway F. *The Forgotten Need for Rehabilitation in Contemporary Mental Health Services: A Position Statement from the Executive Committee of the Faculty of Rehabilitation and Social Psychiatry.* London: Royal College of Psychiatrists; 2005.

27. Steffen S, Kosters M, Becker T, Puschner B. Discharge planning in mental health care: a systematic review of the recent literature. *Acta Psychiatr Scand* 2009;120:1–9.

28. The University of Manchester *The National Confidential Inquiry into Suicide and Homicide by People with Mental Illness. Making Mental Health Care Safer: Annual Report and 20-year Review.* Manchester: University of Manchester; 2016.

29. Caton CLM, Koh SP, Fleiss JL, Barrow S, Goldstein JM. Rehospitalisation in chronic schizophrenia. *J Nerv Mental Dis* 1985;173:139–148.

30. Boydell KM, Malcolmson SA, Sikerbol K. Early rehospitalization. *Can J Psychiatry* 1991;36:743–745.

31. Naji SA, Howie FL, Cameron IM, Walker SA, Andrew J, Eagles JM. Discharging psychiatric in-patients back to primary care: a pragmatic randomized controlled trial of a novel discharge protocol. *Prim Care Psychiatry* 1999;5:109–115.

32. Legislation.gov.uk. National Health Service Act. Section 75. 2006. http://www.legislation.gov.uk/ukpga/2006/41/section/75

33. Croisdale-Appleby D. Re-visioning social work education. An independent review. Department of Health. 2014. https://www.gov.uk/government/uploads/system/uploads/attachment_data/file/285788/DCA_Accessible.pdf

34. Department of Health and Social Care. New Mental Health Act code of practice. 2015. https://www.gov.uk/government/news/new-mental-health-act-code-of-practice

SECTION 3
Medical aspects

10

Initial assessment, ward rounds, the discharge process

Alvaro Barrera

Introduction

The experience of being admitted to an acute psychiatric ward can be extremely distressing (1, 2). Therefore, the ward team must deliver not only effective interventions but do so in a way that promotes dignity, autonomy, and a sense of hope for patients and carers. In this regard, the importance of a ward environment that is predictable, organized, and accountable, and that has clear leadership cannot be overemphasized. Such an environment will, at the very least, not add to the sense of threat and confusion that usually overwhelms patients and their families at the point of admission to hospital.

Wards teams must focus on patients' needs, including mental, physical, and social aspects. In this regard, the Care Programme Approach describes the framework that supports and coordinates effective mental health care for people with severe mental health problems in secondary mental health services (3). The issues to be addressed include mental health, physical health, housing, income (state benefits or else), work, transport, spiritual needs, carers' needs and views, support for carers, a clear description of the patient's relapse signature, a crisis plan including details of who to contact if the relapse signature is identified, as well as written statements of wishes and preferences.

The account provided in this chapter takes place within the wider national, regional, and local institutional framework provided by clinical governance systems. In virtue of these systems, all National Health Service (NHS) professionals and organizations are accountable for their actions and omissions and for continually improving the quality of services and safeguarding high standards of care (4). All efforts of the inpatient team aim at supporting the person admitted to the ward to recover their ability to function independently in the community and therefore, discharge planning must start from the very moment the patient is admitted to hospital. In this chapter, an overview of the medical care provided by an acute inpatient unit for adults is described, following the patient pathway from admission to discharge.

Medical aspects of the hospital admission process

There is a dynamic interaction between the assessment and the treatment process. Although described as consecutive stages (i.e. clerking in, ward rounds, discharge planning, and discharge), the clinical process during the hospital admission is constantly shaped and reviewed by all the information gathered from patients, relatives, friends, statutory and non-statutory agencies, as well as the ongoing assessment by nursing and medical staff, occupational therapists, social workers, and clinical psychologists. In this regard, multidisciplinary work is crucial in the sense that all skills and perspectives must be listened to and considered for the benefit of patients (see Chapter 6).

Pathways to hospital admission

There are three ways in which patients are admitted to a given inpatient ward, namely:

Unplanned hospital admission

Usually outside normal working hours; the patient was not known or was not in contact with services. Most cases are patients admitted under the Mental Health Act 1983, following a situation that involved the police and ambulance services, in circumstances that may have been associated with distress for patients, friends, and relatives.

Planned hospital admission

Usually within normal working hours; the admission has been coordinated by the patient's community mental health team and their general practitioner (GP), following unsuccessful attempts of care in the community through the acute day hospital as well as enhanced community input (through step-up care or crisis and home treatment services).

Patients transferred from other hospitals

Usually from where they had been originally admitted in crisis. This route to admission in England is not used very often, as mental health trusts cover geographically defined areas; this means that trusts are responsible for repatriating those patients from wherever they were admitted to. Overall, every effort is made to admit patients to wards closer to their residence.

Clerking in process

Clerking in a patient just admitted to the acute ward starts the process of assessment, management, and treatment. It is usually completed by a doctor as part of their daytime work or their on-call responsibilities and encompasses a range of actions until the first ward round or multidisciplinary meeting takes place. If thoroughly done, the clerking in will provide invaluable information for the team's biopsychosocial formulation and, as result, a care plan that is individualized and focused on the patient's specific issues.

Psychiatric history

This includes the history of the presenting complaint, personal history including screening for developmental conditions (such as autism spectrum disorder or attention deficit hyperactivity disorder) as well as abuse and neglect, schooling, work history, psychiatric and medical history (documenting any allergies or adverse reactions to medication), family history (nuclear as well as extended), use of alcohol and legal and illegal substances, including novel psychoactive substances, and forensic history.

Third-party information

Third-party or collateral information is usually obtained from a relative (e.g. spouse or parent), close friend, or colleague and it is crucial. Issues regarding patient consent and confidentiality must be carefully considered (5). In most circumstances where risks to self or to others are high, it is considered justifiable and defensible to offer the relative the opportunity to be listened to, providing usually extremely valuable information for the process of assessment and treatment. The third-party perspective and contribution will help to inform the clinical plan, including the risk assessment and management. For example, where a patient had been initially described as 'a bit anxious and worried over financial matters', a spouse may report that there are no financial concerns at all and that the patient has actually been ruminating around extreme feelings of guilt (e.g. stating that he or she has squandered the firm's money and that they must be punished or killed for it). We suggest that the third-party person is given the option of being seen alone, without the patient being present, with the clarification that the admitting doctor will not be able at this stage to share confidential information with that third-party person.

Mental Health Act documentation

A review of all Mental Health Act documentation is performed to clarify the patient's legal status and review the findings of the Mental Health Act assessment that may have preceded the admission to hospital.

Mental state examination: cognitive assessment

This is carried out using either the Addenbrooke's Cognitive Examination (ACE III) (6) or the Montreal Cognitive Assessment (MOCA) (7) and will provide a useful baseline for subsequent assessments.

Physical examination

This includes weight, body mass index, waist circumference, blood pressure, pulse, neurological examination with fundoscopy, signs of alcohol and substance misuse, evidence of self-harm, and more detailed review of some systems depending on the history taken (teeth, thyroid, evidence of intravenous substance misuse, etc.).

Cardiovascular assessment

This includes electrocardiography (ECG) with a focus on the QTc interval, a risk factor for ventricular arrhythmias. The results of the risk assessment for venous thromboembolism and cardiometabolic risk (Q-risk) must be documented.

Blood tests

Some tests are needed to rule out general conditions as well as to provide a baseline for potential side effects of psychotropic medication. The tests include a full blood count, urea and electrolytes, liver function tests, thyroid tests, fasting or random glucose, glycated haemoglobin, lipid profile, and prolactin. Depending on the patient's history (risk behaviour, intravenous drug misuse) screening for blood-borne viruses and sexually transmitted infections may be indicated. In Oxford, patients are being tested for N-methyl-D-aspartate receptor (NMDAr) and other antibodies with a view to rule out autoimmune encephalitis as the aetiology of mental ill health (see Chapter 18).

Pregnancy tests

Mandatory on any female of child-bearing age.

Urine tests

Urine analysis and urine drug screen.

Risk assessment

This involves assessing the risks to self (e.g. suicide, deliberate self-harm, self-neglect, financial or sexual exploitation, emotional or physical abuse, socially or financially reckless behaviour, reputation and social standing, work position, and further deterioration of mental or physical health) and risks to others (e.g. homicide, assault, neglect of children and other dependants, emotional, sexual, or physical abuse of others, threatening behaviour, and reckless or dangerous driving) (8).

Aetiological factors or biopsychosocial formulation

This involves identifying on each level (biological, psychological, and social) the predisposing, precipitating, and maintaining factors that led to the current episode of mental ill health (9). The formulation will initially be tentative and a work in progress to be enriched as the assessment process progresses. At any rate, the precipitating factors will be addressed in the short-term care plan while the predisposing and maintaining factors will need to be addressed in the medium- and long-term care plan.

Initial management plan

The admission process feeds into an initial management plan which should be a multidisciplinary process involving, at the very least in the emergency hospital admission, the admitting doctor and the charge nurse. Depending on the complexity and risks present, the development of the initial management plan may also require input from service managers, social workers, occupational therapists, police, and agencies involved in safeguarding of vulnerable adults and children. The initial plan should specify the following.

Review of communication from the admitting team

This is carried out to ascertain the proposed purpose of admission and management plan if there is one. This handover is of great help and it can be achieved using either a formal Purpose of Admission Form, or documentation on the clinical records of such a plan, or through verbal communication.

Legal status of the patient

Every effort should be made to maximize patients' capacity to validly consent to a voluntary hospital admission. However, 'de facto' detention is to be avoided as it deprives patients of the safeguards of the Mental Health Act. Thus, if the initial plan were to contain recommendations such as 'consider using the Mental Health Act if the patient wants to leave the ward' then the clinical team should consider requesting a formal assessment under the Mental Health Act. Another rather important issue is that of smoking which, with its associated withdrawal syndrome, can escalate leading to conflict and frustration, in particular if factors such as alcohol or benzodiazepines withdrawal are also present. NHS trusts in England are smoking free so it is necessary to inform informal patients that they will not be permitted to smoke on the ward or in the grounds of the hospital during their admission. Of course, all smokers will be offered smoking cessation advice as well as nicotine replacement therapy.

Immediate main risks to be monitored

This include risks of suicide, repeated deliberate self-harm, absconding, exploitation, self-neglect, misuse of alcohol and substances, intimidating others, exploiting others, and risk of verbal or physical aggression.

Physical health observations

Such as pulse, breathing rate, blood pressure, and temperature, including their frequency and any red flags or thresholds on which the nursing team must immediately act upon.

Supportive nursing observations

This is an area of extreme importance and will be discussed in detail in Chapter 22. For some patients, their initial care plan will require a level of support only available on a psychiatric intensive care unit, discussed in Chapter 35.

Physical health monitoring

This includes blood glucose monitoring, risk of falls, temporal or spatial disorientation, snoring, sleep apnoea, generalized or partial seizures, calf pain, chest pain, shortness of breath, hypersalivation, risk of choking, etc.

Withdrawal-related medication

This includes medication to deal with alcohol, nicotine, benzodiazepine, and opiate withdrawal. Caffeine withdrawal may also need to be addressed. The combined effect of withdrawal from caffeine, nicotine, and benzodiazepines should not be underestimated.

Physical health medication

Medication for physical comorbidities that patients may be using regularly includes statins, antihypertensive medication, analgesia, etc. This medication must be checked with the patient's GP to avoid mistakes as well as overprescribing.

As-needed or 'PRN' medication

This refers to when the decision of whether and when to administer a drug is left to the nursing team or the patient. It must include the maximum dose in 24 hours to avoid misuse. *Pro re nata* (PRN) medication usually includes oral and intramuscular lorazepam (maximum dose of 4 mg in 24 hours of oral plus intramuscular), PRN paracetamol, temazepam, or Z-drugs (mainly zopiclone), and it may also include PRN antipsychotic medication, oral or intramuscular. Depending on the patient's presentation and previous history, anticholinergic medication such as procyclidine, oral or intramuscular, may need to be prescribed as PRN. Rapid tranquilization is discussed in Chapter 35.

Psychotropic medication

This is required for the treatment of the presenting mental ill health issue.

Psychotropic-related monitoring

For example, akathisia, acute dystonia, serotonin syndrome, autonomic instability, etc. (see Chapter 12).

Induction to the ward

Induction to the ward for patients and carers involves giving oral and written information including the names of key staff involved in the patient's care, visiting times, visits by under-16 relatives, how to contact senior staff, rules regarding nursing observations and leave from the ward, non-smoking policy, items that can be brought to patients, Mental Health Act issues (including discharge by the Nearest Relative), and how to make a complaint.

At this stage, relatives and friends should be offered direct support by staff, including listening to their account of the circumstances leading to admission and how the process of admission took place. Carers should be given written information on how to access support from statutory and non-statutory groups. Efforts to engage and support carers must continue throughout the hospital admission, including considering their views about discharge planning (see Chapter 26).

The first ward round

The term and practice of holding ward rounds have been criticized for a variety of reasons, not least for an environment and structure that can make patients feel uncomfortable or intimidated. In modern mental health care, every effort must be made to create an atmosphere of respect and partnership (10). Here, we use the term ward round to refer to the process through which the views of the team members as well as those of patients and carers are listened to and discussed to provide a formulation of the main issues and to develop a care plan. Before discussing the content and goals of this first meeting, two specific points of etiquette need to be mentioned. First, it is important to time the ward round a few days in advance to give the patient, carers, and the community team advance warning so everyone can plan to attend. Second, even at the risk of being repetitive, all attendants must introduce themselves with their names and roles.

The first ward round is the first multidisciplinary team (MDT) meeting including the patient and their relatives or friends, if the latter wish to attend and the patient consents. The professionals involved include senior nurses (ward matron or ward manager), the patient's named nurse or their representative, the occupational therapist, the clinical pharmacist, and the clinical psychologist. The consultant psychiatrist, a junior doctor, and usually a medical student, if the patient consents, will be present. If the patient has requested it, an independent advocate will also be present (11, 12), who would have prepared with the patient beforehand the issues the patient wants to discuss. Independent advocates will be able to speak on behalf of patients, asking for clarifications and requesting clear answers from the ward team, making an extremely valuable contribution to the care of patients and the running of ward rounds. Last but not least, the patient's allocated care coordinator will also be in attendance and their role is crucial. Every effort is made to provide continuity of care, which is carried out within the framework of the Care Programme Approach (3) and implemented in practice by the care coordinator who will ideally attend the first ward round and continue until the discharge meeting. However, work load, staffing levels, and travelling time may sometimes understandably prevent care coordinators from being present. Similarly, the same factors can conspire against having all the above-mentioned professionals in attendance.

It is suggested that the first ward round should have the following conceptual structure:

Handover, discussion, formulation

This will include reviewing the reason for the hospital admission, the main points of the clerking in, the risk assessment and risk management, and a nursing handover regarding the patient's behaviour since their arrival on the ward. At this point, it will be clear that further information must be gathered and who and by when this will be done is one of the key outputs of the ward round. The MDT will then generate a working formulation. At this point the patient will be invited to join the meeting and, if appropriate, their relatives or friends.

Discussion with the patient and carers

This includes welcoming the patient to the ward, introducing the team members present, describing the aim and procedure of the ward round, and explaining the legal framework of the hospital admission. This is followed by a discussion about the circumstances leading to the admission, the patient's views about it, as well as clarification of any mental state issues. The goal or objective of the hospital admission is hopefully provisionally agreed as well as the time

frame to achieve it. Also, any possible barriers to discharge are identified, such as accommodation, transport, and vulnerability issues. A range of possible issues and interventions are discussed including diet, exercise, medication, talking therapy, occupational therapy input, and further medical investigations. Given their importance and sensitivity, nursing observations and leave from the ward require discussion on their own merits. Importantly, there will be an assessment of the patient's capacity to consent to the components of the suggested care plan.

Review of the proposed plan by the multidisciplinary team

At this stage, the MDT may need to adjust or change the proposed plan depending on any new information that may have come to light, either through the mental state examination or contextual factors of which the MDT may have not been aware (e.g. a spouse having decided to divorce the patient). The nature of this stage of the ward round will depend on the outcome of the discussion with the patient and carers. If there was full agreement on the formulation of issues, provisional goals, length of admission, and care plan, this stage will be rather brief. On the contrary, if there were disagreements (e.g. an acutely unwell patient bitterly disagreeing with their detention under the Mental Health Act and demanding being immediately discharged) then a careful MDT discussion will take place to put a care plan in place that provides at least some common ground (e.g. that it is in everybody's interest to keep the hospital admission as brief as possible and with the least restrictive interventions) while at the same time competently managing risks (e.g. the patient and the MDT will work on establishing a healthy lifestyle, including physical exercise and occupational therapy activities as well as the use of medication, but with the patient being unable to leave the ward for the time being as well as being on higher levels of nursing observations).

Communication of the reviewed care plan

The content at this stage of the ward round process will depend on the outcome of the previous stage, and it will take place in an environment and circumstances appropriate to maximize dignity and respect as well as keeping potential risks at a minimum. This may require carers to leave the meeting or for this stage of the ward round to take place in a low-stimulation and more secure environment.

First Care Programme Approach meeting

An important step in the process of assessment and discharge planning, the first Care Programme Approach meeting may or not coincide with the first ward round but crucially it must include the patient's care coordinator, who should have been allocated by the corresponding community mental health team shortly after admission. Relatives or friends are also invited, with the patient's consent. The agenda of the meeting is flexible but must follow the principles of the Care Programme Approach, providing an opportunity to address mental, physical, social, legal, financial, housing, spiritual, and other types of need. The main features of the care plan should be agreed, focusing on recovery and working towards the patient's return to the community. Information and support for carers is important at this stage as well as throughout the admission and they will also be offered an independent assessment of their needs (13).

Subsequent ward rounds

During subsequent ward rounds, other issues will be discussed such as accessing appropriate services on discharge, for example, counselling for alcohol or substance misuse or gambling, support to help maintaining a tenancy and paying bills, and activities of social inclusion such as voluntary work, gym attendance, as well as artistic, cultural, and religious activities. Also, referrals to acute day hospital and for increased intensity of support upon discharge (e.g. crisis and home treatment team) to help a smooth transition from hospital to the community will be considered. Finally, the patient, their relatives and friends, the ward team, and the care coordinator should have worked towards identifying the patient's specific relapse signature as well as developing and writing down a crisis plan which should be provided to the patient and, with the patient's consent, to their relatives and friends.

Importantly, all these discussions and decisions should include regular and ongoing assessments of the patient's capacity to consent to admission or treatment and a review as to whether detention under the Mental Health Act is still necessary under the principle of least restrictive practice. There should be documentation made of the patient's involvement in the key decisions and their capacity should be assessed and documented (14).

Discharge as a process

Right from the start of the hospital admission, the ward team, the care coordinator, and the wider community mental health team would have been working in preparation for the patient to be able to return to the community. This requires a great deal of work behind the scenes, liaising with agencies involved in issues such as housing, benefits, debt management, money management, police, courts, solicitors, third sector organizations promoting social inclusion and rehabilitation, and so on. The views of patients must be kept at the centre of the process, the aim of which is to empower them to be able to return to their environment in a safe and stable way. Examples of practice in this area are provided elsewhere (15).

What is the threshold to decide when a patient is ready to leave hospital? There is not a clear-cut answer to this crucial question. Deciding this is a craft that will require the partnership of seasoned clinicians, empowered patients and carers, and the right community support being available at the right time. The issue of readiness for discharge should not be unilaterally dominated by a view focused exclusively on symptoms. Patients can be and are discharged even if they remain presenting symptoms of their disorder. The key issue is that a thorough risk assessment to self and others (i.e. a risk assessment of all the relevant factors involved for this particular patient at this particular time) is carried out and leads to the conclusion that treatment can safely continue with the patient in the community. Similarly, a patient could be asymptomatic, but if the central heating in their flat is currently broken or they do not have electricity, then they will not be in a position to be discharged. It goes without saying that the more robust and consistent the available community

support is, be it in the form of the community team, other agencies, relatives, and friends or their combination thereof, the more likely will be for a patient to be ready for discharge to continue their treatment in the community.

Care Programme Approach discharge meeting

The final Care Programme Approach meeting prior to discharge should be the culmination of a well-conducted hospital admission process. Ideally, the patient's community consultant, if different from the inpatient consultant, and the patient's GP should be able to attend this meeting. However, geographical and time constraints can make this very difficult. Usually, at this meeting there should be no surprises or unexpected changes to the plan. Also, this is not a meeting where new, unsettling avenues of inquiry are opened unless it is strictly necessary. Instead, this should be a meeting where the care plan, the relapse signature, and the crisis plan are reviewed and clarified to everyone.

The role of the care coordinator during the hospital admission is to ensure that continuity of care is achieved via three elements. First, the patient and their relatives meet the care coordinator during the hospital admission and before the discharge meeting. Second, patients and carers receive the details of the team as well as the telephone number of a 24-hour, 7-day a week point of contact should urgent help be needed. Third, the care coordinator will support the safe transfer of information (e.g. medication, risks, relapse signature, and post-discharge care plan) from the inpatient ward to the community team.

Meetings with relatives and friends

We have already mentioned the importance of engaging relatives, friends, and those who provide a significant degree of care to patients. Booklets, leaflets, details of organizations providing support, and so on are all helpful. However, for parents, partners, relatives, and friends, it is very important to have face-to-face contact with the medical team and the consultant psychiatrist. The first point to be discussed usually includes an update of the treatment provided thus far; there should be the opportunity for carers to ask as many questions as they wish. The second point will be obtaining from carers what is usually valuable information about the patient, including developmental, family, and personal history, as well as their account of the circumstances leading to the hospital admission, which may include issues until then unknown to the team. Offering a realistic assessment of the situation along with hope and the explicit commitment of the ward team to try their best in supporting the patient are crucial at this stage. A third point must be addressing the emotional, psychological, medical, social, and occupational impacts of the current episode of mental ill health on the carers themselves. It is not an exaggeration to think of what professionals and services call 'community' as basically tantamount, for many patients, to their partners, parents, siblings, or one or two friends.

One issue that needs consideration is the patient's consent for the clinical team to meet with their carers. The guidance regarding confidentiality from the General Medical Council (5) and the Royal College of Psychiatrist (16) as well as the National Institute for

Health and Care Excellence guidelines on inpatient care (17) must all be closely reflected upon and considered. These are complex issues, the careful management of which may lead to the strengthening of the therapeutic partnership between patient, carers, and the clinical team. However, mishandling of the same issues may lead to disappointment, friction, and complaints. Here, openness, clarity, and interpersonal skills are of the essence.

Barriers to discharge

Unnecessarily prolonged hospital admissions have a clear demoralizing effect on patients so they should be avoided. Also, with the increasing pressure for acute mental health beds, this has become a required feature of well-run services. A range of models have been developed to make sure that the inpatient admission is available at the right time and takes place at the right place, namely close to the patient's home and without delay. One way of maximizing the efficient use of the inpatient beds is to start discharge planning from the moment of admission. This not only prevents delayed discharges of patients due to factors not related to mental health (e.g. a patient's flat needed a deep clean or a patient not having the key to access her flat) but it frames the hospital admission as a process focused on recovery right from the beginning, instilling hope and promoting autonomy. A formal and explicit way of addressing this issue is carrying out 'rapid reviews' on a weekly, twice-weekly, or daily MDT meeting where the focus is on non-clinical barriers to discharge, including accommodation, lack of money, debts, issues involving the police and courts, access to transport, issues to do with dependants (e.g. elderly or children), etc. A rapid review will also inform specific plans allocated to named team members with a duty to report back on progress at the next rapid review. Most of the barriers to discharge will require close liaison between the patient's care coordinator, the ward team, and statuary and non-statutory agencies.

Discharge-related clinical administrative work

Timely communication with the community team, the patient's community psychiatrists, and the patient's GP are tasks of clinical importance, as they ensure that the required information is communicated to all the relevant stakeholders in a way that facilitates a smooth transition to the community, so reducing risks to self and others.

Interim discharge summary

On the same day of discharge, the medical team must send to the patient's GP the interim discharge summary which must contain demographic information, date of admission and discharge, diagnosis, legal status, main findings and outstanding issues, as well as arrangements for follow-up by the care coordinator within 7 days of discharge, contact details of the care coordinator and the community mental health team, any referrals made to the acute day hospital and step-down community care, and medication on discharge. Patients will usually be discharged with a supply of medication for a certain period of time (subject to risk assessment), after which the patient's GP will continue prescribing it.

Discharge summary: part 1

Within the first week of admission, the medical team send this clinical document to the patient's GP. It should include the circumstances leading to the hospital admission, personal, medical and social history, family psychiatric and neurological history (nuclear as well as extended family), alcohol and substance use (legal and illegal), forensic history, mental state examination and risk assessment on admission, physical and neurological examination, as well as admission ECG and blood tests results.

Discharge summary: part 2

Within the first week after discharge from the ward, the ward medical team send this clinical document to the patient's GP. It should include progress on the ward, any relevant findings from assessments, blood tests, ECG, brain imaging, electroencephalography, sleep apnoea assessments, etc, as well as diagnosis, mental state examination, and risk assessment on discharge. Importantly, it should include information about the patient's relapse signature and crisis plan for future reference.

Times of increased risk

Transfer between wards and hospitals

Within the inpatient setting, transfers of patients between wards can also increase risk and distress so it is important to ensure that patients are given sufficient attention by using the following principles:

- There must be a consultant-to-consultant (or between senior nursing staff) dialogue and agreement before a transfer takes place, which is recorded in the case notes.
- The reasons for the transfer should be explained to the service user and their relative or carer(s) in terms that they understand.
- A comprehensive verbal and written handover is necessary along with an updated risk assessment to also reflect any risk associated with transfer.
- Where a transfer to a ward outside a trust is necessary, a comprehensive handover must take place verbally and in writing along with a transfer letter and other applicable documents.
- The receiving ward or unit will be responsible for checking, amending, and updating all documentation.

Discharge from hospital

Poorly coordinated, unresponsive, and difficult-to-access services not only prolong delays but also escalate the risk of suicide post discharge. Services have a responsibility to minimize these potential barriers to care by managing the transfer period robustly. The 2016 National Confidential Inquiry into Suicide and Homicide by People with Mental Illness report (18) noted that a third of patients who died by suicide in England did so within the first week of being discharged from mental health hospitals. Nearly half of those died before their first follow-up appointment. Other risk factors included a hospital stay of less than 1 week, recent adverse socioeconomic events, older age, and coexisting mental health conditions; 43% lived alone. It is important also to recognize the factors associated with a decreased risk so these can be robustly implemented into inpatient practice, including an enhanced period of aftercare, clear communication about a safety plan, and maintaining communication during the transfer period.

Conclusion

Acute mental health inpatient admission can be a bewildering experience for patients and their friends and relatives, usually associated with a sense of chaos and unpredictability. It is important that the ward team staff have a clear sense of what they must do and do it in an orderly and predictable fashion. This may go some way to alleviate the distress associated with a mental health crisis as well as making sure that all relevant biomedical and psychosocial factors are competently addressed.

REFERENCES

1. Hardcastle M, Kennard D, Grandison S, Fagin L. *Experience Mental Health Inpatient Care: Narratives from Service Users, Carers and Professionals*. The International Society for Psychological and Social Approaches to Psychosis Book Series. London: Routledge; 2007.

2. Bowers L, Simpson A, Alexander J, et al. The nature and purpose of acute psychiatric wards: the Tompkins acute ward study. *J Ment Health* 2005;14:625–635.

3. Department of Health. *Refocusing the Care Programme Approach: Policy and Positive Practice Guidance*. London: Department of Health; 2008.

4. James A, Worral A, Kendall T. *Clinical Governance in Mental Health and Learning Disability Services: A Practical Guide*. London: Gaskell; 2005.

5. General Medical Council. *Confidentiality: Good Practice in Handling Patient Information*. London: General Medical Council; 2017.

6. Hsieh S, Schubert S, Hoon C, Mioshi E, Hodges JR. Validation of the Addenbrooke's Cognitive Examination III in frontotemporal dementia and Alzheimer's disease. *Dement Geriatr Cogn Disord* 2013;36:242–250.

7. Nasreddine ZS, Phillips NA, Bédirian V, et al. The Montreal Cognitive Assessment, MoCA: a brief screening tool for mild cognitive impairment. *J Am Geriatr Soc* 2005;53:695–699.

8. Department of Health. *Best Practice in Managing Risk Principles and Evidence for Best Practice in the Assessment and Management of Risk to Self and Others in Mental Health Services*. London: Department of Health; 2000.

9. Campbell WH, Rohrbaugh RM. *The Biopsychosocial Formulation Manual: A Guide for Mental Health Professionals*. Abingdon: Routledge; 2006.

10. Cappleman R, Bamford Z, Dixon C, Thomas H. Experiences of ward rounds among in-patients on an acute mental health ward: a qualitative exploration. *BJPsych Bull* 2015;39:233–236.

11. Carver N, Morrison J. Advocacy in practice: the experiences of independent advocates on UK mental health wards. *J Psychiatr Ment Health Nurs* 200;12:75–84.

12. McKeown M, Ridley J, Newbigging K, Machin K, Poursanidou K, Cruse K. Conflict of roles: a conflict of ideas? The unsettled relations between care team staff and independent mental health advocates. *Int J Ment Health Nurs* 2014;23:398–408.

13. National Institute for Health and Care Excellence (NICE). *Psychosis and Schizophrenia in Adults: Prevention and Management*. Clinical guideline [CG178]. London: NICE; 2014.

14. Perry J, Palmer L, Thompson P, Worrall A, Chittenden J, Bonnamy M (eds). *Standards for Inpatient Mental Health Services*. London: The Royal College of Psychiatrists; 2015.

15. National Institute for Mental Health in England. *A Positive Outlook: A Good Practice Toolkit to Improve Discharge from Inpatient Mental Health Care*. London: National Institute for Mental Health in England; 2007.

16. Royal College of Psychiatrists. *Good Psychiatric Practice: Confidentiality and Information Sharing*. College Report CR160. London: Royal College of Psychiatrists; 2010.

17. National Institute for Health and Care Excellence (NICE). *Service User Experience in Adult Mental Health: Improving the Experience of Care for People Using Adult NHS Mental Health Services*. Clinical guideline [CG136]. London: NICE; 2011.

18. The National Confidential Inquiry into Suicide and Homicide by People with Mental Illness. *Making Mental Health Care Safer: Annual Report and 20-Year Review*. Manchester: University of Manchester; 2016.

11

Physical health care

Mark Toynbee and Valeria Frighi

Introduction

There is a significant disparity between the physical health of individuals with psychiatric illness and the general population. Mortality rates of people with severe mental illness (SMI) are around double those of the general population. Figures from the mid-nineteenth century indicate this is not a new issue: at that time, annual mortality rates in UK asylums were as high as 14% (1). In the early part of the twentieth century, mortality rates for psychiatric inpatients in New York were three to six times greater than the general population (2), and people with mental illness died, on average, 14–18 years earlier. At the same time in the UK, Phillips (3) documented the significant burden of medical comorbidities on individuals in psychiatric units. Regretfully, this gap in morbidity and mortality between individuals with SMI and the general population has been found repeatedly in many different settings worldwide (4, 5) and persists to the present day. The current difference in life expectancy has been variously calculated as between 13 and 30 years (6, 7). Preventable physical illness accounts for the majority of this discrepancy (8, 9).

The endurance and magnitude of the gap in morbidity and mortality reflects the complexity of the issues involved and the barriers to overcoming them. Psychiatric illnesses themselves can affect levels of activity, lifestyle, and engagement with health care services. Some of these lifestyle effects are risk factors for other illnesses, including diabetes mellitus (DM) and cardiovascular disease (CVD). The side effects of many psychotropic medications can contribute to an increased risk of physical ill health. At a societal level, health care systems themselves can hamper individuals with psychiatric illnesses accessing adequate physical health care.

Additionally, psychiatric inpatient units are often separated from other inpatient units, both physically and institutionally. This disconnection has led to inconsistencies in the quality of physical health care on psychiatric inpatient units, and psychiatric care for other inpatients. With the relative number of psychiatric inpatients beds at historically low levels, the threshold for admission has necessarily risen, and the vast majority of individuals on psychiatric inpatient units have severe illnesses. Therefore, admissions should be utilized to address all aspects of both the patient's physical and mental health. In 2015, the Royal College of Psychiatrists in the UK published a set of core standards for mental health services which included a clear focus on physical health issues, particularly in the inpatient setting (10). Along with seven other national bodies representing both physical and mental health experts, they also published a list of essential actions to help improve the physical health of adults with SMI (11). It is clear that physical health care must be the business of all health care professionals on psychiatric inpatient units.

Physical health care

Up to one in five patients admitted to adult psychiatric units have an active and serious medical condition (12), rising to three in four patients in older adult units (13). Physical health comorbidities such as CVD, chronic obstructive pulmonary disease (COPD), cancer, and DM impact negatively on psychiatric symptoms and length of admission. DM is of particular interest, in itself, as some treatments for SMI increase the risk of DM, and it is possible that DM in patients with SMI may differ to some extent from DM in the general population. Additionally, DM is an independent risk factor for other physical illnesses including CVD.

Cardiovascular disease

CVD is responsible for more deaths in individuals with SMI than any another cause. Evidence shows the risk of coronary heart disease is increased in patients with schizophrenia compared to matched controls (14). The risk of cerebrovascular disease is higher in both schizophrenia and depression: the latter is associated with an increased risk of morbidity and mortality from CVD even when adjusted for significant confounders (15) and increases the risk of further morbidity and mortality in patients with established coronary heart disease by at least two times compared to those without depression.

Respiratory disease

Diseases of the respiratory system, including infections and chronic inflammatory disorders, affect around one-quarter of patients with SMI (16), with almost one-fifth having chronic obstructive pulmonary disease; three to four times the rate in the general population (17). A review of patients diagnosed with pneumonia in 2011 found individuals with schizophrenia were also more likely to suffer acute respiratory failure, require admission to an intensive therapy unit, and need mechanical ventilation (18).

Table 11.1 Prevalence of diabetes and of prediabetes in patients with severe mental illness compared to the general population (data from England, years 2009–2013)

Severe mental illness					
Diabetes	20%				
Prediabetes	30%				
Mean age (years)	44±10				
General population					
Diabetes	1.4%	4.6%	10.0%	13.7%	20.3%	19.9%
Prediabetes	2.6%	7.8%	14.4%	18.4%	23.2%	30.4%
Age groups (years)	16–39	40–49	50–59	60–69	70–79	80+

Source data from: Gardner-Sood P, Lally J, Smith S et al; IMPaCT team. Cardiovascular risk factors and metabolic syndrome in people with established psychotic illnesses: baseline data from the IMPaCT randomized controlled trial. *Psychological Medicine.* 2015; 45: 2619–29; and Public Health England 2015. NHS Diabetes Prevention Programme (NHS DPP). Non-diabetic hyperglycaemia. https://www.gov.uk/government/uploads/system/uploads/attachment_data/file/456149/Non_diabetic_hyperglycaemia.pdf. Contains public sector information licensed under the Open Government Licence v3.0.

Infectious disease

Individuals with SMI are at high risk for many communicable diseases including HIV and viral hepatitis (19). This is partly due to increased rates of substance abuse and risk-taking behaviour. Compared to the general population, patients with SMI have an eight times higher rate of HIV, and five to eleven times higher rate of viral hepatitis (20).

Neoplastic disease

SMI is associated with factors that increase the risk of cancer such as smoking and obesity. However, rates of cancers do not appear raised in populations with SMI, but mortality in individuals with cancer is higher. A recent study of mortality in US veterans with lung cancer found individuals with schizophrenia were at increased risk of death (hazard ratio 1.3; 95% confidence interval (CI) 1.2–1.4) (21), and individuals with schizophrenia developed lung cancer at a younger age.

Diabetes mellitus

DM is another major cause of death in people with SMI and leads to mortality rates which are up to six times higher in schizophrenia and four times higher in bipolar disorder compared to the general population (8, 22, 23). Significantly, people with both DM and SMI have a markedly increased risk of death than people with only one of these conditions (22, 24, 25).

The form of diabetes most frequently observed in people with SMI has been consistently classified as type 2 DM (T2DM), although other types may exist in this population. However, even if SMI-associated DM carries a very close phenotypical resemblance to T2DM, the two entities are not identical in their epidemiology, nor the type and prevalence of their risk factors. Additionally, while the clinical course of T2DM is well established, little is known on the natural history of SMI-associated DM. Therefore, prevention and treatment strategies of DM in people with SMI may differ to some extent from those adopted for T2DM in the general population. Ordinary T2DM can obviously exist in patients with SMI but this may not necessarily represent the majority of DM cases.

The estimated overall prevalence of DM in the UK adult population is 7.5% and 90% of this is T2DM (26, 27). Compared to matched general population controls, the relative risk of DM in individuals with schizophrenia and bipolar disorder was 2.5 and 2.0 respectively in two meta-analyses (28, 29). Therefore, a conservative estimate suggests a prevalence of DM in adult patients with SMI in the UK of around 15%. This is supported by a recent study of patients with established psychotic illness, in whom the prevalence of diabetes was 20% (30) and by two large studies, in which DM was found in 17% of 1418 adult schizophrenia patients and 13% of 621 bipolar disorder patients (31, 32).

Although there are no direct comparative studies, the mean age of diabetic patients with SMI seems lower than the age of their general population counterparts. This is suggested by recent UK data (30, 33) (Table 11.1), and by a large meta-analysis in which young people (mean age 14 ± 2 years) exposed to antipsychotics for a minimum of 3 months had an odds ratio of 2.6 for developing DM compared to age- and sex-matched healthy control subjects and of 2.1 compared to psychiatric control subjects not taking antipsychotics (34).

T2DM is generally preceded by impaired glucose tolerance or 'prediabetes': an asymptomatic hyperglycaemic phase defined by a concentration of glycated haemoglobin (HbA1c) of 42–47 mmol/mol (6.0–6.4%), which is more frequent and occurs earlier in patients with SMI compared to the general population (Table 11.1).

Therefore, not only is the prevalence of DM and of prediabetes significantly higher, but the age at onset is lower in SMI patients. According to the latest and/or largest studies, it appears that the combined rates of diabetes and prediabetes in adult SMI patients could be a staggering 30–50% (30–32).

Established risk factors for T2DM in the general population include obesity, advancing age (>40 years for white populations, >25 years for most other ethnic groups), non-white ethnicity, family history, impaired glucose tolerance, unhealthy diet, sedentary lifestyle, and smoking. To these, Diabetes UK, the leading organization for the care and research of diabetes in the UK, has added schizophrenia, bipolar disorder, depression, and antipsychotic medication (35).

Risk factors for T2DM operate on a background of susceptibility conferred by multiple genetic abnormalities, only some of which are known, and which are in absolute terms of lesser importance than obesity (36), the single most powerful risk factor for this disorder. The deleterious effect of obesity is confirmed by the fact that each unit (kg/m²) increase in body mass index (BMI) leads to an 8.4% increase in the risk of T2DM (37). Risk factors for DM in the SMI population have not been sufficiently studied. A recent meta-analysis found the only moderator of DM in individuals with schizophrenia to be increasing age (28), although the authors noted limitations in the primary data that prevented the exploration of other risk factors. However, it must be assumed for practical purposes that T2DM risk factors in the general population would also increase the risk of DM in psychiatric patients. Of these risk factors, obesity, sedentary lifestyle, and smoking stand out, given their disproportionately high prevalence in patients with SMI, which is at least twice as high as in the general population (30, 38–40). Moreover, heavy alcohol consumption, which is highly prevalent in people with SMI, can cause chronic pancreatitis, particularly if associated with other toxins such as cigarette smoke, and this in turn can lead to secondary DM (41).

Nevertheless, one element that differs between patients with SMI and the general population is the use of antipsychotics. The hyperglycaemic potential of these drugs became apparent soon after the introduction of chlorpromazine in the 1950s (42) and led to the creation of the term 'phenothiazine diabetes' in 1968 (43). Yet only over the past 15 years has it been widely accepted that antipsychotics can cause diabetes, as shown by widespread clinical experience and myriad formal studies. These include a meta-analysis of studies in first-episode, untreated and treated patients with schizophrenia which showed a large increase in prevalence of the metabolic syndrome and its components including diabetes in patients on antipsychotics compared to unmedicated patients (44). Despite Sir Henry Maudsley's observation in the late nineteenth century that 'diabetes is a disease which often shows itself in families in which insanity prevails' (45), the search for a relationship between schizophrenia and DM through shared genetic factors has not so far led to reproducible results. Although all the mechanisms by which antipsychotics affect glucose metabolism are not established, one obvious factor is the rapid and marked weight increase caused by this class of drugs, albeit with important differences between specific compounds (46, 47). On the other hand, the fact that DM can at times occur in the absence of any weight gain, together with the immediate development of insulin resistance and other metabolic changes following antipsychotic exposure, underlines the contribution from additional pathophysiological mechanisms (48).

Mortality rates are higher in diabetic patients compared to the general population; however, the gap has narrowed (49). Morbidity has also improved since the publication, and subsequent public health interventions, of large trials showing the benefits of blood glucose, blood pressure, and lipid control in the prevention of diabetic complications, namely macrovascular (cardiovascular, cerebrovascular, and peripheral artery disease) and microvascular disease (nephropathy, retinopathy, neuropathy) (50–54). By contrast, one recent large study (24) in patients with DM and schizophrenia and patients with DM from the general population showed that mortality rates were almost four times higher in those with DM and schizophrenia than in patients with DM alone. It also showed that the incidence of macrovascular complications was 50% higher in the schizophrenia group although the incidence of microvascular complications was similar.

Patients admitted to a psychiatric ward may be known to be diabetic or may be diagnosed with DM during admission screening tests. In the latter case, for patients with hyperglycaemic symptoms (polyuria, polydipsia, weight loss, etc.), one abnormal test will suffice, such as a fasting plasma glucose concentration of at least 7.0 mmol/L, a random plasma glucose concentration of at least 11.1 mmol/L, or a HbA1c concentration of at least 48 mmol/mol (6.5%), although

the HbA1c result would be reliable only if symptoms have been present for a minimum of 2 months. For asymptomatic patients, two abnormal tests on different days are necessary to make a diagnosis of DM. Those in whom the second test did not confirm DM should be considered at risk and managed as patients with prediabetes. In either case, care of diabetic patients should be in collaboration with the diabetes team or the general practitioner (GP).

For patients in whom DM is suspected to be iatrogenic, and who are in a stable condition, the first step would be to consider whether a change in antipsychotic medication could be attempted without adverse effects on the mental state. If a switch is considered safe, knowledge of the metabolic impact of different antipsychotics will help to make a choice: olanzapine and clozapine confer the highest risk of weight gain and an unfavourable metabolic profile; quetiapine, risperidone, paliperidone, and chlorpromazine are intermediate risk; and other antipsychotics are lower risk (47). Case reports and case series have shown that antipsychotic treatment-related DM can be reversed by changing to aripiprazole or, in a few cases, amisulpride (55, 56). However, despite the existence of switching studies to reverse or ameliorate antipsychotic-induced weight gain or dyslipidaemia (57), to our knowledge there are no systematic studies of switching strategies specifically to reverse DM. The limitation of the data available on the degree of reversibility of DM on antipsychotic switching reinforces the need for meticulous attention both to the metabolic parameters and to the patient's mental state whenever attempting a change in medication.

For patients in whom DM, or pre-DM, is thought to be iatrogenic but in whom a change in antipsychotic is unwarranted, current management guidelines should be followed (58–60). However, many factors including alcohol consumption, the ability to recognize and treat hypoglycaemia, the capacity for glucose monitoring and self-management, the possibility of deliberate overdose, the tendency to infections including those of the genital and urinary tracts, and the degree of adherence to treatment will have to be considered in setting the glycaemic target and choosing the treatment for individual patients.

For patients in whom DM is not thought to be iatrogenic, management depends on many factors including the type of DM, and GP and/or specialist advice should be sought as appropriate.

Psychiatrists need to be conversant with acute, life-threatening diabetic emergencies that can arise on the ward, especially if they require immediate management. Diabetic ketoacidosis (DKA), although typical of type 1 DM can also occur in T2DM, is generally triggered by infection or severe intercurrent illness (61). Mortality rates are approximately 2% in the UK (62). Hyperosmolar hyperglycaemic state (HHS), which is typical of T2DM, occurs in the older patient, although presentations at a young age are increasingly observed, and carries a mortality rate as high as 15–20% (63). A large study in a hospital population showed that the incidence of DKA was over ten times higher in patients with schizophrenia treated with antipsychotics compared to patients without schizophrenia (64). A recent review of DKA case reports, found a mortality rate of 7% in patients on atypical antipsychotics (65), which is up to sevenfold higher than in DM patients from the general population (62, 66). DKA and hyperosmolar hyperglycaemic state cannot be managed on a psychiatric ward, and prompt recognition is therefore essential. A blood glucose and ketone meter should be available on all wards (63, 66). For patients in whom DM is suspected to be iatrogenic, in the setting of a life-threatening emergency such as DKA or hyperosmolar hyperglycaemic state, there is no other option than to withdraw the offending antipsychotic until the patient is out of danger. Further management depends on their medical and psychiatric status. Additionally, on all psychiatric wards a 'hypo box' should be available (and regularly checked) and all members of the inpatient team should be instructed on how to recognize and treat hypoglycaemia (67).

Table 11.2 shows the currently available treatments for T2DM in the UK. Many combined formulations also exist, which may aid compliance. Even if discussion of individual therapies is beyond our aims, psychiatrists should be conversant with their salient aspects. As treatment decisions should take into consideration physical and mental well-being as well as the wishes and behavioural characteristics of each individual patient, it may be desirable that psychiatrists become more involved in these decisions, particularly in the inpatient setting. This environment also offers the unique opportunity to review the degree of blood glucose, blood pressure, and lipid control, to screen for diabetic complications, and/or to ensure that periodical screening for such complications and appropriate management is in place (58).

For individuals with prediabetes, intensive lifestyle intervention with diet and exercise reduced the incidence of T2DM by almost 60% in two pivotal clinical trials (68, 69) and by 26% in 'real-world' settings (70). A long-term diet and exercise programme should be started on the ward aiming for an initial 5–10% weight loss over 1 year and for 150 minutes of moderate-intensity physical activity per week (60). The hospital diet should be adapted and education

Table 11.2 Treatments for type 2 diabetes mellitus currently licensed in the UK

Class	Medication or type of surgical procedure	Hypoglycaemia or metabolic surgical complications	Weight change	Notes	Cost
Biguanides	Metformin	–	–/↓	Slow up-titration or use of MR preparation reduces GI side effects. Contraindicated if GFR <30 mL/min. Inappropriate in alcohol excess (risk of hypoglycaemia and of lactic acidosis)	Very inexpensive (standard) to inexpensive (MR)
Sulfonylureas	Gliclazide, glibenclamide, glipizide, glimepiride, tolbutamide	↑↑	↑↑	Caution in renal impairment. Risk of prolonged and recurrent hypoglycaemia. High potential for self-harm	Inexpensive
Meglitinides	Repaglinide, nateglinide	↑	↑	Infrequently used partly due to frequent dosing	Inexpensive
Alpha glucosidase inhibitors	Acarbose	–	–	Infrequently used due to side effects	Expensive
Thiazolidinediones	Pioglitazone	–	↑	Fluid retention, risk of congestive heart failure. Requires liver function monitoring. Small increase in bladder cancer and in fracture risk	Expensive
Dipeptidyl peptidase-4 inhibitors (DPPP-4 inhibitors)	Saxagliptin, alogliptin, linagliptin, sitagliptin, vildagliptin	–	–	Increased risk of pancreatitis	Expensive
Sodium glucose co-transporter 2 inhibitors (SGT2 inhibitors)	Canagliflozin, dapagliflozin, empagliflozin	–	↓	Increased risk of genital and urinary tract infections. Risk of euglycaemic DKA	Expensive
Glucagon-like peptide-1 receptor agonists (GLP-1 RA)	Exenatide, liraglutide, dulaglutide, albiglutide, lixisenatide	–	↓↓	Injectable from once daily to once weekly. Generally transient GI side effects. Increased risk of pancreatitis	Very expensive
Insulin	Vast number of preparations	↑↑ / ↑↑↑	↑↑↑	High potential for self-harm	Variable
Bariatric (weight loss) surgery	Gastric bypass, sleeve gastrectomy, gastric banding	Dumping syndrome	↓↓↓	Can lead to complete and long-term remission of DM. Requires extremely careful patient selection	Very expensive

DKA, diabetic ketoacidosis; DM, diabetes mellitus; GFR, glomerular filtration rate; GI, gastrointestinal; MR, modified release.

should be provided on the food that patients buy out of hospital. Despite the lack of evidence on the effectiveness of any lifestyle intervention programmes on diabetes prevention in SMI patients specifically, the degree of weight loss that has been achieved by adaptation of these programmes to this type of patient is comparable to what has been achieved in the general population (71). Given the relationship between BMI and risk of DM, it may be assumed that weight loss will result in a decreased risk of conversion to DM. Additional metformin could be considered for selected patients, in particular those who do not respond to lifestyle intervention or those who are unable to make lifestyle changes (60).

Risk factors contributing to the disparity in physical health

Smoking

Smoking remains one of the leading preventable causes of death in both the general and SMI populations. Compared to the general population, individuals with a history of mental illness are more likely to have smoked (odds ratio (OR) 2.1; 95% CI 1.9–2.4) or currently smoke (OR 1.9; 95% CI 1.7–2.2) (72). Schizophrenia is the mental illness associated with the highest rates of smoking compared to the general population (OR 5.3; 95% CI 4.9–5.7) (73). Individuals with bipolar disorder are over three times more likely to have previously smoked or currently smoke compared to the general population (74). The higher the number of comorbid psychiatric diagnoses, the higher the risk of heavy smoking. The more severe the psychiatric illness, the more cigarettes are smoked, the deeper they are inhaled, and the greater the resultant morbidity and mortality (38).

A general downward trend in smoking prevalence in the general population has not been matched by a reduction in those with psychiatric diagnoses (38, 75). Up to half of individuals admitted to psychiatric wards are current smokers. The benefits of quitting are not only a decreased risk of premature mortality, but also often a reduction in the severity of psychiatric symptoms (76). Stopping smoking before the age of 40 reduces excess mortality by 90% (77), emphasizing the potential benefit from proactive smoking cessation treatment during inpatient admissions. Smoke-free psychiatric inpatient units reduce smoking rates, at least in the short term (78). However, nicotine withdrawal can be distressing and enforced smoking cessation on admission to a ward without adequate support is likely to negatively impact both the therapeutic relationship and patient outcomes. Nicotine replacement therapy should be considered on admission, particularly as many inpatient units are smoke free. High-intensity behavioural interventions with nicotine replacement therapy and follow-up after discharge improve cessation rates in the general hospital setting (79). The long-term success of attempts to reduce and stop smoking requires consideration of the individual's environment after discharge, with those living with non-smokers more likely to attempt to quit (80).

Obesity

Obesity is associated with an increased risk of CVD, DM, and various types of cancer. Recent UK data show that approximately half of SMI patients are obese (BMI ≥30 kg/m^2), compared to a quarter of general population subjects (30, 81). Obesity, and abdominal obesity

in particular, is a component of metabolic syndrome, a cluster of risk factors for CVD and T2DM which also includes dyslipidaemia, hyperglycaemia, and hypertension (82). The prevalence of the metabolic syndrome in individuals enrolled in the Clinical Antipsychotic Trials of Intervention Effectiveness (CATIE) trial was double that of the general population (83) and one in three patients with schizophrenia or bipolar disorder have metabolic syndrome (84).

Obesity can be addressed during an inpatient admission by tackling diet, physical activity levels, alcohol consumption, sleep patterns, and medications. Particular consideration is necessary with antipsychotics with a significant metabolic impact as previously discussed, and with lithium, valproate, mirtazapine, and paroxetine (85), because iatrogenic weight gain leads to subjective distress, which markedly reduces treatment compliance (86). Switching to drugs with limited or no effect on weight could be tried, if considered safe, but otherwise 'behavioural lifestyle programmes' with diet and exercise should be the fundamental approach to counteract or prevent obesity (87–89). Various drugs have also been tried to mitigate or reverse antipsychotic-induced weight gain (90). Switching to aripiprazole was shown to induce a mean 2 kg difference in weight loss compared to placebo. The difference between metformin, the most extensively studied drug, and placebo was greater at 3 kg, albeit still modest. Metformin should only be used in addition to a diet and exercise programme.

As for other lifestyle interventions, reducing weight and maintaining weight loss is a very difficult process requiring behavioural change, and therefore a long-term approach. The ward environment can offer the initial peer group and professional support required.

Dyslipidaemia

Dyslipidaemia is a powerful CVD risk factor and a lipid profile should be obtained. Cardiovascular risk in patients without a history of coronary heart disease or of stroke/transient ischaemic attack should be evaluated by the QRISK®2-2016 risk calculator (91), bearing in mind that risk will be underestimated in those with SMI, particularly if taking an antipsychotic, as well as patients with hypertriglyceridaemia and in those with a BMI of 40 kg/m^2 or greater (92). Although antipsychotic-induced dyslipidaemia is common (93), to our knowledge, only one study has examined the effectiveness of switching antipsychotic to improve it. This showed that non-high-density lipoprotein cholesterol and triglyceride levels could be reduced in patients treated with olanzapine, quetiapine, or risperidone by switching to aripiprazole (57). Should a decision be made to switch antipsychotic, close attention needs to be paid both to metabolic parameters and mental state. Lipid management independent of antipsychotic switching should follow current guidelines (92). Except in the most uncomplicated cases, lipid management should generally be undertaken in consultation with the GP and/or the local hospital specialist. This also applies to the assessment and management of lipids in patients who already have a history of CVD, and for whom the psychiatry hospital admission may represent the opportunity for a general treatment review.

Hypertension

Hypertension is a significant risk factor for CVD, particularly cerebrovascular disease. Depression is associated with an increased risk of hypertension (94) and patients with schizophrenia are treated for their hypertension less often than the general population (95). Modifiable risk factors for hypertension overlap with many of the other physical health issues discussed in this chapter, and include smoking, physical inactivity, diet, and alcohol intake.

A diagnosis of hypertension should not be made based on a single measurement, particularly in a stressful setting such as acute admission to a psychiatric unit. However, identification and timely management of individuals with a hypertensive emergency (systolic pressure >180 mmHg, diastolic pressure >120 mmHg) is essential, and requires prompt transfer to a general ward or hospital. Exploration of raised but not immediately dangerous readings is also the responsibility of the ward team. Management should be in conjunction with the GP. For known hypertensive patients, review and optimization of their current management should be undertaken.

Alcohol

Alcohol and substance misuse are covered in depth in Chapter 13, however there are important acute physical health care considerations. Up to 1 in 20 alcohol-dependent individuals will develop delirium tremens when alcohol intake is ceased, characterized by confusion and autonomic hyperactivity. Delirium tremens is extremely dangerous with a mortality rate of almost one in three in untreated cases and 5–15% even with treatment. Prompt identification and management of acute intoxication and recent alcohol intake is therefore essential on admission. Deficiency in thiamine (vitamin B1) is relatively common in alcohol-dependent individuals which can lead to Wernicke's encephalopathy and in turn, Korsakoff's syndrome. Therefore, high doses of thiamine should be given during any periods of detoxification. Detoxification attempts should only be considered with support from community services to increase the chances of longer-term abstinence and reduce the risk from recurrent detoxifications.

Other factors impacting on physical health

Individuals with SMI are at increased risk of a number of other diseases and disorders which impact negatively on morbidity and mortality including blood-borne viral infections (19), respiratory infections, and poor dentition. They are also at risk from the side effects of psychotropic medication including extrapyramidal side effects, prolonged QTc, arrhythmias, hyperprolactinaemia, sexual dysfunction, and sedation (96). Each impacts well-being and can affect compliance and psychiatric outcomes as well as physical health outcomes.

Inpatient opportunities

The number of psychiatric beds available in England fell from almost 70,000 in the late 1980s to under 20,000 in 2015, with only just over half of those acute adult NHS beds (97), reflecting trends across the rest of the world. In practice, this means that most admissions are emergencies and outside of normal working hours. This in turn means that coordinated handover from a community team or GP at the time of admission is not possible. Also, the general level of both psychiatric and physical need is likely to be significant. Timely, comprehensive physical health review is therefore indicated.

Admission

Immediate assessment for acute physical issues on admission is essential; initially this can be achieved by appropriately trained staff recording baseline physical observations including heart rate, blood pressure, respiratory rate, oxygen saturations, and blood glucose levels on a standardized chart (such as the National Early Warning Score, as suggested by the Royal College of Physicians) and informing the responsible psychiatrist. The mental state of the individual on admission may initially make attaining a full history, examination, and investigation inappropriate. However, as soon as is suitable these should be completed to identify acute and chronic conditions, current medications (the exact list can be reconciled later), allergies, and any recent alcohol or drug use (to anticipate possible physical withdrawal symptoms). A family history of significant health conditions should be included. Smoking status should be established early and appropriate cessation support started. A full physical assessment should include height, weight, blood tests, and an electrocardiogram (10, 98) (Table 11.3). Other relatively cost-effective and simple admission investigations should include urine tests for infection and recent drug use as indicated. Patients' primary care records, hospital records, and previous investigations should be reviewed to minimize duplication and omission. Together, these data help risk assessment and management planning.

Health promotion

Admission is also an important opportunity to explore individuals' lifestyles and offer appropriate support and health promotion. Essential areas include sleep, diet, smoking, exercise, sexual activity, and substance and alcohol use (11). Issues in these areas have a significant impact on well-being and are often iatrogenic or related to psychiatric illness. Having access to a full multidisciplinary team including psychiatrists, nurses, occupational therapists, physiotherapists, dieticians, psychologists, general physicians, GPs, and oral health practitioners is likely to be a unique opportunity for many individuals with SMI. Various strategies have been proposed to achieve this including dedicated physical health clinics on psychiatric wards, sometimes run by or in conjunction with primary care physicians, as well as 'liaison physicians' providing physical health care advice. Adequate physical space (10) and equipment are vital to achieve this.

Barriers

Mental health nurses are perfectly placed to help both assess and provide management for physical health issues in psychiatric inpatients but unfortunately, they often receive little appropriate training or support (99). This can lead to a lack of confidence, which combined with multiple other demands, can led to physical health monitoring and management being deprioritized. Post-registration training is associated with increased confidence (100). Most providers of psychiatric inpatient care require all their frontline staff to have regular retraining in basic assessment and management of acute physical illness and resuscitation. This 'firefighter' approach is necessary but not sufficient. In some areas, training courses are being developed for health care staff who work in psychiatric wards in assessing medical issues, reflecting a willingness of staff to gain and maintain appropriate skills. Other barriers include negative symptoms impacting the functioning and outcomes of patients with

Table 11.3 Summary of some physical health assessments and interventions that should be considered during inpatient stay based on current recommendations and clinical experience (10, 11, 38, 58-60, 63, 66, 89, 91, 92, 98)

Admission stage	Physical health areas	Assessments and interventions
Immediate	Physical observations	Heart rate, blood pressure, respiratory rate, oxygen saturations, temperature, capillary blood glucose, Glasgow coma scale—on standardized chart, e.g. National Early Warning Score
	Medical history	Venous thromboembolism prophylaxis, document acute physical health issues
	Medications and allergies	Document current medications, over-the-counter medications, and prescribe appropriately, document allergies
	Recent substances/smoking	Alcohol detoxification regime, nicotine replacement therapy, opiate withdrawal management
<24 hours	Full history	Document complete history including family, lifestyle social (accommodation, employment), medication history
	Physical examination	Full systems examination, height, weight, calculate BMI, waist circumference
	Investigations: blood tests	Haematological, renal, hepatic, bone and lipid profiles, fasting plasma glucose, HbA1c and thyroid function. Prolactin in patients due to start antipsychotics Others as indicated by history, physical examination, and other investigation results such folate and B12
	Investigations: electrocardiography	For a baseline and QTc
	Investigations: others	Urine dip, urine drug screen, pregnancy test, imaging as indicated by history and examination
During admission: *Modifiable lifestyle risk factors*	Addictions	'No smoking' policies Nicotine replacement therapy Smoking cessation interventions Alcohol/drug worker liaison
	Activity	Physiotherapy review Occupational therapy review Access to gym/exercise on ward Promotion of activity on ward
	Diet	Dietician review Food policies and review of food provided on ward
	Sleep	Sleep hygiene advice Medication review Consideration of how current social situation is impacting on sleep
System reviews	Cardiovascular	QRISK®2—risk predictor for cardiovascular disease In coordination with primary or secondary care where appropriate start statin and/or antihypertensive treatment
	Respiratory	Asthma review/inhaler technique review Flu vaccine if indicated
	Diabetes	Fasting plasma glucose, Hba1C and lipid profile. Foot examination. Liaise with GP or diabetes team regarding medication for blood glucose, lipid and blood pressure control, and regarding screening for diabetic complications
	Sexual	Menstrual history in women, enquire about sexual dysfunction in men and women Blood tests including prolactin (if on antipsychotics and amenorrhoea or sexual dysfunction), hepatitis, HIV, syphilis Sexual health clinic/nurse
	Oral	Dental nurse/dentist review
	Cancer	Liaise with GP regarding if up-to-date with screening programmes
	Other	As indicated by history, examination, and investigation findings, such as chronic pain or skin conditions and assessing falls risk in older adults
Acute deterioration		National Early Warning Score Basic life support Swift transfer to appropriate care provider
Discharge	Written summary	Written care plan, including summary of history, examination and investigation findings, lifestyle interventions and follow-up plans agreed with patient and care coordinator prior to discharge

chronic schizophrenia and the lack of adequate facilities to allow physical activity and diet to be addressed.

Non-adult wards

Although the acute physical needs of individuals admitted to a child and adolescent mental health services, older adult, learning disability, or forensic inpatient unit may differ, the underlying principles of good physical health care are equally relevant in each setting: a timely and thorough assessment of acute and chronic physical health issues should be undertaken and a cohesive and collaborative management plan produced, including treatments, health promotion, and appropriate follow-up.

Post discharge

The long-term nature of many risk factors for poor physical health outcomes makes the continuation of interventions started during inpatient stays essential. Good communication between inpatient, community, acute services, and GP is required for the benefit of both the patient and the health care system. One way in which this may be achieved is with a written care plan as recommended by the Royal College of Psychiatrists, involving those who will be responsible for care post discharge (e.g. care coordinators) during inpatient stays.

Summary

Unfortunately, the disparity between the health and life expectancy of individuals with SMI and the general population remains as large as ever, and if anything is increasing. Patients with SMI face many disadvantages. These include disease processes that may restrict their ability to engage with support, leading to self-neglect; increased rates and severity of risk factors for physical ill health, such as smoking; treatments which exacerbate some of those risk factors, such as the lack of physical activity during detainment and weight gain and diabetes from some psychotropics; and a fragmented health system which is largely unable to promote a holistic approach to health. Additionally, patients with the severest psychiatric illnesses require more intense management, which generally means a greater risk of physical side effects.

This chapter has highlighted some modifiable factors which contribute to increased morbidity and mortality; however, it must be acknowledged that making significant changes in lifestyle as an individual is extremely hard. Future research should therefore include a focus on making ward environments more conducive to health promotion and integrating this with longer-term community programmes. Development of new medications with greater efficacy on negative symptoms of psychosis and more tolerable side effect profiles could also lead to considerable health improvements. Novel professional roles that could help fill the current gap between mental and physical health care should be investigated.

The primary motivation and goal for admission is the assessment and treatment of psychiatric illnesses that cannot be achieved in the community. However, this need not and should not be the only objective as inpatient care also provides an unrivalled opportunity for the comprehensive review and management of the physical health issues which so negatively affect both physical and mental wellbeing. Arbitrary separations between mental and physical health care are immaterial when viewed from a patient-centred perspective. Thus, given the necessary support, physical health care should be the business of all professionals looking after individuals with SMI.

REFERENCES

1. Smith L. Welcome release: perspectives on death in the early county lunatic asylums, 1810–50. *Hist Psychiatry* 2012;23:117–128.
2. Malzberg B. Life tables for patients with mental disease. *J Am Stat Assoc* 1932;27:160–174.
3. Phillips RJ. Physical disorder in 164 admissions to a mental hospital. *Br Med J* 1937;2:363–366.
4. Fekadu A, Medhin G, Kebede D, et al. Excess mortality in severe mental illness: 10-year population-based cohort study in rural Ethiopia. *Br J Psychiatry* 2015;206:289–296.
5. Walker ER, McGee RE, Druss BG. Mortality in mental disorders and global disease burden implications: a systematic review and meta-analysis. *JAMA Psychiatry* 2015;72:334–341.
6. Chang CK, Hayes RD, Perera G, et al. Life expectancy at birth for people with serious mental illness and other major disorders from a secondary mental health care case register in London. *PLoS One* 2011;6:e19590.
7. Wahlbeck K, Westman J, Nordentoft M, Gissler M, Laursen TM. Outcomes of Nordic mental health systems: life expectancy of patients with mental disorders. *Br J Psychiatry* 2011;199:453–458.
8. Olfson M, Gerhard T, Huang C, Crystal S, Stroup TS. Premature mortality among adults with schizophrenia in the United States. *JAMA Psychiatry* 2015;72:1172–1181
9. Lawrence D, Hancock KJ, Kisely S. The gap in life expectancy from preventable physical illness in psychiatric patients in Western Australia: retrospective analysis of population based registers. *BMJ* 2013;346:f2539.
10. Perry J, Palmer L, Thompson P, Worrall A, Chittenden J, Bonnamy M (eds). *Standards in Inpatient Mental Health Services*. Publication Code: CCQI200. London: Royal College of Psychiatrists; 2015.
11. Working Group for Improving the Physical Health of People with SMI. *Improving the Physical Health of Adults with Severe Mental Illness: Essential Actions*. OP100. London: Royal College of Psychiatrists; 2016.
12. Lyketsos CG, Dunn G, Kaminsky MJ, Breakey WR. Medical comorbidity in psychiatric inpatients: relation to clinical outcomes and hospital length of stay. *Psychosomatics* 2002;43:24–30.
13. Adamis D, Ball C. Physical morbidity in elderly psychiatric inpatients: prevalence and possible relations between the major mental disorders and physical illness. *Int J Geriatr Psychiatry* 2000;15:248–253.
14. Goff DC, Sullivan LM, McEvoy JP, et al. A comparison of ten-year cardiac risk estimates in schizophrenia patients from the CATIE study and matched controls. *Schizoph Res* 2005;80:45–53.
15. Ruo B, Rumsfeld JS, Hlatky MA, Liu H, Browner WS, Whooley MA. Depressive symptoms and health-related quality of life: the Heart and Soul Study. *JAMA* 2003;290:215–221.
16. Jones DR, Macias C, Barreira PJ, Fisher WH, Hargreaves WA, Harding CM. Prevalence, severity, and co-occurrence of chronic physical health problems of persons with serious mental illness. *Psychiatr Serv* 2004;55:1250–1257.
17. Himelhoch S, Lehman A, Kreyenbuhl J, Daumit G, Brown C, Dixon L. Prevalence of chronic obstructive pulmonary disease among those with serious mental illness. *Am J Psychiatry* 2004;161:2317–2319.

18. Chen YH, Lin HC, Lin HC. Poor clinical outcomes among pneumonia patients with schizophrenia. *Schizophr Bull* 2011;37:1088–1094.

19. Hughes E, Bassi S, Gilbody S, Bland M, Martin F. Prevalence of HIV, hepatitis B, and hepatitis C in people with severe mental illness: a systematic review and meta-analysis. *Lancet Psychiatry* 2016;3:40–48.

20. De Hert M, Correll CU, Bobes J, et al. Physical illness in patients with severe mental disorders. I. Prevalence, impact of medications and disparities in health care. *World Psychiatry* 2011;10:52–77.

21. Bradford DW, Goulet J, Hunt M, Cunningham NC, Hoff R. A cohort study of mortality in individuals with and without schizophrenia after diagnosis of lung cancer. *J Clin Psychiatry* 2016;77:e1626–e1630.

22. Davis WA, Starkstein SE, Bruce DG, Davis TM. The interactive effects of type 2 diabetes mellitus and schizophrenia on all-cause mortality: the Fremantle Diabetes Study. *J Diabetes Complications* 2015;29:1320–1322.

23. Crump C, Sundquist K, Winkleby MA, Sundquist J. Comorbidities and mortality in bipolar disorder: a Swedish national cohort study. *JAMA Psychiatry* 2013;70:931–939.

24. Wu CS, Lai MS, Gau SS. Complications and mortality in patients with schizophrenia and diabetes: population-based cohort study. *Br J Psychiatry* 2015;207:450–457.

25. Vinogradova Y, Coupland C, Hippisley-Cox J, Whyte S, Penny C. Effects of severe mental illness on survival of people with diabetes. *Br J Psychiatry* 2010;197:272–277.

26. Diabetes UK. Quality and Outcomes Framework (QOF), 2013–2014. Quoted in: Facts and Stats. 2015. https://www.diabetes.org.uk/Documents/Position%20statements/Facts%20and%20stats%20June%202015.pdf

27. NHS Scotland. Scottish Diabetes Survey 2013: Scottish Diabetes Survey Monitoring Group. 2013. http://www.diabetesinscotland.org.uk/Publications/SDS2013.pdf

28. Stubbs B, Vancampfort D, De Hert M, Mitchell AJ. The prevalence and predictors of type two diabetes mellitus in people with schizophrenia: a systematic review and comparative meta-analysis. *Acta Psychiatr Scand* 2015;132:144–157.

29. Vancampfort D, Mitchell AJ, De Hert M, et al. Prevalence and predictors of type 2 diabetes mellitus in people with bipolar disorder: a systematic review and meta-analysis. *J Clin Psychiatry* 2015;76:1490–1499.

30. Gardner-Sood P, Lally J, Smith S et al. Cardiovascular risk factors and metabolic syndrome in people with established psychotic illnesses: baseline data from the IMPaCT randomized controlled trial. *Psychol Med* 2015;45:2619–2629.

31. Schoepf D, Uppal H, Potluri R, Heun R. Physical comorbidity and its relevance on mortality in schizophrenia: a naturalistic 12-year follow-up in general hospital admissions. *Eur Arch Psychiatry Clin Neurosci* 2014;264:3–28.

32. Schoepf D, Heun R. Bipolar disorder and comorbidity: increased prevalence and increased relevance of comorbidity for hospital-based mortality during a 12.5-year observation period in general hospital admissions. *J Affect Disord* 2014;169:170–178.

33. Public Health England. NHS Diabetes Prevention Programme (NHS DPP). Non-diabetic hyperglycaemia. 2015. https://www.gov.uk/government/uploads/system/uploads/attachment_data/file/456149/Non_diabetic_hyperglycaemia.pdf

34. Galling B, Roldán A, Nielsen RE, et al. Type 2 diabetes mellitus in youth exposed to antipsychotics: a systematic review and meta-analysis. *JAMA Psychiatry* 2016;73:247–259.

35. Diabetes UK. Diabetes risk factors. https://www.diabetes.org.uk/Guide-to-diabetes/What-is-diabetes/Know-your-risk-of-Type-2-diabetes/Diabetes-risk-factors/

36. Langenberg C, Sharp SJ, Franks PW, et al. Gene-lifestyle interaction and type 2 diabetes: the EPIC interact case-cohort study. *PLoS Med* 2014;11:e1001647.

37. Bombelli M, Facchetti R, Sega R, et al. Impact of body mass index and waist circumference on the long-term risk of diabetes mellitus, hypertension, and cardiac organ damage. *Hypertension* 2011;58:1029–1035.

38. Royal College of Physicians. Smoking and mental health. A joint report of the Royal College of Physicians and the Royal College of Psychiatrists. 2013. http://www.ncsct.co.uk/usr/pub/Smoking%20and%20mental%20health.pdf

39. Stubbs B, Ku PW, Chung MS, Chen LJ. Relationship between objectively measured sedentary behavior and cognitive performance in patients with schizophrenia vs controls. *Schizophr Bull* 2017;43:566–574.

40. Vancampfort D, Stubbs B, Sienaert P, et al. A comparison of physical fitness in patients with bipolar disorder, schizophrenia and healthy controls. *Disabil Rehabil* 2016;38:2047–2051.

41. Braganza JM, Lee SH, McCloy RF, McMahon MJ. Chronic pancreatitis. *Lancet* 2011;377:1184–1197.

42. Charatan FB, Bartlett NG. The effect of chlorpromazine (largactil) on glucose tolerance. *Br J Psychiatry* 1955;101:351–353.

43. Thonnard-Neumann E. Phenothiazines and diabetes in hospitalized women. *Am J Psychiatry* 1968;124:978–982.

44. Mitchell AJ, Vancampfort D, De Herdt A, Yu W, De Hert M. Is the prevalence of metabolic syndrome and metabolic abnormalities increased in early schizophrenia? A comparative meta-analysis of first episode, untreated and treated patients. *Schizophr Bull* 2013;39:295–305.

45. Maudsley H. *The Pathology of Mind*. London 1895. Quoted in Holt RIG, Peveler R, Byrne CD. Schizophrenia, the metabolic syndrome and diabetes. *Diabet Med* 2004;21:515–523.

46. Zhang ZJ, Yao ZJ, Liu W, Fang Q, Reynolds GP. Effects of antipsychotics on fat deposition and changes in leptin and insulin levels. Magnetic resonance imaging study of previously untreated people with schizophrenia. *Br J Psychiatry* 2004;184:58–62.

47. Leucht S, Cipriani A, Spineli L, et al. Comparative efficacy and tolerability of 15 antipsychotic drugs in schizophrenia: a multiple-treatments meta-analysis. *Lancet* 2013;382:951–962.

48. Deng C. Effect of antipsychotic medications on appetite, weight and insulin resistance. *Endocrinol Metab Clin North Am* 2013;42:545–563.

49. Lind M, Garcia-Rodriguez LA, Booth GL, et al. Mortality trends in patients with and without diabetes in Ontario, Canada and the UK from 1996 to 2009: a population-based study. *Diabetologia* 2013;56:2601–2608.

50. UK Prospective Diabetes Study (UKPDS) Group. Effect of intensive blood-glucose control with metformin on complications in overweight patients with type 2 diabetes (UKPDS 34). *Lancet* 1998;352:854–865.

51. UK Prospective Diabetes Study (UKPDS) Group. Intensive blood-glucose control with sulphonylureas or insulin compared with conventional treatment and risk of complications in patients with type 2 diabetes (UKPDS 33). *Lancet* 1998;352:837–853.

52. UK Prospective Diabetes Study Group. Tight blood pressure control and risk of macrovascular and microvascular complications in type 2 diabetes: UKPDS 38. *BMJ* 1998;317:703–713.

53. Collins R, Armitage J, Parish S, Sleigh P, Peto R, Heart Protection Study Collaborative Group. MRC/BHF Heart Protection

Study of cholesterol-lowering with simvastatin in 5963 people with diabetes: a randomised placebo-controlled trial. *Lancet* 2003;361:2005–2016.

54. Callaghan BC, Little AA, Feldman EL, Hughes RA. Enhanced glucose control for preventing and treating diabetic neuropathy. *Cochrane Database Syst Rev* 2012;6:CD007543.

55. De Hert M, Hanssens L, van Winkel R, et al. Reversibility of antipsychotic treatment-related diabetes in patients with schizophrenia: a case series of switching to aripiprazole. *Diabetes Care* 2006;29:2329–2330.

56. Arnoldy R, Curtis J, Samaras K. The effects of antipsychotic switching on diabetes in chronic schizophrenia. *Diabet Med* 2014;31:e16–e19.

57. Stroup TS, McEvoy JP, King KD, et al. A randomized trial examining the effectiveness of switching from olanzapine, quetiapine, or risperidone to aripiprazole to reduce metabolic risk: comparison of antipsychotics for metabolic problems (CAMP). *Am J Psychiatry* 2011;168:947–956.

58. National Institute for Health and Care Excellence. Type 2 diabetes in adults: management. NICE guideline [NG28]. 2015. https://www.nice.org.uk/guidance/NG28

59. Cooper SJ, Reynolds GP, Barnes T, et al. BAP guidelines on the management of weight gain, metabolic disturbances and cardiovascular risk associated with psychosis and antipsychotic drug treatment. *J Psychopharmacol* 2016;30:717–748.

60. National Institute for Health and Care Excellence. Type 2 diabetes: prevention in people at high risk. Public health guideline [PH38]. 2012. https://www.nice.org.uk/guidance/ph38

61. Kitabchi AE, Umpierrez GE, Miles JM, Fisher JN. Hyperglycemic crises in adult patients with diabetes. *Diabetes Care* 2009;32:1335–1343.

62. Wright J, Ruck K, Rabbitts R, et al. Diabetic ketoacidosis (DKA) in Birmingham, UK, 2000–2009: an evaluation of risk factors for recurrence and mortality. *Br J Diabetes Vasc Dis* 2009;9:278–282.

63. Joint British Diabetes Societies Inpatient Care Group. The management of the hyperosmolar hyperglycaemic state (HHS) in adults with diabetes. 2012. https://www.diabetes.org.uk/Documents/Position%20statements/JBDS-IP-HHS-Adults.pdf

64. Henderson DC, Cagliero E, Copeland PM, et al. Elevated hemoglobin A1c as a possible indicator of diabetes mellitus and diabetic ketoacidosis in schizophrenia patients receiving atypical antipsychotics. *J Clin Psychiatry* 2007;68:533–541.

65. Guenette MD, Hahn M, Cohn TA, Teo C, Remington GJ. Atypical antipsychotics and diabetic ketoacidosis: a review. *Psychopharmacology (Berl)* 2013;226:1–12.

66. Joint British Diabetes Societies Inpatient Care Group. The management of diabetic ketoacidosis in adults. 2013. http://www.diabetologists-abcd.org.uk/jbds/JBDS_IP_DKA_Adults_Revised.pdf

67. Joint British Diabetes Societies Inpatient Care Group. The hospital management of hypoglycaemia in adults with diabetes mellitus. 2013. https://www.diabetes.org.uk/Documents/About%20Us/Our%20views/Care%20recs/JBDS%20hypoglycaemia%20position%20(2013).pdf

68. Tuomilehto J, Lindström J, Eriksson JG, et al. Finnish Diabetes Prevention Study Group. Prevention of type 2 diabetes mellitus by changes in lifestyle among subjects with impaired glucose tolerance. *N Engl J Med* 2001;344:1343–1350.

69. Knowler WC, Barrett-Connor E, Fowler SE, et al. Diabetes Prevention Program Research Group. Reduction in the incidence of type 2 diabetes with lifestyle intervention or metformin. *N Engl J Med* 2002;346:393–403.

70. Public Health England. A systematic review and meta-analysis assessing the effectiveness of pragmatic lifestyle interventions for the prevention of type 2 diabetes mellitus in routine practice. 2015. https://www.gov.uk/government/uploads/system/uploads/attachment_data/file/456147/PHE_Evidence_Review_of_diabetes_prevention_programmes-_FINAL.pdf

71. Gierisch JM, Nieuwsma JA, Bradford DW, et al. Pharmacologic and behavioral interventions to improve cardiovascular risk factors in adults with serious mental illness: a systematic review and meta-analysis. *J Clin Psychiatry* 2014;75:e424–e440

72. Lasser K, Boyd JW, Woolhandler S, Himmelstein DU, McCormick D, Bor DH. Smoking and mental illness: a population-based prevalence study. *JAMA* 2000;284:2606–2610.

73. de Leon J, Diaz FJ. A meta-analysis of worldwide studies demonstrates an association between schizophrenia and tobacco smoking behaviors. *Schizophr Res* 2005;76:135–157.

74. Jackson JG, Diaz FJ, Lopez L, Leon J. A combined analysis of worldwide studies demonstrates an association between bipolar disorder and tobacco smoking behaviors in adults. *Bipolar Disord* 2015;17:575–597.

75. Lê Cook B, Wayne GF, Kafali EN, Liu Z, Shu C, Flores M. Trends in smoking among adults with mental illness and association between mental health treatment and smoking cessation. *JAMA* 2014;311:172–182.

76. Taylor G, McNeill A, Girling A, Farley A, Lindson-Hawley N, Aveyard P. Change in mental health after smoking cessation: systematic review and meta-analysis. *BMJ* 2014;348:g1151.

77. Pirie K, Peto R, Reeves GK, Green J, Beral V, Million Women Study Collaborators. The 21st century hazards of smoking and benefits of stopping: a prospective study of one million women in the UK. *Lancet* 2013;381:133–141.

78. Stockings EA, Bowman JA, Prochaska JJ, et al. The impact of a smoke-free psychiatric hospitalization on patient smoking outcomes: a systematic review. *Aust NZ J Psychiatry* 2014;48:617–633.

79. Rigotti NA, Clair C, Munafò MR, Stead LF. Interventions for smoking cessation in hospitalised patients. *Cochrane Database Syst Rev* 2012;5:CD001837.

80. Metse AP, Wiggers J, Wye P, et al. Smoking and environmental characteristics of smokers with a mental illness, and associations with quitting behaviour and motivation; a cross sectional study. *BMC Public Health* 2016;16:332.

81. Health & Social Care Information Centre. Health Survey for England 2014: health, social care and lifestyles. Summary of key findings. 2015. http://content.digital.nhs.uk/catalogue/PUB19295/HSE2014-Sum-bklet.pdf

82. Simmons RK, Alberti KG, Gale EA, et al. The metabolic syndrome: useful concept or clinical tool? Report of a WHO Expert Consultation. *Diabetologia* 2010;53:600–605.

83. McEvoy JP, Meyer JM, Goff DC, et al. Prevalence of the metabolic syndrome in patients with schizophrenia: baseline results from the Clinical Antipsychotic Trials of Intervention Effectiveness (CATIE) schizophrenia trial and comparison with national estimates from NHANES III. *Schizophr Res* 2005;80:19–32.

84. Vancampfort D, Vansteelandt K, Correll CU, et al. Metabolic syndrome and metabolic abnormalities in bipolar disorder: a meta-analysis of prevalence rates and moderators. *Am J Psychiatry* 2013;170:265–274.

85. Hasnain M, Vieweg WV. Weight considerations in psychotropic drug prescribing and switching. *Postgrad Med* 2013;125:117–129.

86. Weiden PJ, Mackell JA, McDonnell DD. Obesity as a risk factor for antipsychotic noncompliance. *Schizophr Res* 2004;66:51–57.

87. National Institute for Health and Care Excellence. Psychosis and schizophrenia in adults: prevention and management. Clinical guideline [CG178]. 2014. https://www.nice.org.uk/guidance/cg178?unlid=9196189462016820111340

88. National Institute for Health and Care Excellence. Bipolar disorder: assessment and management. Clinical guideline [CG185]. 2014. https://www.nice.org.uk/guidance/cg185

89. National Institute for Health and Care Excellence. Obesity: identification, assessment and management. Clinical guideline [CG189]. 2014. https://www.nice.org.uk/guidance/cg189/chapter/1-recommendations

90. Mizuno Y, Suzuki T, Nakagawa A, et al. Pharmacological strategies to counteract antipsychotic-induced weight gain and metabolic adverse effects in schizophrenia: a systematic review and meta-analysis. *Schizophr Bull* 2014;40:1385–1403.

91. QRisk2®. QRisk2®-2016 risk calculator. https://qrisk.org/2016/

92. National Institute for Health and Care Excellence. Cardiovascular disease: risk assessment and reduction, including lipid modification. Clinical guideline [CG181] 2014 (last updated 2016). https://www.nice.org.uk/guidance/CG181

93. De Hert M, van Winkel R, Yu W, Correll CU. Metabolic and cardiovascular adverse effects associated with antipsychotic drugs. *Nat Rev Endocrinol* 2012;8:114–126.

94. Meng L, Chen D, Yang Y, Zheng Y, Hui R. Depression increases the risk of hypertension incidence: a meta-analysis of prospective cohort studies. *J Hypertens* 2012;30:842–851.

95. Nasrallah HA, Meyer JM, Goff DC, et al. Low rates of treatment for hypertension, dyslipidemia and diabetes in schizophrenia: data from the CATIE schizophrenia trial sample at baseline. *Schizophr Res* 2006;86:15–22.

96. Young SL, Taylor M, Lawrie SM. 'First do no harm': a systematic review of the prevalence and management of antipsychotic adverse effects. *J Psychopharmacol* 2015;29:353–362.

97. Crisp N, Smith G, Nicholson K (eds). *Old Problems, New Solutions—Improving Acute Psychiatric Care for Adults in England.* London: The Commission on Acute Adult Psychiatric Care; 2016.

98. Shiers DE, Rafi I, Cooper SJ, Holt RIG. *Positive Cardiometabolic Health Resource: An Intervention Framework for Patients with Psychosis and Schizophrenia. 2014 update.* London: Royal College of Psychiatrists; 2014.

99. Blythe J, White J. Role of the mental health nurse towards physical health care in serious mental illness: an integrative review of 10 years of UK literature. *Int J Ment Health Nurs* 2012;21:193–201.

100. Robson D, Haddad M, Gray R, Gournay K. Mental health nursing and physical health care: a cross-sectional study of nurses' attitudes, practice, and perceived training needs for the physical health care of people with severe mental illness. *Int J Ment Health Nurs* 2013;22:409–417.

12

Adverse reactions to medication

Tomasz Bajorek and Jonathan Hafferty

Extrapyramidal side effects

Antipsychotics, whether typical or atypical, reduce dopaminergic activity in the brain. When deemed undesirable, side effects relating to the dopaminergic system are referred to as extrapyramidal side effects (EPSEs). Dopamine receptor (primarily D_2) blockade in the striatum is the most commonly cited mechanism for the neurological side effects of antipsychotic drugs. Anticholinergic and antiparkinsonian drugs are the typical remedy used; however, this postulated anticholinergic–dopaminergic imbalance is undoubtedly an oversimplification.

The four main forms of EPSE are:

* acute dystonia
* pseudoparkinsonism (also known as drug-induced parkinsonism)
* akathisia
* tardive dyskinesia.

Acute dystonia

This is one of the more rapidly occurring EPSEs with a typical onset in the first few hours or days of taking an antipsychotic. It is usually seen as a tonic muscle spasm affecting the tongue, jaw, or neck but any muscle may be affected. The range of presentations is stark (1) (Table 12.1). It can manifest as a mild tongue stiffness or an extremely distressing opisthotonus (a spasm of the muscles causing backward arching of the head, neck, and spine as in Figure 12.1). Some studies suggest the dystonia occurs as the blood levels of antipsychotics are dropping, indicating the possibility of this being a rebound effect as dopamine blockade drops.

The prevalence with typical antipsychotics is around 10% (2) with a higher incidence in the neuroleptic-naïve patient. It is more likely to be encountered with drugs that do not have an antagonistic effect on muscarinic acetylcholine receptors (mAChs) (e.g. butyrophenones such as haloperidol). Conversely, it is less likely in antipsychotics with intrinsic mACh antagonism (e.g. phenothiazines). This occurs because of the reciprocal actions of mACh and dopaminergic systems in the basal ganglia. Other drugs that can cause dystonia include antiemetics such as metoclopramide, antidepressants, anticonvulsants, and cocaine (3).

Dystonias (and EPSEs in general) are, by definition, less likely to be encountered with atypical antipsychotics. This is thought to be due to lower D_2 binding affinity and high 5-hydroxytryptamine (5-HT_2):dopamine receptor binding ratios.

When encountered, a reduction in dose or switch in medication is usually worth considering. Anticholinergic medication is effective and should be given orally, intramuscularly, or intravenously depending on the severity of symptoms (e.g. intravenous if the patient is having swallowing problems). A response is seen within 5–20 minutes of administration (4). Electroconvulsive therapy, repetitive transcranial magnetic stimulation, and botulinum toxin may be helpful in tardive dystonias or where simpler measures have proven unsuccessful (5).

Table 12.1 Abnormal types of movement disorder seen in acute dystonia

Type of dystonia	Detail
Buccolingual crisis	Forced jaw opening, tongue protrusion, and grimacing
Hyper lordosis/scoliosis	Abnormal curvature of the spine
Laryngospasm	Spasm of the laryngeal muscles rendering the individual unable to speak or breathe normally
Oculogyric crisis	Eye movements deviating upwards and sometimes to the side. The affected individual is unable to see properly.
Opisthotonus	Spasm of paravertebral muscles causing backward arching of the head, neck, and spine
Pisa syndrome (aka pleurothotonus)	Truncal flexion towards one side
Torticollis	Spasm of neck musculature such that head and neck twist to the side
Trismus (aka lockjaw)	Reduced opening of the jaw/mouth caused by spasm of muscles of mastication

Adapted from Cunningham-Owen DG. *A guide to the extrapyramidal side-effects of antipsychotic drugs.* Cambridge: Cambridge University Press; 1999.

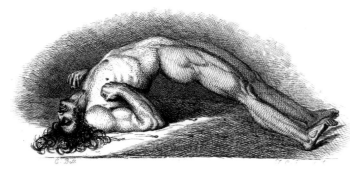

Figure 12.1 The opisthotonic position.
From *Sir Charles Bell's Essays on the Anatomy and Philosophy of Expression* (London: John Muray, 1824), p. 101. (Bethesda, Md.: National Library of Medicine).

Pseudoparkinsonism (drug-induced parkinsonism)

Nigrostriatal blockade of dopamine receptors may result in parkinsonian symptoms including tremor, rigidity, and bradykinesia (1) (Box 12.1). The elderly, those on high-potency antipsychotics, and those who have experienced other EPSEs are at greater risk of developing pseudoparkinsonism (7). Apart from typical antipsychotics, other drugs including certain antiemetics, calcium channel blockers, and atypical antipsychotics may cause the presentation. The symptoms are typically reversible on stopping the offending drug but it may take some weeks or months for this improvement to occur.

Differentiating pseudoparkinsonism from idiopathic parkinsonism can be difficult. The acute presence of bilateral symptoms, in the context of antipsychotic initiation or dose increase, as well as the presence of a postural tremor or orofacial dyskinesia would favour pseudoparkinsonism. A chronic, progressive course, resting tremor, and asymmetrical symptoms would favour Parkinson's disease. Single-photon emission computed tomography imaging can help resolve the matter and will be normal in drug-induced cases.

As with acute dystonias, treatment centres on reducing the dose or potentially switching to an atypical drug (8). There is some data to suggest quetiapine and clozapine ought to be favoured when treating psychosis in Parkinson's disease and with pseudoparkinsonism. The addition of a mACh antagonist (more commonly called an anticholinergic) such as procyclidine or trihexyphenidyl may be helpful

---

Box 12.1 Pseudoparkinsonian symptoms

- Tremor: classically a slow, pill rolling tremor but it is more likely to be bilateral and symmetrical when drug induced. Postural tremors more common than resting. Perioral tremors may be seen.
- Rigidity: cogwheel rigidity.
- Bradykinesia:
  - Shuffling gait
  - Mask-like facies
  - Stooped posture
  - Greater likelihood of concurrent dyskinesia and akathisia (other EPSEs)
- Other: bradyphrenia, salivation.

---

though caution should be exercised given the risk of abuse and other side effects (e.g. urinary retention, exacerbation of cognitive impairment, and precipitation of angle closure glaucoma).

Akathisia

Akathisia is the subjective sense of restlessness often combined with motor manifestations such as pacing, restless legs, rocking, or an inability to sit still (9). Associated symptoms include anxiety and panic. It is particularly distressing and unpleasant for the patient and can be a major factor in non-adherence and serve to elevate suicide risk. Understandably, given the symptom profile, patients are frequently misdiagnosed as having 'deteriorated' or considered to be showing new-onset agitation or even mania. The natural reaction of increasing the medication dosage further will serve only to aggravate the presentation. It is a common side effect especially with higher-potency antipsychotics. It may also be seen with certain antidepressants and metoclopramide. Estimates of prevalence in inpatient settings vary from around 11% to 25% (10).

Withdrawal of, or reductions in, antipsychotic dosage are the simplest yet most effective management options. Sometimes this may worsen the akathisia due to receptor hypersensitivity. Benzodiazepines and beta blockers may be considered as adjunctive strategies in managing the condition (5).

Tardive dyskinesia

Tardive syndromes are serious, often permanent, movement disorders. They are called 'tardive' as their onset is months or years after initiation of treatment. They may manifest as dystonias or akathisia but dyskinesias are more frequently encountered. These are characterized by involuntary movements of, most commonly, facial, tongue, and neck muscles but, as detailed in Table 12.2, any muscle group can in theory be affected (6, 11).

The pathophysiology is not completely understood with a significant incidence noted in those with schizophrenia never treated with antipsychotics. A disruption in the balance of D_1/D_2 receptor stimulation is nonetheless hypothesized to lie behind the condition. Tardive dyskinesia affects around 40–50% of those treated with typical antipsychotics after months to years. It is clear that atypical antipsychotics have a lower risk of inducing tardive dyskinesia but the risk is not negligible (3% vs 7.7% according to a recent review) (12–14). Men and women are equally affected by the condition and risk increases with age. It is more common in those with affective illness and may be associated with neurocognitive deficits and higher mortality (15). Their emergence cannot necessarily be predicted by dose or 'prophylactic' antimuscarinic prescription.

The management of tardive dyskinesia initially (and where possible) centres on stopping any anticholinergic and gradually reducing or indeed withdrawing the causative antipsychotic (5, 16). It is common to observe an initial worsening of the dyskinesia. If a switch is needed, alternative antipsychotics to consider include clozapine and quetiapine (5, 18) as they may aid symptom resolution and have a lesser propensity for causing tardive dyskinesia. It may also be worth considering a trial of benzodiazepine, *Ginkgo biloba*, or tetrabenazine (17), which is the only licensed treatment in the UK and acts by depleting vesicular dopamine. The prospects of

Table 12.2 Common features of tardive dyskinesia

Affected area	Description
Eyes	Blepharospasm, excessive blinking
Face	Grimacing, spasms, tics
Mouth	Chewing, lateral jaw movements, lip smacking, pouting, sucking
Tongue	'Fly catching' tongue, protrusion
Pharynx	Abnormal sounds, excessive or stereotyped swallow
Neck	Retrocollis, torticollis
Trunk	Diaphragmatic jerks, forced retroflexion, pelvic thrusting, rocking
Limbs	Ankle flexion/inversion/eversion, arm ballism, finger movements, foot tapping, toe movements, wrist flexion/extension
Whole body	Generalized rigidity

Box 12.2 Clinical features of neuroleptic malignant syndrome

- Hyperthermia.
- Autonomic dysfunction commonly including:
  - tachycardia
  - labile blood pressure
  - diaphoresis
  - pallor
  - urinary incontinence.
- Fluctuating consciousness/confusion.
- Muscular rigidity: cogwheeling, lead pipe rigidity, dysphagia, dysarthria and infrequently myoclonus.
- It evolves rapidly over 24–72 hours. It may last approximately 7 days after cessation of the causative drug (unless it is depot induced in which case it may be more prolonged).

Investigations
- Raised white cell count.
- Raised serum creatinine phosphokinase (secondary to rhabdomyolysis).

---

improvement are reasonable with around 55% showing remission on dose reduction or switching to clozapine (15).

Neuroleptic malignant syndrome

Coined by Delay et al. in 1960 (19), neuroleptic malignant syndrome (usually referred to simply as NMS) is an infrequent yet potentially life-threatening psychiatric emergency that requires immediate attention and treatment. The tetrad of signs typically seen includes hyperthermia, autonomic dysfunction, fluctuating consciousness, and muscular rigidity (Box 12.2) (20–22).

Important differential diagnoses to consider are central nervous system infection, serotonin syndrome, drug-induced extrapyramidal symptoms, anticholinergic crisis, and lithium toxicity.

An idiosyncratic event, it is most commonly associated with the use of first-generation, high-potency antipsychotics but other drug classes have also been implicated including second-generation antipsychotics, antidepressants, and lithium.

Dopamine blockade is presumed to be the trigger for the development of NMS. Dopamine blockade in the hypothalamic thermoregulatory centres would explain pyrexia, that in hypothalamospinal tract neurons would account for autonomic instability while that in the mesocortical pathways may manifest as altered consciousness or confusion.

The incidence rates estimated range from 0.01% to 2.2% though higher values are generally obtained from earlier studies. Risk factors for NMS include the initiation phase of treatment or recent antipsychotic dose increase, polypharmacy with some antidepressants, lithium, or metoclopramide, dehydration, family or personal history of catatonia or NMS, toxicity, infection, multi-morbidity, and neurological disorders (encephalitis, brain tumour, dementia) (24). Male patients of younger age may also be particularly at risk though this may simply reflect the higher preponderance of antipsychotic use in this group. Excessive skeletal muscle breakdown in NMS can cause a very significantly raised creatine kinase level, as well as myoglobinuria and risk of acute kidney injury.

Management of NMS

NMS is a medical emergency and the causative antipsychotic agent needs to be stopped immediately. Initial treatment is with benzodiazepines (aggressive treatment with high doses, such as up to 24 mg lorazepam daily, may be required). Usually, the patient will need to be admitted to a medical ward or intensive care unit for supportive care. Specifically, this is likely to include careful maintenance of fluid and electrolyte balance. Dantrolene (a muscle relaxant which inhibits calcium release from the sarcoplasmic reticulum thereby reducing muscle rigidity and pyrexia) or bromocriptine (a dopamine receptor agonist) may be required. Complications seen in more severe cases include seizures, myoglobinuria, respiratory depression, and renal failure. The mortality is generally thought to exceed 10% in those that develop the full syndrome and are left untreated (23).

Assuming further treatment with antipsychotics is indicated, allow time for the symptoms of NMS to resolve and restart treatment with a structurally unrelated compound to that which precipitated NMS. A very slow dose titration regimen should be used with close physical monitoring (pulse, blood pressure, temperature, creatinine kinase). Drugs with low dopamine affinity (e.g. clozapine or quetiapine) are generally less likely to precipitate further bouts. High potency, typical antipsychotics, and depots should be avoided (5).

Antipsychotic-induced hyperprolactinaemia

Prolactin is a hormone synthesized in and secreted from lactotroph cells in the anterior pituitary gland (25). Its production and secretion is mainly controlled by dopamine. Normally, dopamine has an inhibitory effect on its release. Hence, a reduction in dopaminergic input to the lactotroph cells results in a rapid prolactin increase.

Prolactin promotes milk secretion. Hyperprolactinaemia, whether physiological (pregnancy and lactation) or pathological (neoplastic, iatrogenic, etc.) can cause breast enlargement and galactorrhoea in both female and male patients (31). It can also inhibit

Box 12.3 Adjunctive treatments for drug-induced sexual side effects

- Amantadine.
- Bupropion.
- Buspirone.
- Cyproheptadine.
- *Ginkgo biloba*.
- Sildenafil.
- Tadalfil.
- Vardenafil.
- Yohimbine.

the pulsatile secretion of gonadotrophin-releasing hormone. This in turn inhibits the release of both luteinizing hormone and follicle-stimulating hormone, thus blocking sex hormone secretion by the ovaries and the testes. Such hypogonadism is characterized by menstrual disturbances, reduced fertility, and sexual dysfunction. In the longer term, it risks osteoporosis and an increased propensity to bone fracture (26–29).

As already stated, dopamine inhibits prolactin release. Dopamine antagonists can therefore be expected to raise serum prolactin levels. Almost all antipsychotics can therefore be expected to cause changes in prolactin levels. The ubiquity of this effect was such with first-generation drugs that the use of the prolactin level to guide adequate dosing of antipsychotics had been considered!

Aside from antipsychotic-induced hyperprolactinaemia, there are other causes of hyperprolactinaemia that ought to be borne in mind as detailed in Table 12.3.

The effects of drug-induced hyperprolactinaemia are extremely variable. Some people with significantly raised prolactin levels

Table 12.3 Causes of hyperprolactinaemia that are important for the psychiatrist

Physiological	Pharmacological	Pathological
Pregnancy	Antipsychotics	Prolactinoma
Lactation	Peripheral dopamine receptor blocking agents (e.g. metoclopramide)	Pituitary or hypothalamic tumours/lesions
Stress	Opiates	Hypothyroidism
Macroprolactin: the presence of these large molecular aggregates lacking biological activity leads to falsely elevated prolactin results	Proton pump inhibitors (e.g. omeprazole)	
	Antidepressants	
	Oestrogens	
	H_2 antagonists (e.g. cimetidine)	
	Calcium channel blockers (e.g. amlodipine and verapamil)	

Adapted from Brown R. & Frighi V., Antipsychotic-induced hyperprolactinaemia, Oxford Health NHS Foundation Trust guideline for identification, monitoring and management. Copyright 2015.

are asymptomatic. Commonly experienced effects however include galactorrhoea, breast enlargement, amenorrhoea, reduced libido, erectile dysfunction, and anorgasmia (29). Fertility is reduced in hyperprolactinaemic women even if they continue to menstruate. Hypogonadism is directly related to the degree of hyperprolactinaemia. It follows that the antipsychotics inducing the most significant increase in prolactin (e.g. amisulpride, risperidone, haloperidol), are those most likely to be cause of amenorrhoea and sexual dysfunction. It is important to remember, however, that sexual dysfunction is very common in mentally ill patients and antipsychotic-induced hyperprolactinaemia is one of many causes.

In the longer term, prolactin-induced hypogonadism risks the development of osteoporosis. Women who are amenorrhoeic should be considered at particularly high risk, especially if it goes on for a prolonged period. In men, a low '9 a.m.' testosterone result would suggest an increased risk of low bone mineral density. Further investigation including dual-energy X-ray absorptiometry scans and an endocrinology opinion may be warranted (30). Particular caution needs to be exercised with younger patients as peak bone mass does not occur until the mid twenties and while prolactin normalization prevents further bone loss, bone mineral density does not generally return to normal. An association between raised prolactin and various types of cancer has been suggested; however, current evidence is weak.

Management of drug-induced hyperprolactinaemia

- Baseline prolactin levels should be obtained prior to initiation of any antipsychotic (Box 12.4).
- Asymptomatic hyperprolactinaemia in those under 25, those with a history of osteoporosis, or those with a history of breast cancer needs to be carefully considered and ideally a non-prolactin-elevating drug used.
- Where baseline prolactin was normal and antipsychotic-induced hyperprolactinaemia occurs but the patient is asymptomatic, a discussion with the patient may be warranted but no action is usually indicated especially with a level of prolactin less than 2500 mIU/L (30).
- Where symptomatic drug-induced hyperprolactinaemia occurs, switching to an alternative, less hyperprolactinaemia-inducing agent (Box 12.5) ought to be considered. If this is not possible, aripiprazole used as an adjunct may reduce prolactin levels. This will be effective at relatively low doses (e.g. 3–6 mg/day). It may prove possible

Box 12.4 Baseline prolactin measurement

- Baseline prolactin levels should be obtained prior to any doses of antipsychotic. Even a single dose can raise prolactin.
- Obtain the sample 1 hour or more after waking or eating.
- Minimize stress during venepuncture.
- Raised baseline levels, in the absence of recent antipsychotic exposure can sometimes be explained by stress.
  - Stress may cause slight increases in prolactin (up to about 700 mU/L in men and 900 mU/L in women).
- Levels higher than those potentially explained by stress, especially if taken prior to the initiation of any antipsychotic, warrant referral to the local endocrinology services for further investigation.

Box 12.5 Non-prolactin-raising antipsychotics

- Aripiprazole
- Asenapine
- Clozapine
- Lurasidone
- Quetiapine.

to subsequently reduce the dose of the offending antipsychotic. Dopaminergic drugs such as amantadine, bromocriptine, and cabergoline can be used under special circumstances though care needs to be exercised given the risk of aggravating psychosis (26–28).

Cardiovascular adverse effects

A number of psychiatric medications produce adverse effects on the cardiovascular system. The most common adverse autonomic effect of antipsychotics is orthostatic hypotension, defined a decrease in systolic blood pressure of at least 20 mmHg or decrease in systolic blood pressure to less than 90 mmHg with upright posture (32). Hypotension is an established adverse effect of a number of atypical antipsychotics and low-potency typical antipsychotics (e.g. chlorpromazine), as well as antidepressants, especially selective serotonin reuptake inhibitors (SSRIs) (33). A likely mechanism is postsynaptic alpha-1 adrenoceptor blockade. Untreated, orthostatic hypotension can result in dizziness, syncope, and falls, especially in the elderly. Hypertension can also result from the same medications blockading presynaptic alpha-2 adrenoceptors, or there can be oscillating hypo- and hypertension (as can be observed for example with clozapine) (5). The judicious choice of medication, related to patient risk history, and slow titration to avoid excess dosage will reduce the incidence of blood pressure-related adverse effects.

Antipsychotic medication has also been associated with an increased risk of venous thromboembolism (34), particularly in elderly or immobile patients. This may be caused or exacerbated by antipsychotic-induced sedation, weight gain, platelet aggregation, and hyperprolactinaemia. The metabolic adverse effects of psychiatric medications (see Chapter 11) also contribute to the established increased risk of coronary artery and vascular disease in psychiatric patients and increased risk of acute coronary syndromes. Additionally, the risk of cerebrovascular adverse events, such as stroke, may be raised as much as threefold in elderly patients with dementia who are prescribed an antipsychotic (35, 36). Particular caution should therefore be used in prescribing antipsychotics to the elderly and especially in the presence of dementia (37).

Cardiac rhythm disturbances are a less common but potentially serious and life-threatening adverse effect of psychiatric medications. Diagnosing these often requires interpretation of the 12-lead electrocardiogram (ECG). On the ECG trace, the QT interval is the length of time between the initiation of the Q wave in the QRS complex (ventricular depolarization) and the end of the T wave (ventricular repolarization) (Figure 12.2). As the QT interval normally shortens with increased heart rate and lengthens with decreasing heart rate, it is summarized by the rate-corrected QTc interval. The normal range of the QT interval is 0.36–0.44 seconds. The QTc is

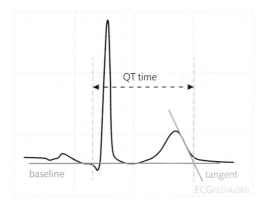

Figure 12.2 Measuring the QT interval on the ECG trace.
CardioNetworks: Googletrans/Wikimedia Commons. Used under the Creative Commons Attribution-ShareAlike 3.0 Unported License (https://creativecommons.org/licenses/by-sa/3.0/).

considered prolonged if it is more than 0.45 seconds in men and 0.47 seconds in women (38). A QTc in excess of 0.5 seconds for either sex should prompt an urgent review of medication (with a view to discontinuation) and referral to cardiology. A prolonged QTc interval is an established (albeit contentious) risk factor for ventricular tachyarrhythmias (although they can occur in the absence of prolonged QTc). A classic example is the potentially life-threatening torsades de pointes, with its characteristic 'twisting' of the QRS complexes on the ECG trace. Prolonged QTc interval is also associated with increase in risk of sudden cardiac death (38) and cardiac arrest during exertion or even sleep. More commonly, it can result in cardiac syncope.

The most commonly used methodology for deriving QTc is the Bazett formula (39), whereby $QTc = QT/\sqrt{RR}$, although this method is thought to overestimate and produce false positives at heart rates outside the 60–80 beats per minute (bpm) range. For faster heart rates (e.g. 80+ bpm) the Friderica correction can be employed, whereby the QT is divided by the cube root of the RR interval ($QTc = QT/\sqrt[3]{RR}$). Other methods such as Framingham and Hodges are also described (39).

QTc prolongation can result from use of both antipsychotics and antidepressants. Among antipsychotics, the evidence for cardiotoxicity is most robust for pimozide (40, p. 64), haloperidol, and sertindole. It is also well established that tricyclic antidepressants are potentially cardiotoxic, especially in those with pre-existing cardiac disease, and may cause left bundle, right bundle, or atrioventricular heart block at high doses (33). Among SSRIs, dose-dependent prolongation of the QT interval has been reported in citalopram and escitalopram, and periodic ECG monitoring should be considered as part of the treatment plan for antidepressant users (41). Antidepressants that increase antipsychotic drug levels via cytochrome P450 interactions (e.g. fluoxetine) (42) may also increase risk of QTc prolongation through this mechanism.

The risk of QTc prolongation and ventricular arrhythmia is increased by a higher dosage of antipsychotics or antidepressants. Other risk factors include older age, female sex, personal or family history of cardiac disorders, personal history of QT prolongation or arrhythmia (or family history of sudden cardiac death), and electrolyte imbalance (e.g. hypokalaemia). Polypharmacy of QTc-increasing medications or medications that produce electrolyte imbalance (e.g. diuretics and corticosteroids) also increases risk.

In the inpatient setting, the best risk reduction measures for arrhythmias are careful history taking of patient risk factors; regular monitoring with a 12-lead ECG, including detailed ECG recording and examination prior to the initiation of therapy; sufficient staff training to recognize abnormalities on the ECG trace and to respond to cardiac emergencies; and instructions to patients and carers to report promptly symptoms such as dizziness or palpitations. If there is significant QTc prolongation, the antipsychotic or antidepressant medication should be discontinued and specialist cardiology advice sought. Torsades de pointes or other ventricular arrhythmias are a medical emergency.

Clozapine has additional important cardiac adverse effects that often occur in the first weeks of treatment. These include persistent tachycardia and potentially lethal myocarditis (which may also occur, although less frequently, with other medications including quetiapine, risperidone, haloperidol, and lithium) (32). Clinical signs of myocarditis include tachycardia, chest pain, dyspnoea, fever, and malaise (43). There may be ECG changes and elevation of blood cardiac and inflammatory markers. Myocarditis is potentially serious and requires discontinuation of clozapine and urgent advice from cardiology. Over the longer term, cardiomyopathy and heart failure can occur.

Sexual side effects

General considerations

Primary sexual disorders are more common than generally appreciated (44). The incidence of sexual dysfunction in those with physical or psychiatric illness, those prescribed medications, and those misusing substances will be higher still (45). An assessment of baseline sexual functioning should probably be conducted in all psychiatric patients especially when psychotropic medication is being considered. Sexual side effects are likely to be an underestimated factor in non-compliance with medication though can also reflect untreated underlying physical or mental illness. Table 12.4 outlines some elements worth addressing in the history and initial investigations to consider when encountering sexual side effects.

Antipsychotics

Sexual dysfunction is extremely common in schizophrenia even during a first episode of psychosis (46). In established illness, its presence is far more common than not. Individuals with psychosis are generally less able to form and maintain good psychosexual relationships. Antipsychotic treatment may in fact improve this. That said, men treated with antipsychotics commonly report reduced desire, inability to achieve or sustain erections, and premature ejaculation. Treated women have reduced fertility.

All antipsychotics have sexual dysfunction as a recognized side effect (5, 47). Studies looking at prevalence are, by and large, poorly controlled. The effects on sexual function are probably mediated through a number of mechanisms. Reducing dopaminergic transmission may reduce libido. The ensuing hyperprolactinaemia is undoubtedly significant in terms of sexual functioning. It is often suggested that the propensity of an antipsychotic to raise prolactin is proportional to its likelihood of causing sexual

Table 12.4 Relevant aspects of patient history and initial investigations in patients reporting sexual side effects

History	Investigations
Physical health	Blood pressure
Psychiatric history	ECG
Medication history	Prolactin levels (≥1 hour after eating/sleep)
Substance misuse	Fasting glucose and lipids
Presence of sexual problems before medication	Thyroid function tests (hypothyroidism may lower libido)
Are the same issues evident when masturbating?	Liver function tests (liver failure can cause sexual dysfunction)
Gynaecomastia	Urea and electrolytes (renal failure can cause sexual dysfunction)
Galactorrhoea	Pregnancy test
Erectile dysfunction, e.g. getting vs maintaining, ability to get morning erections	
Reduced libido	
Ejaculatory problems; premature vs delayed vs absent	
Anorgasmia	
Impact of symptoms on sexual relationship	
Consider menstrual cycle and cause for any abnormalities, e.g. weight/pregnancy	
Consider possible impact of chronic hyperprolactinaemia	

dysfunction. This assertion is not, however, supported by head-to-head trial data such as that from the Cost Utility of the Latest Antipsychotics in Schizophrenia Study (CUtLASS-1) (48). Of the antipsychotics, aripiprazole is comparatively unlikely to cause sexual dysfunction. The anticholinergic action of antipsychotics may reduce arousal while peripheral alpha-1 receptor blockade may be responsible for problems with erection and ejaculation. Antipsychotic-induced weight gain and sedation are also relevant to the aetiology of sexual dysfunction (49). Finally, it is important to counsel patients that individual susceptibility varies and that the effects are reversible.

Figure 12.3 outlines a broad approach to treatment of sexual dysfunction.

Antidepressants

Since the arrival of SSRIs in the 1990s, treatment-related sexual dysfunction has been increasingly recognized as a clinical challenge (50). Drug companies reported an incidence of less than 4% subsuming reduced libido, impotence, delayed ejaculation, and anorgasmia. More recent data, however, report the incidence to be closer to 60–70% for all SSRIs. There is some amelioration in these effects over time (10–21% will resolve even if medication is continued) but such improvement can take months or years. Reasonable first steps may include dose reduction (if appropriate) or 'drug holidays'—that is, missing a dose of shorter-acting SSRIs (e.g. paroxetine/sertraline) in the 24 hours preceding sexual activity (51, 52).

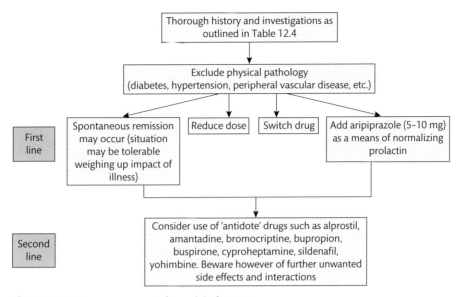

Figure 12.3 The management of sexual dysfunction.

Switching medication is nonetheless commonly required. Agomelatine and bupropion probably pose the lowest risk of sexual dysfunction. Duloxetine, mirtazapine, and trazodone also have more favourable data.

Interventions trialled for drug-induced sexual side effects are listed in Box 12.3. This area is not particularly robustly researched and most of the advice is based on case reports or open-label studies. Findings of the controlled studies are inconclusive. Buspirone (a partial agonist of 5-HT$_{1A}$) may be useful in SSRI-induced sexual dysfunction. Bupropion has been investigated favourably as both an alternative antidepressant with fewer sexual side effects and as an adjunctive treatment, though probably only at higher doses (53).

Sildenafil has been found to be effective in treating SSRI-induced sexual dysfunction despite the observation that SSRI-induced sexual dysfunction is usually decreased libido and delayed orgasm rather than erectile dysfunction. One explanation for this may be the reported improvement in overall sexual satisfaction seen with sildenafil use in both men and women (52).

Cyproheptadine has been observed to reverse SSRI-induced sexual dysfunction but this may be at the expense of their antidepressant and anti-obsessive effects. It is also somewhat sedating.

Conflicting data exist regarding yohimbine, amantadine, amphetamines, and bromocriptine. *Ginkgo biloba*, used at higher doses, has been reported to be of some benefit but the risks of gastrointestinal side effects, bleeding, and confusion probably outweigh the benefits and existing trials have been poorly controlled (52).

Hyponatraemia

Hyponatraemia is the most common electrolyte disorder in clinical practice (54) and is defined as reduction of serum sodium to below 135 mmol/L. Hyponatraemia is often undiagnosed or untreated in psychiatric patients, but it is a potentially life-threatening condition due to risk of cerebral oedema (55, 56). There are numerous medical causes for hyponatraemia, but two special considerations for inpatient psychiatry are (a) hyponatraemia arising as an adverse effect of (psychiatric) medication, and (b) psychogenic polydipsia, the excessive oral intake of fluid in absence of physiological stimulus.

Mild to moderate hyponatraemia (125–135 mmol/L) is often asymptomatic. Symptoms can include lethargy, nausea, headache, dizziness, cramps, confusion, weakness, and—in the case of psychogenic polydipsia—excess drinking and urinary incontinence. When caused by psychiatric medications, hyponatraemia typically occurs during the first few weeks following the onset of treatment. It is not thought to be dose related (5) but the risk increases with polypharmacy of medications that are associated with lowered serum sodium (Table 12.5).

Table 12.5 Medications associated with hyponatraemia

Medication class	Examples
Antidepressants	SSRIs, venlafaxine, duloxetine
Antipsychotics	Amisulpride, aripiprazole, chlorpromazine, clozapine, fluphenazine, haloperidol, olanzapine, pimozide, quetiapine, risperidone, trifluoperazine
Diuretics	Loop diuretics (e.g. furosemide), thiazide diuretics (e.g. amiloride)
Anticonvulsants	Carbamazepine
Antihypertensives	ACE inhibitors Calcium channel antagonists
NSAIDs/COX-2 inhibitors	Celecoxib
Chemotherapy	Vincristine, vinblastine, carboplatin, cisplatin, cyclophosphamide
Opioid analgesics	Tramadol
Proton pump inhibitors	Omeprazole
Antibiotics	Trimethoprim

ACE, angiotensin-converting enzyme; COX, cyclooxygenase; NSAIDs, non-steroidal anti-inflammatory drugs; SSRIs, selective serotonin reuptake inhibitors.

Source data from Guirguis et al. Management of Hyponatraemia: Focus on Psychiatric Patients. *US Pharm.* 2013. 38(11):HS3–HS6.l and Taylor D, Paton C, Kapur S. *The Maudsley prescribing guidelines in psychiatry.* John Wiley & Sons; 2015 Feb 23.

When psychiatric medications induce hyponatraemia, the cause is likely to be the *syndrome of inappropriate antidiuretic hormone secretion* (SIADH). Serotonergic antidepressants, particularly SSRIs, are commonly implicated, but hyponatraemia can arise from antipsychotic use and a number of other medications (Table 12.5). Other risk factors include recent initiation of drug treatment, older age (especially elderly females), low weight, sweating (which is often exacerbated by antidepressants), trauma (especially head trauma), and numerous medical comorbidities (see following paragraphs). Heavy nicotine use and alcoholism, which are common in the psychiatric population, are also associated with hyponatraemia.

Psychogenic polydipsia has an unclear pathophysiology, likely related to abnormal regulation of thirst by the hypothalamus. It is more common in schizophrenia (57) and may also be exacerbated by the dry mouth associated with antipsychotics. In cases of euvolaemic hyponatraemia (see later in this section), it is important for the psychiatrist to distinguish between SIADH-related causes and psychogenic polydipsia. Measurement of serum and urine osmolality enables determination of whether the hyponatraemia is hypovolaemic (low total body water), euvolaemic (normal total body water), or hypervolaemic (excess body water).

Regular monitoring of serum electrolytes is advised for mild to moderate hyponatraemia. In addition to serum electrolytes, the diagnosis of hyponatraemia is based on the investigation of other medical causes, such as dehydration, hypothyroidism, glucocorticoid deficiency, heart failure, renal failure, liver cirrhosis, alcoholism, head injury, and 'pseudohyponatraemia' caused by the metabolic syndrome.

Immediate treatment of hyponatraemia depends on first determining the type and aetiology. Euvolaemic hyponatraemia (including SIADH related) may respond to fluid restriction (e.g. ≤1 L per day). In refractory cases, saline infusion may be recommended, although correction of sodium must not be too rapid due to the risk of cerebral oedema from central pontine myelinolysis. Inhibitors of antidiuretic hormone, such as the tetracycline antibiotic demeclocycline, may be used for SIADH-related hyponatraemia under specialist guidance. Lithium is also an inhibitor of antidiuretic hormone (55); however, in practice, the main consideration for hyponatraemic patients on lithium is careful monitoring for the considerably increased risk of lithium toxicity.

In cases of pharmacologically induced hyponatraemia, discontinuation of the offending medication and fluid restriction is usually sufficient. Rechallenge or commencement of alternative antidepressant/antipsychotic treatment can be attempted when the hyponatraemia has resolved.

Severe hyponatraemia (sodium concentration <120 mmol/L) is a medical emergency and may be accompanied by seizures, coma, and respiratory arrest. Urgent transfer to medical hospital and critical care facilities is recommended.

SSRIs and bleeding

In addition to their effect on the brain, SSRIs also reduce the uptake of serotonin by platelets, which unlike neurons cannot synthesize serotonin and therefore rely on uptake. Serotonin is released by platelets in response to vascular injury and promotes platelet aggregation (58). As a consequence, the risk of haemorrhage, particularly gastrointestinal, increases when SSRIs are commenced (potentially exacerbated by the irritant effect of SSRIs on gastric mucosa through increased gastric acid secretion). This increased risk has been estimated as approximately threefold for upper gastrointestinal bleeds and also other kinds of haemorrhage, such as uterine (59). The absolute risk is, however, relatively low and estimated at 1 in 300 patient years for upper gastrointestinal bleeds, or equivalent to that of a low dose of ibuprofen (60). A meta-analysis has also found that the risk of brain haemorrhage is moderately elevated, although again the absolute risk is low (61). For all forms of SSRI-related haemorrhage, the clinical rather than the theoretical risk is significantly greater in elderly patients and in those with pre-existing haemorrhage risk factors (62).

There is some evidence that antidepressants with particularly high affinity for the serotonin transporter—such as fluoxetine, paroxetine, and sertraline—carry a greater risk than those of more moderate (citalopram, venlafaxine) or low (mirtazapine, nortriptyline, doxepin) affinity (59). The risk of clinically significant haemorrhage is further raised when SSRIs are co-prescribed with other medications associated with bleeding (e.g. aspirin, clopidogrel, warfarin, non-steroidal anti-inflammatory drugs, and corticosteroids).

When commencing a patient on SSRIs, attention should be paid to risk factors for haemorrhage (e.g. older age, alcoholism, peptic ulcer, *Helicobacter pylori* infection, and cirrhosis) (63). Those at increased risk of gastrointestinal bleeding can be considered for lower serotonin affinity antidepressants and also prophylaxis with a proton pump inhibitor or histamine H_2 antagonist. It is not recommended to routinely use gastroprotective agents for those SSRI users not considered at increased risk of haemorrhage (59). A further consideration is whether SSRIs should be continued in the event of major surgery. Current guidance suggests that the risks of stopping antidepressant therapy (withdrawal effects, relapse of illness) outweigh the benefits (64), although this should be calibrated to an individual patient's overall haemorrhage risk.

Serotonin syndrome

Serotonin syndrome is an uncommon but potentially life-threatening psychiatric emergency which results from excess serotonin/5-HT transmission in the central nervous system. It occurs more frequently when multiple serotonergic agents are combined, especially polypharmacy involving a monoamine oxidase inhibitor (MAOI), but any combination of serotoninergic agents (see Table 12.6) could be involved. Use of a single serotonergic agent within therapeutic limits is not usually associated with serotonin syndrome (65).

Serotonin syndrome can present initially with tremor (especially fingers and tongue), stomach upset, and diarrhoea. The presentation tends to be very rapid (e.g. 1 hour) from ingestion of excessive serotonergic agents (65). More advanced cases can lead to agitation and confusion, and on clinical examination there may be pronounced tremor, shivering, hyperthermia, hyperreflexia, rigidity, ataxia, and myoclonus (brief muscular twitching and jerking, especially on ankle dorsiflexion or eye movement). If untreated, these can progress to seizures and death (although mortality occurs in <0.1% cases (66)).

It is important to distinguish serotonin syndrome from NMS, as despite presenting similarly, the two conditions require different management. Both are precipitated by medication use, with serotonergic agents in the case of serotonin syndrome and (usually)

Table 12.6 Medications implicated in serotonin syndrome

Medication class	Examples
Antidepressants	MAOIs, SSRIs, TCAs, SNRIs,
Other psychiatric medications	Lithium, amphetamines, buspirone
Herbal supplements	St John's wort, tryptophan
Opioid analgesics with serotonergic properties	Tramadol, fentanyl, pethidine
Antimigraine medications	Triptans
Antibiotics	Linezolid
Appetite suppressants	Fenfluramine, sibutramine (no longer marketed but may be obtained illicitly)
Illicit substances	MDMA/ecstasy, amphetamines

MAOIs, monoamine oxidase inhibitor; MDNA, 3,4-methyl enedioxy methamphetamine; SNRIs, serotonin and norepinephrine reuptake inhibitors; SSRIs, selective serotonin reuptake inhibitors; TCAs, tricyclic antidepressants.

antipsychotics for NMS. The onset of serotonin syndrome is classically very rapid (hours), whereas NMS progresses more slowly (days/weeks). Serotonin syndrome tends to be characterized by hyperkinesia with moderate muscle rigidity and myoclonus, whereas NMS more usually has severe muscle rigidity and bradykinesia, but no myoclonus (65, 66).

Clinically, mild cases of serotonin syndrome respond within days to cessation of serotonergic medication. Severe serotonin syndrome requires urgent medical attention and intensive care facilities for aggressive supportive therapy, treatment of hyperthermia, and treatment of myoclonus (67). Untreated hyperthermia increases the risk of rhabdomyolysis and multiorgan failure. Intravenous benzodiazepines may be required to control agitation, and other agents such as serotonin receptor antagonists (e.g. intravenous cyproheptadine), intravenous chlorpromazine, and propranolol can be used under specialist guidance (67).

The first risk-reduction step in avoiding serotonin syndrome is recognizing the range of medications that block serotonin reuptake, are serotonin precursors or agonists, or affect serotonin degradation (Table 12.6). Combining these medications requires specialist pharmacist guidance and should be avoided altogether when using MAOIs. When switching from one serotonergic drug to another, an appropriate 'washout' period should be allowed.

Perinatal considerations for psychiatric medications

The decision to continue to prescribe any psychiatric medication during pregnancy involves a careful assessment of the risks to the mother and fetus of the untreated psychiatric illness and potential for relapse (which can be considerable), balanced against the risks to the fetus of adverse effects from the medication, including teratogenicity (first trimester), growth abnormalities, fetal withdrawal reactions, and long-term consequences of fetal drug exposure (68). Close and well-informed partnership between the expectant mother and the prescriber in decision-making is recommended.

The available evidence base for clinical guidance is limited in pregnancy (prospective clinical trials would be unethical) and

continues to evolve, and the clinician is advised to regularly update their clinical knowledge of this area. In discussion with the patient, it may be advisable to continue the current medication regimen with careful monitoring, switch to medications with a better evidence base in pregnancy (always taking stock of the latest advice), or discontinuing the medication and using close nursing support and psychological therapies as appropriate. Up-to-date advice is available from the UK Teratology Information Service (69).

When commencing psychiatric medication in women of childbearing age, it is important to discuss the implications for pregnancy, options for birth control, and obtain a pregnancy test where possible. Women should be encouraged to discuss with their treatment team if they plan to get pregnant. Fertility may be affected by the inhibitory effect of antipsychotics on dopamine's action as a prolactin-inhibiting hormone, which may necessitate a change of antipsychotic if pregnancy is desired.

Sodium valproate and semi-sodium valproate have well-established teratogenicity (including an increase in incidence of spina bifida from 0.005% to 1–2%) (70) and neurotoxicity risks to the fetus (including long-term deficits in cognition and behaviour). Valproate should not be used in women of childbearing age (unless they follow a comprehensive pregnancy-prevention programme) and should not be used in pregnancy unless the woman has a form of epilepsy unresponsive to other antiepileptics (71). Valproate's spina bifida risks are not ameliorated even by high concurrent doses of folic acid.

Carbamazepine is also relatively contraindicated due to significant risks of spina bifida and other malformations (which are nevertheless less than valproate). The fetal risks associated with lamotrigine appear to be closer to the general population, suggesting that lamotrigine is the safest mood stabilizer in pregnancy, although clinical evidence is relatively sparse and specialist guidance is advised. Lithium has been associated with a tenfold increased risk of a congenital abnormality of the tricuspid valve (Ebstein's syndrome), as well as several other malformations. The extent of this risk remains controversial, although lithium use in pregnancy should be avoided if possible, unless antipsychotic medication has not been effective (68). If lithium is used during pregnancy, regular serum level monitoring should be employed (68) and lithium should be discontinued during birth to prevent toxicity (72).

Commonly used antidepressants are not major teratogens (5). There is, however, some evidence that early pregnancy exposure to SSRIs and tricyclic antidepressants, especially paroxetine, is associated with a small increased risk of congenital cardiac defects (73) (absolute risk 1.4% for paroxetine compared with 0.8% in a non-depressed population), although the risk of major congenital deformity overlaps with the general population (74). Among the SSRIs, the best evidence for successful use in pregnancy is available for fluoxetine and sertraline. There is very limited data supporting the use of Serotonin and Noradrenaline Reuptake Inhibitors and mirtazapine in pregnancy, and as such their use cannot currently be recommended over SSRIs. Current clinical guidelines advocate the avoidance of tricyclic antidepressants during pregnancy due to their multiple autonomic side effects which may be harmful to the pregnancy (75), although nortriptyline may be an exception (5).

SSRIs in late pregnancy have been associated with an increased risk of persistent pulmonary hypertension in the newborn, but this is a rare condition (general incidence 0.2% and <1% in neonates exposed to SSRIs in the third trimester), and the relationship remains controversial (74). SSRIs and Serotonin and Noradrenaline Reuptake Inhibitors are associated with a moderate increase in risk of pre-eclampsia, hypertension of pregnancy, and postpartum haemorrhage. Use of SSRIs in late pregnancy has been associated with a neonatal withdrawal syndrome including irritability, tremor, hypotonia, poor sleep, and decreased suckling. This is reportedly more common in short half-life antidepressants (e.g. paroxetine and venlafaxine) (76).

Low-dose first-generation antipsychotics have been in use for decades for treatment of hyperemesis gravidarum, but there is a lack of drug-specific reports of the use of antipsychotics at psychiatric therapeutic doses in pregnancy (74). The evidence for second-generation psychotics is even less complete. For all antipsychotics, there appears to be a modest increase in risk of low birth weight, premature delivery, and gestational diabetes (77), and possible small increased risk of congenital malformations (although first- and second-generation antipsychotics are not considered major teratogens (5)). An antipsychotic withdrawal syndrome has also been reported alongside risk of EPSEs in the newborn. Depot antipsychotics and anticholinergic medications should be avoided during pregnancy. The most comprehensive reproductive safety data are available for quetiapine, olanzapine, risperidone, and haloperidol (5), but pharmacist advice should be sought.

There has been concern that benzodiazepine use in pregnancy is associated with a twofold increased risk of cleft lip and cleft palate, although a meta-analysis of nine studies and 1 million pregnancies found risk overlapped with the general population (odds ratio 1.07; 95% confidence interval 0.91–1.25) (78). There is evidence linking use of benzodiazepines in later pregnancy to preterm birth, low birth weight, and a neonatal withdrawal syndrome. It is therefore recommended to use the lowest possible dose and rapid elimination benzodiazepines (such as lorazepam) if rapid tranquilization or sedation is required for a pregnant inpatient.

When using any psychiatric medication in pregnancy, it is important to pay careful attention to the dosage and the patient's individual relapse signatures—not least because understandable excessive caution on the part of prescribers risks subtherapeutic dosing and resultant relapse.

Many psychiatric drugs taken at therapeutic doses are not thought to be harmful in breastfeeding (79), although this does not include carbamazepine, clozapine, lithium, or benzodiazepines with long half-lives (and also excludes valproate which should not be used in women of childbearing potential). Among antidepressants, fluoxetine and citalopram are excreted in relatively high amounts in breastmilk and are not recommended (44). There is limited information from clinical trial data regarding safety in breastfeeding, and medication manufacturers generally tend to advise against it, but this must be weighed against the significant benefits of breastfeeding to the infant in the early months and the wishes of the mother. National Institute for Health and Care Excellence updated guidelines (72) encourage women with mental health issues to breastfeed, unless they are taking carbamazepine, clozapine, or lithium (also excluding valproate). Among the antipsychotics, olanzapine and sulpiride show relatively small levels of drug excreted in breastmilk. Among antidepressants, sertraline, paroxetine, nortriptyline, and imipramine are among the agents of choice (80). The UK Medicines Information service can provide further information (81).

Further information

In this chapter, we have endeavoured to cover some of the most relevant, concerning, and problematic adverse reactions to psychotropic medications encountered in an inpatient setting. Inevitably, there will be presentations not covered, for example, clozapine-induced neutropenia/agranulocytosis and lithium-induced renal toxicity, but these are well described and their management reviewed in other resources.

In addition to the *British National Formulary*, further information on psychiatric medications and their adverse effects from the respective manufacturers is available from the Electronic Medicines Compendium (https://www.medicines.org.uk/emc). *The Maudsley Prescribing Guidelines in Psychiatry* (David Taylor et al., Wiley Press) is a frequently updated, comprehensive, and well-referenced guide to psychiatric prescribing. The Medicines and Healthcare products Regulatory Agency (MHRA) provides online learning modules on antipsychotics, SSRIs, benzodiazepines, and other medications with details of adverse effects and how to reduce medicines risk (https://www.gov.uk/government/publications/e-learning-modules-medicines-and-medical-devices/e-learning-modules-medicines-and-medical-devices).

The Yellow Card scheme is a system for reporting suspected adverse drug reactions from medicines (and other regulated medicinal substances) in the UK. In the event of encountering a suspected adverse effect of a drug which appears not to have been described in the sources detailed in the preceding paragraph, 'Yellow Cards' can be completed electronically at https://yellowcard.mhra.gov.uk or hard copies can be found at the back of the *British National Formulary* and posted to the MHRA.

REFERENCES

1. Gervin M, Barnes TR. Assessment of drug-related movement disorders in schizophrenia. *Adv Psychiatr Treat* 2000;6:332–341.
2. American Psychiatric Association. Practice guideline for the treatment of patients with schizophrenia. III. Treatment principles and alternatives. *Am J Psychiatry* 1997;154:7–34.
3. van Harten PN, Hoek HW, Kahn RS. Acute dystonia induced by drug treatment. *BMJ* 1999;319:623.
4. Casey DE. Neuroleptic-induced acute dystonia. In: Lang AE, Weiner WJ (eds), Drug-Induced Movement Disorders, pp. 21–40. Mount Kisco, NY: Futura; 1992.
5. Taylor D, Paton C, Kapur S. *The Maudsley Prescribing Guidelines in Psychiatry*. Chichester: John Wiley & Sons; 2015.
6. Cunningham-Owen DG. *A Guide to the Extrapyramidal Side-Effects of Antipsychotic Drugs*. Cambridge: Cambridge University Press; 1999.
7. Thanvi B, Treadwell S. Drug induced parkinsonism: a common cause of parkinsonism in older people. *Postgrad Med J* 2009;85:322–326.
8. Nguyen N, Pradel V, Micallef J, Montastruc JL, Blin O. Drug-induced Parkinson syndromes. *Therapie* 2003;59:105–112.
9. Barnes TR. The Barnes Akathisia rating scale—revisited. *J Psychopharmacol* 2003;17:365–370.
10. Halstead SM, Barnes TR, Speller JC. Akathisia: prevalence and associated dysphoria in an in-patient population with chronic schizophrenia. *Br J Psychiatry* 1994;164:177–183.
11. American Psychiatric Association. *Tardive Dyskinesia: A Task Force Report of the American Psychiatric Association*. Washington, DC: American Psychiatric Publishing; 1992.

12. Correll CU, Schenk EM. Tardive dyskinesia and new antipsychotics. *Curr Opin Psychiatry* 2008;21:151–156.

13. Woods SW, Morgenstern H, Saksa JR, et al. Incidence of tardive dyskinesia with atypical versus conventional antipsychotic medications: a prospective cohort study. *J Clin Psychiatry* 2010;71:463–474.

14. Peritogiannis V, Tsouli S. Can atypical antipsychotics improve tardive dyskinesia associated with other atypical antipsychotics? Case report and brief review of the literature. *J Psychopharmacol* 2010;24:1121–1125.

15. Caroff SN, Davis VG, Miller DD, et al. Treatment outcomes of patients with tardive dyskinesia and chronic schizophrenia. *J Clin Psychiatry* 2011;72:295–303.

16. Simpson GM. The treatment of tardive dyskinesia and tardive dystonia. *J Clin Psychiatry* 1999;61:39–44.

17. Leung JG, Breden EL. Tetrabenazine for the treatment of tardive dyskinesia. *Ann Pharmacother* 2011;45:525–531.

18. Glazer WM. Expected incidence of tardive dyskinesia associated with atypical antipsychotics. *J Clin Psychiatry* 2000;61:21–26.

19. Delay J, Pichot P, Lemperiere T, Elissalde B, Peigne F. A non-phenothiazine and non-reserpine major neuroleptic, haloperidol, in the treatment of psychoses. *Ann Med Psychol (Paris)* 1960;118:145.

20. Guzé BH, Baxter LR Jr. Neuroleptic malignant syndrome. *N Engl J Med* 1985;313:163–166.

21. Jahan MS, Farooque AI, Wahid Z. Neuroleptic malignant syndrome. *J Natl Med Assoc* 1992;84:966.

22. Stübner S, Rustenbeck E, Grohmann R, et al. Severe and uncommon involuntary movement disorders due to psychotropic drugs. *Pharmacopsychiatry* 2004;37:54–64.

23. Shalev A, Hermesh H, Munitz H. Mortality from neuroleptic malignant syndrome. *J Clin Psychiatry* 1989;18:25–50.

24. Medicines and Healthcare products Regulatory Agency. 3.2.3 Neuroleptic malignant syndrome. 2018. http://www.mhra.gov.uk/antipsychotics-learning-module/con155606?useSecondary=&showpage=16

25. Barrett KE, Barman SM, Boitano S, Brooks H. *Ganong's Review of Medical Physiology*, 25th edition. New York: McGraw-Hill Medical Publishing Division; 2015.

26. Bostwick JR, Guthrie SK, Ellingrod VL. Antipsychotic induced hyperprolactinemia. *Pharmacotherapy* 2009;29:64–73.

27. Haddad PM, Wieck A. Antipsychotic-induced hyperprolactinaemia. *Drugs* 2004;64:2291–2314.

28. Holt RI, Peveler RC. Antipsychotics and hyperprolactinaemia: mechanisms, consequences and management. *Clin Endocrinol* 2011;74:141–147.

29. Nelson JC, Bell PM, Guy ST. Hyperprolactinaemia and antipsychotics. *BJPsych Adv* 2015;21:240–241.

30. Brown R, Frighi V. Antipsychotic-induced hyperprolactinaemia – Oxford Health NHS Foundation Trust guideline for identification, monitoring and management. 2015. http://www.oxfordhealthformulary.nhs.uk/docs/AntipsychoticinducedhyperprolactinaemiaguidelineJuly2015.pdf?UNLID=2082094120151222131512

31. Melmed S, Casanueva FF, Hoffman AR, et al. Diagnosis and treatment of hyperprolactinemia: an Endocrine Society clinical practice guideline. *J Clin Endocrinol Metab* 2011;96:273–288.

32. Mackin P. Cardiac side effects of psychiatric drugs. *Hum Psychopharmacol* 2008;23:3–14.

33. Marano G, Traversi G, Romagnoli E, et al. Cardiologic side effects of psychotropic drugs. *J Geriatr Cardiol* 2011;8:243–253.

34. Thomassen R, Vandenbroucke JP, Rosendaal FR. Antipsychotic medication and venous thrombosis. *Br J Psychiatry* 2001;179:63–66

35. Committee on Safety of Medicines. Atypical antipsychotic drugs and stroke: message from Professor Gordon Duff, Chairman, Committee on Safety of Medicines. 2004. http://webarchive.nationalarchives.gov.uk/20141206131857/http://www.mhra.gov.uk/home/groups/pl-p/documents/websiteresources/con019488.pdf

36. Schneider LS, Dagerman KS, Insel P. Risk of death with atypical antipsychotic drug treatment for dementia: meta-analysis of randomized placebo-controlled trials. *JAMA* 2005;294:1934–1943.

37. Gareri P, De Fazio P, Manfredi VG, De Sarro G. Use and safety of antipsychotics in behavioural disorders in elderly people with dementia. *J Clin Psychopharmacol* 2014;34:109–123

38. Strauss SM, Kors JA, De Bruin ML, et al. Prolonged QTc interval and risk of sudden cardiac death in a population of older adults. *J Am Coll Cardiol* 2006;47:362–367

39. Vandenberk B, Vandael E, Robyns T, et al. Which QT correction formula to use for QT monitoring? *J Am Heart Assoc* 2016;5:e003264.

40. Puri BK. *Drugs in Psychiatry*. Oxford: Oxford University Press; 2013.

41. Dodd S, Mitchell PB, Bauer M, et al. A consensus statement for safety monitoring guidelines for major depressive disorder. *Aust N Z J Psychiatry* 2011;45:712–725.

42. Bleakey S. Antidepressant drug interactions: evidence and clinical significance. *Prog Neurol Psychiatry* 2016;2016:21–27.

43. Knoph KN, Morgan III RJ, Palmer BA, et al. Clozapine-induced cardiomyopathy and myocarditis monitoring: a systematic review. *Schizophr Res* 2018;199:17–30.

44. Healy D. *Psychiatric Drugs Explained*, 6th edition. Edinburgh: Elsevier Health Sciences; 2016.

45. Lewis RW, Fugl-Meyer KS, Bosch R, et al. Epidemiology/risk factors of sexual dysfunction. *J Sex Med* 2004;1:35–39.

46. Montejo ÁL, Majadas S, Rico-Villademoros F, et al. Frequency of sexual dysfunction in patients with a psychotic disorder receiving antipsychotics. *J Sex Med* 2010;7:3404–3413.

47. Serretti A, Chiesa A. A meta-analysis of sexual dysfunction in psychiatric patients taking antipsychotics. *Int Clin Psychopharmacol* 2011;26:130–140.

48. Peluso MJ, Lewis SW, Barnes TR, Jones PB. Non-neurological and metabolic side effects in the Cost Utility of the Latest Antipsychotics in Schizophrenia Randomised Controlled Trial (CUtLASS-1). *Schizophr Res* 2013;144:80–86.

49. Serretti A, Chiesa A. Sexual side effects of pharmacological treatment of psychiatric diseases. *Clin Pharmacol Ther* 2011;89:142–147.

50. Baldwin DS. Sexual dysfunction associated with antidepressant drugs. *Expert Opin Drug Saf* 2004;3:457–470.

51. Serretti A, Chiesa A. Treatment-emergent sexual dysfunction related to antidepressants: a meta-analysis. *J Clin Psychopharmacol* 2009;29:259–266.

52. Taylor MJ, Rudkin L, Bullemor Day P, Lubin J, Chukwujekwu C, Hawton K. Strategies for managing sexual dysfunction induced by antidepressant medication. *Cochrane Database Syst Rev* 2013;5:CD003382.

53. Clayton AH, Croft HA, Horrigan JP, et al. Bupropion extended release compared with escitalopram: effects on sexual functioning and antidepressant efficacy in 2 randomized, double-blind, placebo-controlled studies. *J Clin Psychiatry* 2006;67:736–746.

54. Adrogué HJ, Madias NE. Hyponatraemia. *N Engl J Med* 2000;342:1581–1589.

55. Reynolds RM, Padfield PL, Seckl JR. Disorders of sodium balance. *BMJ* 2006;332:702.

56. Guirguis E, Grace Y, Seetaram M. Management of hyponatraemia: focus on psychiatric patients. *US Pharm* 2013;38: HS3–HS6.

57. Dundas B, Harris M, Narasimhan M. Psychogenic polydipsia review: etiology, differential and treatment. *Curr Psychiatry Rep* 2007;9:236–241.

58. Skop BP, Brown TM. Potential vascular and bleeding complications of treatment with selective serotonin reuptake inhibitors. *Psychosomatics* 1996;37:12–16.

59. Paton C. SSRIs and gastrointestinal bleeding. *BMJ* 2005;331:529–530.

60. de Abajo FJ, Rodríguez LA, Montero D. Association between selective serotonin reuptake inhibitors and upper gastrointestinal bleeding: population based case control study. *BMJ* 1999;319:1106–1109.

61. Hackham DG, Mrkobrada M. Selective serotonin reuptake inhibitors and brain haemorrhage: a meta-analysis. *Neurology* 2012;79:1862–1865.

62. Topiwala AG, Chouliaras L, Ebmeier KP. Prescribing selective serotonin reuptake inhibitors in old age. *Maturita* 2013;77:118–123.

63. Mehta D, Hafferty J. Selective serotonin reuptake inhibitors learning module. MHRA; 2015. http://www.mhra.gov.uk/ssri-learning-module/con146583?usesecondary=&showpage=25

64. Mrkobrada M, Hackam DG. Selective serotonin inhibitors and surgery: to hold or not to hold, that is the question: comment on "Perioperative use of selective serotonin reuptake inhibitors and risks for adverse outcomes of surgery". *JAMA Intern Med* 2013;173:1082–1083.

65. Buckley NA. Serotonin syndrome. *BMJ* 2014;348:1626.

66. Semple D, Smyth R. *Oxford Handbook of Psychiatry*. Oxford: Oxford University Press; 2005.

67. Pedavally S, Fugate JE, Rabinstein AA. Serotonin syndrome in the intensive care unit: clinical presentations and precipitating medications. *Neurocrit Care* 2014;21:108–113.

68. Chisolm MS, Payne JL. Management of psychotropic drugs during pregnancy. *BMJ* 2015;351:h5918.

69. UK Teratology Information Service. Homepage. http://www.uktis.org/

70. Galbally M, Roberts M, Buist A, Perinatal Psychotropic Review Group. Mood stabilizers in pregnancy: a systematic review. *Aust N Z J Psychiatry* 2010;44:967–977.

71. Wieck A, Jones S. Dangers of valproate in pregnancy. *BMJ* 2018;361:k1609.

72. National Institute for Health and Care Excellence. Antenatal and postnatal mental health: clinical management and service guidance. Clinical guideline [CG192]. 2014 (last updated 2018). https://www.nice.org.uk/guidance/cg192

73. Ban L, Gibson JE, West J, et al. Maternal depression, antidepressant prescriptions, and congenital anomaly risk in offspring: a population-based cohort study. *BJOG* 2014;121:1471–1481.

74. Vitale SG, Laganà AS, Muscatello MR, et al. Psychopharmacotherapy in pregnancy and breastfeeding. *Obstet Gynecol Surv* 2016;71:721–733.

75. Scottish Intercollegiate Guidelines Network. Management of perinatal mood disorders: a national clinical guideline. 2012. https://www.guideline.gov/summaries/summary/36811

76. Stiskal JA, Kulin N, Koren G, Ho T, Ito S. Neonatal paroxetine withdrawal syndrome. *Arch Dis Child Fetal Neonatal Ed* 2001;84:F134–F135.

77. Reis M, Källén B. Maternal use of antipsychotics in early pregnancy and delivery outcome. *J Clin Psychopharmacol* 2008;28:279–288.

78. Enato E, Moretti M, Koren G. The fetal safety of benzodiazepines. *J Obset Gynaeco Can* 2011;33:46–48.

79. Anderson IA, McAllister-Williams RH (eds). *Fundamentals of Clinical Psychopharmacology*, 4th edition. Boca Raton, FL: CRC Press; 2016.

80. di Scalea TL, Wisner KL. Antidepressant medication use during breastfeeding. *Clin Obstet Gynaecol* 2009;52:483–497.

81. UK Medicines Information. Homepage. http://www.ukmi.nhs.uk/

13

Substance misuse disorders on the psychiatric ward

Gail Critchlow and Theodoros Bargiotas

Introduction

The focus of this chapter is the management of substance misuse and addiction on the psychiatric ward in patients who have presented with a psychiatric disorder. Some patients will display other forms of addictive behaviour such as gambling, sexual activity, or Internet use. Where this is not the primary focus, the same principles of broad-based biopsychosocial management apply.

There are a number of guidelines available, such as those from the Department of Health (the 'Orange Book') (1) and the National Institute for Health and Care Excellence (2–5), and prescribing advice, such as the British Association for Psychopharmacology guidelines (6) and *The Maudsley Prescribing Guidelines in Psychiatry* (7), that are useful references for the treatment of patients with substance misuse disorders and addiction.

This chapter does not seek to replicate this advice, but does include useful and common scenarios that will be encountered on the general psychiatric ward.

Epidemiology and nosology

Abuse of psychoactive substances is commonplace and prevalent around the world. Addiction disorders are considered to be psychiatric disorders in their own right and share biopsychosocial factors in common with other mental disorders. As the issues presented are multifactorial and complex, the approach requires a dual diagnosis or comorbidity model of management.

Treating a dual diagnosis patient can be challenging in the acute psychiatric ward environment and patients will present with varying motivation to engage in treatment. However, it is important to also note that interventions for substance misuse are evidence based and effective.

Drug misuse is common in the UK. The most recent report (8) estimates that 34.7% of 16–59-year-olds have used an illicit drug at least once during their lifetime. There has been a general decrease in drug use over the last 10 years in the UK but an increase in the use of novel and new psychoactive substances (previously referred to as 'legal highs'). Excluding tobacco and alcohol, cannabis is the most common drug with a prevalence of 3.7% in 16–59-year-olds. This is followed by cocaine and 3,4-methylenedioxymethamphetamine (MDMA).

More than 9 million people drink more than the recommended daily and weekly limits of alcohol (9).

Substance misuse has a wide range of forms and severity, depending on variables such as drug of choice, monosubstance or polysubstance use, amount and frequency of use, length of use, social circumstances and impact of drug use, functional impairment, the presence of dependence, and withdrawal.

The international classification for psychiatric diagnosis of substance misuse disorders (10) covers mental and behavioural disorders due to a variety of substances or polysubstance with criteria for substance intoxication, harmful use, and dependence. See Table 13.1 for features of dependence (11).

Table 13.1 Features of dependence syndrome

Salience	Use of the substance is prioritized, otherwise known as primacy
Compulsion to use	Lack of personal control over use, manifested by repeated unsuccessful efforts to cut down, use despite harmful consequences
Tolerance	Using more over a period of time to achieve intoxication or control of withdrawals
Withdrawal	A combination of physical or psychological symptoms on reduction of use
Relief use	Using substance to reverse withdrawals
Narrowed repertoire	Stereotyped pattern of use with forgoing of alternative activity
Reinstatement	Resurgence of features of dependence when using after a period of abstinence.

Source data from Edwards, G and Gross, M. (1976) Alcohol Dependence: Provisional Description of a Clinical Syndrome. *British Medical Journal*, 1: 1058–106.

The problem of dual diagnosis

The prevalence of substance misuse among psychiatric populations is high; this has long been recognized and referred to as dual diagnosis. Approximately 40% of patients with psychosis misuse substances at one point in their lifetime, with approximately one-third suffering from harmful use or dependence (12–14).

Common comorbidities include cannabis abuse in patients with depression, attention deficit hyperactivity disorder, or anxiety; alcohol dependence in patients with social anxiety, depression, or personality disorder; and novel psychoactive substances and amphetamines in patients with psychosis.

Inpatient psychiatric populations lie at the most severe end of the spectrum of psychiatric populations. Dual diagnosis is associated with hospitalization, poorer outcomes, poorer physical health, and higher cost:

- *Increased risk.* The relationship between substance abuse, crime, violence, and mental illness is well established. Less well understood is the relationship of particular substances and patterns of use to offending. Alcohol (and possibly crack cocaine) has an association with domestic violence. Substance misuse is generally associated with repeated offending (8).
- *Stigma, discrimination, and therapeutic nihilism.* Staff may perceive the patient as unworthy of care and treatment as they are seemingly making a choice to damage themselves and 'disobey' ward rules. Drug users are generally socially disadvantaged and suffer high rates of social hardship such as homelessness, criminalization, and unemployment.
- *Increased treatment failure* due to synergistic effects between mental illness and substance misuse. For instance, a suspicious and paranoid psychotic patient may be less likely to engage with addiction programmes; side effects of psychotropic drugs may sedate the patient and reduce their ability to participate in meaningful activity. Patients who are acutely mentally unwell generally have difficulties with attention, judgement, and decision-making which will further undermine their ability to evaluate their substance use and engage in treatment. Negative symptoms will also interfere with treatment engagement.
- *Patients may harbour incorrect beliefs* about the role of substance misuse in their mental illness. For example, that the escapist qualities of alcohol will help the depressed patient feel better whereas the opposite is actually true.

There are specific issues of dual diagnosis on the acute ward. Addiction may be missed, and symptoms of intoxication wrongly attributed to other forms of psychiatric disorder. There is a risk of untreated withdrawals from alcohol, opiates, or benzodiazepines that are a risk to health. Psychiatric assessment and clerking can fail to adequately assess and treat addictions aspects of presentation, with inaccurate assessment and recording of the substance misuse elements. There may be poor engagement of the patient with a lack of shared goals and ongoing substance misuse in the ward. Attribution errors may occur where improvement from a period of abstinence is mistaken as evidence for psychiatric treatments and medication.

Models of dual diagnosis

Dual diagnosis is best thought of within a model of shared vulnerability with complex causality and significant genetic and familial influences (15). Therefore, a joint biopsychosocial understanding of the conditions is preferable to a parallel model.

In the UK, service delivery for psychiatry is generally organized and commissioned separately from that of addictions. This division of services and knowledge can therefore be problematic in attempts to jointly manage dual diagnosis. Expertise and knowledge in assessing and treating addiction disorders is essential in the inpatient ward. The ward can seek specialist advice from addiction services.

Some patients (e.g. those who require ongoing opioid substitution therapy) will need ongoing input from addiction services. Addiction services should be involved in management of the patient via the Care Programme Approach (12) with the psychiatric team providing care coordination.

Substance misuse treatment has a variety of approaches ranging from abstinence focused to harm reduction or 'minimization', depending on the needs of the patient. There has been an emphasis away from long-term opioid substitution therapy and maintenance to more 'recovery'-focused approaches within the last few years (16). Similarly, there are still programmes such as needle exchange and hepatitis immunization which are not focused on drug misuse per se but reduce some of the risks of using and are useful contacts to encourage engagement into longer-term treatment. Psychiatric wards should always consider harm reduction strategies (such as hepatitis immunization) as valid interventions.

General principles of assessment of substance misuse problems in the dual diagnosis patient

On the ward, there should be a biopsychosocial assessment with detailed information about the substance misuse pattern (suggest recording a 'typical day' and the last 3 days of use in detail with pattern of use, association with symptoms, quantity and route of use, and any combinations).

The past substance misuse and psychiatric history should be taken in detail noting age of first use, relationship to psychiatric illness, and any periods of abstinence. Patients with severe psychiatric problems may find communication difficult so use of collateral information, such as medical records and third-party information, is essential as is careful assessment and observation of the patient in the ward environment.

Motivation and stage of change (17) should be assessed in order to target interventions at the right level. Patients may move between a state of pre-contemplation to various levels of insight and ambivalence before they garner a recovery (so-called action and maintenance). Motivation is changeable dependent on circumstances and approach to treatment and staff should see themselves as active participants in helping the patient move forward.

Physical history and examination is crucial. Substance misuse patients (particularly injectors or those with severe alcohol problems) may present with a medical emergency such as acute Wernicke's encephalopathy, bacterial endocarditis, or refeeding syndrome.

Table 13.2 Suggested assessment for substance misuse patients

Treat emergency first	Note overdose and poisoning, adverse drug reaction (such as MDMA), acute agitation with stimulants, acute delirium, acute infection, deep vein thrombosis, fits
Establish that the patient uses drugs or alcohol	Observe signs of acute intoxication or withdrawal, e.g. smelling of alcohol, urine drug screen, breathalyser, history, examination, collateral information, and notes
Drug and alcohol history	Note pattern of using, route, and amount of use Symptoms of dependence: assess 'typical day' or last 3 days' use, age of using, any periods of abstinence? Any complications present such as overdose?
Mental state examination	Note intoxication and withdrawal
Physical examination	Stigmata of use, e.g. low weight, intravenous sites Full systems examination and review
Investigations	Liver, full blood count, general profile, ECG (note QTc prolongation risk especially with methadone and psychiatric drugs), others investigations such as magnetic resonance imaging as clinically indicated
Withdrawal scales and response to treatment	Use scales to assess withdrawals and response to treatment such as CIWA-Ar scale for alcohol, COWS for opioids
Collateral information	GP summary including hepatitis immunization Communicate with pharmacy if on medication; particularly confirm any supervised consumption of opioid substation therapy
Family and children	Note names, date of birth, and school of children, associated with patient, any social services involvement or concern

Source data from Department of Health (England) and the devolved administrations (2007). *Drug Misuse and Dependence: UK Guidelines on Clinical Management.* London: Department of Health (England), the Scottish Government, Welsh Assembly Government and Northern Ireland Executive. Contains public sector information licensed under the Open Government Licence v3.0 http://www.nationalarchives.gov.uk/doc/open-government-licence/version/3/.

Particular drugs are associated with some common ill effects listed in the following section. If in doubt, seek specialist toxicological and addictions advice.

Drug testing should be available on the ward via both near-patient testing (using a ward-based test often for drugs such as opioids, benzodiazepines, cocaine, amphetamines, and cannabis) and access to some specialist tests for novel drugs. There are specialist analysis laboratories that are able to test for a battery of new psychoactive substances if this is considered to be clinically important. Note that drug intoxication can also be *observed*. Table 13.2 outlines a supplementary assessment to the 'general psychiatric clerking' and Table 13.3 outlines some commonly encountered harmful effects of drugs.

Treatment of substance misuse problems on wards

Alcohol

Untreated or undertreated alcohol withdrawal has a number of dangerous and unwanted consequences. If there are complications such as Wernicke's encephalopathy, alcohol withdrawal seizures, and delirium tremens the patient should be treated in the general hospital. Patients who misuse alcohol may also present with other serious medical conditions such as pancreatitis or acute cardiomyopathy and these also require urgent medical intervention.

General features of alcohol withdrawal

These features include fear, low mood, anxiety, sensitivity to sound, light, and touch, fleeting hallucinations, tremor, agitation, hypertension, and tachycardia. There is a risk for delirium tremens which presents with marked disorientation and confusion, hallucinosis and delusions, and a mortality risk of around 10%. Assisted alcohol

Table 13.3 Some harmful effects of drugs

Type of drug	Drug examples	Possible harmful effects
Hallucinogens or cannabinoids	LSD Psilocybin Mescaline Cannabis and 'spice'	Acute confusion and accidents Psychosis Tobacco smoking risks
Stimulants, modified amphetamines, and other drugs combining reality distortion and excitement	Amphetamine Mephedrone Cocaine 'Ecstasy' (MDNA) Novel psychoactive substances	Acute psychosis Depression and anxiety Insomnia Overheating, dehydration Hypertension and related complications Weight loss
Unpredictable drugs; causing excitement, reality distortion, and drowsiness	Ketamine (K) Phencyclidine GHB and GBL	Acute thought disorder and poor judgement Overdose, analgesic injury Bladder problems (K)
Opioids	Heroin, methadone, buprenorphine	Overdose Injecting complications (e.g. viral disease, infections, deep vein thrombosis) Note: Methadone: prolonged QTc
Alcohol and benzodiazepines	Wine, beers and spirits, alcopops, diazepam	Depression Delirium and dementia Hallucinosis Fits
Image- and performance-enhancing drugs	Anabolic steroids, Botulinum toxin and 'melanotan' Modafinil or 'smart drugs'	Injecting complications Depression and anxiety, hypertension

detoxification should be offered for all patients either experiencing or at risk of developing acute alcohol withdrawal who consume over 15 units per day or have an Alcohol Use Disorders Identification Test (AUDIT) score over 20 (18).

Alcohol detoxification as an inpatient can be either fixed dose or symptom triggered as there are staff available to monitor and assess the severity of withdrawal in real time. Benzodiazepines or carbamazepine can be used for alcohol detoxification but clomethiazole should only be used in a supervised environment as it increases the risk of overdose and other complications.

For fixed dose schedules, starting doses of benzodiazepine (e.g. diazepam or chlordiazepoxide) are determined by the expected severity of withdrawal and other factors such as the age of the patient (lower doses for elderly) and comorbidities such as liver disease. Patients with liver disease should be given lower doses of benzodiazepines to prevent toxicity. Oxazepam can be used as it has a shorter half-life.

Starting doses should be observed and titrated so that medication is adequate to cover withdrawal but does not incapacitate and intoxicate the patient. The dosing should also generally be 'front loaded' to adequately medicate the patient at the time of peak complications. An example withdrawal schedule is given in Table 13.4.

Symptom-triggered detoxification relies on a formal measure of alcohol withdraw such as the Clinical Institute Withdrawal Assessment for Alcohol, revised (CIWA-Ar) (19). The advantage here is that dosing is titrated to severity, overall fewer drugs are used, and peak control of symptoms is derived at the highest risk time for complications, generally front-loading plasma levels (20). The protocol is to administer 20 mg diazepam every 2 hours for each CIWA-Ar score over 11 and stop when there are two consecutive scores over 11. Maximum dose is usually under 200 mg in 24 hours, but could be extended by a specialist in cases of severe withdrawals.

Acamprosate, naltrexone, nalmefene, and disulfiram

Acamprosate is a useful addition to alcohol detoxification as it reduces alcohol use and craving over the longer term but also has a putative neuroprotective effect during acute detoxification (21). It is generally well tolerated and has few side effects. Naltrexone and nalmefene (22) are opioid receptor antagonists which have been shown to have efficacy in reducing alcohol misuse and should be offered in combination with psychological interventions for dependent drinkers. Disulfiram can also be used but in conjunction with specialist services. It is contraindicated in psychosis, severe depression, and personality disorders so is not suitable for many inpatients. It causes an aversive reaction when combined with alcohol and is associated with enforcing abstinence.

Table 13.4 Suggestion of a fixed dose schedule using diazepam

	09.00	12.00	17.00	22.00
Day 1 (mg)	20–30	10	10	10
Day 2 (mg)	10	10	10	10
Day 3 (mg)	10	–	10	10
Day 4 (mg)	5	–	5	10
Day 5 (mg)	5	–	–	5
Day 6 (mg)	–	–	–	5

Box 13.1 Patients at risk of thiamine deficiency complications

- Severe alcohol withdrawal and dependence.
- Poor diet.
- Vomiting or other gastrointestinal disturbance.
- Patients being treated in a hospital setting.
- Patients at risk of refeeding syndrome (monitor potassium).
- Comorbidity and long-term conditions.

Thiamine and vitamins

Parenteral thiamine and vitamin prophylaxis should generally be used in inpatient settings. The dose is *one* pair of ampoules of Pabrinex® daily for 5 days (7) and to continue with oral thiamine (300 mg daily) and multivitamins until discharge. Those at chronic risk of relapse and malnutrition on discharge should be continued on 100 mg thiamine daily indefinitely in the community. See Box 13.1 for risk factors.

Patients requiring opioid withdrawal stabilization

Symptoms of opioid withdrawal should be assessed using a scale such as the Clinical Opioid Withdrawal Scale (COWS) (23) to ascertain severity of withdrawal: mild, moderate, or severe. Special consideration should be made of the pre-existing risk profile, significant mental health problems (note psychiatric inpatients will usually present with psychiatric risk), injecting drug use, and overdose history. Opioid substitution therapy using buprenorphine or methadone has favourable effects on reducing drug-related risk and reducing illicit opioid misuse (16).

General features of opioid withdrawal

The features of opioid withdrawal include anxiety, aching, restlessness, sweating, yawning, large pupil, gooseflesh, diarrhoea, tachycardia, tears, and runny nose.

Ward scenarios

Existing treatment: a patient admitted to the ward is already under treatment for opioid dependence using opioid substitution therapy (using methadone, buprenorphine, or Suboxone® (buprenorphine–naloxone))

Suggested treatment: contact community drug team and general practitioner (GP) to confirm treatment history. Contact community pharmacy to ascertain last dose of *supervised* consumption. If within 3 days and patient compliant for the preceding 7 days, continue with the same dose. If the patient has missed doses for more than 3 consecutive days, the dose needs to be re-titrated as per titration guidelines (see 'Titration guideline onto opioid substitution therapy'). Importantly, failure to take into account lowered tolerance could result in a fatal opioid overdose on the ward.

Low-risk patient or mild withdrawal

This includes occasional heroin smokers and over-the-counter misuse of opioid-containing medications.

Suggested treatment—offer the patient symptomatic relief as follows:

- Abdominal cramps: hyoscine butylbromide 20 mg four times a day.
- Diarrhoea: loperamide 4 mg initially, then 2 mg with each loose stool.

- Muscle and joint pain: ibuprofen 400–600 mg three times a day; paracetamol 500 mg–1 g four times a day.
- Anxiety and agitation: diazepam 5 mg four times a day.

Lofexidine 400 micrograms twice a day can be used as an adjunct for control of withdrawal as long as the QTc interval is within normal limits on the electrocardiogram (ECG).

Moderate to severe withdrawals in heroin users (smoking or injecting) with significant mental health history

Suggested treatment: titrate onto buprenorphine or methadone and stabilize dose; suggest period of maintenance treatment before planning structured detox via specialist drug services if the patient stabilizes.

Severe withdrawals in high-risk patient (such as opioid overdose and injecting with viral transmission risk behaviours)

Suggested treatment: methadone maintenance treatment (unless contraindicated) at adequate dose, supervised on ward, and plan for supervised consumption via pharmacy on discharge. Joint working with specialist drug services.

Titration guideline onto opioid substitution therapy

Titration using buprenorphine

Assess severity of opioid withdrawal. If definite withdrawal symptoms present, issue 4 mg buprenorphine. If equivocal or very mild symptoms, issue 2 mg.

As buprenorphine is a partial agonist it can precipitate worsening withdrawals if the patient has recently used methadone or heroin. If this happens, suspend the titration and use symptomatic relief until rechallenge. See Table 13.5 for a suggested induction.

Titration using methadone

Methadone is toxic in opioid-naïve or low-level dependent patients and should be used on the ward with caution. Methadone can also lengthen the QTc interval and cause fatal arrhythmias. An ECG should be performed before use and then repeated on the ward once titrated. However, methadone remains the gold standard for opioid replacement therapy (5) as it has beneficial effects in preventing drop-out from treatment.

Suggested treatment: assess severity of withdrawal. If definite withdrawals present, then issue 20 mL methadone mixture, 1 mg per 1 mL. Reassess the patient in 2 hours. If significant and objectively observed withdrawals persist, issue a further 10 mg methadone. Maximum dose on day 1 is 40 mg but this requires careful assessment and monitoring and ideally the involvement of a specialist.

Methadone has a half-life which can be in excess of 24 hours so it accumulates in plasma during the first week of treatment. This should be considered when ascertaining dose levels; generally increases should only be done weekly unless by a specialist. Target

dose range is between approximately 60 mg and 120 mg methadone daily. This may not be achieved until several weeks have elapsed.

Naltrexone

Naltrexone is an opioid antagonist that can be used to assist a period of abstinence from opioids. It should be used after specialist assessment generally for well-motivated and informed patients who understand the risks of lowered tolerance in relapse.

Benzodiazepine dependence

Patients may be dependent on illicit or prescribed benzodiazepines. Some may exhibit symptoms of benzodiazepine withdrawals. It must be kept in mind that illicit users can overestimate their daily consumption to maximize prescribing. Illicit benzodiazepine misuse increases risk in polydrug users (such as overdose) and there is no evidence that substitute prescribing alters this risk.

Ward scenarios

Existing treatment in long-term prescribed user, no alcohol misuse, and no illicit drug misuse. No evidence of missed doses, dose under 30 mg diazepam or equivalent daily.

Suggested treatment: confirm prescription with GP and continue prescribed dose, look to negotiate reduction when patient is mentally well. Observe response to initial dose including any symptoms of intoxication or withdrawal. Alter dose accordingly if problems.

Existing treatment for drug misuser via GP or drug service. It is now rare that substance misuse patients are prescribed benzodiazepines as the risks (such as diversion and abuse of medication) are well recognized. A safe starting dose and reduction regimen should be discussed with the treating team and the patient. This dose should usually be under 30 mg diazepam equivalent; the response to dose should be observed and adjusted and be reduced under supervision by the ward.

Illicit benzodiazepine misuse: the patient should be monitored for benzodiazepine withdrawal (using a scale such as the Clinical Institute Withdrawal Assessment for Benzodiazepines (CIWA-B) (24)) and prescribed diazepam only if symptoms of withdrawal are observed. If there are concerns about withdrawal seizures, carbamazepine could be considered instead. If diazepam is prescribed, the dose should be the lowest to control withdrawals and not exceed 30 mg diazepam. The medication should be reduced during the inpatient stay. No drugs should be given to take away on discharge. If there is an excess on discharge, consider issuing as a supervised daily dose in conjunction with the community drugs team.

Rate of reduction: for genuine long-term benzodiazepine dependence, a safe rate of reduction is approximately 1/15 to 1/10 dose every 2 weeks (25). However, for short-term or binge users the time should be reduced and most reductions can be achieved within 2 weeks (refer to https://www.benzo.org.uk for more detailed advice).

Intoxication or withdrawals from stimulants, cannabis, or novel psychoactive substances

Symptoms should be assessed on a case-by-case basis. Symptomatic relief can be used including a short course of benzodiazepine to reduce agitation and anxiety. Consider advice from addictions services and toxicology services.

Table 13.5 Suggested induction schedule for buprenorphine

	Day 1	Day 2	Day 3	Days 4–7
Buprenorphine dose	4–8 mg	6–12 mg (day 1 plus 2–4 mg)	8–16 mg (day 2 plus 2–4 mg)	8–16 mg (day 3 plus 2–4 mg)

For some drugs, such as ketamine or cannabinoids ('spice'), patients will present either in acute intoxication or with a more prolonged period of psychosis perhaps lasting a number of days. In these cases, there is a clear relationship between substance misuse and symptomatology. Longitudinal assessment, use of collateral history, and observation will usually lead to a clear diagnosis. Generally, psychosis that is chronic and debilitating despite some drug use tends to be a process of illness and indicative of a true comorbidity such as schizophrenia or bipolar disorder, rather than so-called drug-induced psychosis.

Hepatitis A and B immunization and harm reduction

Patients at risk of hepatitis C (such as intravenous drug users and crack smokers) should have the accelerated course of Twinrix® combined hepatitis A and B immunization if they have not received this already. Patients may wish to undergo viral testing but this is not required before immunization. Patients should have advice on viral transmission (including safer sex) and be encouraged not to inject. If they do inject they should use clean needles and be put in touch with needle exchange programmes. Some drug services train users in life support and the use of naloxone for overdose.

Psychiatric medication and substance misuse

Drugs of misuse cause unwanted effects and harms both directly and as a result of drug interactions with psychiatric drugs. Some of these are common and important drug interactions. Substance misuse generally decreases the efficacy of psychiatric treatment (such as drinking while on antidepressants). Attention should be paid to drug interactions and potential toxicity, obtaining specialist pharmacological advice (26).

Patients with major psychiatric disorders should not be denied psychiatric drug treatment because they have substance misuse problems. However, drug interactions, efficacy, and toxicity should be considered in the treatment of choice and monitored closely. See Table 13.6 for some drug interactions.

Psychological therapies for patients with substance misuse

On the ward, psychosocial interventions can be delivered by general ward staff, such as nurses and psychologists. The interventions offered will depend on the stage of change and the severity

Table 13.6 Common significant drug interactions

Tobacco and cannabis smoking	Increase clearance and decrease plasma levels of antipsychotics, particularly significant of clozapine
Stimulants and MDMA Ketamine	Increase risk of serotonin syndrome with antidepressants, lower fit threshold in combination with antipsychotics. QTc prolongation. MAOI hypertensive crisis All cause acute psychosis that is not reversed by antipsychotics
Alcohol	Increases cocaine toxicity (coca-ethanol), decreases efficacy of antidepressants, drowsiness with antipsychotics
Opioids and methadone (illicit or prescribed)	QTc prolongation in combination with antipsychotic, antidepressant, mood stabilizers MAOI drug toxicity

Table 13.7 A decisional balance sheet: 'My use of crack cocaine'

Good things about using	Bad things about using
Excitement, a buzz, using with friends, escapism, more energy	No money, get arrested, family upset, end up in hospital, lose too much weight
Good things about not using	**Bad things about not using**
Feel better and healthier, more money, more interests	Get bored, lack confidence, worried about losing friends

of the patient's problems. There are a number of interventions including residential rehabilitation available for patients with addictions. These interventions are beyond the scope of the general psychiatric ward but can be accessed via referral to drug and alcohol teams.

The inpatient ward can offer the following types of intervention:

* Psychoeducation about drugs, alcohol, and risk/complications.
* Brief interventions using FRAMES (27): Feedback, Responsibility, Advice, Menu of options, Empathy, and promote Self Efficacy.
* Brief motivational interventions such as drawing up a motivational balance sheet (with pros and cons of using and not using).
* Referral into day programmes, local assessments for residential rehabilitation, Alcoholics Anonymous and Narcotics Anonymous facilitation, and referral into other evidence-based interventions such as cognitive behaviour therapy/relapse prevention.
* Ward-based interventions and group programmes to develop psychological skills such as 'handling difficult emotions', 'assertiveness', or 'anxiety management'.
* Referral into assessment for other specialist programmes such as complex needs and therapeutic community programmes for people with personality disorders. Table 13.7 is an example of a decisional balance in a crack cocaine user.

Evidence for specific dual diagnosis treatment

It is generally accepted that addiction treatment is effective with a combination of psychosocial interventions (such as brief interventions and motivational enhancement therapy) and pharmacological treatments (such as opiate substitution therapy and craving modifying drugs, such as acamprosate) when such treatment exists for a specific substance.

In terms of specific treatment for dual diagnosis, there is some evidence for clozapine in treating patients who have a dual diagnosis with treatment-resistant schizophrenia, albeit if substance misuse is continued there is a greater occurrence of drug interactions (28). Clozapine treatment has been shown to reduce the number of drinking days in alcohol-dependent patients and may have a direct effect on the pathophysiology of addiction via dopamine-mediated effects.

There have been several attempts to produce bespoke programmes for dual diagnosis and some limited evidence for benefits of integrated approaches such as combining psychiatric treatment, motivational enhancement, cognitive behaviour therapy, and family intervention (Motivational Interventions for Drug and Alcohol use in Schizophrenia (MIDAS) trial (29, 30)).

The legal framework and the use of drugs

Wards are required to have robust policies and procedures when dealing with illicit drug misuse. If the ward is seen as allowing drug abuse on the premises there can be legal consequences for staff under Section 8 of the Misuse of Drugs Act 1971 (31). In the Wintercomfort case, charity workers were jailed for not taking reasonable steps to prevent heroin dealing (32). Similarly, there have to be procedures for confiscation, disposal, and declaration of any drug found on the ward on patients. This includes procedures for searching wards and possessions, the use of drug testing, and in some cases even sniffer dogs.

Patients who are dependent on drugs should not drive until they have been stable and abstinent (including on stable prescribed treatment) in most cases for a year but there are variations which lengthen this period, for instance, comorbid conditions and the driving regulator such as the Driver and Vehicle Licensing Agency (DVLA) (33) should be notified. The patient should be fully involved in these discussions and be encouraged to engage with the process. If a patient is using drugs or drinking and driving and not informing the DVLA there is an onus on services to inform them for public safety. The police should be involved if an offence has been or is about to be committed.

The Mental Health Act 1983 (34) makes an exception for drug and alcohol use as a reason for detention but patients with coinciding mental disorder and substance misuse, including psychiatric symptoms as a result of substances, are covered. Note again that substance misuse can increase the risk of harm to self and others for patients with other illnesses such as psychosis.

Safeguarding concerns and domestic violence

Patients with substance misuse problems are more likely than others to be perpetrators or victims of domestic abuse and violence. The Domestic Abuse, Stalking and Honour Based Violence Risk Identification Model (DASH) (35) should be used if there is domestic violence and staff should be trained in its use. The V-DASH which is self-administered can also be used. This both promotes awareness and stratifies response (including the police) in conjunction with a multiagency approach. Safeguarding concerns about children (note that all contacts should be fully recorded at assessment) or adults should have formal referral via local safeguarding arrangements such as Multi Agency Safeguarding Hubs (MASHs).

Implications for psychiatric wards

The divide between addictions and generic mental health services has meant that there is a growing gap both in service provision and knowledge about addictions and substance misuse. There is a need for training in substance misuse and dual diagnosis for psychiatrists, but also training in the recognition of dual diagnosis for GPs and substance misuse workers.

Wards should actively involve substance misuse services via the Care Programme Approach and seek to build bridges, for instance in training, wherever they can. Staff on wards should also be encouraged that substance misuse treatment works, whether it is aimed at abstinence or harm reduction, and that careful assessment and monitoring of dual diagnosis patients both protects their health and the security of the ward.

Conclusion

Dual diagnosis is common both within wards and in community psychiatric patients. Generic staff on wards should have knowledge and skills in treating dual diagnosis patients and being able to coordinate and collaborate with specialist agencies as required. Dual diagnosis is complex and an integrated approach to treatment is required. Treatment for substance misuse problems has evidence of efficacy. However, targeted or combined approaches for dual diagnosis are still being developed. Wards should seek to positively engage substance users in treatment.

REFERENCES

1. Department of Health and Social Care. *Drug Misuse and Dependence: UK Guidelines on Clinical Management*. London: Department of Health and Social Care; 2017.
2. National Institute for Health and Care Excellence. Alcohol-use disorders: diagnosis, assessment and management of harmful drinking and alcohol dependence. Clinical guideline [CG115]. 2011. https://www.nice.org.uk/guidance/cg115
3. National Institute for Health and Care Excellence. Alcohol use disorders: diagnosis and management of physical complications. Clinical guideline [CG100]. 2010. https://www.nice.org.uk/guidance/cg100
4. National Institute for Health and Care Excellence. Drug misuse in over 16s: opioid detoxification. Clinical guideline [CG52]. 2007. https://www.nice.org.uk/guidance/cg52
5. National Institute for Health and Care Excellence. Methadone and buprenorphine for the management of opioid dependence. Technology appraisal guidance [TA114]. 2007. https://www.nice.org.uk/guidance/ta114
6. Lingford-Hughes A, Welch S, Peters L, et al. BAP updated guidelines: evidence-based guidelines for the pharmacological management of substance abuse, harmful use, addiction and comorbidity: recommendations from BAP. *J Psychopharmacol* 2012;26:899–952.
7. Taylor D, Paton C, Kapur S. *The Maudsley Prescribing Guidelines in Psychiatry*, 12th edition. Oxford: Wiley Blackwell; 2015.
8. European Monitoring Centre for Drugs and Drug Addiction. Country Report UK 2014/15. 2016. http://www.emcdda.europa.eu
9. Alcohol Concern. Alcohol statistics. 2016. https://www.alcoholconcern.org.uk/alcohol-statistics
10. World Health Organization (WHO). *International Statistical Classification of Diseases and Related Health Problems (ICD-10)*. Geneva: WHO; 1992.
11. Edwards G, Gross M. Alcohol dependence: provisional description of a clinical syndrome. *Br Med J* 1976;1:1058–1106.
12. Department of Health. *Mental Health Policy Implementation Guide: Dual Diagnosis Good Practice Guide*. London: Department of Health; 2002.
13. Weaver T, Madden P, Charles V, et al. Comorbidity of substance misuse and mental illness in community mental health and substance misuse services. *Br J Psychiatry* 2003;183:304–313.

14. Pickard H, Fazel S. Substance abuse as a risk factor for violence in mental illness: some implications for forensic psychiatric practice and clinical ethics. *Curr Opin Psychiatry* 2012;4:249–354.

15. Kendler KS, Davis CG, Kessler RC. The familial aggregation of common psychiatric and substance use disorders in the National Comorbidity Survey: a family history study. *Br J Psychiatry* 1997;170:541–548.

16. National Treatment Agency. *Recovery-Orientated Drug Treatment: An Interim Report by Professor John Strang, Chair of the Expert Group.* London: National Treatment Agency; 2013.

17. Prochaska JO, DiClemente CC. Trans-theoretical therapy—toward a more integrative model of change. *Psychotherapy* 1982;19:276–288.

18. Saunders JB, Aasland OG, Babor TF, et al. Development of the Alcohol Use Disorders Identification Test (AUDIT): WHO Collaborative Project on Early Detection of Persons with Harmful Alcohol Consumption – II. *Addiction* 1993;88:791–804.

19. Sullivan JT, Sykora K, Schneiderman J, Naranjo CA, Sellers EM. Assessment of alcohol withdrawal: the revised Clinical Institute Withdrawal Assessment for Alcohol scale (CIWA-Ar). *Br J Addict* 1989;84:1353–1357.

20. Day E, Patel J, Georgiou G. Evaluation of a symptom-triggered front-loading detoxification technique for alcohol dependence: a pilot study. *Psychiatr Bull* 2004;28:407–410.

21. De Witte P, Littleton J, Parot P, Koob G. Neuroprotective and abstinence-promoting effects of acamprosate: elucidating the mechanism of action. *CNS Drugs* 2005;19:517–537.

22. National Institute for Health and Care Excellence. Nalmefene for reducing alcohol consumption in people with alcohol dependence. Technology appraisal guidance [TA325]. 2014. https://www.nice.org.uk/guidance/ta325

23. Wesson DR, Ling W. The Clinical Opiate Withdrawal Scale (COWS). *J Psychoactive Drugs* 2003;35:253–259.

24. Busto UE, Sykora K, Sellers EM. A clinical scale to assess benzodiazepine withdrawal. *J Clin Psychopharmacol* 1990;9:412–416.

25. Ashton CH. How to withdraw from benzodiazepines after long-term use. In: Benzodiazepines: how they work and how to withdraw (aka The Ashton Manual). 2002. http://www.benzo.org.uk/manual/bzcha02.htm

26. Dean A. Illicit drugs and drug interactions. *Aust Pharm* 2006;25:685–689.

27. Henry-Edwards S, Humeniuk R, Ali R, et al. *Brief Intervention for Substance Use: A Manual for Use in Primary Care. (Draft Version 1.1 for Field Testing).* Geneva: World Health Organization; 2003.

28. Marin-Major M, Lopez-Alvarez J, Lopez-Munoz F, et al. Clozapine use in dual diagnosis patients. *J Clin Med Res* 2014;1:11–20.

29. Barrowclough C, Haddock G, Tarrier N, et al. Randomised controlled trial of cognitive behavioural therapy plus motivational intervention for schizophrenia and substance use. *Am J Psychiatry* 2001;158:1706–1713.

30. Barrowclough C, Haddock G, Wykes T, et al. Integrated motivational interviewing and cognitive behavioural therapy for people with psychosis and comorbid substance misuse: randomised controlled trial. *BMJ* 2010;341:c6325.

31. Legislation.co.uk. Misuse of Drugs Act 1971, Chapter 38. https://www.legislation.gov.uk/ukpga/1971/38

32. Weale S. The unlikely criminals. *The Guardian* 2010;10 July. https://www.theguardian.com/society/2000/jul/10/homelessness

33. Driver and Vehicle Licencing Authority. Assessing fitness to drive: a guide for medical professionals. 2016. https://www.gov.uk/government/publications/assessing-fitness-to-drive-a-guide-for-medical-professionals

34. Department of Health. *Reference Guide for the Mental Health Act 1983.* London: Department of Health; 2015.

35. DASH Risk Checklist. DASH risk model. http://www.dashriskchecklist.co.uk

14

Electroconvulsive therapy

Emad Sidhom and David Welchew

Historical background

Electroconvulsive therapy (ECT) can be defined as the passage of a brief electric current through the brain, with the intention of inducing a seizure. It has been established that having a seizure is a prerequisite for effective treatment; however, not every seizure means that ECT has been performed effectively—the ultimate measure is clinical improvement, as reported by the patient and observed by the treating clinician.

From a taxonomic point of view, ECT belongs to the group of physical treatments in psychiatry, and predates all current pharmacological treatments by a decade or more. Current physical treatments all involve direct or indirect stimulation of the brain, and can be subclassified in various ways—for example, cephalic and noncephalic, electric and magnetic, convulsive and non-convulsive, and invasive and non-invasive (Table 14.1).

The predecessors of ECT in psychiatry included chemical convulsions induced by camphor oil or pentylenetetrazol (Metrazol®). These were effective, but difficult to control, and were profoundly unpleasant for patients (1). Non-convulsive electrotherapy was briefly in vogue during the second half of the nineteenth century (2) and its use declined by the 1920s (3), due to concerns about its lack of efficacy (4). ECT was first administered to humans in April 1938, and rapidly superseded the earlier treatments due to its efficacy, tolerability, and ease of administration. Following its introduction, ECT went through a period of development in two main domains—effective stimulation and safe administration.

Initially, ECT delivered sine wave stimuli (50–60 Hz), similar to an attenuated version of the 'wall-socket' supply. Various modifications were proposed, and the form of the stimulus was refined over time. Brief-pulse ECT (0.5–2 ms pulses) was first suggested in the 1940s by Lieberman, and by the 1970s this had become the dominant wave form, due to its superior efficacy in eliciting a seizure and lower incidence of side effects. This rectangular-shaped stimulus provides a steep rise in electric current as compared to the slow rise of the sine wave, and has provided a platform for the emergence of calculated electric doses.

Most modern, non-urgent ECT involves a process of tailoring the dose to the individual patient. The ECT pioneer Cerletti noted that different people have different seizure thresholds and hence require variation in the electric dose, with higher electric doses associated with better improvement but more pronounced side effects. Dose titration is the concept of establishing the minimum dose sufficient to induce a seizure, and then increasing by multiples of this dose to optimize the balance of efficacy and side effects.

The safety of early ECT was compromised by reports of fractures and dislocations, resulting from the expression of a motor convulsion at full strength. The introduction of muscle relaxants overcame this, and necessitated the use of general anaesthesia to avoid distress (the administration of a convulsive electric stimulus to the head is not in itself a painful procedure, as it causes an almost instantaneous loss of consciousness). In the UK, the Bolam case (5) highlighted the unacceptable risks of 'unmodified' (awake) ECT, and accelerated the introduction of anaesthesia. The use of muscle relaxants made observation of the motor seizure less reliable, and spurred the introduction of electroencephalographic (EEG) monitoring, which is now the gold standard for confirming that a seizure has ended.

Indications and contraindications for electroconvulsive therapy

The National Institute for Health and Care Excellence (NICE) states that ECT can be used in severe depressive illness and it can be also considered in moderate depression that has not responded to multiple treatments. The use of 6–12 ECT treatments has a (Ia) level of evidence for efficacy in depression, particularly when associated with psychosis or significant suicidal ideation, where it can achieve remission rates of 80–95% (6). NICE also suggests that ECT can be used to achieve rapid (short-term) relief of symptoms in severe or prolonged mania, and for catatonia (of any cause), where these are either life-threatening, or have proved resistant to other treatments (7). For these conditions, ECT can be life-saving, and it should not be considered only as a last choice treatment (6). ECT can achieve

Table 14.1 Brain stimulation in psychiatry

Treatment	Site	Type of stimulation	Convulsiveness	Invasiveness
Electroconvulsive therapy	Cephalic	Electric	Convulsive	Non-invasive
Magnetic seizure therapy	Cephalic	Magnetic	Convulsive	Non-invasive
Deep brain stimulation	Cephalic	Electric	Non-convulsive	Invasive
Repetitive transcranial magnetic stimulation	Cephalic	Magnetic	Non-convulsive	Non-invasive
Vagus nerve stimulation	Non-cephalic	Electric	Non-convulsive	Non-invasive

full recovery in 80% of patients with catatonia, and in 73% of those with bipolar depression (8).

The World Health Organization reported that ECT is probably more effective than drug treatments in depression (9). The American Psychiatric Association (10) and the guidelines of British Columbia (11) classify the use of ECT into primary use in depression, mania, and schizophrenia (especially where there is an abrupt onset of positive symptoms), and secondary indications including motor symptoms of Parkinson's disease and intractable seizure disorder. The NICE technology appraisal guidance on ECT also states that it is occasionally used in schizophrenia (12), but at the time of the updated appraisal, there was insufficient evidence to recommend its use. ECT was used effectively to augment non-clozapine antipsychotic medication in patients with treatment-resistant schizophrenia (13). Subsequent randomized controlled trials lend a degree of support to the use of ECT to augment clozapine in patients with intractable positive symptoms of psychosis (14–16). ECT can also be considered in pregnant women who suffer severe mood disorders that put the health of the mother or fetus at serious risk, although particular caution is required due to the anaesthetic and procedural risks of pregnancy.

There are also reports with varying levels of evidence describing ECT having been used successfully in first-episode psychosis (17), schizoaffective disorder (18), neuroleptic malignant syndrome (which some authors consider as a variant of malignant catatonia) (19), Parkinson's disease (for both motor (20) and depressive symptoms (21)), and as a treatment of last resort in status epilepticus (22), delirium, and acute confusional states (23). There are case reports on the use of ECT in treatment-resistant delusional disorder (24), and it has been prescribed in excited states following cocaine, amphetamine, and LSD (lysergic acid diethylamide) intoxication (25).

There are no absolute contraindications to ECT, and the procedure has been used safely in children and adolescents (26) and in adults as old as 102, as well as in pregnancy and the puerperium (27). However, extreme caution has to be taken in cases of cardiovascular instability, increased intracranial pressure, recent cerebral infarction, unstable chronic obstructive pulmonary disease, and in general for cases with an unfavourable American Society of Anesthesiologists physical status grade (25). There are other less severe risks such as dental damage, gastro-oesophageal reflux disease (GORD), and GORD during pregnancy. These will rarely lead to a decision against using ECT, but are worth addressing to minimize the risks being weighed against the benefits of ECT.

It is important to weigh the benefits of ECT against the individual risks for the patient, and to explain this process to the patient in a straightforward way if their condition allows. Close liaison between prescribing psychiatrists and ECT anaesthetists can help determine whether the risks are justified, and whether they can be ameliorated prior to treatment.

Prescribing electroconvulsive therapy: consent and patient information

In the UK, best practice in ECT requires that patients who have the capacity to do so provide written and informed consent, regardless of whether they are subject to involuntary detention in hospital. Information given to the patient must include an estimate of its efficacy in their case, information about general anaesthesia, a discussion of side effects, and any reasonable alternatives to ECT (including their risks) (28). The Royal College of Psychiatrists has developed an information leaflet about ECT, and many ECT services can support referrers by providing locally tailored information in various formats. Some patients (and their carers) may also appreciate the opportunity to visit their local ECT suite, both to ask questions of the ECT team and to familiarize themselves with the facility.

In England, where an adult patient is subject to detention in hospital under a Section of the Mental Health Act 1983 that allows involuntary treatment, their informed consent should still be sought if they have the capacity to give this. In addition to locally agreed consent forms, this consent is also recorded on the statutory Form T4. Where the patient lacks capacity to accept or refuse ECT, the opinion of a 'Second Opinion Appointed Doctor' must be sought. If ECT must begin before this opinion can be given to save the patient's life or prevent a serious deterioration in their condition, this can be authorized by the patient's Responsible Clinician under Section 62 of the Act.

Prescribing electroconvulsive therapy: dose and route

ECT is a generalized brain treatment that does not offer localization over a specific brain region. It was originally given bilaterally, however, concerns regarding cognitive side effects led to the emergence of unilateral electrode placement, which was intended to minimize cognitive side effects. Other placements have been developed, but have not entered into widespread use, such as bifrontal (29) and left anterior right temporal (30). The use of bilateral ECT has been associated with better efficacy across different diagnoses, capacity to delay rehospitalization (31), but also with more pronounced cognitive side effects, relative to unilateral electrode placement (32).

Seizure threshold varies according to patient factors such as age, sex, body mass index (33), and head anatomy (34). It can be increased by medications such as barbiturates, benzodiazepines, and antiepileptics, making it harder to induce a seizure, or even preventing seizures altogether, as can occur with valproate (35). The seizure threshold can be lowered by antipsychotics (particularly clozapine) and antidepressants. Recent ECT treatment may also increase the seizure threshold. Empirical stimulus dose titration is a way of providing a personalized electric dose to each individual, as the many interacting variables make accurate prediction of the threshold impractical, but will delay the first effective treatment in patients with a high threshold.

Where the situation is not immediately life-threatening, a prescriber should usually request that titration be carried out, and the protocol will be determined by the local ECT service. Any such protocol represents a trade-off between clinical efficacy, speed of obtaining an effect, and adverse effects. Other variables that should be considered include of the choice of unilateral or bilateral ECT, and to what extent the ECT team should consider restimulation at higher electric doses in cases of inadequate seizures. Relevant patient variables include illness severity, and whether the psychiatric disorder poses a threat to the life of the patient. Comorbid medical disorders are also taken into consideration. Due to the complex interplay of these factors, the decision is usually made collaboratively between the treating doctor and the lead ECT clinicians.

In brief, during the first session, titration begins by the team administering up to three small but increasing electric doses and observing for seizures. Seizure threshold is (arbitrarily) inferred as the smallest electric charge sufficient to induce a seizure.

In the second session, the electric charge administered will be a multiple of the assumed seizure threshold. In bilateral ECT, a moderately suprathreshold stimulus is used (usually 1.5 times the seizure threshold), whereas for unilateral ECT a markedly suprathreshold stimulus is administered (typically six times the seizure threshold). In bilateral ECT, administering ECT at a moderately suprathreshold stimulus is a trade-off between efficacy and side effects—however, for unilateral ECT, the markedly suprathreshold stimulus is necessary for efficacy. After this, the electric dosage continues so long as an adequate seizure is elicited. Over the years, various arbitrary cut-off points have been taken to represent an 'adequate' seizure—for example, a minimum of 15 seconds of motor seizure. More recently, this approach has been challenged on the basis of lack of correlation between seizure duration and clinical improvement. The EEG findings including postictal voltage suppression and changes in EEG waveform features may provide more robust correlation between seizure adequacy and clinical improvement (36), but the most important point is for the referring team to closely document and communicate to the ECT team the patient's progress, and the extent of any side effects, to accurately guide the course of treatment.

In cases where rapid improvement can be life-saving, as in malignant catatonia, neuroleptic malignant syndrome, or severe suicidality due to depression, the use of preselected dosage strategy or protocols that are based on age and sex, or age alone, may be justified as the clinical need for urgent improvement supersedes the concern about short-term side effects. In one example of age-based dosing, the bilateral dose is estimated as 2.5 times age (in millicoulombs) (37). This 'half-age'[1] method seems to induce seizure more robustly in patients who are not receiving benzodiazepines (38).

Monitoring a course of electroconvulsive therapy

Monitoring a course of ECT entails observing the interplay of clinical improvement, adverse effects, and dose parameters. Proper assessment can lead to safer practice, and more effective treatment. Clinical improvement is the definitive outcome of ECT. A satisfactory assessment of outcome requires serial assessments at baseline, during treatment, and after the end of an ECT course. The use of assessment scales may help to provide a structure for comparing different points in treatment, especially where more than one clinician will be involved in the process. Some scales can be used across various diagnoses, such as the Clinical Global Impressions Scale (39). For depression, the Beck Depression Inventory or Montgomery–Åsberg Depression Rating Scale can be used. In catatonia, the Bush–Francis Catatonia Rating Scale (40) has been one of the most widely used scales for monitoring of catatonia (41). In psychoses, the Brief Psychiatric Rating Scale may be used. The use of psychometric assessment scales is not, however, a substitute for full clinical assessment before, during, and after the ECT course.

The side effects of ECT are broadly classified as cognitive and non-cognitive (35). Cognitive side effects are usually short-lived, subsiding within a few weeks after ECT (35). These include impairment of anterograde, visuospatial, and retrograde autobiographical memory. In practice, this means that patients may have only patchy recall of the period of an acute course of ECT after it finishes. Partial retrograde amnesia for events immediately preceding treatment is not uncommon, but does not usually extend beyond 6 months into the past. Some patients do report loss of autobiographical memories earlier than this, and estimates in the literature are wide, in part due to the intrinsically subjective nature of the complaint (42).

The detection of cognitive side effects can be confounded by the impact of the underlying illness, as depression, catatonia, and mania can all cause cognitive impairment. In addition, there are the side effects of psychotropic medications, especially those with anticholinergic effects (43). A commonly used battery of assessment of cognitive side effects is the Montreal Cognitive Assessment (44); previously, the Mini-Mental State Examination (and modified forms of it) has been used. Naturally, the sensitivity of the assessment tool will influence sensitivity to cognitive side effects. Some studies have suggested the use of oral thiamine and donepezil in management of ECT-induced cognitive impairment (45), although this is not yet in widespread use.

Given that severe depression can cause profound impairment of memory, patients being treated for this may also report an improvement in memory following treatment (46). Baseline assessment of cognitive function is essential where the patient can engage with this. Time to reorientation following each treatment is a strong

---

[1] Half-age is so-called because the dosage setting on a certain widespread ECT machine will be half the patient's age to achieve the required dose in millicoulombs.

predictor of post-ECT retrograde amnesia (47, 48), and this should be tracked in the ECT suite's recovery room if possible.

ECT can cause damage to the teeth, due to the supraphysiological bite cause by direct electrical stimulation of the masseter muscles. Pretreatment assessment of dentition is essential, and where problems are identified, or where a patient has orthodontic implants or prostheses, a dental opinion should be sought on how to best reduce the risk (if the patient's clinical state allows); careful use of bite guards, and if necessary a switch from bilateral to unilateral paddle placement, can also reduce these risks. Headache is a common side effect of ECT, which is usually transient and responsive to simple analgesia. Where the headache is recurrent and severe, pretreatment with ibuprofen (30, 49) is helpful, and for particularly treatment-resistant headache the use of topiramate has been suggested (50). Myalgia, nausea, and transient ocular inflammation (51) are also observed in some patients, and are usually short-lived. ECT is ten times safer than childbirth, and the death rate by ECT has been calculated to be smaller than the spontaneous death rate in the general population (52). In one study, the mortality rate was 0.19 per 10,000 treatments (53).

During a course of ECT, the frequency of sessions, electrode placement, and stimulus intensity may change to allow for an adequate seizure and to address clinical improvement and side effects, in order to provide an optimized personalized treatment. On the ward, it is recommended that medications that increase the seizure threshold be reduced or stopped prior to treatment if possible. The patient should have nil by mouth the night before ECT. The nursing care plan needs to take account of this, and an appropriate level of observation is of paramount importance to ensure the safety of patients, as inadvertent or deliberate eating or drinking prior to treatment may carry the risk of aspiration under anaesthesia.

The presence of a clearly written protocol or pathway as well as checklists can help to improve the standardization of monitoring of a course of an ECT. Auditing this process on a regular basis helps to guard against attrition or deviation from the protocol, as well as provoking discussions regarding improving and updating local protocols.

When to continue or discontinue electroconvulsive therapy

ECT is usually stopped as soon as remission is achieved. Patients who have not responded to psychopharmacological interventions may benefit from continuing with ECT. Continuation ECT (C-ECT) is defined as the administration of ECT to prevent relapse of symptoms, following an index course of ECT, and can last up to 6 months (54). Maintenance ECT (M-ECT) is defined as prophylactic treatment against recurrence of the illness following a period of remission (10). In some instances, these terms are used interchangeably, such as in the NICE guidance, which currently takes a neutral position regarding C-ECT and M-ECT (35). There is no consensus regarding the frequency and intensity in C-ECT and M-ECT. However, there is a tendency to reduce the frequency of ECT as compared to the index ECT course. One recently-developed alternative is the Symptom-Titrated, Algorithm-Based Longitudinal ECT (STABLE) algorithm, which varies the weekly treatment schedule (between zero and two

treatments) based on that week's Hamilton Depression Rating Scale score (55).

There is no preset number of sessions that would define an 'ECT course', although in the UK the modal range is 6–12 treatments. ECT is best delivered as a dynamic and tailored treatment where clinical response and side effects determine the direction of the treatment.

Where there has been no response to ECT after six adequate treatments, it is important to re-evaluate the clinical situation. In particular, the diagnosis should be reconfirmed, the presence of any untreated comorbid problems evaluated, medications affecting seizure threshold reviewed, and the EEG quality of the seizures re-examined, along with the electric dose. Consideration should also be given to switching from unilateral to bilateral treatment. For patients experiencing a severe depressive episode, 40% of patients with no response after six treatments will still go on to achieve remission (35). The decision whether to continue in the face of lack of effect is generally based on the severity of the underlying condition, the presence of medication that can interfere with ECT efficacy (and whether this can safely be stopped), the degree to which treatment can be further optimized, the potential to augment ECT with medication, and the availability of any adequate alternative treatments. It has been proposed that provided that all conditions are optimal, it is unlikely that a patient will show a response if there is no observable improvement after 12 sessions (35).

Use of medication during electroconvulsive therapy

Benzodiazepines, antiepileptic medication, and barbiturates tend to reduce the seizure duration (56). Zopiclone was shown to attenuate the motor-seizure duration in animal models (57), but the clinical significance of this is unclear. With respect to lithium, it seems that patients on lithium take longer to recover from ECT in a manner that is directly correlated with its serum level (58), although the evidence for increased potential for confusion is conflicting (56). It is probably safest to keep the serum level of lithium as low as possible during the course of ECT if lithium is indicated.

Antipsychotics, antidepressants, and central nervous system stimulants (59) may increase seizure duration. Caution may be required with higher serum levels of clozapine, as it may prolong seizure duration (46). Augmentation of ECT with antipsychotic medication or antidepressants is generally well tolerated. A few studies have examined ECT augmentation with psychotherapy with promising outcomes in depression (60), and so ECT should not be considered an absolute contraindication for therapy. Methylxanthine derivatives such as aminophylline, caffeine, and theophylline may increase the seizure duration (61), although deliberate use of these drugs to 'improve' seizure length is not recommended (35).

Selecting and working with an electroconvulsive therapy suite

An ECT suite is a prime example of a multidisciplinary team in action. A typical ECT team is composed of a lead ECT psychiatrist, lead ECT nurse (and deputies), anaesthetist, operating department practitioner, recovery nurses, and healthcare assistants. ECT is one of the few procedural skills in psychiatry. Core Psychiatry Trainees in the UK are expected to receive training in ECT as part of the requirements of the Core Training Curriculum, and should provide evidence that they have done so in their portfolios. The Royal College of Psychiatrists has developed a knowledge and skills-based assessment framework for doctors at every level from their Foundation Programme years to consultanthood. However, there is currently no guidance on the expected level of practical involvement in ECT for grades other than Core Psychiatry Trainee and clinical lead.

The Electroconvulsive Therapy Accreditation Service (ECTAS) is the body that governs the quality of ECT across England, Wales, Northern Ireland and the Republic of Ireland (62), and forms part of the Royal College of Psychiatrists College Centre for Quality Improvement. In NHS Scotland, The Scottish ECT Accreditation Network (SEAN) audits the quality of ECT (63). ECTAS standards cover the ECT clinic and facilities, staff and training, assessment and preparation, consent, anaesthesia, administration of ECT, and recovery. These standards ensure quality by auditing ECT services and by detailing both minimum and aspirational standards with respect to ECT machines, EEG monitoring, staff requirements, and even the physical structure of the ECT suite, which must be designed to allow patients to be treated in a calm and dignified way. The standards are updated on regular basis, and participating suites are reviewed every 3 years by a team appointed by ECTAS. ECTAS-accredited clinics are also expected to audit their practice regularly; comparable measures were also set by SEAN.

Future directions for electroconvulsive therapy and neural stimulation in psychiatry

ECT is not the only form of brain stimulation or physical treatment contributing to the psychiatric armamentarium. Emerging treatments usually delivered by an ECT service include repetitive transcranial magnetic stimulation and intravenous ketamine (64) infusions for treatment-resistant depression, and intravenous lorazepam for catatonia. The ECT suite is a natural environment for these intravenous treatments within mental health facilities, due to the mixture of anaesthetic and mental health skills within the team.

ECT itself is developing in the direction of minimizing cognitive side effects. The use of unilateral ECT, ultra-brief pulse width, and low pulse amplitude ECT (65), and focal electrically administered seizure therapy (FEAST) (66) are a few examples of key areas of development in ECT. Advances in anaesthesia have made ECT available for more patient groups, and the high quality of nursing care has increased levels of patient satisfaction with ECT (67).

Challenging prevailing views

ECT is an outstanding example of how stigma can hinder the availability and utilization of an evidence-based and effective treatment. Antipsychiatry movements, the news media, literature, and films have tended to focus on a negative portrayal of ECT as an instrument of torture, punishment, and repression (68, 69). One review

of British press depictions of ECT showed them to be more negative than positive (70). There are a few exceptions to the rule in fiction (71) and autobiographies where ECT is depicted in a more positive light (72, 73). To engage with these critical views of ECT, we must acknowledge the role of past medical practice in entrenching them—'regressive ECT' and 'depatterning' (74) are examples of theories that were put into practice without sufficient weighing of the potential risks.

The discrepancy between the depiction of ECT in the media on one hand and its actual administration on the other is probably best addressed by exposure; experience with ECT seems to have a positive effect on reducing stigma among patients and carers (75). By the same token, more exposure of medical students and student nurses (along with other healthcare professionals) may help to neutralize any prevailing negative ideas of ECT, to return it to its definition and role as a routine and safe minor medical procedure.

REFERENCES

1. Shorter E, Healy D. *Shock Therapy: A History of Electroconvulsive Treatment in Mental Illness*. Brunswick, NJ: Rutgers University Press; 2007.
2. Beverdige A, Renvoize EB. Electricity: a history of its use in the treatment of mental illness in Britain during the second half of the 19th century. *Br J Psychiatry* 1988;153:157–162.
3. Gilman S. Electrotherapy and mental illness: then and now. *Hist Psychiatry* 2008;29:339–357.
4. Alexander L. *Treatment of Mental Disorders*. Philadelphia, PA: Saunders; 1953.
5. Kirby M. Patients' rights—why the Australian courts have rejected 'Bolam'. *J Med Ethics* 1995;21:5–8.
6. Maxiner D, Taylor M. The efficiency and safety of electroconvulsive therapy. In: Tyrer P, Silk R (eds), *Cambridge Textbook of Effective Treatments in Psychiatry*, pp. 57–82. Cambridge: Cambridge University Press; 2008.
7. Soares M, Moreno R, Moreno D. Electroconvulsive therapy in treatment-resistant mania: case reports. *Rev Hosp Clin Fac Med Sao Paulo* 2002;57;31–38.
8. Dabrowski M, Parnowski T. Clinical analysis of safety and effectiveness of electroconvulsive therapy. *Psychiatr Polska* 2012;46: 345–360.
9. Möller H, Henkel V. *What are the Most Effective Diagnostic and Therapeutic Strategies for the Management of Depression in Specialist Care?* Copenhagen: World Health Organization, Health Evidence Network; 2005.
10. American Psychiatric Association. *The Practice of Electroconvulsive Therapy: Recommendations for Treatment, Training and Privileging (Task Force Report)*, 2nd edition. Washington, DC: American Psychiatric Association Publishing; 2001.
11. Acton M, Burgi P, Chan P, et al. Electroconvulsive therapy: guidelines for health authorities in British Columbia. British Columbia Ministry of Health; 2000. https://www.health.gov.bc.ca/library/publications/year/2002/MHA_ect_guidelines.pdf
12. National Institute of Health and Clinical Excellence. Guidance on the use of electroconvulsive therapy. Technology appraisal guidance [TA59]. 2003 (last updated 2009). http://www.nice.org.uk/guidance/ta59
13. Zheng W, Cao XL, Ungvari G, et al. Electroconvulsive therapy added to non-clozapine antipsychotic medication for treatment resistant schizophrenia: meta-analysis of randomized controlled trials. *PLoS One* 2016;11:1–13.

14. Hasan A, Falkai P, Wobrock T, et al. World Federation of Societies of Biological Psychiatry (WFSBP) guidelines for biological treatment of schizophrenia, part 1: update 2012 on the acute treatment of schizophrenia and the management of treatment resistance. *World J Biol Psychiatry* 2012;13:318–378.

15. Petrides G, Malur C, Braga R, et al. Electroconvulsive therapy augmentation in clozapine-resistant schizophrenia: a prospective, randomized study. *Am J Psychiatry* 2016;172:52–58.

16. Lally J, Tully J, Robertson D, Stubbs B, Gaughran F, MacCabe J. Augmentation of clozapine with electroconvulsive therapy in treatment resistant schizophrenia: a systematic review and meta-analysis. *Schizophr Res* 2016;171:215–224.

17. Kellner C. *Brain Stimulation in Psychiatry ECT, DBS, TMS and Other Modalities.* Cambridge: Cambridge University Press; 2012.

18. Benzoni O, Fazzari G, Placentino A, Marangoni C, Rossi A. Treatment of resistant mood and schizoaffective disorders with electroconvulsive therapy: a case series of 264 patients. *J Psychopathol* 2015;21:266–268.

19. Semple D, Smyth R. *Oxford Handbook of Psychiatry*, 3rd edition. Oxford: Oxford University Press; 2013.

20. Fregni F, Simon D, Wu A. Non-invasive brain stimulation for Parkinson's disease: a systematic review and meta-analysis of the literature. *J Neurol Neurosurg Psychiatry* 2005;76:1614–1623.

21. Borisovskaya A, Bryson W, Buchholz J, Samii A, Borson S. Electroconvulsive therapy for depression in Parkinson's disease: systematic review of evidence and recommendations. *Neurodegener Dis Manag* 2016;6:161–176.

22. Lambrecq V, Villéga F, Marchal C, et al. Refractory status epilepticus: electroconvulsive therapy as a possible therapeutic strategy. *Seizure* 2013;21:661–664.

23. Nielsen RM, Olsen KS, Lauritsen AO, Boesen HC. Electroconvulsive therapy as a treatment for protracted refractory delirium in the intensive care unit – five cases and a review. *J Crit Care* 2014;29:881.

24. Uezato A, Yamamoto N, Kurumaji A, et al. Improvement of asymmetrical temporal blood flow in refractory oral somatic delusion after successful electroconvulsive therapy. *J ECT* 2012;28:50–51.

25. Fink M. *Electroshock: Restoring the Mind.* Oxford: Oxford University Press; 2009.

26. Ghaziuddin N, Walter G. *Electroconvulsive Therapy in Children and Adolescents.* Oxford: Oxford University Press; 2013.

27. Power J, Hiscock R, Galbally M, Walker S, Rolfe T. ECT in pregnancy and the postpartum. In: Braddock K (ed), *Electroconvulsive Therapy: Clinical Uses, Efficacy and Long Term Health Effects*, chapter 2. New York: Nova Science Publishers; 2014.

28. Mankad M. Informed consent for electroconvulsive therapy—finding balance. *J ECT* 2015;31:143–146.

29. Mankad M, Beyer J, Weiner RD, Krystal A. *Clinical Manual of Electroconvulsive Therapy.* Arlington, VA: American Psychiatric Publishing Inc.; 2010.

30. Swartz C. *Electroconvulsive and Neuromodulation Therapies.* Cambridge: Cambridge University Press; 2009.

31. Little J, Munday J, Atkins M, Khalid A. Does electrode placement predict time to rehospitalization? *J ECT* 2004;20:213–218.

32. Sidhom E, Youssef N. Ultra-brief pulse unilateral ECT is associated with less cognitive side effects. *Brain Stimul* 2014;7:768–769.

33. Chung K, Wong S. Initial seizure threshold of bilateral electroconvulsive therapy in Chinese. *J ECT* 2001;17:254–258.

34. Peterchev A, Rosa M, Deng ZD, Prudic J, Lisanby S. ECT stimulus parameters: rethinking dosage. *J ECT* 2010;26:159–174.

35. Waite J, Easton A. *The ECT Handbook*, 3rd edition. London: The Royal College of Psychiatrists; 2013.

36. Lalla F, Milroy T. The current status of seizure duration in the practice of electroconvulsive therapy. *Can J Psychiatry* 1996;41:299–304.

37. Abrams R. *Electroconvulsive Therapy.* Oxford: Oxford University Press; 2002.

38. Yasuda K, Kobayash K, Yamaguchi M, et al. Seizure threshold and the half-age method in bilateral electroconvulsive therapy in Japanese patients. *Psychiatry Clin Neurosci* 2014;69:49–54.

39. Busner J, Targum S. The Clinical Global Impressions Scale: applying a research tool in clinical practice. *Psychiatry (Edgmont)* 2007;4:28–37.

40. Bush G, Fink M, Petrides G, Dowling F, Francis A, Catatonia. I. Rating scale and standardized examination. *Acta Psychiatr Scand* 1996;93:129–136.

41. Kirkhart R, Ahuja N, Lee J, et al. The detection and measurement of catatonia. *Psychiatry (Edgmont)* 2007;4:52–56.

42. Fraser L, O'Carroll R, Ebmeier K. The effect of electroconvulsive therapy on autobiographical memory: a systematic review. *J ECT* 2008;24:10–17.

43. Porter R, Douglas K, Knight R. Monitoring of cognitive effects during a course of electroconvulsive therapy: recommendations for clinical practice. *J ECT* 2008;24:25–34.

44. Nasreddine Z, Phillips N, Bédirian CS, et al. The Montreal Cognitive Assessment, MoCA: a brief screening tool for mild cognitive impairment. *J Am Geriatr Soc* 2005;53:695–699.

45. Bazire S (ed). *Psychotropic Drug Directory 2012: The Professionals' Pocket and Aide Memoire.* Malta: Lloyd-Reinhold Communications; 2012.

46. Mohn C, Rund B. Maintained improvement of neurocognitive function in major depressive disorders 6 months after ECT. *Front Psychiatry* 2016;7:200.

47. Martin D, Gálvez V, Loo C. Predicting retrograde autobiographical memory changes following electroconvulsive therapy: relationships between individual, treatment, and early clinical factors. *Int J Neuropsychopharmacol* 2015;18:pyv067.

48. Donel M, Gálvez V, Loo C. Predicting retrograde autobiographical memory changes following electroconvulsive therapy: relationships between individual, treatment, and early clinical factors. *Int J Neuropsychopharmacol* 2015;18:pyv067.

49. Leung M, Hollander Y, Brown GR. Pretreatment with ibuprofen to prevent electroconvulsive therapy-induced headache. *J Clin Psychiatry* 2003;64:551–553.

50. Ye L, Karlapati S, Lippmann S. Topiramate for post-electroconvulsive therapy headaches. *J ECT* 2013;29:e49.

51. Wang ZY, Waldeck K, Grundemar L, Håkanson R. Ocular inflammation induced by electroconvulsive treatment: contribution of nitric oxide and neuropeptides mobilized from C-fibres. *Br J Pharmacol* 1997;120:1491–1496.

52. Abrams R. The mortality rate with ECT. *J ECT* 1997;13:125–127.

53. Kramer B. Use of ECT in California, revisited: 1984–1994. *J ECT* 1999;15:245–251.

54. Petrides G, Tobias K, Kellner C, Rudorfer M. Continuation and maintenance electroconvulsive therapy for mood disorders: review of the literature. *Neuropsychobiology* 2011;64:129–140.

55. Lisanby S, Sampson S, Husain M, et al. Towards individualized post-ECT care: piloting the Symptom-Titrated Algorithm-Based Longitudinal ECT (STABLE) intervention. *J ECT* 2008;24:179–182.

56. Taylor D, Paton C, Kapur S. *The Maudsley Prescribing Guidelines in Psychiatry*, 12th edition. Chichester: Wiley-Blackwell; 2015.

57. Andrade C, Reddy K, Srihari B, Sudha S, Chandra J. Effects of zopiclone and lorazepam on ECT seizure duration: clinical implication of findings from an animal model. *Indian J Psychiatry* 2000;42:308–311.

58. Thirthalli J, Harish T, Gangadhar B. A prospective comparative study of interaction between lithium and modified electroconvulsive therapy. *World J Biol Psychiatry* 2011;12:149–155.

59. Zolezzi M. Medication management during electroconvulsant therapy. *Neuropsychiatr Dis Treat* 2016;12:931–939.

60. McClintock S, Brandon A, Husain M, Jarrett R. A systematic review of the combined use of electroconvulsive therapy and psychotherapy for depression. *J ECT* 2011;27:236–243.

61. Kemp M, Allard J, Pâquet M, Marcotte P. Impact of an oral theophylline loading dose pre-electroconvulsive therapy: a retrospective study in patients with missed or inadequate seizures. *J ECT* 2015;31:37–42.

62. Buley N, Hailey E, Hodge E. *ECT Accreditation Service (ECTAS): Standards for the Administration of ECT*, 13th edition. London: Royal College of Psychiatrists; 2016.

63. Scottish ECT Accreditation Network. *SEAN Standards*. Report No. 2.0. Edinburgh: NHS Scotland; 2013.

64. Diamond P, Farmery A, Atkinson S, et al. Ketamine infusions for treatment resistant depression: a series of 28 patients treated weekly or twice weekly in an ECT clinic. *J Psychopharmacol* 2014;28:536–544.

65. Peterchev A, Krystal A, Rosa M, Lisanby S. Individualized low-amplitude seizure therapy: minimizing current for electroconvulsive therapy and magnetic seizure therapy. *Neuropsychopharmacology* 2015;40:2076–2084.

66. Nahas Z, Short B, Burns C, et al. A feasibility study of a new method for electrically producing seizures in man: focal electrically administered seizure therapy [FEAST]. *Brain Stimul* 2013;6:403–408.

67. Navidian A, Ebrahimi H, Keykha R. Supportive nursing care and satisfaction of patients receiving electroconvulsive therapy: a randomized controlled clinical Trial. *Iranian Red Crescent Med J* 2015;17:e27492.

68. Matthews A, Rosenquist P, McCall V. Representation of ECT in English-language film and television in the new millennium. *J ECT* 2016;32:187–191.

69. Sienaert P. Based on a true story? The portrayal of ECT in international movies and television programs. *Brain Stimul* 2016;9:882–891.

70. Euba R, Crugel M. The depiction of electroconvulsive therapy in the British press. *J ECT* 2009;25:265–269.

71. Bishop C. *Micah Found It: A Shock Treatment Short Story, Part One*. Boston, MA: Emerson Publishing; 2014.

72. Dukakis K, Tye L. *Shock: The Healing Power of Electroconvulsive Therapy*. New York: Penguin Group; 2006.

73. Fisher C. *Shockaholic*. New York: Simon and Schuster; 2011.

74. Cameron D, Lorhenz J, Handcock K. The depatterning treatment of schizophrenia. *Compr Psychiatry* 1962;3:65–76.

75. Aoki Y, Yamaguchi S, Ando S, Sasaki N, Bernick P, Akiyama T. The experience of electroconvulsive therapy and its impact on associated stigma: a meta-analysis. *Int J Soc Psychiatry* 2016;62:708–718.

15

Prevention and management of violence and aggression

Alyson Price and David Price

Historical influences

The management and treatment of patients who present with acute mental distress, accompanied by disturbed behaviour, may include restraint if staff are unable to successfully verbally de-escalate a situation. This may represent the only intervention capable of protecting the patient and others from harm.

Currently, inpatient services in the UK use physical restraint, which involves the restriction of movement by holding the limbs (as opposed to mechanical restraint where a device is used to restrict movement) (1).

Health and safety legislation in the UK (2, 3) imposes a duty on employers to do all that is reasonably practicable to ensure a safe place of work (1). Where there is a possible risk of violence, staff must be supplied with the appropriate information, instruction, and training to manage the risk. Staff may be required to use physical interventions and the employer thereby must ensure that this training is provided and is fit for purpose.

Training in physical intervention skills is now widespread within the UK and is influenced by good practice guidance and research (which has been more abundant in recent years). Historically staff learned these skills through unofficial on-the-job training or ad hoc training sessions (4).

More structured training was offered to staff working in the high secure hospitals which were then part of the prison service, and health services adopted the 'control and restraint' (C&R) system from the prison service (4).

C&R was assimilated into mental health care through training offered by the prison service instructors to the 'special hospitals' in the 1980s (5). Although the term C&R was in widespread use, there was no formal training programme for the health service, although general adult acute mental health services did adopt the approach (5).

Initial programmes were governed by the prison service but were allowed to proliferate, independently of any central regulation, throughout the National Health Service (NHS) from the special hospitals. This led to a number of training providers offering different training systems—with most having their roots in some form of martial arts. Physical interventions were often delivered without training in prevention (6)—violence was seen as something to be managed reactively by physical force rather than relationship building, collaborative working, and establishing a therapeutic culture. The underlying perception was of a skill which needed to be taught rather than an intervention for a service user which considered violence prevention.

There has since been a shift in practice and language, moving forward to collaborative working with the introduction of mandatory training in the non-physical interventions training programme—'Promoting Safe and Therapeutic Services' (7)—for all frontline mental health staff. It was designed to promote a cultural change due to NHS trusts having to ensure that the theoretical underpinnings of violence and aggression were a component part of the training they provided in PMVA. Although NHS Protect was disbanded from 1 April 2017 (8), the legacy is likely to remain in light of the other guidance which has superseded it.

Finally, the connotations of C&R are not suited to the present era in mental health settings where the emphasis is on partnership and recovery, and the culture change and best practice influences on this are discussed in the following sections.

Recent influences

Since the death of David Bennett in 1998, the management of violence and aggression in mental health care has been under increasing scrutiny, and has remained at the centre of a number of national initiatives (6, 7, 9–14). Mr Bennett died as a result of positional asphyxia (which will be discussed in detail later in this chapter) while being restrained in the prone position following a violent altercation with a staff member. However, not only was he restrained in the prone (face-down) position, additional pressure (of up to five staff at one point) was placed on him during the restraint procedure in order to control his position on the floor.

Any death such as this is a tragedy and many issues arose from this enquiry including the encouragement to look more deeply at what led to the restraint being necessary: what caused the aggressive and violent behaviour in the first instance and What preventative measures were in place to try and minimize the risk of this type of situation occurring? Why did staff have the perception of the situation which led them to go against what they had been taught in training? Mr Bennett was an Afro-Caribbean man who had been experiencing a high level of racial abuse from a fellow patient on the unit. Mr Bennett also had a long history of violent behaviour towards staff and others, and as a result had significant contact with forensic and secure mental health services.

Staff were unaware of the corrosive and cumulative effect of the racist abuse, and their lack of understanding of the impact of the abuse on Mr Bennett. The subsequent lack of intervention to address these issues ultimately influenced the occurrence of the violent incident which led to the restraint (15).

The enquiry called for a time limit to be set on the length of restraint in the prone position and highlighted the significant risks of prone restraint. It also highlighted that institutional racism was a significant concern for the NHS along with making negative assumptions regarding a person's behaviour and how that is managed, based on their ethnicity (16). The need to focus on understanding and prevention has been the central focus of several guidance documents which were published in the immediate aftermath of this report (6, 7, 9, 11). Indeed, around the same time as the Blofeld report was published (15), the United Kingdom Central Council for Nursing, Midwifery and Health Visiting (now the Nursing and Midwifery Council) (6) had already highlighted in their audit that there was a significant inconsistency in training provision across the NHS and very little information was given consistently to staff around prevention and de-escalation strategies.

However, it was following a report into the care and treatment of patients with learning disabilities at Winterbourne View (17), which was particularly focused around abuse and restraint issues, that the drive to ensure these principles were embedded into practice gathered significant momentum. The publication of the Mind report (13) which focused on the overall use of restraint procedures, and criticized the 'overreliance' of mental health staff in the use of restraint and in particular prone restraint, branding it a 'barbaric' procedure which carried a high risk of death, led to a call for a total ban on the procedure.

Equally, it brought into stark reality that in order to change outcomes and improve care, promotion of primary prevention was necessary to reduce the risk, occurrence, and impact of such incidents. Training is a significant part of this and must reflect a move away from reactive management, towards proactive prevention; however, as the work of Colton (18) and Huckshorn (19) identifies, this is only one aspect of the change required, and will be referred to later in the chapter.

Risks associated with restraint and the prone restraint debate

As already identified, the ideal is to avoid any physical restraint, as such interventions risk the possibility of physical and psychological trauma (20). However, at times, physical restraint may represent the only interventions available to staff to protect the patient and/ or others from a violent incident. Nevertheless, the intervention of restraint is not risk free, and both serious injuries and deaths have been reported in the UK and other countries (1).

The available evidence (1, 21, 22) suggests a number of factors in combination may increase a person's susceptibility to death during restraint such as obesity, physical ill health, prescribed medication, and illicit drug use (23). In addition, restraint is likely to involve significantly increased levels of exertion and thereby increased demand on respiratory and cardiac function. As Lancaster et al. (21, p. 307) state, 'physical restraint is the only non-medical intervention in mental health with the potential to directly cause severe and even fatal injury to patients'.

There are different ways of restraining patients and some positions carry more risk than others; indeed it has been suggested by policymakers that certain restraint positions (especially prone) should be avoided (13, 14, 24).

The Mental Health Act Code of Practice (24, para. 26.70) states: 'Unless there are cogent reasons for doing so, there must be no planned or intentional restraint of a person in a prone position (whereby they are forcibly laid on their front) on any surface, not just the floor'.

Thus, the position of the body during restraint has been noted as a factor in the small number of patients who have died either during or immediately following a restraint (1). Early research pointed to the idea that being restrained in the prone position particularly resulted in a significant restriction of respiration and may be fatal—giving rise to the term 'positional asphyxia' as proposed by Reay et al. (25, 26). The concept was used to explain such deaths suggesting that this body position can limit movement of the ribs and diaphragm to a degree that asphyxia results. Respiratory function involves the 'respiratory triad'—an unobstructed open airway, adequate gas exchange between the alveoli and the pulmonary vascular system, and a functional ventilatory pump (or bellows) to produce airflow in and out of the lungs (1).

The restraint asphyxia hypothesis proposed that when a patient is placed in the prone position, the bellows aspect of the respiratory triad may be compromised (22), and contraction of the diaphragm may be prevented. The effect may be exacerbated if the person is obese or pressure is applied downwards on the patient's back by staff.

A number of reports supported this idea of restraint-related asphyxia; however, later research and subsequent studies questioned the extent of this effect and direct causality of death due to the prone position (27), and expressed doubt that levels of restriction on lung function demonstrated in these studies was sufficient to cause death.

One such study (26) found that there was a reduction of lung function in the prone restraint position, but went on to suggest that the reductions were not sufficient to be fatal. They went on to say that participants in their study, who were restrained in a prone position but included the body weight of those restraining them placed upon them, did show a significant decrease in lung function. The National Institute for Health and Care Excellence (NICE) guidance (11) following the death of David Bennett concluded that there was no clear evidence that prone restraint presented a significantly greater risk than other restraint positions (27).

The Parkes et al. (27) study concluded that some but not all prone restraint positions cause a significant reduction in lung function and that positional asphyxia is inferred in the absence of any other identifiable cause of death. It is clear from Parkes et al. (26, 27) and Aiken et al. (23) that deaths have occurred in other restraint positions, for example, seated but bent forward (Jimmy Mubenga and Gareth

Myatt are examples of two such cases in recent years), and this position can cause a more significant reduction in lung function and should be considered to have a significant potential risk of harm, particularly when coupled with a higher body mass index (>25 kg/m²). Additionally, supine restraint can also carry a risk of choking and inhalation of vomit (23).

In considering all of the above information, the potential clinical significance for staff is that PMVA training should have a focus not only on reducing and minimizing the need for restraints but importantly having a full and detailed understanding of the risks involved in carrying out every one of the numerous restraint procedures available to them, and how to avoid or minimize these risks. The restraint position should be considered a risk factor for sudden death and that some restraint positions may present a greater risk to patients than others, and staff must apply these as effectively and safely as possible. Of paramount importance within this is ensuring staff have a full understanding of any of the aforementioned additional risk factors for particular restraint procedures, the signs to be aware of in relation to respiratory distress, and how to respond to a medical emergency in these situations.

Monitoring of the physical condition of the patient is obviously paramount in circumstances whereby restraint is utilized and in the UK, NICE (12) and NHS England (29) have issued clear guidance related to this.

'Positive & Safe'—the restraint reduction agenda

In introducing this next section it is important to note all current guidance directs us towards promoting dignity and respect, understanding the nature and function of behaviour, and utilizing a public health approach to its management and planning, thereby minimizing the need to utilize any restrictive practices. The most influential of these are the *Positive and Proactive Care* (14) guidance and NICE guideline NG10 (12).

One of the key actions for NHS trusts in the UK from the *Positive and Proactive Care* (14) guidance is the creation of 'Individualised support plans, incorporating behaviour support plans, [which] must be implemented for all people who use services who are known to be at risk of being exposed to restrictive interventions' and indeed UK NHS trusts are required to audit and report on the quality and implementation of these.

The Department of Health (14) identifies that individualized recovery-based approaches should be used, that is, a human rights-based approach, which works with individuals to improve their clinical and social outcomes by enhancing independence, promoting choice, and increasing social inclusion—and the approach recommended is the Positive Behaviour Support (PBS) model.

PBS provides a framework that seeks to understand the context and meaning of behaviour in order to inform the development of supportive environments and skills which enhance a person's quality of life and by doing so potentially reduce the prevalence of challenging behaviours and thus the potential for assaultive behaviour to occur; the knock-on effect of this is subsequently to reduce the need to utilize restrictive interventions.

PBS recognizes that individuals engage in challenging behaviours because they have challenging or complex individual needs which are not being met, they are exposed to challenging environments, and they may have an impoverished quality of life as a result of their illness.

It is noted that much of the evidence base for PBS lies in the field of learning disabilities, autistic spectrum disorders, and neurodisabilities rather than mental health services or dementia care (30). Nevertheless, the principles of PBS do have an evidence base and Skills for Care and Skills for Health (30) recognize that other models of care may be prevalent across different settings (e.g. the recovery model), and as long as the core principles of a public health approach are incorporated, this satisfies the proactive workforce strategy.

Behaviour support planning

Risk management plans related to management of violence and aggression should ensure that the functional assessment of behaviour gives rise to effective behaviour support plans, identifying primary preventative strategies (identifying and meeting needs and minimizing potential for distress), secondary prevention (de-escalation, diffusion, and distraction strategies), and tertiary interventions (physical intervention strategies), for when behaviour escalates and risks cannot be managed in any other way. These must include patient input where appropriate and should identify a post-incident review process (12).

The public health approach to violence

In recent reports and audits of violence (6, 7, 14, 15), the health sector has frequently been accused of working largely reactively in relation to the management of violence and aggression. Violence, however, is a complex phenomenon and needs to be addressed in a more comprehensive and holistic manner. Indeed, in some cases (although not all) the variable and poorly regulated training in this field has contributed to this approach.

Earlier in the chapter the historical and current influences on PMVA training in the UK were discussed, the most recent being NICE (12), Department of Health (14), and Skills for Care and Skills for Health (30), and the core of how we should be working in relation to management of violence and aggression sits with the public health model.

Public health places emphasis on preventing disease or injury from occurring or reoccurring, rather than on treating the health consequences: 'Public Health is above all characterized by its emphasis on prevention. Rather than simply accepting or reacting to violence, its starting point is the strong conviction that violent behaviour and its consequences can be prevented' (31, p. 4).

As far as violence is concerned, the starting point should be that violent behaviour and its consequences, if they can be understood, can also be prevented. Therefore it is important to gain an understanding of the risk factors for violence and where they emerge from.

There is no single factor to explain why one person and not another behaves in a violent manner; violence is an extremely complex phenomenon that has its roots in the interaction of many factors—biological, social, cultural, economic, and political.

The *World Report on Violence and Health* (31) uses an ecological model to try to understand the multifaceted nature of violence. The model assists in examining factors that influence behaviour—biological and personal history, social relationships (family, friends, partners, peers), community/social environment, and broad societal factors that all influence how individuals behave and increase their likelihood of becoming a victim or perpetrator of violence.

Care planning

Besides helping to clarify the causes of violence and their complex interactions, the ecological model also suggests that in order to prevent violence, it is necessary to implement actions/develop strategies across all areas using the following levels of intervention (14, 24, 31):

Primary prevention

Strategies which support the creation of environments, attitudes, activities, and cultures aimed at reducing the potential for conflict.

This means addressing the underlying triggers and causes of violence and aggression before it happens, both on an organizational level (acting on research, local audit, etc.) and on an individual level (completing mental health and risk assessments), looking at an individual's past history, and attempting to predict when and how violence may occur.

Secondary prevention

Are actions, such as crisis resolution and de-escalation skills, to resolve conflict and avoid violence when it is perceived to be imminent. It necessitates an awareness of the signs of increased agitation and the potential for escalation of behaviour, internal and external triggers specific to the individual, and knowledge of the individualized strategies that have effective previously.

Indeed primary and secondary levels of intervention are where the Safewards interventions established by Bowers et al. (32) are utilized (see Chapter 24 for more details).

Tertiary intervention

This is the reactive physical response (breakaway, restraint, seclusion, rapid tranquillization) to a situation where violence is occurring/has occurred and after (post-incident review). The care plan must reflect hierarchical levels of physical intervention and any physical risks identified.

Staff need to recognize that on occasion, a restrictive intervention may be unavoidable to minimize risk and maintain safety of all; it should, however, be viewed as an emergency procedure and absolute last resort (12, 14, 24).

After an incident has occurred whereby restrictive interventions have been utilized, a post-incident review should occur (12, 14). This is to ensure the individuals involved in the incident can learn from the experience, and any changes to practice and future interventions can be implemented—thus feeding back into the hierarchical cycle.

Risk assessment

This section will discuss the interaction and relevance of particular factors and considerations in identifying how and why someone may become aggressive and how this supports development of appropriate care plans to reduce behaviour and manage risk. Staff must understand the importance of good formulation (see Chapter 16) and should identify any historical, static, clinical, situational factors,

triggers, and protective factors. Importantly, however, mental health services have in the past taken a paternalistic approach to risk management (33–35)—making decisions and plans in the best interests of the patient. However, the recovery model being utilized currently in mental health services in the UK is designed to work collaboratively with patients to identify their perception of their illness, how it impacts them, their strengths and skills, and what strategies to manage their risk and relapse are meaningful for them (34, 35).

If we are to truly utilize a public health approach, the collaborative approach is vital in understanding and being able to identify good primary and secondary prevention strategies.

Our starting point for looking at restraint reduction and prevention must be to gain some understanding around why people become aggressive and perspectives on how staff manage this, so as to promote an environment, training, and practices which reduce the need for any restrictive practices to occur. As such, Duxbury and Whittington (36) provide us with that initial insight; they studied staff and patient perspectives on the underlying causes of violence and aggression and found that there was a disparity between staff and patient perceptions of these incidents. Staff tended to see patient aggression as a behaviour related to their mental illness, whereas patients felt that the environment, staff behaviour, and poor communication were precursors. However, staff did also identify that the inpatient environment could have a negative impact. This highlights a very complicated interaction between different variables in relation to causation—and they discuss three models related to this—internal (the association between mental illness and aggression), external (the environmental factors which influence the prevalence of aggression), and situational/interactional (negative staff/patient interactions/relationships). This provides a basis for identifying different influences in the decision-making process in relation to restraints also. Duxbury and Whittington (36) point out that if staff label patients as 'mad' or 'bad', this will influence the treatment they then decide to respond with, and this is clearly borne out in their findings in relation to responses to aggression, which seem to suggest an element of 'control'. They identified that a model is required which focuses on the complexity of the interaction between all these factors.

Similarly, Van der Schaaf et al. (37) identified that we have to consider the complex interaction of the contextual characteristics (such as the ward environment), staff characteristics, and patient characteristics—the ward environment being particularly relevant.

McCue et al. (38) appear to support the hypothesis that there is a complex interaction. In their study which identified a programme to reduce restraint in a psychiatric inpatient service, they identified strategies which worked on nurses' non-physical skills and understanding of crisis situations and also on providing patients with stress and anger management sessions. Interestingly, they also identified a review process post incident to discuss the progress of the situation and how it was managed, in order to assist learning—a strategy that has been long promoted in best practice guidance (11, 12, 14).

Papadopulos et al. (39) equally identified that if services want to enable staff to manage situations more preventatively, they need a more detailed understanding of why these incidents occur. In this meta-analysis of the antecedent themes which occur in incidents of violence and aggression, across 71 studies they identified 59 themes which occurred, and these were further categorized into nine 'higher-level' themes. These included staff–patient interaction, patient–patient interaction, patient conflict behaviours, external/personal themes (personal matters external to the ward), structural themes (related to the physical ward environment), patient behavioural cues, patient emotional/mood cues, and patient symptoms. No clear cause was also a theme, where the antecedent was not recognized or none was present.

Similarly to Duxbury and Whittington (36), this study seems to identify the importance of staff–patient interactions; they found that the most common antecedent to aggressive or violent behaviour was staff–patient interaction, accounting for 39% of all antecedent profiles. This included limiting patient's freedoms, placing restrictions, denying requests, and understanding and meeting of needs—essentially staff exercising some form of power and control over the patient. Papadopoulos et al. (39) suggest therefore that any interventions to reduce violence and aggression cannot ignore the influence of the nurse–patient interaction and must enhance it.

Leading on from this, Bowers et al. (32, 40) and Bowers (41) have made a significant contribution to the literature relating to understanding conflict situations, the interaction of particular variables in conflict and containment situations, and restraint reduction strategies overall both in terms of understanding the causes of conflict and containment and the development of strategies to minimize the occurrence of such events, culminating in the development of the 'Safewards' model (41). The Department of Health directive, through the *Positive and Proactive Care* guidance (14), for all mental health trusts nationwide to implement the 'Safewards' model, is testament to the value of this research.

In the last 10–15 years, NICE (11) and NHS Protect (7) have made significant headway in attempting to provide us with a framework to tackle this issue of awareness, understanding, early intervention, and prevention and yet inpatient mental health services still find ourselves in a position whereby our reactive approach is still called into question (12–14). However, those working in mental health inpatient services will identify that there has been a culture shift in how we work as suggested by significant changes in the prevalent ethos in inpatient mental health services, and evidence of very positive quality improvement initiatives which have demonstrated significant progress (42), but there is still work to do. Significant changes to culture have occurred, but our challenge is maintaining consistency in our approach to truly understand and reduce violence and aggression and ultimately reduce restraint. This will be covered specifically later in the chapter; however, we next need to turn our attention to the practical considerations for managing restraint situations.

Practical considerations in managing restraint situations

Decision-making in restraint situations

In order to have any significant impact in changing the practice of restraint, particular attention should be paid to how people make decisions when they are involved in a situation whereby restraint may be required.

Whittington et al. (43) provide us with a good starting point of considering the different restraint options and identify the factors which increase or decrease the likelihood of staff deciding to use them.

This study found that the decision-making process is highly subjective, and certain factors seemed to correlate with the use of either floor or seated/standing restraint strategies—for example, increased vocal volume prior to the incident or the patient being detained under Section 2 of the Mental Health Act tended to increase the likelihood of floor (prone or supine) restraint; whereas perceived rational causation for the aggression or being an older person tended to reduce the likelihood. Fundamentally, however, the decision-making should match the level of risk and likelihood of harm in all situations, and therefore a critical component in the decision-making process is the perception of threat and imminent danger, which is the highly subjective component and will be influenced by a range of psychological, experiential, and environmental factors.

Whittington et al. (43) consider the importance of 'cognitive appraisal' of situations (43, 44) and highlighted that the decision to use a floor restraint response may be made unnecessarily if the risk is overestimated and the staff members also underestimate their capacity to control the situation. This could be linked to a variety of factors including environmental resources such as de-escalation areas, staffing levels and skills mix, previous experience, and knowledge of the patient—a whole host of potential internal and external factors may be influencing the process. Core questions therefore are raised and must be addressed into understanding decision-making in these situations and also understanding where and how we may be able to provide the correct environments, support, and training to staff in an attempt to attenuate the impact of some factors where possible.

The importance of this cannot be overestimated as it provides some links back to key issues raised by the Blofeld report (15) into David Bennett's death, and suggests that staff may have used excessive force due to their perception of their ability to manage him.

Other studies since the Blofeld report (15, 45–49) indicate a variety of factors around the same themes generally related to the decision to restrain or not, rather than how they appraise what level of intervention to utilize. They provide some useful insights into decision-making processes which potentially may assist in developing a model to understand how and why situations may be perceived in a particular way and therefore how to help staff more effectively through training and support mechanisms.

Laiho et al. (45), identified four areas of assessment that are relevant to decision-making: patient-related cues, personnel-related cues, previous experiences of the use of seclusion and restraint (both staff and patients), and organizational cues.

Lindsey (46) points out that nurses appear to choose low-level de-escalation and medication with greater frequency; however, more experienced nurses were more likely to restrain patients. Moylan and Cullinan (50) also identified that those nurses who had been injured in the process of restraint previously were less likely to restrain early in the de-escalation process, instead waiting until later in the progression of aggression (Figure 15.1).

Training

Crucially, for training in this field there has never been a clear diktat which specifies exactly what must be included in physical interventions training or the content and ethos of the physical

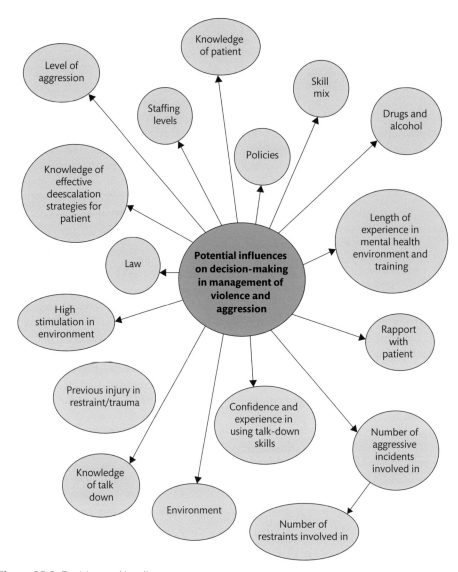

Figure 15.1 Decision-making diagram.

skills. NHS Protect (7) specified non-physical skills training content for mental health and learning disability services, and was tasked with monitoring the implementation of this, and at the time there were discussions around a similar profile for physical skills content; and although the National Institute for Mental Health in England (9) got as far as producing a draft consultation document, unfortunately this never came to fruition. Training providers with appropriate governance structures should provide staff with a detailed understanding of the risks associated with restraint, how to manage these appropriately, and the theoretical underpinnings related to understanding, therapeutic engagement, prevention, and least restrictive management. There should be an additional focus on 'talk down' (32, 40, 41) as an essential secondary prevention tool, which staff should be confident and competent in utilizing.

Lavelle et al. (51) identified that de-escalation was frequently successful when preceded by lower-level conflict events. However, patients with a history of violence brought specific challenges and the de-escalation process was less likely to be successful, suggesting that nurses may lack confidence in using talk-down skills when the risk/perception of risk of violence is greater. This appears to support the assertion that cognitive appraisal of the events (43) and perceived capacity to manage the situation successfully is significant. Lavelle et al. (51, p. 1) also suggest that 'providing evidence based staff training may improve confidence in the use of this potentially powerful technique'.

Legislation relevant to the use of restraint

Using restraint can place health care staff in a difficult situation—application of an inappropriate restraint may result in being held accountable for assault; failing to intervene to protect the patient or others may result in being held to account for negligence (52); therefore it is important that legislation provides a framework when a restraint may be required either as an emergency response or a planned intervention. This section provides a brief overview of the relevant legislation in the UK in the management of violence in the inpatient setting.

Following devolution, the constituent countries in the UK have differing mental health legislation:

- England and Wales:
  - Mental Capacity Act 2005 (53).
  - Mental Health Act 1983 (amended 2007) (54).
- Scotland:
  - Mental Health (Care and Treatment) (Scotland) Act 2003 (55).
  - Adults with Incapacity (Scotland) Act 2000 (56).
- Northern Ireland:
  - The Mental Health (Amendment) (Northern Ireland) Order 2004 (57).
- All three jurisdictions:
  - Human Rights Act 1998 (58).

Human Rights Act 1998

The Act (58) requires public authorities, including the NHS, to act in accordance with the European Convention on Human Rights (59). Articles 3 (Prohibition of Torture) and 8 (Right to Respect for Private and Family Life) acknowledge that there may be a need to restrain a person. Article 3 is not compromised where restraint is used in treatment and its therapeutic necessity exists (60). Any infringement, such as restraint, on a person's Article 8 rights needs to be legitimate (justified) and proportionate (61). It can be seen that human rights law allows for restraint, but places some limitations on its use in practice, which to some extent are principles emulated in the Mental Capacity Act 2005.

Mental Capacity Act 2005 and the Code of Practice

There are conditions where restraint is legitimate, namely where staff reasonably believe that restraint is necessary to prevent harm to the person who lacks capacity, and that it is a proportionate response to the likelihood of the person suffering harm (53, Section 6).

In relation to restraint, Section 6 acknowledges that there may be occasion to restrain a person who lacks capacity. Restraint is defined as 'the use or threat of use of force, and restricts a person's liberty of movement, whether or not a person resists'.

The staff need only have a 'reasonable belief' that a restraint was necessary; to justify the restraint, reasoning needs to be recorded, identifying the rationale as to why it was used (62). For the restraint to be necessary, staff need to show that harm would be suffered unless there was a proportionate forcible intervention and that the restraint used represented the minimum amount of force for the shortest time possible. By proportionate response, it is meant the least intrusive and restrictive and minimum period of time to receive the desired outcome in the best interests of the person who lacks capacity.

If a person is required to be frequently restrained, it may amount to a deprivation of liberty, and if this is the case, authorization should be sought under the Deprivation of Liberty Safeguards, from the appropriate supervisory body (59).

The Adults with Incapacity (Scotland) Act 2000 (58), is similar to the Mental Capacity Act (53) in relation to violence and states that the use of force is not authorized unless it is immediately necessary

and only for as long as necessary (59). There is no current equivalent legislation in Northern Ireland.

Mental Health Act 1983 (amended 2007)

When a person is detained under the Mental Health Act 1983, appropriate treatment needs to be available; Section 62 allows for treatment that is immediate and necessary and of minimum interference to prevent a patient from behaving violently (24) and may include the use of restraint strategies.

Chapter 26 of the Mental Health Act Code of Practice (24)—'Safe and therapeutic responses to disturbed behaviour'—offers extensive guidance and strategies for responding to violence and applies to all people receiving care and treatment for a mental disorder in a hospital, who present with behaviour disturbance whether or not they are detained under the Act (24).

Recommendations for disturbed behaviour are put forward and concur with those outlined in other best practice guidance (12, 14).

The code outlines specifically what is meant by restrictive interventions: 'acts that restrict a patient's movement in order to take immediate control of a dangerous situation where there is a real possibility of harm if no action is taken and to end or reduce the danger to patients or others' (24, p. 290).

Common reasons although not an exhaustive list to utilize restraint might include physical assault, threatening/destructive behaviour, self-harm, extreme overactivity that is likely to lead to physical harm or exhaustion, and attempts to abscond. However, restrictive interventions should also not be used to punish or to intend to inflict pain.

The code goes on to state that where there is restriction of movement or force is used then it should:

> Be used for no longer than necessary to prevent harm to the person.
> Be a proportionate response to that harm and be the least restrictive option.

Regarding prone restraint, patients should not be deliberately restrained in a way that impacts their airway, breathing, or circulation. The mouth and/or nose should not be covered and there should be no pressure to the neck region, ribcage, or abdomen (24). Unless there are cogent reasons for doing so, there must be no planned or intentional restraint of a person in the prone position (24, para. 26.70). A question for inpatient staff is therefore around what cogent means; there may be a situation whereby a patient has expressed a preference within their care plan for prone over supine restraint (and there are no additional risk factors for utilizing this type of restraint). If a person is not detained under the Act but restraint is necessary, for example, emergency management of a violent situation where failure to intervene would result in serious risk of harm, then restraint should take account of best practice guidance, such as that from NICE (12) and Department of Health (14), or there should be consideration as to whether the criteria in Sections 5 and 6 of the Mental Capacity Act apply.

Ultimately, it is important for staff to be clear on the legal principles guiding their decision-making, and training and local policy must provide clarity about the implications of implementing the variety of strategies at staff's disposal.

The future of prevention and management of violence and aggression: reducing violence, reducing restraint

Getting it right—developing the right ethos, culture, environment, resources, training, and support

In the bid to promote organizational change, researchers such as Huckshorn (19) (*Six Core Strategies for Reducing Seclusion and Restraint Use*) have identified essential steps to achieving restraint reduction.

Right ethos and culture

It is the responsibility of mental health professionals to actively seek to reduce the incidence of violence and restraint in our services. Bell and Gallacher (42), using a quality improvement methodology, achieved a sustained 50% reduction in restraints through focusing effects on changing training structure and content, promoting an environment for utilizing seated over floor restraints, adapting data collection methods, and implementing a staff post-incident review strategy following restraint.

Environments

Conducive to de-escalation and reducing emotional arousal—de-escalation suites and space for meaningful activity.

Resources

Much of the staff considerations mentioned previously potentially link to cognitive appraisal—discussed earlier—however, we can begin to impact this organizationally by providing the resources staff need to do their job effectively:

- Staffing—if not regular at least consistent regular agency staff that the organization has invested in training wise to support the ethos of the wards and to work consistently with regular staff and understand the importance of this.
- Time—to engage, to notice when individuals are struggling, distressed, and conflicts may arise.

Training

The right training, by the right providers, with clinical credibility and appropriately updated and monitored in line with best practice (30). Our training and frameworks for restraint reduction should ideally be designed to address the influences on decision-making for staff mentioned earlier in the chapter. Knowing these influences gives us a solid platform to impact practice organizationally. If the right information, ethos, skills, and confidence are not being provided in training, then this will affect how the skills are utilized in practice.

Training needs to focus on risk assessment and care planning, risk management strategies based on the public health approach, and the communication skills required to support this. Following the work begun by the National Institute for Mental Health in England (9) over a decade ago, the Department of Health is once again consulting on the potential value of more robust monitoring and possible accreditation of training provision in the UK, in order to ensure the appropriate culture is embedded across NHS services.

Support structures

The area of post-incident support is poorly researched and there is a lack of consistency in approachs across services. NICE (12) identified that 'After using a restrictive intervention, and when the risks of harm have been contained, conduct an immediate post-incident review, including a nurse and a doctor, to identify and address physical harm to service users and staff, ongoing risks, and the emotional impact on service users and staff, including witnesses'.

In order to give support effectively, staff need to feel supported; in order to give care effectively they need to feel cared for and to give compassion, they need to feel compassion—unless we provide this for our staff in inpatient services, we are never likely to fully achieve the desired outcome of significantly reducing restraint.

Conclusion: looking to the future

PMVA raises a number of issues and dilemmas for staff involved in this intervention. This chapter has reviewed the historical roots of PMVA and the shifting emphasis from an intervention carried out on a person to more collaborative working between staff and those being restrained, with an overall aim of restraint reduction.

There is a complex area of decision-making in restraint situations and the important factors that play a part in this—from the risks involved to those being restrained and the legal framework that informs the use of restraint.

There have been a number of recent key influences concerning PMVA within a mental health setting—notably NICE (12), the Department of Health (14), and the Mental Health Act Code of Practice (24), which all work towards a proactive, preventative public health approach to reducing restraint.

The future of PMVA is changing, with ever-evolving training packages and restraint reduction strategies being implemented across mental health trusts in the UK, informed by an ever-growing body of good practice guidance, policy directives, and research.

This chapter has sought to highlight and clarify some of those key considerations with a view to supporting inpatient mental health staff to better understand the PMVA in their settings, hopefully making these complex issues more straightforward and overall reducing the need for such interventions.

REFERENCES

1. Paterson B, Bradley P, Stark C, Saddler D, Leadbetter D, Allen D. Deaths associated with restraint use in health and social care in the UK. The results of a preliminary survey. *J Psychiatr Ment Health Nurs* 2003;10:3–15.
2. Legistation.co.uk. Health and Safety at Work etc. Act 1974. https://www.legislation.gov.uk/ukpga/1974/37/contents
3. Legistation.co.uk. The Management of Health and Safety at Work Regulations 1992. http://www.legislation.gov.uk/uksi/1992/2051/contents/made
4. Winship G. Further thoughts on the process of restraint. *J Psychiatr Ment Health Nurs* 2006;13:55–60.
5. Turnbull J, Aitken I, Black L, Patterson B. Turn it around: short-term management for aggression and anger. *J Psychosoc Nurs Ment Health Serv* 1990;28:6–9.

6. Wright S, Gray R, Parkes J, Gournay K. *The Recognition, Prevention and Therapeutic Management of Violence in Acute In-patient Psychiatry—A Literature Review and Evidence Based Recommendations for Good Practice.* London: United Kingdom Central Council for Nursing, Midwifery and Health Visiting; 2002.

7. NHS Protect. *Promoting Safer and Therapeutic Services: Implementing the National Syllabus in Mental Health and Learning Disability Services.* London: Department of Health; 2005.

8. Hanks T. Department of health to remove NHS staff safety body. *The Mancunion* 2017;15:6. https://mancunion.com/2017/02/16/department-of-health-to-remove-nhs-staff-safety-body/

9. National Institute for Mental Health in England. *Mental Health Policy Implementation Guide: Developing Positive Practice to Support the Safe and Therapeutic Management of Aggression and Violence in Mental Health In-Patient Settings.* Leeds: Department of Health; 2004.

10. NHS Protect. *Meeting Needs and Reducing Distress: Guidance on the Prevention and Management of Clinically Related Challenging Behaviour in NHS Settings.* London: Department of Health; 2013.

11. National Collaborating Centre for Nursing and Supportive Care. *Violence: The Short Term Management of Disturbed/Violent Behaviour in In-Patient Psychiatric Settings and Emergency Departments.* London: Royal College of Nursing; 2005.

12. National Institute for Health and Care Excellence. Violence and aggression: short term management in mental health, health and community settings. NICE guideline [NG10]. 2015. https://www.nice.org.uk/guidance/ng10

13. Mind. *Mental Health Crisis Care: Physical Restraint in Crisis. A Report on Physical Restraint in Hospital Settings in England.* London: Mind; 2013.

14. Department of Health. *Positive and Proactive Care: Reducing the Need for Restrictive Interventions.* London: Department of Health; 2014.

15. Blofeld J. *The Independent Inquiry into the Death of David Bennett.* Cambridge: Norfolk, Suffolk and Cambridgeshire Strategic Health Authority; 2003.

16. Bradby H. Institutional racism in mental health services: the consequences of compromised conceptualisation. *Sociol Res Online* 2010;15:8.

17. Department of Health. *Transforming Care: A National Response to Winterbourne View Hospital.* London: Department of Health; 2012.

18. Colton D. *Checklist for Assessing Your Organization's Readiness for Reducing Seclusion and Restraint.* Staunton, VA: Commonwealth Center for Children and Adolescents; 2004.

19. Huckshorn KA. *Six Core Strategies for Reducing Seclusion and Restraint Use.* Alexandria, VA: National Association of State Mental Health Program Directors; 2006.

20. Bonner G, Lowe T, Rawcliffe D, Wellman N. Trauma for all: a pilot study of the subjective experience of physical restraint for mental health in-patients and staff in the UK. *J Psychiatr Ment Health Nurs* 2002;9:465–473.

21. Lancaster G, Whittington R, Lowe S, Riley D, Meehan C. Does the position of restraint of disturbed psychiatric patients have any association with staff and patient injuries? *J Psychiatr Ment Health Nurs* 2008;15:306–312.

22. Patterson B. Restraint related deaths in health and social care in the UK: learning the lessons. *Ment Health Pract* 2003;6:10–17.

23. Aiken F, Duxbury J, Dale C, Harbinson I. *Review of the Medical Theories and Research Relating to Restraint Related Death.* Lancaster: UCLAN; 2011.

24. Department of Health. *Mental Health Act 1983: Code of Practice.* Norwich: The Stationery Office; 2015.

25. Reay DT. Suspect restraint and sudden death. *FBI Law Enforc Bull* 1996;65:22–25.

26. Parkes J, Thake D, Price M. Effect of seated restraint and body size on lung function. *Med Sci Law* 2011;51:177–181.

27. Parkes J, Carson R. Sudden death during restraint: do some positions affect lung function. *Med Sci Law* 2008;48:137–141.

28. Morrison L, Moore C, Nathanson-Shinn A. *The Lethal Hazard of Prone Restraint: Positional Asphyxiation.* Oakland, CA: Protection & Advocacy, Inc.; 2001.

29. NHS England. *Patient Safety Alert Stage One: Warning. The Importance of Vital Signs During and After Restrictive Interventions/ Manual Restraint.* NHS/PSA/W/2015/011. London: NHS England; 2015.

30. Skills for Care, Skills for Health. *A Positive and Proactive Workforce: A Guide to Workforce Development for Commissioners and Employers Seeking to Minimise the Use of Restrictive Practices in Social Care and Health.* Leeds: Skills for Care, Skills for Health; 2014.

31. World Health Organization. *World Report on Violence and Health.* Geneva: World Health Organization; 2002.

32. Bowers L, Stewart D, Papadopoulos C, DeSanto Iennaco J. Correlation between levels of conflict and containment on acute psychiatric wards: the City 128 Study. *Psychiatr Serv* 2013;64:423–430.

33. Department of Health. *Best Practice in Managing Risk: Principles and Evidence for Best Practice in the Assessment and Management of Risk to Self and Others in Mental Health Services.* London: Department of Health; 2007.

34. Gilbert H. Evidence and principles for service user involvement. In: Whittington R, Logan C (eds), *Self Harm and Violence: Towards Best Practice in Managing Risk in Mental Health Services*, pp. 119–141. Chichester: Wiley Blackwell; 2011.

35. Whittington R, Logan C (eds). *Self Harm and Violence: Towards Best Practice in Managing Risk in Mental Health Services.* Chichester: Wiley Blackwell; 2011.

36. Duxbury J, Whittington R. Causes and management of patient aggression and violence: staff and patient perspectives. *J Adv Nurs* 2005;50:469–478.

37. Van der Schaaf PS, Dusseldorp E, Keuning FM, Janssen WA, Noorthoorn EO. Impact of the physical environment of psychiatric wards on the use of seclusion. *Br J Psychiatry* 2013;202:142–149.

38. McCue RE, Urcuyo L, Lilu Y, Tobias T, Chambers MJ. Reducing restraint use in a public psychiatric inpatient service. *J Behav Health Serv Res* 2004;31:217–224.

39. Papadopulos C, Ross J, Stewart D, Dack C, James K, Bowers L. Meta-analysis: the antecedents of violence and aggression within psychiatric in-patient settings. *Acta Psychiatr Scand* 2012;125:425–439.

40. Bowers L, Van Der Merwe M, Paterson B, Stewart D. Manual restraint and shows of force: the City 128 study. *Int J Ment Health Nurs* 2012;21:30–40.

41. Bowers L. Safewards: a new model of conflict and containment on psychiatric wards. *J Psychiatr Ment Health Nurs* 2014;21:499–508.

42. Bell A, Gallacher N. Succeeding in sustained reduction in the use of restraint using the improvement model. *BMJ Qual Improv Rep* 2016;5:u211050.w4430.

43. Whittington R, Lancaster G, Meehan C, Lane S, Riley D. Physical restraint of patients in acute mental health carer settings: patient, staff and environmental factors associated with the use of the horizontal restraint position. *J Forens Psychiatry Psychol* 2006;17:253–265.

44. Lazarus RS, Folkman S. *Stress, Appraisal and Coping.* New York: Springer; 1984.

45. Laiho T, Kattainen E, Astedt-Kurki P, Putkonen H, Lindberg N, Kylma J. Clinical decision making involved in secluding and restraining an adult psychiatric patient: an integrative literature review. *J Psychiatr Ment Health Nurs* 2013;20:830–839.
46. Lindsey PL. Psychiatric nurses decision to restrain—the association between empowerment and individual factors. *J Psychosoc Nurs* 2009;47:41–49.
47. Larue C, Dumais A, Ahern E, Bernheim E, Mailhot MP. Factors influencing decisions on seclusion and restraint. *J Psychiatr Ment Health Nurs* 2009;16:440–446.
48. Goethals S, Dierckx de Casterle B, Gastmans C. Nurses decision making in cases of physical restraint: a synthesis of qualitative evidence. *J Adv Nurs* 2011;68:1198–1210.
49. Casterle BD, Goethals S, Gastmans C. Contextual influences on nurses' decision-making in cases of physical restraint. *Nurs Ethics* 2015;22:642–651.
50. Moylan LB, Cullinan M. Frequency of assault and severity of injury of psychiatric nurses in relation to the nurses' decision to restrain. *J Psychiatr Ment Health Nurs* 2011;18:526–534.
51. Lavelle M, Stewart D, James K, et al. Predictors of effective de-escalation in acute inpatient psychiatric settings. *J Clin Nurs* 2016;25:2180–2188.
52. Griffith R. Using restraint—legal and professional considerations. *Br J Neurosci Nurs* 2016;12:94–95.
53. Legistation.co.uk. Mental Capacity Act 2005. https://www.legislation.gov.uk/ukpga/2005/9/contents
54. Legistation.co.uk. Mental Health Act 1983. https://www.legislation.gov.uk/ukpga/1983/20/contents
55. Legistation.co.uk. Mental Health (Care and Treatment) (Scotland) Act 2003. https://www.legislation.gov.uk/asp/2003/13/contents
56. Legistation.co.uk. Adults with Incapacity (Scotland) Act 2000. https://www.legislation.gov.uk/asp/2000/4/contents
57. Legistation.co.uk. The Mental Health (Amendment) (Northern Ireland) Order 2004. https://www.legislation.gov.uk/nisi/2004/1272/contents
58. Legistation.co.uk. Human Rights Act 1998. https://www.legislation.gov.uk/ukpga/1998/42/contents
59. Khwaja M, Beer D. *Prevention and Management of Violence: Guidance for Healthcare Professionals.* London: Royal College of Psychiatrists; 2013.
60. *Herczegfalvy* v. *Austria*, 15 E.H.R.R. 437, 1992 E.C.H.R. 58 (1993).
61. *PS, R (On the Application Of)* v *Responsible Medical Officer & Anor*, Court of Appeal—Administrative Court, 10 October 2003, [2003] EWHC 2335 (Admin).
62. Department for Constitutional Affairs. *Mental Capacity Act 2005: Code of Practice.* London: The Stationery Office; 2007.

16

Assessment and management of vulnerable patients

Sophie Behrman and Dorcas Dan-Cooke

Introduction

Staff working on mental health wards are well accustomed to assessing and managing vulnerable patients. With the current organization of mental health care in the UK, where only 5.7% of patients in contact with mental health services received inpatient care in a year (1), only the most unwell and/or complex patients are seen on mental health wards. These patients may well have numerous vulnerabilities, which require assessment and management as part of the holistic treatment of the patient during their admission and for discharge planning. This chapter discusses who these particularly vulnerable patients are, examines what sort of vulnerabilities patients might experience, and suggests possible management strategies.

Who is a vulnerable patient?

The Safeguarding Vulnerable Groups Act 2006 (2) defines all patients receiving 'any form of health care' as 'vulnerable'. Additional indicators of vulnerability mentioned in the Act are adults in residential accommodation or sheltered housing, receiving domiciliary care or any welfare payments, being detained in lawful custody (i.e. in a form of prison or as an asylum seeker) or under a court order, or requiring 'assistance in the conduct of his own affairs'. Hence, patients admitted to a mental health ward may well be 'vulnerable' in several respects.

The term 'vulnerable person' has evolved through recent judgments following the introduction of the Mental Capacity Act 2005 in 2007 (3), which broaden the designated population to which the Act applies from those 'mentally incapacitated' to include those who are 'vulnerable' (and thus likely to have capacity to make pertinent decisions) (4). This definition of 'vulnerability' is an objective finding based on the circumstances and risks that person may face, rather than an understanding of what it might feel subjectively to be 'vulnerable' (4).

Admission itself may expose previously masked or non-existent vulnerabilities. For example, a patient with mobility problems may be more vulnerable to falls in a new environment; another patient may struggle to eat in a strange environment; and all patients are at risk of becoming institutionalized through their admission. Admission also places a patient in a specialist environment, which may not suit all their needs. For example, a patient with significant mental health comorbidities will be more vulnerable on a ward primarily managing physical health care and vice versa.

Vulnerable adults are protected by several pieces of legislation in England. The Safeguarding Vulnerable Groups Act 2006 ensures that professionals working with vulnerable adults are adequately vetted, currently through the Disclosure and Barring Service procedure. The Care Act 2014 (5) places the onus on local authorities to ensure physical, mental, and emotional well-being of people under their care, including protection from abuse and neglect. There is no specific legislation covering how vulnerable adults should be managed within the National Health Service (NHS), but the NHS England 'Safeguarding policy' (6) recognizes that 'safeguarding is everybody's business and that the safety and well-being of those in vulnerable circumstances is at the forefront of our business'. It is recommended that health services work closely with social services in order to promote well-being of vulnerable people through the Safeguarding Adults Boards.

Ill treatment of vulnerable patients within the health service is a criminal offence. Originally specified in the Mental Health Act 1983 (Section 127) (7) to protect patients with mental disorders, it was subsequently also made an offence to ill-treat or wilfully neglect a patient who lacks capacity to make relevant decisions (3). More recently, the Berwick report (8), commissioned by the government following the poor care exposed in the Mid-Staffordshire NHS Foundation Trust, proposed to 'place wilful or reckless neglect or mistreatment of all NHS patients on a par with the offence that currently applies to vulnerable people under the Mental Capacity Act'. Although the legal onus of protecting vulnerable adults falls on social care, there is a duty of care in the health service and the 'Government Policy on Adult Safeguarding' states that 'safeguarding is everybody's business' (9).

The term 'vulnerable adult' must be used with caution. There is a danger that patients with such a label will be stigmatized and perhaps be assumed to lack the ability to make decisions, resulting in a lack of empowerment. Conversely, if patients are not recognized to be 'vulnerable', there is a danger that they will not receive sufficient support.

As all patients admitted to a mental health ward are likely to be vulnerable in some sense, for the purposes of this chapter, we will consider the assessment and management of patients who are particularly vulnerable within the inpatient population.

Who is particularly vulnerable on admission to a mental health ward?

There is no definitive list of who will be most vulnerable, but it could be argued that the most vulnerable patients on a ward will have conditions or difficulties outside or on the periphery of the spectrum of expertise of the ward staff and environmental set-up. The nature of specialist wards means that patients requiring admission may have specialist treatment for one condition perhaps at the expense of another. For example, a patient admitted to a mental health ward with an acute psychotic episode may find their comorbid diabetes is less well managed than it was in the community. It is the responsibility of ward staff to be aware of their limitations as a team and to seek external support and advice where required. The 'silo mentality' of specialist services occurs within mental health services as well, where patients are slotted into a service based on (perhaps) geographical location, age, and diagnosis and little information is shared between services or teams, for example, between general services and specialist services such as learning disability and older adult psychiatry. Even if the patient technically meets the ward's admission criteria, they will be more vulnerable if the ward staff are less familiar with working with people with similar conditions. Furthermore, it is not uncommon for people to be admitted to inappropriate wards (e.g. an elderly patient admitted to a general ward) in an emergency when a more appropriate bed is not available. A patient being cared for on a ward that is not geared towards their age and/or diagnosis is vulnerable to receiving potentially substandard and/or unsafe care (10). This might include delayed discharge if the ward staff are unfamiliar with his/her condition and associated issues, and potential harm from other patients and from being cared for in an inappropriate environment (e.g. heavy doors on a general ward may harm a frail elderly person).

Demographic characteristics

Age

Wards' admission criteria are typically guided by age. Those at both ends of the age spectrum may be more vulnerable on a general ward. The Royal College of Psychiatrists recognizes that an 'adult ward cannot automatically provide safe or effective care for young people' (11) and advises that patients under 18 year of age are admitted to specialist child and adolescent mental health units where possible. Similarly, frail elderly people are seen to be at increased risk on a general adult ward (12). Despite these recommendations, there has been a trend towards 'ageless services' in psychiatry in the UK; in some areas, elderly patients with functional illness (as opposed to dementia) are admitted to wards shared with younger adult patients (13).

Gender

The Department of Health directed trusts to eliminate mixed-sex accommodation in 2009 (14), which eradicated some of the vulnerabilities patients faced on mixed-sex wards. There is still some element of vulnerability with regard to transgender patients, who should be 'accommodated according to their presentation: the way they dress, and the name and pronouns that they currently use'. Transgender people may be vulnerable to stigma as health care systems and staff may intentionally or unintentionally (through lack of understanding) mistreat or offend (15). In a psychiatric ward, this may manifest as staff treating the patient differently, perhaps making the patient less willing to seek help. Conversely, staff may be overly sensitive to the patient's gender and are at risk of misattributing all symptoms, including common medical problems, to the patient's gender dysphoria.

Ethnicity

Black and minority ethnic (BME) people are known to face more difficulties during a hospital admission due to both sociocultural difficulties (e.g. different health beliefs) and systemic problems (e.g. culturally insensitive mental health services) (16). Improving the inpatient experience of BME groups is a priority for the Royal College of Psychiatrists. With individual, holistic assessments by culturally aware staff members, it is hoped that any vulnerabilities experienced by BME patients will be minimized.

Language barrier

People who do not speak English well will be vulnerable to their needs not being met as swiftly as patients who are better able to communicate with ward staff. Even people who usually communicate well in English, although it is not their mother tongue, may struggle to communicate effectively when highly stressed or anxious, as they might be on admission to a ward. In emergency situations, the onus of translating may be put on a family member or individual staff member (where one is available with a common language) and this may subsequently affect family or team dynamics and the relationship between the patient and the person translating. Where professional translators are available, they are often not effectively used (17) and the time constraints mean the conversation may be prematurely curtailed.

Sexuality

The effect of sexuality on a patient's inpatient care has not been examined. Lesbian, gay, and bisexual (LGB) individuals have high levels of mental disorder, which may be linked to perceived discrimination (18). LGB individuals are likely to report negative experiences of accessing mental health care, with concerns that clinicians are uncomfortable or inexperienced when dealing with issues relating to sexuality, or over-attributing psychopathology to the patient's sexuality (19). It is possible that this would make LGB patients more vulnerable on a mental health ward.

Physical health problems

Sensory problems

A mental health ward is an alien and, at times, unnerving environment even for people without sensory impairment. Patients with sensory impairment may feel particularly vulnerable during an admission.

Hearing-impaired patients may use sign language and require an interpreter (see 'Language barrier' for difficulties with translators). Patients with hearing impairment may find conversations in a large group difficult (e.g. ward round, discharge planning meetings) and may miss key information or feel unable to participate.

Visually impaired patients may feel vulnerable on a mental health ward, not being able to orientate themselves in a new environment and not recognizing others around them.

Delirium

A patient with delirium will be subjectively and objectively confused and may struggle to make their needs known. The recognized adverse outcomes of delirium include falls, pressure sores, infections, and malnutrition (20), which are all indicative of the vulnerability of a patient with delirium in any environment. Delirium is a medical emergency and often related to an underlying physical illness; there is a risk on a psychiatric ward that the patient's symptoms of delirium are misattributed to a mental illness and the physical illness is not recognized or effectively treated.

Other physical health problems

The relationships between comorbid physical and mental health conditions are complex and multifactorial. It is well recognized that people with mental illnesses are likely to receive substandard physical health care and there are campaigns to address potential barriers to accessing treatment (21). In a psychiatric ward environment, a patient who is acutely mentally unwell may be less adept at managing their own physical health conditions, leading to a potential decline in physical health. Similarly, patients with mental illness admitted to medical wards are at risk of deterioration of their mental health during their admission and are more vulnerable to other associated adverse outcomes (21).

Mental health problems

As discussed earlier, any mental health problem that is beyond the usual remit of the ward may lead to a patient being particularly vulnerable. All mental illnesses carry particular risks, which may increase a patient's vulnerability: for example, a patient with depression may be at risk of not maintaining sufficient oral intake, and a patient with dementia may be at risk of falls. These risks associated with mental illnesses are specific to each individual patient and will result in some patients being more vulnerable than others.

What vulnerabilities might a patient experience?

In order for an admission to be deemed helpful and necessary, in most cases it will have been agreed that the risk of a patient remaining in the community outweighs the potential risks and undesirable aspects of admission. Identifying and managing risk is a huge part of a psychiatric assessment and is beyond the scope of this chapter. Risks and vulnerability are interlinked, but for the purposes of this chapter we will consider a subsection of patients with vulnerabilities that augment and/or compound the more standard 'risks' associated with mental illness.

Some vulnerability may occur because of mental illness (e.g. a patient with an affective disorder may self-medicate with alcohol and develop alcohol dependence). Some vulnerability may contribute to

mental disorder (e.g. a patient may be more likely to develop depression if they lose employment). Some vulnerabilities may be unrelated to a patient's mental disorder.

Vulnerabilities specific to being on a ward

Iatrogenic harm

There is scope for a patient coming to harm when accessing health care whether in the community or in a ward. Perhaps the most pertinent incidents of iatrogenic harm in hospital are medication errors, where (for example) a patient is accidentally given a medication they have not been prescribed. Some patients may be more vulnerable to such errors, if they are unable or unwilling to engage with their treatment plan or if they feel unable to question staff. Empowering patients to 'speak up' has been identified as a key factor in maximizing patient safety in the Berwick report, which concludes that 'patient safety improves when patients are more involved in their care and have more control' (8). Active participation of individual inpatients in their care has been shown to reduce the risk of adverse events (22).

Accidents

Even with a move towards clinical environments designed and built to optimize safety, accidents happen. Falls are a common accident both in and out of hospital and risk factors have been well characterized in medical wards (23), but there is a dearth of evidence to suggest who may be more vulnerable to falls on a psychiatric ward (24). Falls are a particular problem in the elderly population and older adult psychiatric wards commonly have a 'falls pathway' which triggers a multidisciplinary assessment of patients prone to falls to ensure that all potential risk factors are minimized (e.g. a physiotherapy assessment, a review of medication and medical comorbidities, and a review of any sensory impairment).

Ward environment

The ward environment may be disorientating and precipitate or worsen an acute confusional state, particularly in older patients with medical comorbidities. Similarly, a younger patient with acute paranoid symptoms may experience a transient worsening of symptoms on admission.

Loss of appetite is a symptom of many mental health conditions, and this symptom may be worsened on admission to a ward, as a patient will not be accustomed to the ward regime and hospital food. If not detected and managed, this may lead to malnutrition. The Royal College of Nursing has issued guidance as to how nutrition should be assessed and managed in a ward environment (25).

Risk from other patients

Even with good care and a well-managed ward (26), there remains a risk of a patient being assaulted or otherwise abused by other patients. There is no evidence to suggest which patient groups may be more at risk of being on the receiving end of such abuse. Where abuse is suspected, or has occurred, staff are advised to follow the safeguarding process (see later sections).

Risk from staff

Fortunately, incidents of staff abusing patients on psychiatric wards are very rare, but less severe violations of professional relationships do occur more frequently, when the clinician–patient relationship blurs into one of friendship (27). A patient may be more vulnerable to violations of the boundary of a therapeutic relationship on a ward where staff and patients spend more time together than they would do in the community. Patients may develop an overdependence on certain staff members as professional roles blur; this may lead to later distress and potential future mistrust of professionals. There is detailed guidance available on how to manage therapeutic professional relationships with vulnerable patients (27).

Vulnerabilities from the wider community ongoing through admission

A patient with a mental health crisis may well have ongoing psychosocial stressors while on the ward. Admission may have been precipitated by a crisis and/or may compound ongoing social problems, such as housing and employment difficulties. Relationships with friends and families may be strained or even pathological. Emotional, physical, and financial abuse may continue through an admission. A thorough, sensitive, and compassionate assessment on the ward should enable the staff to develop a holistic picture of the patient and their relationships and help to identify and manage any vulnerabilities through an admission.

Why do we assess vulnerability?

The subjective experience of vulnerability may cause or exacerbate stress and anxiety, which affect physiological, psychological, and social functioning. The relationship between vulnerability and well-being is examined in the stress vulnerability model developed by Zubin and Spring (28). The model suggests that individuals become unwell when the stress they face exceeds their coping skills. Individuals have unique biological, psychological, and social vulnerabilities and strengths that interact when faced with a stressful situation. When vulnerabilities exceed strengths, there is the risk of development or exacerbation of mental illnesses or disorders. Using this model, it is possible to argue that the greater an individual's level of vulnerability, the less stress is required to trigger the symptoms of a mental illness or poverty in their overall well-being (29). Stress is known to have a negative effect on physical health: stress slows down wound healing and impairs recovery from surgery (30). In order to minimize the effects of stress on patients' physical and mental health, it is necessary for patients' vulnerabilities to be identified and, where possible, addressed.

Health professionals' failure to identify and respond effectively to these vulnerabilities can increase the effects of stress and lead to poor clinical outcomes, such as worsening of the illness and death, as was found to be the case in the Mid Staffordshire NHS Foundation Trust. The Francis report published in 2013 was the result of a public inquiry into the role of commissioning, supervisory, and regulatory bodies in the monitoring of the Mid Staffordshire NHS Foundation Trust between January 2005 and March 2009 (31). Findings uncovered reports of staff treating patients and their families with indifference and a lack of basic kindness. An independent report found that up to 1200 people had died as a result of 'unacceptable' neglect or maltreatment (31).

Health care professionals have also been found not to identify and manage vulnerable patients at risk of abuse during their care. In 2015, the publication of a further 34 NHS investigations found

evidence to support allegations of a prolific history of sexual abuse on hospital premises, after the Jimmy Savile inquiry (32). Lampard and Marsden (33) identified a very fragmented approach to managing reports of abuse and vulnerable patients, where patients were not empowered to make choices about their care, and neglect and abuse arose in the absence of effective prevention and early warning systems. Revelations of this kind have led professionals to question what measures should be put in place to prevent a repeat of such scandals, and what the role of health care professionals should be in identifying and managing vulnerable adults.

Organizational role in managing vulnerability

Following the Francis report and the Jimmy Savile investigations (see 'Why do we assess vulnerability?'), strategies for organizational reform have been identified (7, 30). Firstly, a cultural change is required in order for patients, and their families and friends, to feel confident to identify when something is not right and speak to relevant authorities. This may manifest as a change in staff attitudes to accepting criticisms and complaints, or perhaps systems put in place to facilitate people speaking up. Secondly, frontline staff should be supported to foster change through their individual responsibilities, behaviours, and values, and by working effectively together in strong teams. Thirdly, the leadership teams within the NHS are to have the principal responsibility of ensuring that care in their organizations is safe and that those who use their services are treated as individuals, with dignity and compassion. Fourthly, the external structures surrounding each individual organization, including commissioners, regulators, professional bodies, local scrutiny bodies, and government, must support this and tackle any areas of poor performance rapidly and decisively. These reforms were realized with the publication of the Care Act 2014 (5) which provides a legal framework of principles and duties for local authorities and in turn the health services and professionals within them to reduce the risk of abuse and neglect (34).

A key principle within this legislation is the concept of safeguarding. The Care Act 2014 (5) explains safeguarding as protecting an adult's right to live in safety, free from abuse and neglect. It is about people and organizations working together to reduce the risks of abuse and neglect, while at the same time making sure that the adult's well-being and autonomy are promoted. This is translated into local safeguarding processes, where health care professionals can raise a 'safeguarding alert', which triggers a review of the situation and involves the relevant agencies to ensure the risks are adequately assessed and managed appropriately.

How to assess the vulnerable patient and their needs

When undertaking any safeguarding assessment, professionals should uphold principles of positive risk management, working to promote autonomy, support well-being, and also maximize safety.

There are six key principles that underpin safeguarding (9):

1. Empowerment—presumption of person-led decisions and informed consent.

2. Prevention—it is better to take action before harm occurs.
3. Proportionality—proportionate and least intrusive response appropriate to the risk presented.
4. Protection—support and representation for those in greatest need.
5. Partnerships—local solutions through services working with their communities.
6. Accountability—accountability and transparency in delivering safeguarding.[1]

A vulnerable patient may be able to identify their vulnerabilities themselves and discuss this with their health care professionals, and such information can be used to draw up a timeline of suspected and reported risks and other pertinent events. As well as the vulnerabilities to harm, a patient's strengths and coping resources may be added to complete a holistic and individual assessment. Any ongoing safeguarding interventions should also be noted and their efficacy reviewed regularly.

Involving the vulnerable person in decision-making

There is a danger that the term 'vulnerable adult' may be stigmatizing and lead to discrimination; in particular, it may lead to a paternalistic system, with a tendency for the vulnerable person to be less involved in decisions regarding their health and social care. The 'Statement of Government Policy on Safeguarding Adults' addresses this to some extent by its first principle: 'Empowerment – presumption of person-led decision and informed consent' (9). This resonates with the Mental Capacity Act 2005 principle: 'a person must be assumed to have capacity unless it is established that he lacks capacity' (3).

Under the Mental Capacity Act 2005, a decision made on behalf of a person who lacks capacity will be done in his/her 'best interests', but the person making the decision must 'permit and encourage the person to participate … as fully as possible in any act done for him and any decision affecting him'. Regardless of whether a person has capacity or not to make a decision, they should be involved as much as possible in the decision-making process. Special care may be needed to encourage a vulnerable person to involve themselves in the process, particularly as it may be simpler and faster for well-meaning professionals to take a paternalistic stance.

How to manage the vulnerable patient and their needs

On admission to a ward, a patient will undergo assessment by a variety of professionals, including doctors, nurses, occupational therapists, psychologists, and social workers. Any professional may uncover aspects of the patient's history or presentation which they may consider to be 'vulnerabilities'. Should these vulnerabilities be considered serious enough to reach the threshold for safeguarding,

it is the responsibility of the professional involved to report using local procedures, for example, an incident form, to ensure the safeguarding team are aware of the risk and appropriate agencies are contacted. The professional will devise an immediate care plan to manage this risk and ensure the patient's notes and risk assessment are updated. The safeguarding procedure will examine the case using the guiding principles mentioned previously and amend the plan as needed. If the vulnerabilities concerned do not require the raising of a safeguarding alert, the case can be purely managed within the multidisciplinary team, with ward and community teams working together to share information and decision-making about how to manage the vulnerabilities through admission to discharge.

Throughout admission, the principles of safeguarding can be used as prompts for managing vulnerabilities, even if they do not reach a threshold for raising a safeguarding alert (9).

• Empowerment: what does the person want? How can they be best involved in decision making? What rights need to be respected? Are there duties to act—are others at risk of harm?
• Prevention: can acting now prevent problems occurring later?
• Protection: is this person a 'vulnerable adult'? What support do they need? Is capacity an issue? Should others, such as a carer (relatives, friends), be involved?
• Proportionality: have risks been weighed up? Does the nature of the concern require referral through multi agency procedures? In some areas, multiagency safeguarding hubs manage major safeguarding risks and ensure that relevant agencies including (where appropriate) police, health, mental health, and social care share information and collaborate to manage risk.
• Partnership: what is the view of others involved? How do multiagency procedures apply?
• Accountability: is the decision well made? Have all relevant factors and viewpoints been considered and documented? Is it defensible? Is it in line with appropriate legislation? Have local procedures been followed and documentation completed?[2]

All assessments and discussions need careful documentation in the clinical notes, including the rationale for any decisions made, particularly if they are made in the patient's best interests. At all points during the patient's care, there should be opportunities to review and reflect on decisions made. This may be used for individual learning and development opportunity, but also to consider wider organizational themes and identify possibilities for systemic quality improvement.

What is the professional responsibility to support and prevent risk to vulnerable adults?

It is the responsibility of individual professionals to acquaint themselves with local protection policies and procedures and understand their professional role in identifying and managing safeguarding concerns. In an inpatient setting, health care professionals must

[1] Social Care Policy. *Statement of Government Policy on Adult Safeguarding*. Department of Health 2013. Contains public sector information licensed under the Open Government Licence v3.0. http://www.nationalarchives.gov.uk/doc/open-government-licence/version/3/.

[2] Social Care Policy. *Statement of Government Policy on Adult Safeguarding*. Department of Health 2013. Contains public sector information licensed under the Open Government Licence v3.0. http://www.nationalarchives.gov.uk/doc/open-government-licence/version/3/.

endeavour to open dialogues with patients and carers to ensure an open and honest culture. Patients and carers must also feel empowered to report maltreatment and abuse, and it is the role of the professionals to ensure pathways to speaking up are clear and accessible; this may include supplying literature in different formats (e.g. for the visually or hearing impaired, and in different languages).

The assessment and management of vulnerable patients and the safeguarding process are topics that should be covered in individual reflective practice and supervision, which may be informed by requesting feedback from colleagues and patients. Professional bodies such as the Nursing and Midwifery Council and General Medical Council set the culture and professional standards (35, 36), and, when required, act where professionals may have abused or neglected people in their care.

Clinical vignettes

John

John is a 35-year-old man with an acquired brain injury following an accident 10 years ago. John usually lives independently with daily support from his family and friends. He has a history of depression following his accident and was admitted to the ward in a depressive episode as he was unable to manage his self-care, was not eating and drinking, and had suicidal thoughts. John was considered to have capacity to consent to his admission and treatment.

Vulnerabilities experienced by John

- Difficulties when interacting with other patients, leading to potentially violent arguments.
- Difficulties when interacting with ward staff unaccustomed to patients with brain injuries.
- Epilepsy, requiring medication. Vulnerable to potential drug errors.
- Risk of not being involved in decision-making due to brain injury, even though he has capacity to consent to his current treatment.
- Social support network breaking down while in hospital.
- Poor oral intake.

Possible management strategies

- Regular nursing observations on admission while patient acclimatizes to the ward and to monitor interactions with other patients.
- Training for ward staff in managing patients with brain injuries.
- Pharmacist and medical staff to review his medication.
- Appropriate family/friend or independent patient advocate to support John at ward rounds and other key meetings.
- Involvement of friends and family (as appropriate) in discharge planning.
- Occupational therapy assessment with regard to self-care skills.
- Food and fluid chart to monitor oral intake.

Frederick

Frederick is a 68-year-old man with a history of chronic alcohol abuse and some mild cognitive impairment. He is admitted acutely to a general adult ward under the Mental Health Act 1983 as there are no older adult beds. Frederick is believed to be psychotic as he believes his wife is having an affair, which she denies to the assessing team. Through the admission, it transpires that Frederick's wife *is* having an affair and Frederick is *not* psychotic and his cognitive impairment improves while abstinent from alcohol. While Frederick is in hospital, his wife withdraws a substantial sum of money from their joint account.

Vulnerabilities experienced by Frederick

- Wife abusing the health care system to have Frederick detained.
- Frederick's account not 'believed' by the assessing team, perhaps influenced by his known cognitive impairment.
- General adult staff unaccustomed to managing an older patient with cognitive impairment.
- Financial abuse by family.

Possible management strategies

- Open a safeguarding alert and discuss urgently with safeguarding lead. This is likely to require police/court involvement.
- Incident report around original assessment and analysis of situation that led to Frederick being detained with a view to assessing if further staff training may help.
- Older adult's team to assess if Frederick would be more suitable on an older adult ward and, if not, to advise the general adult ward team on management strategies.

Leah

Leah is a 25-year-old woman brought to A&E by police who found her acting strangely at a train station. No physical health problem was identified and she is subsequently detained under the Mental Health Act 1983. She is acutely psychotic and thought disordered on admission to the ward. No information is known about her and staff are not even sure they have the correct name.

Vulnerabilities experienced by Leah

- Lack of information means any number of vulnerabilities could be present and unidentified.
- Bizarre behaviour associated with thought disorder may make Leah vulnerable to difficult interactions with other patients.

Possible management strategies

- Search of belongings in order to try to find out her identity and potential leads to gain collateral/background information.
- Careful and sensitive assessment to see if Leah can give any further information about her identity and/or background. Leah may be more forthcoming when her psychosis is treated.
- Check police missing person reports to see if the patient can be identified.
- Nursing observations on the ward to monitor for interpersonal difficulties with other patients.

Charlotte

Charlotte is a 34-year-old lady, admitted with a manic episode on a background of bipolar affective disorder. Charlotte is known to become trusting and rather promiscuous when manic and has given money and keys to people she does not know well. A new male 'friend' is keen to be involved in her care and visits the ward frequently.

Vulnerabilities experienced by Charlotte

- Risk of financial exploitation as Charlotte has given away money and access to her property.
- Potential risk of sexual exploitation/risk of pregnancy and sexually transmitted infections.
- The status of the relationship with the new 'friend' needs to be assessed and the input in her care must be approached with caution.

Possible management strategies

- Open safeguarding with regard to potential financial and sexual exploitation.
- Ensure property is secure (may need to have locks changed).
- Review status of bank cards, if possible.
- Pregnancy test and encouragement to attend genitourinary medicine clinic to screen for sexually transmitted infections.
- Ongoing assessment of capacity to consent for information to be shared with her new friend. While she lacks capacity, staff to monitor the friend's visits for any potential abuse.
- Liaising with carers, relatives, friends, and professionals who may have information about Jasmine's behaviour when euthymic and when unwell.

Conclusion

As part of a full comprehensive assessment on admission to a ward, health care professionals will identify patients who are more 'vulnerable' and those specific vulnerabilities will be outlined. Some vulnerabilities identified may require the formal safeguarding process and a discussion with the trust safeguarding lead in order to maintain the safety of the patient and/or others. Some vulnerabilities identified may be due to the ward staff's lack of expertise; in these cases, it is the responsibility of the staff to seek advice from other professionals or seek further training, as appropriate. The assessment and management of vulnerabilities is likely to be ongoing through admission and after discharge and will be most nuanced and thorough if it involves input from all members of the multidisciplinary team.

REFERENCES

1. Health & Social Care Information Centre. Mental health bulletin, annual statistics 2014–2015. 2015. https://digital.nhs.uk/data-and-information/publications/statistical/mental-health-bulletin/mental-health-bulletin-annual-report-2014-15
2. Legislation.gov.uk. Safeguarding Vulnerable Groups Act 2006. 2006. http://www.legislation.gov.uk/ukpga/2006/47/contents
3. Legislation.gov.uk. Mental Capacity Act 2005. 2005. http://www.legislation.gov.uk/ukpga/2005/9
4. Dunn MC, Clare ICH, Holland AJ. To empower or to protect? Constructing the 'vulnerable adult' in English law and public policy. *Legal Studies* 2008;28:234–253.
5. Legislation.gov.uk. Care Act 2014. 2014. http://www.legislation.gov.uk/ukpga/2014/23/contents/enacted
6. NHS England. Safeguarding policy. Version 2. 2015. https://www.england.nhs.uk/wp-content/uploads/2015/07/safeguard-policy.pdf
7. Legislation.gov.uk. Mental Health Act 1983. 1983. http://www.legislation.gov.uk/ukpga/2005/9
8. Berwick D, National Advisory Group on the Safety of Patients in England. 2013. A promise to learn – a commitment to act. https://assets.publishing.service.gov.uk/government/uploads/system/uploads/attachment_data/file/226703/Berwick_Report.pdf
9. Social Care Policy. Statement of government policy on adult safeguarding. Department of Health; 2013. https://assets.publishing.service.gov.uk/government/uploads/system/uploads/attachment_data/file/197402/Statement_of_Gov_Policy.pdf
10. Goulding L, Adamson J, Watt I, Wright J. Patient safety in patients who occupy beds on clinically inappropriate wards: a qualitative interview study with NHS staff. *BMJ Qual Saf* 2012;21;218–224.
11. O'Herlihy A, Lelliott P. *Safe and Appropriate Care for Young People on Adult Mental Health Wards. Pilot Programme Report.* London: Royal College of Psychiatrists; 2009.
12. Pinner G, Hillam J, Branton T, Ramakrishnan A. *Inpatient Care for Older People Within Mental Health Services.* Faculty Report FR/OA/1. Faculty of the Psychiatry of Old Age of the Royal College of Psychiatrists. London: Royal College of Psychiatrists; 2011.
13. Warner J, Jenkinson J. Psychiatry for the elderly in the UK. *Lancet* 2013;381:1985.
14. Beasley C, Flory D. Eliminating mixed sex accommodation in hospitals. PL/CNO/2009/2. Department of Health; 2009. https://assets.publishing.service.gov.uk/government/uploads/system/uploads/attachment_data/file/200215/CNO_note_dh_098893.pdf
15. White Hughto JM, Reisner SL, Pachankis JE. Transgender stigma and health: a critical review of stigma determinants, mechanisms and interventions. *Soc Sci Med* 2015;147:222–231.
16. Fitch C, Wilson M, Worrall A. *Improving In-Patient Mental Health Services for Black and Minority Ethnic Patients.* Occasional Paper 71. London: Royal College of Psychiatrists; 2009.
17. Tribe R. Working with interpreters in mental health. *Int J Cult Ment Health* 2009;2:92–101.
18. Warner J, McKeown E, Griffin M, et al. Rates and predictors of mental illness in gay men, lesbians and bisexual men and women. *BJPsych* 2004;185:479–485.
19. King M, McKeown E. *Mental Health and Social Wellbeing of Gay Men, Lesbians and Bisexuals in England and Wales: A Summary of Findings.* London: Mind; 2003.
20. British Geriatrics Society and Royal College of Physicians. *Guidelines for the Prevention, Diagnosis and Management of Delirium in Older People.* Concise Guidance to Good Practice Series, No. 6. London: Royal College of Physicians; 2006.
21. BMA Board of Science. *Recognising the Importance of Physical Health in Mental Health and Intellectual Disability: Achieving Parity of Outcomes.* London: BMA; 2014.
22. Weingart SN, Zhu J, Chiappetta L, et al. Hospitalized patients' participation and its impact on quality of care and patient safety. *Int J Qual Health Care* 2011;23:269–277.
23. Oliver D, Daly F, Martin FC, McMurdo MET. Risk factors and risk assessment tools for falls in hospital in-patients: a systematic review. *Age Ageing* 2004;33:122–130.
24. Bunn F, Dickinson A, Simpson C, et al. Preventing falls among older people with mental health problems: a systematic review. *BMC Nurs* 2014;13:4–18.
25. Royal College of Nursing. Nutrition and hydration. https://www.rcn.org.uk/clinical-topics/nutrition-and-hydration
26. Royal College of Psychiatrists. *Do the Right Thing: How to Judge a Good Ward. Ten Standards for Adult In-Patient Mental Healthcare.* Occasional Paper 79. London: Royal College of Psychiatrists; 2011.
27. Milavic G, Adshead G, Jarrett P. *Vulnerable Patients, Safe Doctors; Good Practice in our Clinical Relationships,* 2nd edition. College Report 180. London: Royal College of Psychiatrists; 2013.

28. Zubin, J, Spring B. Vulnerability: a new view on schizophrenia. *J Abnorm Psychol* 1977;86:103–126.

29. Goh C, Agius M. The stress-vulnerability model how does stress impact on mental illness at the level of the brain and what are the consequences? *Psychiatr Danub* 2010;22:198–202.

30. Mavros MN, Athanasiou S, Gkegkes ID, et al. Do psychological variables affect early surgical recovery? *PLoS One* 2011;6:e20306.

31. Francis R. *Report of the Mid Staffordshire NHS Foundation Trust Public Inquiry, Volume 1*. London: The Stationery Office; 2013.

32. Lampard K. Independent oversight of NHS and Department of Health investigations into matters relating to Jimmy Savile. An assurance report for the Secretary of State for Health. 2014. https://www.gov.uk/government/publications/nhs-jimmy-savile-investigation-assurance-report

33. Lampard K, Marsden E. Themes and lessons learnt from NHS investigations into matters relating to Jimmy Savile. Independent report for the Secretary of State for Health. 2015. https://assets.publishing.service.gov.uk/government/uploads/system/uploads/attachment_data/file/407209/KL_lessons_learned_report_FINAL.pdf

34. Chisnell C, Kelly C. *Safeguarding in Social Work Practice: A Lifespan Approach*. London: SAGE Publications Ltd; 2016.

35. The Nursing and Midwifery Council. The code: professional standards of practice and behaviour for nurses and midwives. 2015. https://www.nmc.org.uk/globalassets/sitedocuments/nmc-publications/nmc-code.pdf

36. General Medical Council. Good medical practice. 2013. http://www.gmc-uk.org/guidance/good_medical_practice/contents.asp

17

People with personality disorders and developmental conditions on an inpatient ward

Steve Pearce and Gail Critchlow

Introduction

People with personality disorders (PDs) incur high costs ((1), attract negative judgements (2, 3), and evoke defensive practice (4). Most psychiatric patients with PDs suffer from borderline personality disorder (BPD) (5) and accordingly most of the research in PD management and treatment has focused on this condition. People with BPD constitute the majority of patients presenting with repeated suicidality (6), and are among the most difficult to manage on psychiatric wards.

The debate about whether there is an effective treatment for PDs, and in particular BPD, is now over. A range of psychosocial treatments have demonstrated effectiveness in outpatient settings, mostly over long treatment periods. One has also demonstrated persisting gains (7). The progress in this area answers one of the reasons for the neglect of PD by psychiatrists and mental health treatment services. Very few studies, however, have examined the impact of inpatient treatment, or addressed the problems of attempting to help patients with this diagnosis in an inpatient setting. Patients with BPD in psychiatric inpatient wards represent a more disabled and higher-risk group than those in the community (8); they have high rates of suicide (9), and can be difficult to discharge. Patients with BPD suffer from long-term intractable disability even after symptom remission (10). Inpatient admissions often occur out of hours, reflecting both the urgent and episodic nature of the distress that characterizes the disorder, and difficulties in implementing a consistent management plan. Patients with BPD tend to be more severely ill but are admitted less often than other psychiatric patients presenting out of hours, of which they constitute almost 10% (11). Nevertheless, even emergency admissions can be viewed as an opportunity: to rationalize medication, clarify management strategies, and sometimes to have a positive impact on the trajectory of the patient's interactions with services.

Patients admitted with PD often suffer from other comorbid mental disorders, which may complicate management (such as varieties of dissociation, (12); substance misuse; eating disorders; and depression and anxiety (13)). Those admitted because of a psychotic or affective disorder often suffer from comorbid PD. This is important because comorbid PD is underdiagnosed, increases risks and makes other disorders more difficult to treat (14, 15).

The value of psychiatric admission for patients with PD, in particular those with BPD, has been questioned. Expert opinion regards this question has settled (16). Although admission to psychiatric inpatient care can cause iatrogenic harms (outlined below), there are situations in which it is the only feasible way to manage risk. Other indications for admission are less common but a policy of never admitting patients with PD without comorbid axis I pathology is likely itself to cause harms (17).

Guidelines for inpatient treatment suffer from a lack of research, and tend to be vague or difficult to implement. Most of the literature concerns BPD, as it presents the most difficulties in management. Most of the conclusions we outline from this literature are applicable to patients identified as personality disordered on psychiatric wards who may suffer from other PDs manifesting interpersonal difficulties, at times with accompanying abnormal illness behaviour. In this chapter, we review the evidence that exists for inpatient treatment of people with BPD, and draw conclusions about the management of inpatients with PD more widely.

The developmental conditions autism spectrum disorder (ASD) and adult attention deficit hyperactivity disorder (ADHD) can pose similar problems of splitting, negative staff attitudes, and pessimism. ASD can impact concordance with treatment planning, and interpersonal difficulties can make effective management and discharge difficult, to which is added the problem that an effective psychiatric treatment is not available. Adult ADHD is a controversial diagnosis. Although the prevalence of symptoms drops off sharply after the age of 18, some symptoms can persist. Faraone et al. (18) found in a meta-analysis that significant symptoms of ADHD persist in 15% of 25-year-olds diagnosed with ADHD in childhood to the extent that they could be diagnosed with adult ADHD. Research to date has focused on defining and consolidating the concept, and on medication. Some of the symptoms of ADHD are similar to those of BPD, and ADHD is common in the childhoods of people who go on to suffer BPD (19). The overlap between the diagnoses in adulthood is high, and ADHD symptoms have been proposed as differentiating an impulsive subtype of BPD from an affective subtype (20). Patients with ADHD symptoms in adulthood should receive stimulant medication as the evidence base evolves to support improved long-term outcomes or short-term benefits. Some issues of management that arise on inpatient units are likely to mirror those in BPD.

Personality disorder

Research on medication

Patients with BPD may be prescribed medication for comorbid mental illness, but those both with and without significant comorbidity are often prescribed multiple medications without a clear rationale (5). In one survey of outpatient treatment of people with BPD, 94% of patients were given medication, most commonly antidepressants, followed by antipsychotics, mood stabilizers, and benzodiazepines. There is no indication that these prescriptions were for comorbid disorders (21). On a secure ward, a survey found 80% of patients with BPD were receiving psychotropic medication, with almost half receiving more than one, mostly 'off-label' medications, meaning they were prescribed for a disorder for which the drugs are not licensed (22). The most commonly prescribed psychotropic in this forensic setting was clozapine.

Evidence for the effectiveness of medication is weak (23), which has led to the National Institute for Health and Care Excellence (NICE) recommending that it not be used except for comorbid conditions (24). This conclusion does not do justice to the occasional usefulness of psychotropic medication for individuals. Trials of medication in BPD have shown modest results, and suffered from low numbers and short follow-ups (23), and so the data available to guide prescribing is of low quality. Medication nevertheless seems to be useful in a proportion of patients. Apart from the low trial quality this might be due to heterogeneity in the population of people with BPD, as requiring five or more out of nine symptom criteria to reach caseness leads to 256 possible criteria combinations, groups of which may constitute subcategories of BPD.

Many clinicians tailor medication in BPD to observed symptoms, prescribing antipsychotics for impulsivity and cognitive perceptual disturbances, and antidepressants or mood stabilizers for mood instability and dysthymia. Given the lack of evidence for the effects of medication being clearly linked to the correction of neurochemical abnormalities in mental illness generally (25), this may be a reasonable approach, although placebo arms of trials of medication in BPD have produced significant improvement (26), which underlines the psychological aspects of prescribing (27). Lieb (23) recommends a trial of mood stabilizers and possibly second-generation antipsychotics for affective dysregulation, mood stabilizers for behavioural dyscontrol/impulsivity, and second-generation antipsychotics for cognitive perceptual symptoms. Most studies have looked at second-generation antipsychotics, and for this reason and their side effect profile, first-generation drugs should be avoided (28). Clozapine has gained popularity in secure settings (22) and there are early indications that it may be useful (29) but its effectiveness has not been convincingly examined. Antidepressants, despite being the most commonly prescribed medication in BPD, are probably only effective for comorbid depression and anxiety (28), and possibly affective dysregulation (26). Although some studies have

indicated that selective serotonin reuptake inhibitors might reduce impulsiveness, anger, and possibly deliberate self-harm, this is not a consistent finding (23). The frequency of antidepressant prescription in BPD may be explained by their use for comorbid conditions, and the relatively benign side effect profile and safety in overdose of the majority of modern antidepressants.

Benzodiazepines and 'Z drugs' are often used for emergency and sometimes longer-term sedation during episodes of anger, distress, and agitation, and for sleep. They can be useful in this context, but care should be taken due to their tendency to rapidly lose effectiveness after a short period of treatment (30), the tendency of benzodiazepines to impair the formation of emotional memory (31) and cognitive function more generally (32), making it difficult to use the admission to facilitate the acquisition of prosocial skills or alternative coping strategies, and the difficulties patients often experience while withdrawing. Withdrawal may prove more difficult in patients with BPD because of their interpersonal sensitivity, and so should normally be completed before discharge. Long-term benzodiazepine use is associated with persisting cognitive deficits beyond eventual withdrawal (33).

In addition to what may be specific effects on symptom clusters, many psychotropics dampen down behaviour through general sedation, emotional distancing, and cognitive slowing (34). This may provide a justifiable rationale for prescription as long as the risks and benefits have been carefully considered and documented, but is only likely to be ethical when acute risks are high or for a short period while waiting for an element of the management plan to become available, for example, specialist psychosocial treatment.

The best advice is that if a medication results in sustained improvement for a particular individual with BPD it can be continued, but medication often leads to transient improvement (possibly through the psychological impact of a new prescription (27)) which is not sustained. Because stopping medication can lead to withdrawal effects, and when cessation is due to lack of efficacy it tends to be disappointing, symptoms can worsen when medication is withdrawn. The withdrawal of medication might also be misinterpreted as a withdrawal of care (27). For this reason, many patients end up taking large numbers of psychotropic drugs without evidence of their ongoing effectiveness, with the attendant risks of side effects and stockpiling.

Research on psychosocial interventions

Psychosocial interventions have increasingly been shown to have a beneficial impact on BPD. Staff should be familiar with the local availability of specialist psychological interventions, and patients with PD should be referred for longer-term specialist treatment. Patients and families should be provided with information about local services and resources. NICE guidance recommends that family and friends (carers) services are available; these are often attached to specialist PD treatment teams (35).

Some of the techniques and understanding gleaned from specialist approaches can be used by untrained inpatient staff. Successful interventions for BPD can be divided into cognitive and behavioural, psychoanalytic, and interpersonal.

Cognitive and behavioural interventions

The intervention with the greatest evidence base at the time of writing is dialectical behaviour therapy, a skills-based intervention which teaches patients mindfulness, self-soothing and distraction techniques, and interpersonal effectiveness (36). These skills, normally taught in a group, appear to be effective when delivered without other elements of the formal therapy, such as individual therapy and 24-hour phone support (37), and can be delivered to inpatients. There is some limited evidence that formal dialectical behaviour therapy delivered to inpatients may be effective (38). A similar programme consisting only of group-based skills classes also appear to be effective and could be delivered simply to inpatients (39).

Psychoanalytic interventions

Although individual psychoanalytic approaches have shown some effectiveness (40), the most useful method from this tradition is mentalization-based therapy, which has demonstrated long-term effectiveness in day patients with BPD (7). Applications of the method in inpatients are dealt with elsewhere in this chapter.

Interpersonal interventions

One of the earliest interventions for patients with PD was democratic therapeutic community treatment. It has demonstrated effectiveness in outpatients with a range of PDs (41), and has given rise to the milieu approaches discussed here. The principles of empowerment, joint decision-making, and peer support derived from democratic therapeutic community technique are now widespread. Democratic therapeutic community research demonstrates the importance of the structured and purposeful activity recommended in inpatient guidelines such as Accreditation for Inpatient Mental Health Services (AIMS) for patients with PD, and the importance of services such as inpatient occupational therapy.

In addition to techniques and approaches derived from PD-specific therapies, staff should be aware of a range of other resources that might be helpful to these patient groups. Dissociation is common in BPD, and staff should have resources available to help patients manage their symptoms. Grounding techniques for dissociation and flashback experiences; relationship management skills such as interpersonal effectiveness from dialectical behaviour therapy and assertiveness; psychoeducation regarding the causes, nature, and course of PD, ASD, and ADHD symptoms; and advice on avoiding overexposure or isolation should all be made available, and staff should be trained in their delivery. Peer relationships are important in many mental disorders (42) but may be particularly important in BPD, in which prosocial skills can be difficult to acquire (43). Training to implement consistent empathic care adhering to the principles of PD care more generally (16) has shown beneficial effects in outpatients (44) and in emergency departments (45). This approach, known either as structured clinical management or good psychiatric management, uses group skills sessions along with regular supervision and can be implemented on inpatient wards.

Joint (coproduced) crisis plans are widely used in an attempt to mitigate risk and are recommended in spite of a lack of evidence in outpatients (46).

The impact of the inpatient environment in borderline personality disorder

There are inherent challenges of inpatient treatment for patients with BPD. Acute wards can be demanding for patients and staff, with high acuity and constant shift changes. There may also be staff coming from outside, such as agency workers, which increases disturbance and potentially decreases the consistency of approach.

This makes for an unpredictable environment and milieu, which can interact badly with the patient's already fragmented sense of self and boundary.

Consistent care and an understanding of the nature of reinforcement are particularly important in inpatient units, as both negative and positive attention can be reinforcing. A patient who becomes settled on a ward after a period of high risk or destructive behaviour may experience a decrease in activity from staff as lack of care or interest. This acts as an incentive to recreate the destructive behaviour. Patients also learn strategies from one another for keeping staff involved (47). For this reason, staff should take care to spend time with patients no matter how distressed or unwell they are, and should try to avoid interactions which might reinforce self-destructive or aggressive behaviours. Safety behaviours, such as remaining in a bedroom for fear of social interaction, should be challenged gradually and consistently as part of a shared plan of graded exposure, drawn up according to the resilience and history of the patient. Wards must have expertise available from psychological practitioners to aid in the construction of such plans.

Staff on wards also have variable attitudes and feelings towards patients with PDs and even those who are generally reflective and supportive can experience unhelpful countertransferences given the particular interpersonal challenges that this patient group brings (Box 17.1). Patients with BPD can both seek out and provoke negative attention, and test out issues of trust in the system. A tit-for-tat situation of negative attention can quickly turn into a destructive escalation. Splitting can lead to schisms within and between staff groups, often with allegiances forming along existing hand offs (for instance, community versus ward) as well as splits between ward staff (some overprotecting and others rejecting the patient) and splits in the internal psychic experience of staff who may feel dissonant positive and negative views about the same patient simultaneously.

Self-harm and suicide, accidental or planned, are risks for PD patients on wards. A particularly challenging decompensation related to breakdown of the therapeutic milieu has been called malignant alienation, malignant because of the association of the breakdown of clinical judgement with suicide (and self-harm). In this scenario, the patient who does not straightforwardly convey their needs (they may well act out or say one thing and think another) is perceived as difficult or not deserving of care. Again, the staff viewpoint here is polarized; staff may start off as protective and zealous but then become rejecting and negative, with conscious or unconscious hatred projected onto the patient (48).

Box 17.1 Problems on wards for management of patients with personality disorders

- Inconsistent milieu and environment.
- Splitting between and within staff groups.
- Interpersonal countertransference problems.
- Wards can foster dependence and escapism.
- Negative attention and escalation of destructive behaviour; alienation.
- Trust-based mistakes and interpersonal issues.
- Abuse on wards.
- Symptom triggering, for example, flashbacks, dissociation, and self-harm.
- Staff group may be seen by patient as lacking feedback credibility.

Another facet of splitting, idealizing the care environment, is just as dangerous as alienation. Here the patient may make dangerous trust-based mistakes (49), for instance, testing out trust in relationships with staff by committing acts of serious self-harm to see if they will be rescued. Inappropriate personal boundaries and sexual abuse may occur out of similar dynamics.

Positive approaches to management of patients with personality disorders

Wards are already set up to field adverse reactions and problems within their organization and governance structures, such as the issues outlined in earlier sections. Clinical leadership, supervision, and reflective practice are all mechanisms to help manage these challenges on the ward. The patient with PD can be seen as offering a 'stress test' for existing structures.

The ultimate aim is to help staff retain a realistic and boundaried but optimistic approach. In this way, they can develop open and trusting relationships with personality disordered patients that are non-judgemental and reliable but not rescuing or fostering dependence. It is important to remember that patients with BPD may well have suffered past trauma and abuse, and sometimes suffer ongoing stigmatization and abuse, at times within the psychiatric system. This can cause patients to re-experience trauma leading to symptom provocation such as repeated self-harm, flashbacks, and dissociation. Thought should be given to reducing the potential harms on the ward for personality disordered patients, for example, not expecting patients to repeat their history to every new staff member, challenging negative or stigmatizing views towards them and their family, and talking to patients directly, with respect, but not 'treading on egg shells' or trying to please.

Patients with BPD may have difficulty crystalizing and expressing their feelings and thoughts (in terms of purposeful mental states such as needs, desires, feelings, beliefs, goals, purposes, and reasons), and skills-based interventions to improve the patient's understanding of their own mental state and behaviour and the reciprocal mental states of others (mentalization) have demonstrated some evidence of effectiveness as noted earlier. Crucially, loss of mentalizing in one person can lead to a lack of mentalizing in another, as it is more difficult to see things from the point of view of someone who cannot see your point of view (50). A primary task of staff on mental health wards is therefore to develop and maintain a 'mentalizing' milieu. Ways of achieving this are summarized in Box 17.2. A short skills-based course in mentalization (MBT-S) has been found to empower

staff and promote empathy as a response to instances of self-harm, and can contribute to removing the potential of a vicious cycle of iatrogenic harm (51).

Clinical supervision, both informal and formal, and even support over a cup of tea, are essential components in management of a successful ward milieu, as is the non-punitive support of management in staffing, skill mix, understanding of incidents and complaints, emotional support, and understanding (52).

The effects of admission: institutionalization and self-efficacy

BPD has been called a disorder of agency (53) (to be differentiated from the disorders of agency in schizophrenia, referring to passivity phenomena). This means that, along with substance misuse, adult ADHD, some other PDs, and some other mental health conditions, the diagnosis depends mainly upon actions or omissions, and recovery depends at least in part upon the patient no longer engaging in the behaviour. Many mental disorders demonstrate low self-efficacy—the feeling that the patient is not energetically engaged in their own recovery, and has difficulty taking responsibility for their part in it. This may be related to the more or less ubiquitous association of mental disorders with childhood victimization and adversity (54), which can produce persisting feelings of powerlessness via the sense of an external locus of control. In BPD, these features are often particularly prominent, and attention must be paid to encouraging empowerment and promoting responsible agency. This is recognized in NICE guidance (24), which advises consistently promoting autonomy and choice, with a focus on the consequences of the treatment decisions patients make and ensuring they remain actively involved in finding solutions to their problems.

The nature of disorders of agency means that although progress may depend on changes at an emotional level, effort is always required to adopt more healthy methods of coping and emotional regulation. Patients who have the sense of an external locus of control will tend to feel hopeless (if they regard their future as mostly dependent upon chance), victimized (if they attribute it to the actions of antagonistic or neglectful others), or passive and entitled (if they attribute it to the actions of staff). Staff should make efforts to understand the nature of the internal process that leads to these attitudes, asking how a patient sees the world that leads to these behaviours and attitudes, and how these attitudes might have developed in terms of their history. An external locus of control and its associated low self-efficacy should be addressed explicitly if patients are to be engaged as an active participant in their own recovery. Brief interventions that can be implemented on inpatient wards, such as the milieu approach, mentalization, and motivational interviewing styles, specifically target a deficit in self-efficacy, but encouraging it should be part of routine interactions between all such patients and staff.

Institutionalization generally acts to promote an external locus of control, and is probably one of the reasons that people with PD can deteriorate on inpatient wards. Key personal tasks are normally taken over by the institution. This includes shopping, cooking, and cleaning, but institutional living also reduces a patient's control over their living conditions more generally, making it difficult to control who they see and who enters their private area, and places restrictions on what activities they can undertake. This can lead to the accentuation of hopelessness and sense of victimhood, particularly

---

Box 17.2 Ways of increasing mentalizing on inpatient wards

- Keep arousal contained, step back if overwhelmed.
- Supportive and empathetic stance.
- Curiosity: questioning, clarifying, elaboration, explicit, what, why, how, and when.
- Use humour where appropriate.
- Point out feelings and patterns.
- Skills-based training for staff in mentalization.
- Regular supervision and reflective practice.
- Knowledge and training about BPD.

Source data from Bateman A, Fonagy P. Mentalization based treatment for borderline personality disorder. *World Psychiatry* 2010;9(1):11–15.

if a patient is detained or subject to frequent observations. Efforts should be made to minimize these negative effects of the ward environment. This can be done through adopting some variation of a milieu approach, elements of which are now incorporated into the College Centre for Quality Improvement AIMS framework and the 'Enabling Environments' award, both based at the Royal College of Psychiatrists in the UK (55–57).

Milieu approaches

In the past, attention focused on the ward environment as a mediator of change (e.g. Ellsworth et al. (58)). With the deinstitutionalization of many patients and the closure of the large asylums, the number of patients and length of stay dropped and the focus shifted to medication management and rapid discharge. More recently, with concern over the state of psychiatric inpatient wards (59), and unacceptable levels of overcrowding and violent assaults (60), attention has returned to the impact of the ward environment on patient recovery and staff morale.

Two broad approaches were common: the therapeutic community-derived milieu, and the use of token economies. In addition to the changes to inpatient care outlined earlier in this chapter, the latter appears to have fallen into disuse at least partially through staff resistance and legal and ethical challenges (61), despite early indications of usefulness. Therapeutic community-derived milieu approaches similarly declined despite positive early results. The therapeutic community milieu approach to inpatient psychiatric care includes the following elements:

1. Structured group activities, generally including some kind of productive work and skills acquisition.
2. Regular community meetings to which all patients were invited, sometimes with an element of devolved decision-making around housekeeping arrangements on the ward.
3. The principle of examined living. In therapeutic community milieu approaches, the examination would typically be by the group as a whole (62), whereas in other milieu environments this would usually have been by the staff, and the nature of their observations and conclusions may not have been communicated to the patients. This principle often extended to the examination of intrastaff dynamics through such innovations as staff sensitivity (or support) groups. Behaviour was regarded as a means of communication, and verbal communication between staff and patients, and between patients, was promoted.

The impact of these innovations was unclear, but they have informed the recent development of initiatives to improve inpatient environments. The AIMS programme includes a section entitled 'Therapeutic milieu', and recommends staff support groups, that staff be trained in group methods, a patient community meeting, shared decision-making, and spontaneous staff–patient activities (5) (Box 17.3).

Similar principles have been applied to wider initiatives which set a higher bar for paying attention to the environmental impact on both patients and staff. The 'Enabling Environments' project makes awards to units that adhere to therapeutic principles, some of which are shared with AIMS (e.g. engagement and purposeful activity is encouraged), but many of which go beyond AIMS (e.g. power and authority are open to discussion). Enabling Environment principles (Box 17.4), which are historically closer to therapeutic community

---

> **Box 17.3** Therapeutic milieu
>
> - A minuted patient community meeting takes place at least once per week.
> - The therapeutic value of positive relationships is recognized, and these are promoted both on and off the ward.
> - Staff recognize that all behaviour is a form of communication.
> - There are opportunities for staff and patients to engage in spontaneous activities together.
> - Both staff and patients are involved in making decisions about and maintaining the physical environment.
> - Engagement and purposeful activity is actively encouraged.
> - Staff and patients are supported to ask questions and challenge decisions about care.
> - There are forums to promote peer-support for both staff and patients.

milieu principles, have given rise to two additional milieu-based interventions, 'Psychologically Informed Environments' in hostels for the homeless, and 'Psychologically Informed Planned Environments' which apply milieu principles to prison environments (63, 64).

Crisis, admission, and the balance of risks

Given the potential pitfalls of hospital admission for patients with BPD, the mainstay of treatment programmes are voluntary psychotherapeutic programmes in the community. Before admission is considered, a number of tests and checks need to be factored into the treatment system. NICE guidelines (24) state that before admission the clinician should ensure that the decision is based on an explicit, joint understanding of the potential benefits and likely harm that may result from admission, and the proposed treatment plan and length of stay. Alternatives to admission such as crisis interventions and use of non-hospital placements such as crisis houses or community crisis services (including services such as home treatment, day hospital or 'crisis cafés') should be explored and used if at all possible as preferable to but not excluding admission. Reasons for admission for patients with BPD are summarized as follows:

> **Box 17.4** A positively enabling environment is an environment
>
> - in which the nature and the quality of relationships between participants or members is recognized and highly valued
> - where the participants share some measure of responsibility for the environment as a whole, and especially for their own part in it
> - where all participants—staff, volunteers and service users alike—are equally valued and supported in their particular contribution
> - where engagement and purposeful activity is encouraged
> - where there are opportunities for creativity and initiative, whether spontaneous or shared and planned
> - where decision-making is transparent, and both formal and informal leadership roles are acknowledged
> - where power or authority is clearly accountable and open to discussion
> - where any formal rules or informal expectations of behaviour are clear; or if unclear, there is good reason for it
> - where behaviour, even when potentially disruptive, is seen as meaningful, as a communication to be understood.
>
> Reproduced from Johnson R, Haigh R. Social psychiatry and social policy for the 21st century: new concepts for new needs – the 'Enabling Environments' initiative. *Mental Health and Social Inclusion* 2011;15(1):17–23.

Reasons for admission

- Crisis intervention, particularly to reduce risk of suicide or violence to others.
- Comorbid psychiatric disorder such as depression or a brief psychotic episode.
- Chaotic behaviour endangering the patient and the treatment alliance (aggression/violence).
- To stabilize medication regimens.
- Review of the diagnosis and the treatment plan.
- Full risk assessment.

Above all, the unit must have the capacity, in terms of skills, staffing, and clinical pressures, to manage the admission

Practical considerations for personality disorder treatment on wards

As already stated, the intention of treatment, the goals and potential length of admission, and any risks should be explicit before any admission for patients with BPD. A practical approach to treatment planning is outlined by Fagin (65) who gives the following advice:

- Early care plan with specified goals agreed and communicated to all staff and the patient, paying special attention to perceived or real inconsistencies. Anticipation of crises, especially about impulsive discharge, self-harm, drug use, sexual promiscuity or aggression, and establishment of an agreed multidisciplinary response.
- A focus on immediate needs, mostly of a practical nature.
- Treatment of axis I (non-PD psychiatric) symptoms with medication when necessary.
- Clear boundaries regarding tolerable behaviour, including aggression, suicidal gestures, use of illicit substances or alcohol, and absconding.
- Effective use of inpatient groups, with checks on oversharing.
- Staff support groups and supervision looking at countertransference reactions, particularly of junior staff, who may become overinvolved.

Should there be a breakdown of protective mechanisms, a decision to discharge despite increasing risk on the ward may need to be made, taking into account the purpose of admission, the importance of long-term engagement, and the balance of risks. There is a, probably small, group of patients who react to the restrictions and disempowering nature of inpatient treatment with an escalation in risk. For this group, a careful assessment of the impact of ward-based treatment may lead to a decision to discharge despite escalating risk, if the escalation is judged to be related to inpatient treatment. In these cases, the ward environment and staff training should be examined to ensure they are not contributing unnecessarily to the patient's deterioration (16).

Patients with autism spectrum disorder

Patients with autism are more likely to access psychiatric inpatient care and develop comorbid psychiatric conditions than the general population (66). The prevalence of autism in inpatients during a 2013 census was 30 times that of the general population, with 20% in general adult beds (67). There was an association with comorbid mental illness, challenging behaviour, long length of stay, higher levels of physical restraint and deliberate self-harm, and high cost.

The general psychiatric setting is not adapted to the needs of patients with ASD and there is a need to establish and evaluate specialized approaches to health care to meet their needs. There are currently no research-based guidelines covering adults with ASD. The majority of experience comes from child and adolescent services, including a best practice consensus (68). There is also guidance from the National Autistic Society highlighting the impact of the hospital environment with attendant issues of sensory overload and consequent challenging behaviours (69).

Assessment of patients with autism spectrum disorder

Some patients access hospital care with a pre-existing diagnosis of autism or ASD having undergone rigorous assessment using standardized expert assessment. However, the availability of assessments remains patchy and many patients have a limited medical assessment or no diagnosis at all. Psychiatric services should have access to specialist autism services who can advise on diagnosis and offer assessment. Obtaining a good quality developmental history is a standard part of inpatient assessment.

After making the diagnosis, further assessment is needed to understand the factors associated with the admission. Possible factors are given in Table 17.1.

The inpatient approach to autism

Patients with autism should have individualized care incorporated into the care plan, taking into account the perspectives of carers, relatives, and the multidisciplinary team. Using a personal design of care plan such as using pictures or diagrams can also be helpful. In general, minimizing the length of stay (or using community

Table 17.1 Factors associated with behaviour disturbance in autism

Environmental factors	Sensory overload, e.g. loud noises, particular smells, colours, and touch Sensory underload, e.g. inadequate stimulation leading to self-harm Change of physical environment and routine Change of schooling
Interpersonal and relationship factors	New carers and associates Bereavement and loss of caregiver Caregiver new relationships or marriage Inadvertent reward of unwanted behaviours New teacher or teaching method Bullying Abuse
Illness	Psychiatric disorder, e.g. depression or psychosis Medication and side effects Physical illness and symptoms, e.g. pain, constipation
Communication factors	Expectation of verbal interaction as standard Lack of or difficult to understand explanations Misunderstandings more generally

management if at all possible) and planning as much as possible in advance are strategies to avoid or lessen negative impact.

The environment

The ward poses problems for the autistic patient and proactive design of the environment can ease the disruption of admission. Consideration should be given to the position of the patient's room, minimizing loud noises such as sirens and buzzers and disruptive or disturbed patients, with attention to meal and visitors times. Ask the patient if they want to eat somewhere else, giving them choice over meals. Clothing can be an issue and again patient choice is important here, the person may, for example, prefer a certain feeling of cloth or have their own weighted blanket.

Communication factors

The usual expectation on wards is that the currency for communication is predominantly verbal and based on open questions. These are issues that autistic patients can struggle with. The care plan should use strategies to ease communication. Examples are using flashcards or emoticons, and drawing up a timetable to let the person know what to expect during the day (e.g. ward round). Closed and yes/no questions work well with autistic patients who are likely either not to answer at all or to become overwhelmed in the face of a reflective open question.

Increased observation levels

The best way to deal with behaviour disturbance is to avoid it. If self-harm and 'meltdowns' become an issue (or severely compromise safety), consider high-level observations. The initial aim of observations may be safety but observations can also be used to intensively observe the environment and triggers, and engineer the social environment of the ward to prevent problems (to organize time, help interactions with other patients, and engender a sense of security in a difficult environment).

Management of 'meltdowns'

If there is any acute behaviour disturbance then a plan to deal with this should be in the care plan. The design of the plan is individual but may involve the following elements: use of a low-stimulus area, using a distraction or mindfulness task, and behavioural management such as engaging the patient in a positive activity once the disturbance has passed. Careful use of medication may be appropriate. Interventions should be least restrictive and use physical intervention and restraint as a last resort.

Attention deficit hyperactivity disorder

ADHD in adults is likely to be underdiagnosed in the UK when compared to rates expected from childhood prevalence (70). It is therefore likely that a combination of diagnosed and undiagnosed patients will be admitted to wards either because of a comorbid condition or in psychosocial crisis (Box 17.5).

There are now a number of guidelines in the UK to assist with the assessment and treatment of patients with ADHD (70–72). All psychiatrists should have skills in developmental assessment but there

---

Box 17.5 Comorbidity in attention deficit hyperactivity disorder

- Autism spectrum disorder.
- Learning disability and specific difficulties such as dyslexia.
- Tourette's syndrome.
- Personality disorders.
- Substance misuse disorders.
- Medical conditions (e.g. petit mal epilepsy, hearing and visual issues, hypothyroidism).
- Mood disorders.
- Psychosis.

---

should also be access to specialist assessment and treatment services which also provide ongoing treatment via protocols such as shared care with general practitioners.

Ward approach to patients with attention deficit hyperactivity disorder

Broad biopsychosocial assessment and monitoring including drug screening and cardiovascular examination and investigations with electrocardiography are standard procedures on wards and should be offered to all inpatients with ADHD. As substance misuse is a common comorbidity, and the prescribed medications for ADHD are prone to abuse and diversion, attention to these issues is important, although having an addiction history should not be a complete bar to pharmacological treatment for ADHD. Where there is significant comorbidity, before starting ADHD treatments it may be necessary to optimize existing treatments and weigh up the potential risks of starting ADHD medication. However, if underlying ADHD is not addressed, the patient will retain both unpleasant symptoms and risks for further comorbidity to arise.

Diagnosis of ADHD is a clinical diagnosis but useful screening tools are available, such as the Adult ADHD Self-Rating Scale (73). Treatment should only be started on the ward after careful longitudinal assessment, and not in a crisis situation.

Patients with ADHD may struggle with a distracting ward environment, and the ward milieu should be designed to take this into account. The care plan should be individualized to consider the individual's needs but in addition, strategies should be introduced to optimize stimulation (e.g. engaging the patient with interests that they can concentrate on in a low-stimulus area). Generally, information should be clear and in a format accessible to the patient (Table 17.2).

Patients with ADHD can benefit from psychosocial interventions such as individual or group cognitive behavioural therapy (71) and

---

Table 17.2 Some strategies to improve communication for patients with attention deficit hyperactivity disorder

Discuss one thing at a time	Get the persons attention first
Take turns in speaking	Keep on topic
Plan in advance (i.e. for ward round)	Use memory aids or notes
Make a simple timetable	Consider an intervention e.g. cognitive behaviour therapy

with some possibly minor modifications can be enabled to join in with general ward groups and activities.

Defensive practice, staff attitudes, and burnout

The abnormal attachment status of patients with BPD (74, 75) reflected in the first two diagnostic criteria in the fifth edition of the *Diagnostic and Statistical Manual of Mental Disorders* (DSM-5) (frantic efforts to avoid abandonment and a pattern of unstable and intense relationships alternating between idealization and devaluation) can make staff–patient relationships difficult. This can also become a problem in patients with ASD and ADHD, who along with PD patients may be thought of as 'not ill'. The tendency to idealize or denigrate patients (internal splitting) is often mirrored in staff attitudes becoming polarized between becoming allied to the patient and thinking of other staff or the system as failing them or being cruel or unresponsive, or thinking of them as less deserving of care or to blame for their problems. This can be thought of as adopting a rescuing or persecuting stance ('drama triangle' (76)), and represents a failure of professional objectivity. Disagreements among the staff team can represent external splitting, the acting out of the internal splits that can lead to breakdowns in trust and cooperation between staff members.

Patients come to be seen as difficult gradually. Early markers include pessimism among staff, a tendency to blame the patient for their problems which are seen as moral as well as or instead of psychiatric, and passive treatment or withdrawal of care (77). Withdrawing care from people with PD tends not to have a beneficial long-term outcome; long-term health costs for people with BPD exceed those for people with major depressive disorder (1). In England, this has been recognized in government guidance advising that patients with PD not be excluded from services as a consequence of the diagnosis. The journey from unusual care-seeking behaviour to chronic problematic care-seeking behaviour is marked by ineffective professional interventions (77). These patients do not all suffer from the problems covered here, nor do they all have psychiatric problems, but patients with PD in particular are stigmatized (3, 78), and patients perceived as difficult may be labelled as personality disordered (79).

Defensive practice (practice primarily for the benefit of the clinician rather than the patient) can be common when working with the subgroup of patients who pose a high risk, particularly when the risk varies or is difficult to mitigate. A 2006 survey found 85% of psychiatric clinicians stated they had acted in this way in the previous year towards patients with BPD (4). Admissions can lengthen without evidence of benefit, bringing the dangers of institutionalization and reinforcing abnormal care-seeking behaviour. Early in the admission, the nature (acute or chronic), reality (has the patient carried out any acts for which there is evidence of long-term harm), and modifiability of the risk should be clearly defined, and the action plan formulated accordingly. Chronic risks that are not modifiable by inpatient care should not be used to justify admission, neither should they discourage discharge. Sometimes patients who threaten suicide, or report suicidal acts without third-party corroboration through emergency department records or family report, are wrongly admitted for long periods due to perceived risk. A careful appraisal of the nature of reported suicidal acts should be undertaken to inform the risk assessment, but short-term professional risk taking (positive risk taking) is at times necessary to ensure that management is in the best interests of the patient (80).

Developing methods of improving mentalizing in inpatient teams is likely to improve management. Particular attention should be paid to the tendency to blame patients for their problems (2). The emphasis on agency and self-efficacy outlined here might be expected to exacerbate this. The normal response to someone who engages in negative or upsetting behaviour is to excuse them, which in a psychiatric setting often involves assuming they are unable to do otherwise, or hold them responsible and therefore blameworthy. People with PD are normally included in the latter group. The link between responsibility and blame is close, and in normal life appears to be adaptive in moderating social interactions. In clinical work, particularly when excusing behaviour on the basis of incapability is countertherapeutic, as is the case in PD, the link is counterproductive. It is possible, and desirable, for staff to be taught to separate the attribution of responsibility—the communicated belief that the patient has some control over their behaviour in the sense that they could do otherwise—and the emotional reaction of blaming the patient for their behaviour. The former is a cognitive element; the latter is an affective one with behavioural consequences. Blaming leads to stigmatization, dismissiveness, and poor care, and is probably related to malignant alienation, discussed elsewhere in this chapter. With proper training and supervision, it is possible to establish a culture of responsibility without blame, and avoid the pitfalls of blaming while maintaining the advantages of the promotion of self-efficacy and empowerment (81).

Transparency, stigma, and diagnosis

Problems sometimes arise when a patient is opposed to a diagnosis on the grounds of perceived stigma or blame. This would more commonly occur in an outpatient setting, where most diagnoses are established and communicated, but in complex cases and when inpatient stays are prolonged, diagnoses may be made for the first time or revised on an inpatient ward. Staff may be reluctant to be transparent for fear of complaints or damage to the therapeutic alliance. The diagnosis of PD and factitious disorder are commonly affected. PD still carries the idea of blame, and has a particularly problematic stigma attached which probably exceeds that of other mental disorders (2, 78). Factitious disorder carries the idea of dishonesty which patients may be keen to avoid.

Studies show that making a diagnosis of PD, like other diagnoses, has beneficial effects, and patients tend to find it empowering and comforting in the context of an empathic clinical encounter (82). An accurate diagnosis which is communicated appropriately makes treatment more likely to be effective, promotes transparency in staff–patient relationships, avoids the pitfalls of secret communication between professionals which excludes patients, and can mobilize patient resources. Similarly, in factitious disorder, successful treatment involves negotiation and agreement of the diagnosis with the patient (83).

Summary

Patients with PDs, ASD, and ADHD constitute an important group of inpatients who require different management strategies and skills to patients with affective and psychotic disorders. Their behaviours can be difficult to manage, and the inpatient environment requires careful attention to avoid iatrogenic harms following admission. For these reasons, admission is often avoided in these groups, but with careful management and adequate staffing and training, admission can promote recovery, manage risks, and avoid harms.

REFERENCES

1. Bender DS, Dolan RT, Skodol AE, et al. Treatment utilization by patients with personality disorders. *Am J Psychiatry* 2001;158:295–302.

2. Lewis G, Appleby L. Personality disorder: the patients psychiatrists dislike. *Br J Psychiatry* 1988;153:44–49.

3. Markham D, Trower P. The effects of the psychiatric label 'borderline personality disorder' on nursing staff's perceptions and causal attributions for challenging behaviours. *Br J Clin Psychol* 2003;42:243–256.

4. Krawitz R, Batcheler M. Borderline personality disorder: a pilot survey about clinician views on defensive practice. *Australas Psychiatry* 2006;14:320–322.

5. Paton C, Crawford MJ, Bhatti SF, Patel MX, Barnes TR. The use of psychotropic medication in patients with emotionally unstable personality disorder under the care of UK mental health services. *J Clin Psychiatry* 2015;76:512–518.

6. Peterson LG, Bongar B. Repetitive suicidal crises: characteristics of repeating versus nonrepeating suicidal visitors to a psychiatric emergency service. *Psychopathology* 1990;23:136–145.

7. Bateman A, Fonagy P. 8-year follow-up of patients treated for borderline personality disorder: mentalization-based treatment versus treatment as usual. *Am J Psychiatry* 2008;165:631–638.

8. Coid J, Yang M, Bebbington P, et al. Borderline personality disorder: health service use and social functioning among a national household population. *Psychol Med* 2009;39:1721–1731.

9. Pompili M, Girardi P, Ruberto A, Tatarelli R. Suicide in borderline personality disorder: a meta-analysis. *Nord J Psychiatry* 2005;59:319–324.

10. Zanarini MC, Frankenburg FR, Reich DB, Fitzmaurice G. Attainment and stability of sustained symptomatic remission and recovery among patients with borderline personality disorder and axis II comparison subjects: a 16-year prospective follow-up study. *Am J Psychiatry* 2012;169:476–483.

11. Pascual J, Corcoles D, Castano J, et al. Hospitalization and pharmacotherapy for borderline personality disorder in a psychiatric emergency service. *Psychiatr Serv* 2007;58:1199–1204.

12. Sar V, Akyuz G, Kugu N, Ozturk E, Ertem-Vehid H. Axis I dissociative disorder comorbidity in borderline personality disorder and reports of childhood trauma. *J Clin Psychiatry* 2006;67:1583–1590.

13. Grant BF, Chou SP, Goldstein RB, et al. Prevalence, correlates, disability, and comorbidity of DSM-IV borderline personality disorder: results from the Wave 2 National Epidemiologic Survey on Alcohol and Related Conditions. *J Clin Psychiatry* 2008;69:533–545.

14. Tyrer P, Seivewright N, Ferguson B, Murphy S, Johnson AL. The Nottingham study of neurotic disorder. Effect of personality status on response to drug treatment, cognitive therapy and self-help over two years. *Br J Psychiatry* 1993;162:219–226.

15. Moran P, Walsh E, Tyrer P, Burns T, Creed F, Fahy T. Does comorbid personality disorder increase the risk of suicidal behaviour in psychosis? *Acta Psychiatr Scand* 2003;107:441–448.

16. Bateman AW, Tyrer P. Services for personality disorder: organisation for inclusion. *Adv Psychiatr Treat* 2004;10:425–433.

17. Tyrer P, Merson S, Onyett S, Johnson T. The effect of personality disorder on clinical outcome, social networks and adjustment: a controlled clinical trial of psychiatric emergencies. *Psychol Med* 1994;24:731–740.

18. Faraone SV, Biederman J, Mick E. The age-dependent decline of attention deficit hyperactivity disorder: a meta-analysis of follow-up studies. *Psychol Med* 2006;36:159–165.

19. Philipsen A, Limberger MF, Lieb K, et al. Attention-deficit hyperactivity disorder as a potentially aggravating factor in borderline personality disorder. *Br J Psychiatry* 2008;192:118–123.

20. Ferrer M, Andión O, Matalí J, et al. Comorbid attention-deficit/hyperactivity disorder in borderline patients defines an impulsive subtype of borderline personality disorder. *J Pers Disord* 2010;24:812–822.

21. Knappich M, Horz-Sagstetter S, Schwerthoffer D, Leucht S, Rentrop M. Pharmacotherapy in the treatment of patients with borderline personality disorder: results of a survey among psychiatrists in private practices. *Int Clin Psychopharmacol* 2014;29:224–228.

22. Haw C, Stubbs J. Medication for borderline personality disorder: a survey at a secure hospital. *Int J Psychiatry Clin Pract* 2011;15:270–274.

23. Lieb K, Vollm B, Rucker G, Timmer A, Stoffers JM. Pharmacotherapy for borderline personality disorder: Cochrane systematic review of randomised trials. *Br J Psychiatry* 2010;196:4–12.

24. National Institute for Care and Health Excellence. Borderline personality disorder: recognition and management. Clinical guideline [CG78]. 2015. https://www.nice.org.uk/guidance/cg78

25. Yeomans D, Moncrieff J, Huws R. Drug-centred psychopharmacology: a non-diagnostic framework for drug treatment. *BJPsych Adv* 2015;21:229–236.

26. Vita A, De Peri L, Sacchetti E. Antipsychotics, antidepressants, anticonvulsants, and placebo on the symptom dimensions of borderline personality disorder: a meta-analysis of randomized controlled and open-label trials. *J Clin Psychopharmacol* 2011;31:613–624.

27. Adelman SA. Pills as transitional objects: a dynamic understanding of the use of medication in psychotherapy. *Psychiatry* 1985;48:246–253.

28. Stoffers J, Völlm BA, Rücker G, Timmer A, Huband N, Lieb K. Pharmacological interventions for borderline personality disorder. *Cochrane Database Syst Rev* 2010;6:CD005653.

29. Beri A, Boydell J. Clozapine in borderline personality disorder: a review of the evidence. *Ann Clin Psychiatry* 2014;26:139–144.

30. Moore N, Pariente A, Bégaud B. Why are benzodiazepines not yet controlled substances? *JAMA Psychiatry* 2015;72:110–111.

31. Buchanan TW, Karafin MS, Adolphs R. Selective effects of triazolam on memory for emotional, relative to neutral, stimuli: differential effects on gist versus detail. *Behav Neurosci* 2003;117:517–25.

32. Stewart SA. The effects of benzodiazepines on cognition. *J Clin Psychiatry* 2005;66(Suppl 2):9–13.

33. Barker MJ, Greenwood KM, Jackson M, Crowe SF. Persistence of cognitive effects after withdrawal from long-term benzodiazepine use: a meta-analysis. *Arch Clin Neuropsychol* 2004;19:437–454.

34. Moncrieff J, Cohen D. Rethinking models of psychotropic drug action. *Psychother Psychosom* 2005;74:145–153.

35. Sanders S, Pearce S. The Oxford Friends and Family Empowerment (OFAFE) service: support and education for those affected by

friends or family with personality disorder. *Ment Health Rev J* 2010;15:58–62.

36. Kliem S, Kröger C, Kosfelder J. Dialectical behavior therapy for borderline personality disorder: a meta-analysis using mixed-effects modeling. *J Consult Clin Psychol* 2010;78:936–951.

37. McMain SF, Guimond T, Barnhart R, Habinski L, Streiner DL. A randomized trial of brief dialectical behaviour therapy skills training in suicidal patients suffering from borderline disorder. *Acta Psychiatr Scand* 2017;135:138–148.

38. Bohus M, Haaf B, Simms T, et al. Effectiveness of inpatient dialectical behavioral therapy for borderline personality disorder: a controlled trial. *Behav Res Ther* 2004;42:487–499.

39. Blum N, John DS, Pfohl B, et al. Systems Training for Emotional Predictability and Problem Solving (STEPPS) for outpatients with borderline personality disorder: a randomized controlled trial and 1-year follow-up. *Am J Psychiatry* 2008;165:468–478.

40. Doering S, Horz S, Rentrop M, et al. Transference-focused psychotherapy v. treatment by community psychotherapists for borderline personality disorder: randomised controlled trial. *Br J Psychiatry* 2010;196:389–395.

41. Pearce S, Scott L, Attwood G, et al. Democratic therapeutic community treatment for personality disorder: randomised controlled trial. *Br J Psychiatry* 2017;210:149–156.

42. Mahlke CI, Buck T. Peer to peer support in severe mental disorders: affective disorders, psychosis and personality disorder—a randomized controlled trial. *Eur Psychiatry* 2015;30:165.

43. Zanarini MC, Frankenburg FR, Reich DB, Fitzmaurice G. The 10-year course of psychosocial functioning among patients with borderline personality disorder and axis II comparison subjects. *Acta Psychiatr Scand* 2010;122:103–109.

44. Bateman A, Fonagy P. Randomized controlled trial of outpatient mentalization-based treatment versus structured clinical management for borderline personality disorder. *Am J Psychiatry* 2009;166:1355–1364.

45. Hong V. Borderline personality disorder in the emergency department: good psychiatric management. *Harv Rev Psychiatry* 2016;24:357–366.

46. Borschmann R, Barrett B, Hellier JM, et al. Joint crisis plans for people with borderline personality disorder: feasibility and outcomes in a randomised controlled trial. *Br J Psychiatry* 2013;202:357–364.

47. Bandura A. *Social Learning Theory*. Englewood Cliffs, NJ: Prentice-Hall; 1977.

48. Watts D, Morgan G. Malignant alienation: dangers for patients who are hard to like. In: Adshead G, Jacob C (eds), *Personality Disorder: The Definitive Reader*, pp. 89–97. London: Jessica Kingsley; 2009.

49. Saunders K, Goodwin G, Rogers R. Borderline personality disorder, but not euthymic bipolar disorder, is associated with a failure to sustain reciprocal cooperative behaviour: implications for spectrum models of mood disorders. *Psychol Med* 2015;45:1591–1600.

50. Bateman A, Fonagy P. Mentalization based treatment for borderline personality disorder. *World Psychiatry* 2010;9:11–15.

51. Warrender D. Staff nurse perceptions of the impact of mentalization-based therapy skills training when working with borderline personality disorder in acute mental health: a qualitative study. *J Psychiatr Ment Health Nurs* 2015;22:623–633.

52. Bland AR, Rossen EK. Clinical supervision of nurses working with patients with borderline personality disorder. *Issues Ment Health Nurs* 2005;26:507–517.

53. Pickard H. Responsibility without blame: philosophical reflections on clinical practice. In: Fulford K, Davies M, Gipps R, et al. (eds), *The Oxford Handbook of Philosophy and Psychiatry*, pp. 1134–1154. Oxford: Oxford University Press; 2013.

54. Kessler RC, McLaughlin KA, Green JG, et al. Childhood adversities and adult psychopathology in the WHO World Mental Health Surveys. *Br J Psychiatry* 2010;197:378–385.

55. Baskind R, Kordowicz M, Chaplin R. How does an accreditation programme drive improvement on acute inpatient mental health wards? An exploration of members' views. *J Ment Health* 2010;19:405–411.

56. Cresswell J, Beavon M, Robinson H. *Standards for Acute Inpatient Services for Working-Age Adults*, 5th edition. London: Royal College of Psychiatrists; 2014.

57. Johnson R, Haigh R. Social psychiatry and social policy for the 21st century: new concepts for new needs – the 'Enabling Environments' initiative. *Ment Health Soc Inclus* 2011;15:17–23.

58. Ellsworth R, Maroney R, Klett W, Gordon H, Gunn R. Milieu characteristics of successful psychiatric treatment programs. *Am J Orthopsychiatry* 1971;41:427–441.

59. Crisp N, Smith G, Nicholson K. *Old Problems, New Solutions—Improving Acute Psychiatric Care for Adults in England*. London: The Commission on Acute Adult Psychiatric Care; 2016.

60. Virtancn M, Vahtera J, Batty GD, et al. Overcrowding in psychiatric wards and physical assaults on staff: data-linked longitudinal study. *Br J Psychiatry* 2011;198:149–155.

61. Glynn SM. Token economy approaches for psychiatric patients. Progress and pitfalls over 25 years. *Behav Modif* 1990;14:383–407.

62. Main T. The concept of the therapeutic community: variations and vicissitudes. *Group Anal* 1977;10:S2–S16.

63. Freestone M, Vandevelde S, Bond N, Gemmell L. Experiences of prison officers on a Lifer Psychologically Informed Planned Environment. *Ther Communities* 2014;35:84–94.

64. Haigh R, Harrison T, Johnson R, Paget S, Williams S. Psychologically informed environments and the "Enabling Environments" initiative. *Housing Care Support* 2012;15:34–42.

65. Fagin L. Management of personality disorders in acute in-patient settings. Part 1: borderline personality disorders. *Adv Psychiatr Treat* 2004;10:93–99.

66. Bhaumik S, Tyrer F, McGrother C, Ganghadaran S. Psychiatric service use and psychiatric disorders in adults with intellectual disability. *J Intellect Disabil Res* 2008;52:986–995.

67. Public Health England. *People with learning disabilities or autism in psychiatric hospitals in September 2013: Secondary analysis by the Public Health England Learning Disabilities Team*. London: Public Health England; 2015.

68. McGuire K, Erickson C, Gabriels RL, et al. Psychiatric hospitalization of children with autism or intellectual disability: consensus statements on best practices. *J Am Acad Child Adolesc Psychiatry* 2015;54:969–971.

69. National Autistic Society. Professionals. https://www.autism.org.uk/professionals.aspx

70. Bolea-Alamañac B, Nutt DJ, Adamou M, et al. Evidence-based guidelines for the pharmacological management of attention deficit hyperactivity disorder: update on recommendations from the British Association for Psychopharmacology. *J Psychopharmacol* 2014;28:179–203.

71. National Institute for Care and Health Excellence. *Attention Deficit Hyperactivity Disorder: Diagnosis and Management*. Clinical guideline [CG72]. London: National Institute for Care and Health Excellence; 2016.

72. Royal College of Psychiatrists in Scotland. ADHD in Adults—Good Practice Guidelines. 2017. https://www.rcpsych.ac.uk/pdf/ADHD_in_AdultsFINAL_GUIDELINES_JUNE2017.pdf

73. Kessler RC, Adler LA, Gruber MJ, Sarawate CA, Spencer T, Van Brunt DL. Validity of the World Health Organization Adult ADHD Self-Report Scale (ASRS) Screener in a representative sample of health plan members. *Int J Methods Psychiatr Res* 2007;16:52–65.

74. Scott LN, Levy KN, Pincus AL. Adult attachment, personality traits, and borderline personality disorder features in young adults. *J Pers Disord* 2009;23:258–280.

75. Levy KN. The implications of attachment theory and research for understanding borderline personality disorder. *Dev Psychopathol* 2005;17:959–986.

76. Karpman S. The drama triangle. Fairy tales and script drama analysis. *Transact Anal Bull* 1967;7:26.

77. Koekkoek B, Hutschemaekers G, van Meijel B, Schene A. How do patients come to be seen as 'difficult'?: a mixed-methods study in community mental health care. *Soc Sci Med* 2011;72:504–512.

78. Bodner E, Cohen-Fridel S, Iancu I. Staff attitudes toward patients with borderline personality disorder. *Compr Psychiatry* 2011;52:548–555.

79. Moran P, Rendu A, Jenkins R, Tylee A, Mann A. The impact of personality disorder in UK primary care: a 1-year follow-up of attenders. *Psychol Med* 2001;31:1447–1454.

80. Krawitz R, Jackson W, Allen R, et al. Professionally indicated short-term risk-taking in the treatment of borderline personality disorder. *Australas Psychiatry* 2004;12:11–17.

81. Pickard H. Responsibility without blame: empathy and the effective treatment of personality disorder. *Philos Psychiatr Psychol* 2011;18:209–223.

82. Bilderbeck AC, Saunders KE, Price J, Goodwin GM. Psychiatric assessment of mood instability: qualitative study of patient experience. *Br J Psychiatry* 2014;204:234–239.

83. Bass C, Halligan P. Factitious disorders and malingering: challenges for clinical assessment and management. *Lancet* 2014;383:1422–1432.

18

Autoimmune-related psychosis

Belinda Lennox

Clinical vignette

A 22-year-old female accountant presented to psychiatric services with a 2-week history of paranoid beliefs and auditory hallucinations. The episode had an abrupt onset, and she described how she had the sudden realization that her boyfriend was being unfaithful to her, and she was hearing multiple voices talking to her and to each other saying the same thing. She had insomnia, sleeping for 2 hours per night, and would pace around the house looking for evidence of his infidelity. She was brought for assessment after challenging her boyfriend and attacking him physically, hitting and scratching him. On assessment, she appeared dishevelled and perplexed and it was not possible to assess her cognition in detail. Her speech was limited, with evidence of echolalia and echopraxia. She had no insight into the possibility that she might be unwell. She was admitted to the psychiatric inpatient unit under Section 2 of the Mental Health Act 1983.

She was started on risperidone 1 mg with a working diagnosis of first-episode psychosis. One hour after the first dose, she was observed to collapse with loss of consciousness for 30 seconds. She complained of feeling faint and dizzy. Her blood pressure was 80/50 mmHg and her pulse was 120 beats/min. The risperidone was therefore discontinued and olanzapine was started, with diazepam in view of symptoms of catatonia. She was investigated further and electroencephalography (EEG) revealed slow waves over frontal regions. Magnetic resonance imaging (MRI) was normal. Over the next 2 weeks she became progressively more catatonic. She became mute, and was observed to hold fixed postures for prolonged periods of time. At other times, she was overactive and running through the ward, screaming, and taking her clothes off. At this point, *N*-methyl-D-aspartate receptor (NMDAR) antibody test results were reported as positive in serum.

She was transferred to the neurology ward where she was treated with high-dose intravenous methylprednisolone and plasma exchange, which involved a central line. Pelvic MRI was normal. She continued to be episodically disturbed on the neurology ward. The hospital porters were called to provide special observations, and to stop her leaving the side room, she pulled her central line out. After this, she was given a general anaesthetic to administer the plasma exchange. She then made a rapid recovery from her psychosis over the next 2 weeks, such that she was able to be discharged home from the

neurology ward. Olanzapine and diazepam were stopped. She was maintained on steroids for a further 6 months, during which time she made a gradual recovery back to her premorbid state.

Overview

Autoimmune encephalitis is a neuropsychiatric disorder. While it is generally managed by neurologists in the United Kingdom, many of the presenting symptoms and most of the challenges in management are psychiatric. The description of psychiatric symptoms as part of the presenting symptoms of encephalitis dates back to the first descriptions of the disorder. The more recent discovery of autoimmune causes of encephalitis has particular relevance for psychiatry: there is significant overlap between the initial presentation of encephalitis with other core psychiatric disorders such as depression and psychosis. The particular challenge for inpatient psychiatry is to screen and detect these disorders early. The current evidence indicates that the rapid detection and delivery of immunotherapy, rather than the use of psychiatric treatments, is associated with better long-term outcomes for patients. Conversely, the risks of not detecting encephalitis are of long-term disability, or even death in a proportion of patients.

This chapter describes the evolution in understanding of autoimmune encephalitis, the characteristics associated with particular antibodies, and the investigations and management of patients with autoimmune encephalitis from a psychiatric perspective.

History of autoimmune encephalitis

Limbic encephalitis is a syndrome characterized by subacute memory disturbance, seizures, and disturbance of mood and hallucinations, in association with inflammation of the medial temporal lobes (1).

Autoimmune encephalitis was originally described in association with malignancy. Antibodies are produced as a response to tumour antigens which then have molecular mimicry against autoantigens, thereby causing the neurological syndrome. A number of different antibodies associated with different tumour sites have been described: anti-Hu associated with lung cancer (2), anti-Ma2 associated with testicular cancer (3), and anti CRMP5/CV2 in thymoma (4). However, while explaining the aetiology of the encephalitis, the removal of the antibody is usually not associated with a dramatic treatment response. The antibodies identified are intracellular, and therefore not amenable to immunotherapy. The primary treatment for paraneoplastic limbic encephalitis is through the removal and treatment of the malignancy.

The important breakthrough in the diagnosis and treatment of autoimmune encephalitis was in the discovery of neuronal cell surface antibodies as a cause for a proportion of cases. The implication of being on the neuronal cell surface is that the antibodies are amenable to removal, without killing the neuron. The disorders are therefore treatable, and patients with disabling neuropsychiatric symptoms have the potential to receive treatments that can provide a cure for their illness, for the first time.

Voltage-gated potassium channel-complex antibodies

The first neuronal cell surface antibodies (NSAbs) to be discovered in association with encephalitis was voltage-gated potassium channel (VGKC)-complex antibodies in 2001 (5), with evidence of treatment response in the form of a description of the association between removal of the antibody and improvement in memory in 13 patients in 2004 (6).

These initial case descriptions were of a progressive neuropsychiatric syndrome with abnormalities of mood, sleep, and cognition recognized alongside the neurological symptoms of seizures, and autonomic instability. Most patients also had low sodium and abnormal high-signal change in the medial temporal lobes on MRI.

The understanding of the pathogenic nature of VGKC-complex antibodies has further advanced since 2010 with the discovery that VGKC antibodies are not usually antibodies against the VGKC subunits themselves, but instead to proteins that are complexed with the potassium channel, in particular leucine-rich glioma-inactivated 1 protein (LGI1) and contactin associated protein-2 (CASPR2) (7). Antibodies against these proteins have been associated with particular, although overlapping clinical phenotypes, each also including neuropsychiatric features.

Further recent examination of the antigenic targets of VGKC-complex antibodies indicates that there are a range of targets, a proportion of which are intracellular (8). The interpretation of a positive VGKC antibody test in the absence of LGI1 or CASPR2 antibodies is therefore not straightforward and the relevance of the antibodies in these cases remains controversial, with no randomized controlled trials to guide treatment decisions.

Furthermore, the clinical syndromes associated with VGKC-complex antibodies have broadened considerably over the last 15 years, with cases of patients with chronic pain, dementia, seizures, or psychosis being described, some of which respond to treatment with immunotherapy (reviewed by Prüss and Lennox (9)).

However, an influential study examined patients presenting to a large neurology centre, who were found to have VGKC antibodies, in the absence of LGI1 or CASPR2 antibodies. The study compared the outcomes of patients who received immunotherapy with those who did not receive treatment, and found no difference in outcome between the two groups (10). This has led many clinicians to stop testing for VGKC antibodies, instead testing for LGI1 or CASPR2 antibodies.

N-methyl-d-aspartate receptor antibody encephalitis

In 2007, a new syndrome was described almost exclusively in young women with ovarian teratoma presenting with psychiatric disturbance, amnesia, seizures, dyskinesia, autonomic disturbance, and respiratory failure. Patients were found to have antibodies directed against the NR1 and NR2 subunits of the NMDAR (11).

Since its discovery, this syndrome has been found to be one of the most common forms of autoimmune encephalitis and even surpassing several viral aetiologies (12). More recent case series have broadened the demographics, with NMDAR antibody encephalitis recognized in a wide age range, and not restricted to women. It is not invariably paraneoplastic (13, 14).

The clinical characteristics of NMDAR antibody-mediated encephalitis are of a multistage, invariably progressive disorder. In a fifth of cases, the disorder starts with a viral illness. It is then followed by predominantly psychiatric symptoms (particularly psychosis, mood disorder, and personality change), along with amnesia, confusion, and seizures, although these are not usually prominent. The next stage occurs after 3–4 weeks and is characterized by movement disorders, classically an orofacial dyskinesia, and catatonia. There is demonstrable autonomic disturbance (e.g. cardiac dysrhythmia, hyperthermia, unstable blood pressure, hyperhidrosis and sialorrhoea, and altered respiratory rate) and reduced consciousness levels. At this point, the disorder becomes life-threatening, and unless appropriate supportive treatment is given, may lead to death.

Patients with anti-NMDAR encephalitis generally have good responses to treatment with immunotherapy, especially if diagnosed and treated promptly. In the European case series of over 400 patients with NMDAR antibody encephalitis, treatment with immunotherapy in less than 6 weeks was associated with a far better long-term prognosis (14). In addition, aggressive treatment, with first- and second-line immunotherapy, plus removal of any teratoma, if present, is also associated with better outcomes (15).

It is important to note that psychiatric symptoms, predominantly psychosis, are the most common presenting symptom of anti-NMDAR antibody encephalitis in adults, with the first large case series of 100 patients reporting 80% presenting to psychiatric services (16) and recently a larger series has reported a similar high level of 65% (15). Furthermore, almost all the symptoms of NMDAR antibody encephalitis are also associated with schizophrenia (Table 18.1), such that the clinical presentation is not distinct, and can easily be missed.

The opportunities for early detection of NMDAR antibody encephalitis are in psychiatric units. The recognition of this disorder at an early stage, while under psychiatry, will result in a better outcome for those patients, and will save lives.

Furthermore, there are some studies to suggest that NMDAR antibodies are seen in patients with a purely psychiatric presentation, with

Table 18.1 Overlap in clinical symptoms seen in autoimmune encephalitis and psychiatric disorders

Clinical sign/symptom	In autoimmune encephalitis	In psychiatric diagnoses
Seizures	Observed in association with most NSAbs	Epilepsy overrepresented in patients with schizophrenia (odds ratio 11.1) (Makikyro et al., 1998) Kraepelin observed in his original description of dementia praecox: 'as in dementia praecox epileptiform seizures occur, the malady may be taken for epilepsy'
Cognitive dysfunction	Observed in association with most NSAbs. Memory function is most often and severely affected, with different profiles associating with different NSAbs	Observed in schizophrenia across a range of domains. Associated with poor function and clinical outcome
Movement disorders	Observed in association with most NSAbs	9% of antipsychotic-naive patients with schizophrenia have spontaneous dyskinesias; 17% have spontaneous parkinsonism (Pappa and Dazzan, 2009)
Catatonia	Most marked in NMDAR but observed in cases of AE associated with VGKC complex antibodies and GABA-A antibodies	Prevalence in psychiatric patients ranges from 7.6% to 38%. 10–15% of patients with catatonia have a schizophrenia diagnosis (Taylor and Fink, 2003)
Language disorders	Most marked in NMDAR and AMPA-R. Catatonic speech signs like echolalia and palilalia are also common	'Formal thought disorder' is a cardinal feature of psychotic disorders and manifests in disordered speech, sometimes called 'schizaphasia'—in some cases not distinguishable from neurological dysphasia
Autonomic dysfunction	Can be observed in association with most NSAbs. Can be life-threatening in NMDAR	Ambulatory patients with schizophrenia have mean reduced body temperature of 0.2°C. (Shiloh et al., 2009) Meta-analytical evidence of reduced heart rate variability in psychotic disorders (Alvares et al., 2016)
Hyponatraemia	Observed in association with LGI1 antibodies in particular	Occurs in 6% of chronic psychiatric patients (Elmsley et al., 1990); polydipsia present in 3–17% of psychiatric patients (de Leon et al., 1994); 40% of psychotic patients admitted with unexplained hyponatraemia are not taking antipsychotic medication (Williams and Kores, 2011)
Antipsychotic sensitivity including rhabdomyolysis	Observed in NMDAR in particular	Neuroleptic malignant syndrome (rigidity, catatonia, confusion, hyperthermia and rhabdomyolysis) occurs in up to 0.07–2.2% of patients taking antipsychotics. Rhabdomyolysis can occur with water intoxication and hyponatraemia
Insomnia	Observed in association with most NSAbs. Particularly marked in NMDAR-AE	Reported in 30–80% of patients with schizophrenia (Cohr, 2008). Consistent findings include increased sleep-onset latency, diminished slow wave sleep time, decreased REM latency

See original publication for references.

AE, autoimmune encephalitis; LGI1, leucine-rich glioma inactivated protein 1; NMDAR, *N*-methyl-d-aspartate receptor; NSAb, neuronal cell surface antibody; REM, rapid eye movement.

Reproduced from Al-Diwani A, Pollak TA, Langford AE and Lennox BR, *Front Psychiatry* 8:1, Synaptic and Neuronal Autoantibody-Associated Psychiatric Syndromes: Controversies and Hypotheses. 3 © 2017 Al-Diwani, Pollak, Langford and Lennox. Used under the Creative Commons Attribution 4.0 International Public License (https://creativecommons.org/licenses/by/4.0/).

diagnoses of schizophrenia or psychosis, who do not progress on to develop the fulminant syndrome of encephalitis. Studies suggest that 2–3% of patients with psychosis have antibodies against NMDAR antibodies (17, 18). However, some studies also show that there is no increased rate of NMDAR antibodies in psychosis when compared with control groups (19, 20), and there are no randomized controlled studies of immunotherapy in patients with NMDAR antibodies with purely psychiatric presentations, and so treatment of these patients should currently only be undertaken in the context of a research programme.

Other antibodies

There are case descriptions of other antibodies associated with autoimmune encephalitis, detailed in Table 18.2.

Many of these are also associated with psychiatric symptoms, although will also have other prominent neurological symptoms, such

as seizures. There are currently insufficient data to support the routine screening for these other antibodies in those with primary psychiatric presentations.

Patients with anti-AMPAR antibodies are comparatively rare (predominantly in women and are often paraneoplastic) and mostly have a relapsing course, with prominent psychosis in addition to the other limbic encephalitis symptoms (21). Gamma aminobutyric acid type B receptor (GABA$_B$R) antibody-mediated encephalitis is usually paraneoplastic (often small cell lung cancer) with prominent seizures (22).

Various neurological disorders such as stiff-person syndrome, complex partial seizures, limbic encephalitis, and cerebellar ataxia have been described in patients with high-titre anti-glutamic acid decarboxylase antibodies (>1000 U/mL) (23). Most patients have a chronic non-remitting course but immunotherapies and plasma exchange may have some benefit.

Table 18.2 Clinical characteristics of syndromes due to antibodies against neuronal cell membrane antigens

Antigenic target	Psychiatric symptoms	Neurological symptoms	Tumour associations	Treatment response and prognosis
NMDAR	Psychosis, catatonia, mutism, depression, insomnia	Reduced consciousness, seizures, cognitive impairment	Ovarian teratomas (<50%); occasionally other tumours in patients >45 years	Early tumour removal and immunosuppression associated with good prognosis
LGI1 (VGKC-complex)	Depression, insomnia	Amnesia, seizures, faciobrachial dystonic seizures, encephalopathy, hyponatraemia	Rare	Good response to early immunotherapy. Usually monophasic illness
CASPR2 (VGKC-complex)	Insomnia	Encephalopathy, autonomic disturbance, pain, amnesia	Thymoma, small cell lung cancer	In the absence of tumours, good response to immunotherapy and also spontaneous improvement in some
AMPAR	Psychosis,	Amnesia, seizures	Thymoma, breast, or lung (50%)	Good response to immunosuppression
GABA$_B$R	Not described	Limbic encephalopathy, seizures	Thymoma and lung (80%)	Some patients respond to immunosuppression. Good response with tumour removal
GABA$_A$R	Psychosis, catatonia	Encephalopathy, seizures	Lymphoma (16%)	Treatment response not known
GAD65	Not described	Complex partial seizures, cognitive impairment, stiff person syndrome, cerebellar degeneration	Rare	Poor response to immunotherapy in some
GlyR	Not described	Stiffness, exaggerated startle reflexes, rigidity, rarely cognitive impairment	Rare	Response to early immunotherapy described in some
mGluR5	Not described	Confusion, encephalitis	Lymphoma	Improve with removal lymphoma
DPPX	Not described	Memory loss, seizures, and confusion, exaggerated startle, myoclonus, rigidity, hyper-reflexia	Lymphoma	Improve with removal lymphoma
D2R	Emotional lability, attention deficit and psychosis	Basal ganglia encephalitis	Not known	Not known

AMPAR, 2-amino-3-(3-hydroxy-5-methyl-isoxazol-4-yl)-propanoic acid; CASPR-2, contactin associated protein 2; DPPX, dipeptidyl peptidase-like protein-6; GABA$_B$R, gamma amino butyric acid (GABA) type B receptor; GAD, glutamic acid decarboxylase; Gly R, glycine receptor; LGI1, leucine-rich glioma inactivated protein 1; NMDAR, N-methyl-d-aspartate receptor.

Diagnosis and treatment of autoimmune encephalitis

Who to test

- All people with first-episode psychosis, with less than 3 months' duration.
- Abrupt onset of illness, or rapid deterioration.
- Prodromal headache or temperature prior to onset of psychosis.
- Psychosis and cognitive impairment (short-term memory, disorientation).
- Catatonia, particularly orofacial dyskinesia.
- Autonomic disturbance (hypo/hyperthermia, unstable blood pressure, raised respiratory rate, tachycardia).
- Neuroleptic sensitivity or suspected neuroleptic malignant syndrome.
- Hyponatraemia.
- Altered consciousness level.

What should be tested

Inpatient psychiatry teams should request and coordinate all of these investigations. Currently in the United Kingdom, lumbar punctures are not undertaken in mental health settings. However, this is routine practice in other countries, and is a required investigation to make a diagnosis in these cases. The author would advocate that this is enabled, to allow the adequate investigation of acute psychiatric presentations.

Serum

Test for anti-NMDAR antibodies and LGI1 antibodies. Other antibodies (AMPAR, GABA$_B$, GABA$_A$, glycine, or D2) are also available, but current understanding is that these are not associated with isolated psychiatric presentations, and should only be requested if other neurological symptoms are present.

Other serum inflammatory markers (C-reactive protein or erythrocyte sedimentation rate) are usually normal in both conditions.

Serum sodium should be measured, as hyponatraemia is associated with VGKC antibodies in particular.

Lumbar puncture

Definitive diagnosis of autoimmune encephalitis requires detection of antibodies in CSF. Evidence of inflammation (pleocytosis, oligoclonal bands) would support diagnosis and early treatment. Some studies indicate that antibodies can be seen in cerebrospinal fluid, even when negative in serum (24). Therefore, serum testing alone will result in under-detection of patients.

Electroencephalography

EEG is a useful investigation if there is a suspicion of encephalitis. EEG may show epileptiform activity or slow waves. In more fulminant NMDAR encephalitis, the 'extreme delta brush pattern' is characteristic.

Magnetic resonance imaging

MRI may also be useful in establishing the diagnosis and guiding early treatment. Hyperintensity in medial temporal regions would support a diagnosis of encephalitis, although a normal MRI does not exclude the diagnosis.

Investigations in antibody-positive patients

In those with a positive antibody test, it is usually important to screen for an underlying malignancy, initially using a whole body CT and if negative, a positron emission tomography (PET) scan. MRI scans are useful in young women, since occasionally teratomas may be missed by CT and PET scans and also to reduce radiation exposure (15). The exception would be in those with long histories of illness, where a malignancy is highly unlikely.

Neurological treatment

The evidence for treatment of patients with the classical presentations of NMDAR encephalopathy and LGI1 encephalitis is now well established through clinical practice worldwide, rather than any randomized controlled trial data. The clinical consensus is that these disorders should be treated early and aggressively (25). Treatment involves an initial acute treatment to remove the antibodies from the body, either through plasma exchange or intravenous immunoglobulin, and is followed by maintenance immunosuppression with steroids or steroid-sparing agents such as mycophenolate mofetil or azathioprine. In patients with underlying neoplasia, the underlying tumour should also be removed. (25). Further second-line treatments, such as cyclophosphamide or rituximab are then used as required.

These treatments are currently only possible in secondary acute hospital centres, with the availability of specialist neurology and blood and transfusion centres. However, there are considerable difficulties with treating patients who may be paranoid, catatonic, and confused in these settings. There is often a lack of mental health nursing expertise in general hospital settings, and as a result the patient can become more distressed during treatment, and even pose a risk to safety. It is important that there is a nursing risk assessment for patients being transferred to acute hospital sites for treatment of encephalitis. If possible, hospital liaison psychiatry services should be closely involved in reviewing patients while in the acute hospital, and if necessary, one-to-one mental health nursing should be arranged. In many cases it is possible to treat patients on a day case basis, travelling from an inpatient psychiatric unit.

If there is any concern about a progressive encephalopathic illness, patients will need to be in close proximity to neurological intensive care units. However, if this is not an issue, and certainly once the acute treatment has been undertaken, patients are usually more appropriately managed in a psychiatric inpatient unit. Given the nature of the treatments required and the clinical presentations of patients, discussions and decisions about management should ideally be made jointly between psychiatric and neurological teams specializing in these disorders.

Psychiatric treatments

There is little evidence base to guide the use of antipsychotic treatments in autoimmune encephalitis. There are case series to suggest that there is a higher incidence of an adverse response to antipsychotics, particularly with autonomic instability following their use (26). However, it is impossible to separate the effect of the antipsychotic from the underlying encephalitis in these situations. It is also possible that antipsychotics are helpful in the treatment of encephalitis, possibly through an immunosuppressant effect (27).

Pragmatically, a sedative antipsychotic, such as olanzapine, is often used in the short term, and this is then titrated off after the antibody is removed and the level of disturbance has improved. Benzodiazepines are also used, either as required or regularly, over the period of acute treatment. Care should be taken to monitor autonomic function with both of these treatments, with the risk of exacerbating the autonomic instability that is seen in NMDAR encephalitis.

Caution should also be taken when prescribing with plasma exchange. Most antipsychotics are plasma bound, and will therefore be cleared out of the body with exchange. Doses should be withheld until after treatment. Amisulpride is the most lipid bound of the antipsychotics and so would be a good choice of antipsychotic if this is required.

Antipsychotic treatments are being used for symptom control; they are not being used to treat the underlying disorder, and there is no indication that they provide any benefit for longer-term use, after the acute episode of illness. Indeed, they may contribute to the sedation and cognitive processing difficulties that people with encephalitis may experience.

There are also some case studies where electroconvulsive therapy has been used in the treatment of autoimmune encephalitis, with apparent good effect (28).

Psychiatric consequences of neurological treatments

Some of the treatments used for the neurological treatment of autoimmune encephalitis can have psychiatric effects in their own right, and sometimes it can be difficult to disentangle side effects from symptoms relating to underlying disease process.

Corticosteroids in particular commonly have psychiatric side effects, including insomnia, depression, anxiety, and even psychosis. These side effects are dose dependent, and the aim should always be to use corticosteroids for as short a time as possible, and at as low a dose as possible. An alternative can be to give steroids on alternate days. Cardiometabolic side effects are also common, and require regular monitoring, in particular in those who are also on antipsychotic medication because of the high risk of metabolic syndrome.

Intravenous immunoglobulin, rituximab, mycophenolate mofetil, and azathioprine are normally well tolerated with no commonly described psychiatric side effects. Anticonvulsants may be used for symptomatic treatment of seizures in autoimmune encephalitis; most do not have psychiatric side effects, and indeed are used in their own right as mood stabilizers. However, caution should be taken with the use of levetiracetam (Keppra®) which can cause anxiety, depression, and paranoia as side effects.

Outcome

The case series evidence indicates that without intensive immuno-suppression with first- and second-line treatments, patients often remain hospitalized for several months, with invasive respiratory support and very slow recovery, with 25% experiencing death or severe ongoing disability (15).

By contrast, with early and assertive treatment most patients improve dramatically, achieving remission over a period of a few months. It is unknown how long immunotherapy should be maintained for, but current evidence indicates that relapses, where they occur, tend to be within the first year of follow-up, and in about 30% of cases (14). If the serum antibody is removed with treatment, and remains absent with the titration off immunosuppression, then the chances of relapse are very low.

If a patient with psychosis and any other features of encephal-opathy, such as reduced consciousness level, seizures, autonomic instability, catatonia, or investigations to support an encephalitis such as an abnormality in EEG or MRI or cerebrospinal fluid, then they should be treated as other patients with encephalopathy, with assertive immunotherapy. However, in the absence of other features of encephalitis it is not known whether patients with anti-bodies and psychosis should be treated with immunotherapy, or antipsychotics.

A challenge to psychiatry and neurology

Throughout most of the twentieth century, neurology and psychiatry have developed parallel narratives to describe neuropsychiatric syndromes, and the idea that 'one man's schizophrenia is another man's encephalitis' goes back to at least the 1920s (29). With the advent of biomarkers to diagnose cases of autoimmune encephaltiis amongst those presenting with psychosis, there is the opportunity for the two disciplines to share skills and language to improve patient care, bringing together the traditional strengths of neurology (in molecular biology and the phenomenology of physical symptoms) with those of psychiatry (assessment and management of complex behaviours). We advocate the shared management of people with these conditions between neurologists and psychiatrists.

REFERENCES

1. Corsellis JA, Goldberg GJ, Norton AR. "Limbic encephalitis" and its association with carcinoma. *Brain* 1968;91:481–496.
2. Graus F, Cordon-Cardo C, Posner JB. Neuronal antinuclear antibody in sensory neuronopathy from lung cancer. *Neurology* 1985;35:538–543.
3. Voltz R, Gultekin SH, Rosenfeld MR, et al. A serological marker of paraneoplastic limbic and brain stem encephalitis in patients with testicular cancer. *N Engl J Med* 1999;340:1788–1795.
4. Antoine JC, Honnorat J, Anterion CT, et al. Limbic encephalitis and immunological perturbations in two patients with thymoma. *JNNP* 1995;58:706–710.
5. Buckley C, Oger J, Clover L, et al. Potassium channel antibodies in two patients with reversible limbic encephalitis. *Ann Neurol* 2001;50:73–78.
6. Vincent A, Buckley C, Schott JM, et al. Potassium channel antibody-associated encephalopathy: a potentially immunotherapy responsive form of limbic encephalitis. *Brain* 2004;127:701–712.
7. Irani SR, Alexander S, Waters P, et al. Antibodies to kv1 potassium channel-complex proteins leucine-rich, glioma inactivated 1 protein and contactin-associated protein-2 in limbic encephalitis, Morvan's syndrome and acquired neuromyotonia. *Brain* 2010;133:2734–2748.
8. Lang B, Makuch M, Moloney T, et al. Intracellular and non-neuronal targets of voltage-gated potassium channel complex antibodies. *J Neurol Neurosurg Psychiatry* 2017;88:353–361.
9. Prüss H, Lennox BR. Emerging psychiatric syndromes associated with antivoltage-gated potassium channel complex antibodies. *J Neurol Neurosurg Psychiatry* 2016;87:1242–1247.
10. van Sonderen A, Schreurs MW, de Bruijn MA, et al. The relevance of VGKC positivity in the absence of LGI1 and Caspr2 antibodies. *Neurology* 2016;86:1692–1699.
11. Dalmau J, Tuzun E, Wu HY, et al. Paraneoplastic anti-N-methyl-D-aspartate receptor encephalitis associated with ovarian teratoma. *Ann Neurol* 2007;61:25–36.
12. Granerod J, Ambrose HE, Davies NW, et al. Causes of encephalitis and differences in their clinical presentations in England: a multicentre, population-based prospective study. *Lancet Infect Dis* 2010;10:835–844.
13. Dalmau J, Lancaster E, Martinez-Hernandez E, Rosenfeld MR, Balice-Gordon R. Clinical experience and laboratory investigations in patients with anti-NMDAR encephalitis. *Lancet Neurol* 2011;10:63–74.
14. Irani SR, Bera K, Waters P, et al. N-methyl-D-aspartate antibody encephalitis: temporal progression of clinical and paraclinical observations in a predominantly non-paraneoplastic disorder of both sexes. *Brain* 2010;133:1655–1667.
15. Titulaer MJ, McCracken L, Gabilondo I, et al. Treatment and prognostic factors for long-term outcome in patients with anti-NMDA receptor encephalitis: an observational cohort study. *Lancet Neurol* 2013;12:157–165.
16. Dalmau J, Gleichman AJ, Hughes EG et al. Anti-NMDA-receptor encephalitis: case series and an analysis of the effects of antibodies. *Lancet Neurol* 2008;7:1091–1098.
17. Pollak TA, McCormack R, Peakman M, Nicholson TR, David AS. Prevalence of anti-N-methyl-D-aspartate (NMDA) receptor antibodies in patients with schizophrenia and related psychoses: a systematic review and meta-analysis. *Psychol Med* 2014;44:2475–2487.
18. Lennox BR, Palmer-Cooper EC, Pollak T, et al. Prevalence and clinical characteristics of serum neuronal cell surface antibodies in first-episode psychosis: a case-control study. *Lancet Psychiatry* 2017;4:42–48.
19. Dahm L, Ott C, Steiner J, et al. Seroprevalence of autoantibodies against brain antigens in health and disease. *Ann Neurol* 2014;76:82–94.
20. deWitte LD, Hoffman C, van Mierlo HC, et al. Absence of N-methyl-D-aspartate receptor IgG autoantibodies in schizophrenia: the importance of cross-validation studies. *JAMA Psychiatry* 2015;72:731–733.
21. Graus F, Boronat A, Xifro X, et al. The expanding clinical profile of anti-AMPA receptor encephalitis. *Neurology* 2010;74:857–859.
22. Lancaster E, Lai M, Peng X, et al. Antibodies to the GABA(b) receptor in limbic encephalitis with seizures: case series and characterisation of the antigen. *Lancet Neurol* 2010;9:67–76.
23. Saiz A, Blanco Y, Sabater L, et al. Spectrum of neurological syndromes associated with glutamic acid decarboxylase antibodies: diagnostic clues for this association. *Brain* 2008;131:2553–2563.

24. Gresa-Arribas N, Titulaer MJ, Torrents A, et al. Antibody titres at diagnosis and during follow-up of anti-NMDA receptor encephalitis: a retrospective study. *Lancet Neurol* 201413:167–177.

25. Graus F, Titulaer MJ, Balu R, et al. A clinical approach to diagnosis of autoimmune encephalitis. *Lancet Neurol* 2016;15:391–404.

26. Lejuste F, Thomas L, Picard G, et al. Neuroleptic intolerance in patients with anti-NMDAR encephalitis. *Neurol Neuroimmunol Neuroinflamm* 2016;3:e280.

27. O'Sullivan D, Green L, Stone S, et al. Treatment with the antipsychotic agent, risperidone, reduces disease severity in experimental autoimmune encephalomyelitis. *PLoS One* 2014;9:e104430.

28. Braakman HM, Moers-Hornikx VM, Arts BM, et al. Pearls & Oysters: electroconvulsive therapy in anti-NMDA receptor encephalitis. *Neurology* 2010;75:44–46.

29. Rogers D. *Motor Disorder in Psychiatry: Towards a Neurological Perspective*. Chichester: John Wiley and Sons; 1992.

19

Rehabilitation wards

Karen Dauncey and Janet Patterson

Introduction

Inpatient psychiatric rehabilitation in the UK has evolved significantly in the last 50 years, in tandem with changes on overall provision of psychiatric care. In the 1980s, the emphasis in rehabilitation practice at that time was still on the resettlement of patients who had been resident in the large asylum hospitals that had been built mainly in the nineteenth century. Projects such as the Team for the Assessment of Psychiatric Services (TAPS) explored the process, and recorded how the cohorts of patients who left hospital had increasingly complex problems, and needed increasingly complex systems to support them in the community, such as the development of group homes and hospital hostels (1). These large hospitals in the UK are now almost all closed. Psychiatric rehabilitation practice has moved on, embracing the concept of recovery (2), in working to support individuals to regain their lives, to develop purpose and meaning, while still acknowledging the presence of severe mental disorder.

Modern rehabilitation practice in the UK

Definition

A whole system approach to recovery from mental ill health which maximizes an individual's quality of life and social inclusion by encouraging skills, promoting independence and autonomy in order to give them hope for the future and which leads to successful community living through appropriate support.[1]

This definition recognizes the need for a wide range of facilities and services, of which inpatient rehabilitation is only part of the patient pathway. Psychiatric rehabilitation can be carried out in all settings from the high security hospitals to people who are living rough or on the street.

This chapter describes our experience and knowledge of working within general adult rehabilitation services in England: neither of us has worked for any length of time in other countries or under

other legislation. We believe that all mental health services in the UK should have rehabilitation provision as a core requirement at district level.

Rehabilitation facilities and function

A recent study of rehabilitation facilities in the UK found that there is variation in the characteristics of inpatient rehabilitation units and their target patient group. Variations include the following:

- The site of the unit may be either on the hospital site or a stand-alone unit in the community.
- The expected length of admission can vary from 1 to 5 years or more.
- The level of security needed varies.
- Some units specialize in working with people with brain injury, autism spectrum disorder, or severe personality disorder.
- The functional ability of the patient group varies, and therefore the level of support and the therapeutic aims of the unit also vary. In some units, the focus may be to support patients to develop community living skills *in situ*. In others, the service provides more support with the opportunity/expectation of the individual to develop individual skills. Still others may encourage patients to play some part, but full 'hotel services' are provided.
- Recovery goals vary from independent living, or moving to a highly staffed home.

An outline of the different types of unit is given by Davies and Killaspy (3).

Psychiatry is a medical discipline using a biopsychosocial framework, especially in rehabilitation practice. As doctors using a medical model of illness, we pay attention to the origins of a disorder, its development, and its maintenance. We also seek to understand the individual who experiences this disorder and their circumstances. We explore how we can minimize the impact of a disorder on an individual and those around them and how to support the individual to reach their goals, even if, to some, these goals may seem unrealistic. We also seek to modify the physical and social environment to support the individual.

We start from a point of positive expectation and therapeutic optimism, that an individual who is admitted to a psychiatric

[1] Reproduced from Killaspy, H., Harden, C., Holloway, F., et al. (2005). What do mental rehabilitation services provide and what are they for? A national survey in England. *Journal of Mental Health* 14: 157–165.

rehabilitation ward will have a positive experience and improve their outcome. These expectations may be small or large, but must be realistic and pragmatic: schizophrenia is, after all, a highly disabling illness.

In order to carry out such work, inpatient rehabilitation units need to have their role understood, accepted, and supported throughout the system in which they are based. They cannot work if expected to function in exactly the same way as an acute ward: there are different reasons and expectations of admission, different approaches to management, and staff skills and attitudes can differ significantly. Therefore, management and system support for the unit and its practices must be well established and maintained.

The need for psychiatric rehabilitation

There remains ample evidence that even when there are complex and sophisticated mental health services such as those that exist within the National Health Service (NHS) in the UK, there is a steady flow of patients who need a period of inpatient treatment that is longer, more complex, and more intensive than that which acute services can provide.

This is echoed by the finding from Poole and colleagues (4), working in the North of England, who noted that 18.6% of acute psychiatric beds were occupied by people with delayed discharge, where these patients were defined as delayed discharge on the primary criterion that a senior health professional believed they that they would be better cared for elsewhere. These patients were thus receiving expensive (acute inpatient), but not optimal, care. Of this group, the older inpatients (approximately 24%) were white, diagnosed with dementia, and experienced relatively short admissions. The younger people with delayed discharge were often of black and minority ethnic background with psychosis, long service contact, and they sometimes experienced very long admissions. The whole cohort was socially isolated and marginalized, and frequently had comorbid alcohol use. Looking at the numbers, about 25% of the total adult inpatient group under the age of 65 had delayed discharge.

Reasons for delay included:

- waiting for a bed in a specialist facility
- difficulty in identifying appropriate placement for some types of specialist care (e.g. a unit combining skills and facilities to manage both mental illness and substance misuse problems or autism spectrum disorder)
- waiting for assessment for housing or other specialist provision
- funding problems
- waiting for appropriate care packages
- patients/families exercising choice over placement.

The authors of the paper (4) stated that there was:

> Nothing in our findings to suggest that lack of effort among staff contributed to delayed discharges … yet they continued to devise processes to reduce delayed discharges. The majority of the younger adult delayed discharge group … appeared to be in need of psychiatric rehabilitation. What is more distressing is the clear evidence that people with these problems can recover in the right environment.

Where we work

We work in a mental health NHS Trust in a fairly affluent part of England, covering the counties of Oxfordshire and Buckinghamshire: this is a mixed urban/semirural setting with total population of approximately 1 million. It includes some pockets of deprivation and a small transient population. Compared to other services in England it has a relatively small number of acute and rehabilitation psychiatric beds per head of population.

Local study of patients with delayed discharge on acute psychiatric wards

In our own brief review of services in our Trust, we found there was a cohort of patients who remained in hospital for longer periods: the point prevalence over a period of 18 months of patients in hospital for 6 months or more was a remarkably consistent 23–24% (5).

We used the patient record system to identify all patients on the six acute and one psychiatric intensive care unit (PICU), excluding those on extended Section 17 leave, who had been in hospital for longer than 6 months on a specific date. We then reviewed their clinical records. We identified 27 patients out of a total of 115 acute and 13 PICU beds, and a further 23 patients were identified as being continuously in hospital for over 3 months. Their characteristics are shown in Table 19.1.

Table 19.1 Characteristics of our patients in hospital longer than 6 months occupying acute psychiatric beds

	Male	Female
Total	11	16
Primary diagnosis ICD10		
Schizophrenia	9	11
Schizoaffective	1	2
Bipolar affective	0	2
ASD	0	1
Emotionally unstable PD	0	1
Don't know	1	0
Secondary diagnosis		
Drug and alcohol related	8	1
Depression		1
Learning disability		1
Physical diagnoses (some patients more than one diagnosis)		
Breast cancer		2
Diabetes mellitus		4
Hypothyroidism		1
Asthma		1
Cor pulmonale		1
Polycystic ovaries		1
Pregnant		1
COPD		1
Angina		1
Delay in discharge		
Mental health	5	12
Social care	5	4
Don't know	1	

ASD, autism spectrum disorder; COPD, chronic obstructive pulmonary disease; PD, personality disorder.

Clinical staff were asked to comment on the barriers to their discharge. These comments are presented as follows:

Our medication options were limited by her pregnancy.

Discharge was delayed by the lack of CBT [cognitive behavioural therapy] and getting a support worker allocated who could carry through behavioural work at home.

… needs psychology to try to address fixed delusions refractory to treatment.

It's been very difficult to maintain her stable physical health. [The patient had severe cardiac and lung problems]

Funding is available but she needs a nursing home that can deal with both her physical and mental health needs.

We need more skills in managing ASD [autism spectrum disorder] in inpatient settings.

Perhaps inreach from drug misuse services would have helped.

The opportunity to speak directly to housing dept. would help.

Psychology input supervised by the [specialist rehabilitation ward] psychologist was helpful.

… needs a more thorough IQ and ASD assessment.

Providers of community services and accommodation can be reluctant to accept individuals with increasingly complex problems, or decline their return after a period of inpatient care. Hence some people with severe and enduring illnesses become 'stuck' on acute admission wards with no immediate prospect of discharge. Community placements may no longer be sustainable and tenancies can be lost because of unacceptable behaviour and associated risk, drug use, and non-payment of rent.

In the past, many of these individuals might then have lived for a long time on the 'back wards' of large mental hospitals. However, these facilities, which were not geared to preparing individuals for community living and had been much criticized for institutional practices, have closed down and continuing care facilities are not generally available in modern British mental health care.

The local inpatient rehabilitation unit

Context

We describe an inpatient rehabilitation service which we believe is typical of a 'district-sized' service in England and exists within a system also providing acute inpatient care and low secure forensic services to meet the needs of adults with severe mental illness. It has to cater for the needs of a disparate group of patients who have complex and widely varying/competing needs and comorbidities. More specialist inpatient services are typically provided 'out of area', a situation which is less than ideal.

We attempt to make our system functional by using support from low secure services and community-based social care rehabilitation units and housing projects. The range and availability of specialist housing varies widely across our catchment area. From discussions with our fellow rehabilitation consultants across the country, the resulting complexity and disparity within our system seems very typical of the situation in England at present.

Physical environment

Our one rehabilitation ward in Oxford Health NHS Foundation Trust has 20 beds, 10 male and 10 female. The physical environment of our ward is not ideal as it was originally commissioned to provide acute care but has been adapted to include a rehabilitation kitchen and multitherapy areas. Bedrooms are well designed with en-suite shower rooms. The level of physical security is similar to local acute wards, having a locked door, and de-escalation and seclusion suites, but is lower than a 'low secure' forensic ward. The vast majority of patients are detained under the Mental Health Act 1983 and use of leave is closely tailored to community rehabilitation care plans. It is, nevertheless, a challenge to provide homeliness and personalization of patient living areas, as this has to be balanced against infection control standards and risk management such as the reduction of ligature points, and having good sight lines.

Standards

The Royal College of Psychiatrists runs an inpatient accreditation service, Accreditation for Inpatient Mental Health Services (AIMS) (6), via its Centre for Quality Improvement. We recommend that any inpatient rehabilitation ward should work towards 'AIMS for Rehabilitation', a version of AIMS tailored for rehabilitation wards. This supports physical environmental standards, service quality, and future development. We also operate within the statutory authority of the Care Quality Commission, which carries out regular detailed inspections.

Our inpatient unit is accredited to AIMS standards. The programme provides rolling review, an online support forum, access to academic conferences, and a variety of developmental opportunities. On a local level, improvements to our care and treatment have been incremental and broad. Some examples include improvements to the physical environment, improved access to psychological therapies, and faster access to out-of-hours junior doctor review in emergencies. As our local acute wards also achieve AIMS status we can share good practice and visit other AIMs-accredited rehabilitation services to support benchmarking and share innovative ideas.

Staffing

Skilled but generically trained psychiatric nurses provide the majority of individualized care planning, and with health care assistants deliver care and many rehabilitation interventions. They manage much of the risk using relational risk management techniques and take responsibility for environmental risk management. They manage medication and concordance and facilitate patients developing self-medication skills. The monitoring of physical health is primarily a nursing role. In our ward, the 'Recovery Star' (7) is usually used to develop and guide initial care plans with the aim of achieving specific goals. Low scoring domains on the 'Recovery Star' can be discussed to support a new plan and goals, with higher scoring areas providing valuable positive feedback

The consultant psychiatrist is trained and experienced in the care of patients with complex psychosis. As rehabilitation wards decrease in number, the opportunity for training the next generation of psychiatrists reduces. The Royal College of Psychiatrists expect psychiatrists to achieve a year in higher training to fulfil an endorsement in rehabilitation. Consultant psychiatrists traditionally offer clinical leadership to the team, expertise in the treatment of mental disorder, neuropsychiatry, psychiatric risk management, and physical health problems. They also need to be expert in the Mental Health Act 1983 and Mental Capacity Act 2005 and be able to fulfil the 'Responsible Clinician' role. To maintain training, they need to offer educational and clinical supervision to trainee psychiatrists, General Practice trainees and Foundation doctors. At present, our ward offers posts to first year Foundation doctors, Core psychiatric trainees, and occasionally Senior trainees.

Clinical psychologists provide expertise in psychological assessment and treatment. In rehabilitation settings, the mainstay of treatment is the provision of a range of cognitive behaviour therapies. Assessments to support diagnosis and treatment include those of mental state, autism spectrum disorder (ASD), neuropsychological assessment, IQ, and personality. Treatments may be delivered individually, in groups, or by supervising the work of an assistant psychologist or other team members. Psychoeducation around the purpose of rehabilitation and the nature of symptoms supports cognitive behavioural therapy and behavioural interventions.

Occupational therapists in mental health are core to developing an ethos of rehabilitation and recovery. They provide functional assessments and occupational and activity-based interventions, and deliver individualized plans of occupation and activity. For example, a recent patient with very severe obsessive–compulsive disorder has a stepwise plan combining graded exposure work with practical tasks of everyday living: this aims to combine a specific behavioural intervention with relearning occupational tasks that she has not been able to achieve for several years. This approach has led her now to consider a goal of semi-independent living rather than returning home to live with her mother in a stressful home environment.

Wellness recovery action planning (WRAP) (8) is used to develop individual relapse prevention plans. An example of a WRAP in practice involved the ward occupational therapist developing a relapse prevention plan with a patient who had persistent command hallucinations instructing her to kill herself. They worked together on a combination of an activity plan to fill her day, with a back-up relapse prevention plan of structured contact over the day by phone, with family members. This allowed her to be reassured by contact with her family, without the previous excessive intrusion into her children's lives. This simple approach in combination with medication changes and family interventions has allowed her to be discharged home after an extremely long hospital admission.

The occupational therapists also supervise the work of activity support workers and assist nurses with care planning.

Social workers have good understanding of the limitations of housing, and the skills of support workers, and this places them in a unique position to help commission appropriate community care. On the ward, they lead on supporting staff to raise safeguarding concerns. They are also experts in the law relating to mental health, mental capacity, and community care. Using this knowledge, alongside their social care skills, they work to identify care needs which need to be met once patients leave hospital.

Specialist pharmacists play a key role in supporting medical and nursing staff with safe and effective prescribing and medicines management. This includes prescribing for mental and physical health problems, education for patients, concordance therapy, and support to access local and national guidelines.

The referral process

We would expect referrals to the rehabilitation ward to be made by care coordinators after consultation with the current inpatient team, patient, and carers. Referrers need to understand that a rehabilitation

---

Box 19.1 Additional problems typically experienced by patients referred to an inpatient psychiatric rehabilitation service

Patients admitted to a typical rehabilitation ward have complex problems, including severe mental illness especially schizophrenia, bipolar disorder, schizoaffective disorder, plus any combination of the following:

- Negative symptoms often evident.
- Misuse of alcohol and/or non-prescribed drugs.
- Offending/risky/challenging behaviour.
- Vulnerability to abuse/exploitation, especially financial and sexual.
- Poor cooperation with treatment/management.
- Treatment-resistant illness and resultant polypharmacy.
- Broken social networks.
- Complex family problems.
- Comorbidity: for example, learning disability, ASD, obsessive–compulsive disorder, personality disorder, post-traumatic stress disorder, or severe physical illness.
- Homelessness.

---

referral should be seen as a positive intervention, not just a transfer of care for an individual with whom they feel therapeutically 'stuck'.

Most of our referrals come from local acute, forensic, or other rehabilitation wards. Our ward also monitors patients being cared for in specialist 'out of area' rehabilitation placements and these patients may need to return to the local service as and when appropriate. The characteristics of people likely to be referred for admission to our rehabilitation unit are provided in Box 19.1.

Admissions from the community are rare, although we have found a notable exception to be some patients with very severe obsessive–compulsive disorder, where harm to others and acute risk to self is very rare but where vulnerability and level of disability can grow quietly and insidiously.

There should be a single point of contact in the rehabilitation ward team to receive referrals: ours is a designated senior clinician (our referrals coordinator), who presents the case of the individual to a regular multidisciplinary team meeting. Here the referrals are reviewed and there is a standard time to respond, assess the individual, and feed back to the referring team. We try to see patients within 2 weeks and feed back to the referring team in 4 weeks.

If the outcome of assessment is to decline a referral, then the reasons must be made clear; for example, an individual with a sexual offending risk cannot be managed on our mixed-sex ward. Wherever possible, we make positive recommendations regarding specific interventions and alternative referral pathways. The rehabilitation team is willing to come back and review patients and to keep an open mind as the situation may change.

If patients are accepted but a long wait for a bed is anticipated, it is important that the patient starts, or continues, an active plan of rehabilitation in their current ward. Where our own staffing allows, we aim to offer inreach to all such patients to work on care plans and rehabilitation goals with the acute team prior to transferring the patient. An example is of a young man on an acute ward where our ward occupational therapist visited and developed a rehabilitation plan with the inpatient team, although this was difficult to implement. When a bed eventually became available, a member of our nursing team visited to discuss and plan his transfer as there were concerns about challenging behaviour. The eventual move was facilitated in a manner which maximized his engagement with the process, and was completed without incident.

The referral process should also include a clear system to record unmet need regarding referrals, collate data, and have a system to feed back both to managers and health commissioners in order that future service development can be supported by coherent information.

Initial assessment

When assessing new referrals, we start with the assumption that the rehabilitation team has something positive to offer: decisions should not be based only on past problems and preconceptions. It is crucial to liaise with the current inpatient team, community team, and family/carers when gathering information. Given the broad range of inpatient rehabilitation wards in the country, no standardized assessment tool would cover all options. Services may benefit from developing a local tool or checklist which supports individual circumstances.

Decisions depend on risk assessment as well as clinical state. Security, staffing levels, physical environment, and gender mix vary far more on rehabilitation wards than in the more standard settings found in acute admission wards or forensic units.

Who should assess? The choice of professional to conduct the assessment will depend on the needs of the individual referred. For example, if challenging behaviour is a major concern, a senior nurse is appropriate. If the individual has a significant physical disability, an occupational therapist's skill may be required. Complex diagnostic assessment requires the involvement of a psychiatrist. A multidisciplinary assessment provides a more comprehensive picture of an individual's mental health and functioning and allows for the training of less experienced staff.

Transfer to the rehabilitation unit

Managing the transfer of patients from one ward to another needs to be planned: for example, there needs to be consideration as to whether planning a visit in advance to the unit would be helpful, or disruptive. For example, individuals with ASD who find change especially difficult need an individualized approach, based on the knowledge of the current treating team.

Rehabilitation goals should be developed while waiting for transfer, based on past ability and potential, but more crucially on the patient's aspirations. Poor prognostic indicators include a degree of negative symptoms, while the presence of good insight and clear goals and opinions are a positive indicator. It is fundamental in rehabilitation work to be hopeful, to expect patients to make progress, and to 'set the bar high' about the degree of recovery expected.

Assessment on the rehabilitation ward

At the point of admission, a full physical examination is completed by a ward doctor; contact is made with the patient's general practitioner (GP) and a standardized assessment is incorporated into the electronic patient record. This includes a focus on cardiovascular risk factors, lifestyle choices and interventions, particularly diet and weight management, and monitoring of physical health screening interventions, for example, for breast, cervical, and bowel cancers. Risks should be reviewed, along with ward leave arrangements and the level of observations. This is because the person will be in a new and unfamiliar environment, sharing it with a different and unknown group of individuals, possibly in a new geographic location.

A nursing and occupational therapy assessment should be carried out, the Model of Human Occupation Screening Tool (MOHOST) (9) would be commonly used by the occupational therapist and we commonly use a 'Recovery Star' (7) assessment to help initial care planning by nursing staff. The 'Recovery Star' was initially developed as a tool for working with homeless individuals with complex problems, and it provides a framework for a holistic assessment of need. It is very useful as the basis for developing a detailed care plan with the individual patient. It has now been more widely adopted within adult mental health in England, both within inpatient and community settings.

Psychological screening and interventions will vary depending on diagnosis and need, but there is an expectation that ward-based interventions are at least psychologically informed, even if not delivered directly by a psychologist.

Review of mental state should be ongoing and optimization of medication can be done with pharmacist advice.

From the point of admission to the rehabilitation ward, future discharge is planned. Previous difficulties in the community need to be understood in detail, for example, ongoing symptoms, inadequate or inappropriate support, or whether drug and alcohol problems have impacted the individual's ability to manage a tenancy. Our ward-based social worker liaises with housing providers to assist in this process. Abstinence from illicit drugs and safe use of alcohol is often crucial to future offers of housing so patients are referred to specialist drug and alcohol services.

An early Care Programme Approach review meeting is held in the first 2–4 weeks with the community care coordinator, patient, and carers to review this initial assessment and agree on goals and the focus of the care plan.

Treatment

Evidence-based treatment is delivered in a therapeutic environment which includes an atmosphere of hope, mutual respect, and personalized care. Measures to support and develop the therapeutic environment are beginning to appear. The Quality Indicator for Rehabilitative Care (QuIRC) (10) is a tool developed across a number of European countries, identifying components of care which support recovery in a variety of institutionalized settings, and our previous rehabilitation ward was used to trial it.

Many patients have treatment resistant disorders, and the evidence base for their effective management is limited. In these instances, we seek a second opinion from colleagues, 'Second Opinion Approved Doctors' where a second opinion on a patient's treatment plan is legally mandated, and occasionally outside specialist assessment (e.g. the National Psychosis Unit at South London and Maudsley Trust).

Recent evidence confirms a significantly lower life expectancy for people with severe and enduring mental illness and setting up good-quality liaison with secondary medical care and primary care is essential. The audit of physical health assessment and interventions is embedded into practice onto psychiatric wards. This also includes the training of medical and nursing staff. A well-being clinic has been established on the ward which on subsequent review has increased engagement in positive lifestyle changes. The impact of some of our most effective antipsychotics on weight gain and metabolic syndrome can be substantial, and early use of treatment with metformin to help manage weight gain, in the absence of diabetes mellitus, may be needed in addition to lifestyle changes.

Psychological and occupational therapy can be delivered in groups and individually. With difficult-to-engage patients, one-to-one treatments may be necessary for significant periods of time. Cognitive behavioural therapy-based treatments have the best evidence base and target symptoms may be very specific, but need to be chosen to have the greatest impact on function or risk reduction. Examples are the treatment of chronic command hallucinations, self-harm, and help with debilitating anxiety related to paranoia.

Discharge planning

A discharge plan should be developed on admission, and refined over time. It should meet the goals set by the patient with the multi-disciplinary team. These could include the maintenance of good mental and physical health, maximizing independence, occupation, and meaningful activity, family contact, and the development and maintenance of relationships. Eventually it should include a specific destination for living in the community and the support needed to maintain recovery.

However, we know from years of experience that in reality, plans are often not delivered in a timely fashion and the choices that we are able to offer our patients can be limited. In these circumstances, we have to maintain hope and optimism, and extend our role to being strong advocates for patients and their families.

Appropriate and safe housing is the first requirement for discharge: if a patient is going to their own home or pre-existing tenancy then delays to discharge are few. However, the majority of patients from our rehabilitation setting need specialist supported living. Care coordinators often need help to negotiate the complex discharge processes involved in dealing with Local Authority and social services funding. Each geographical area will be different: the most important factor is to acknowledge the problem, and start planning early and with expert help from an experienced social worker.

Supported living will provide care in a variety of settings. In England, the Local Authority/Council holds responsibility for assessing need. Housing associations provide supported tenancies in a variety of settings and shared supported living. There is a significant growth in the provision of care from a variety of private providers and a consequent need to continually work with social care colleagues to monitor standards.

Rehabilitation teams may also be a position to work with providers to develop services. In the last 2 years, our staff team has worked with a housing provider in Oxfordshire to develop two bespoke housing services. One of these is for young men with autism and comorbid mental illness, and another is for young women with psychosis who are particularly vulnerable in the community. Four of our patients have been discharged to these units so far with no re-admissions but at present it is too soon to be clear about longer-term outcomes.

Health care after discharge

Care coordinators remain involved throughout the patient's admission but full clinical responsibility is returned to the community team and its consultant psychiatrist on discharge, with the community consultant taking on any required Mental Health Act role. The Mental Health Act can provide structure and safety around discharge and it is common to use continued compulsion in the community by the use of trial Section 17 leave and community treatment orders if a longer period of compulsion in the community is necessary.

Primary health care responsibility will return to the patient's GP or the patient may need to be registered with a new GP if living at a new address. If the patient's needs are particularly complex, we would ensure that a direct handover, usually by phone, is made at the point of discharge.

Special consideration has to be given to assisting our patients to engage with primary health care. Once discharged, care coordinators need to have clear and assertive care plans to ensure ongoing engagement with primary care or with community team well-being clinics. Such clinics exist within our local service and are becoming increasing common and necessary, as we acknowledge the poor state of health of patients with psychosis and other severe and enduring mental disorders, and as the challenges for primary care rapidly increase with our ageing population.

Social care

Even within supported living environments, patients may require high levels of individualized care, sometimes from specialist providers, for example, patients with ASD. In our area, the Kingwood Trust is able to provide support staff with expertise in working with people with ASD. Organizing home-based social care may be the only way in which a patient can return home or to their family. The commissioning of such care packages is becoming increasingly common, particularly as specialist health-based rehabilitation teams are disappearing. This is becoming a major pressure on social care provision and often a reason why discharges are slowed down. The quality of home care also needs to be carefully monitored and care coordinators need training and support to understand their role and responsibilities in this area.

Other health environments

Even with the most diligent care and treatment some patients may not progress to a point where discharge is either safe or desirable. In our current NHS configuration, there is virtually no provision for long-term hospital care in mental health or for very specialist care, for example, neuropsychiatry with challenging behaviour. Instead, such provision has largely fallen to the private sector hospitals and nursing homes. Funding for such care usually sits with Clinical Commissioning Groups or may be devolved to mental health Trusts. Care coordinators, and often rehabilitation inpatient teams, take on the roles of monitoring care at a distance. It has been recognized that this can be deeply unsatisfactory for the patients and their carers (11) and is often a considerable drain on trust financial resources.

Carers

Without the support of family and friends, large numbers of people with mental health problems would find independent or semi-independent living virtually impossible. Providing carers with support, information, education, and individualized care of their own allows them to carry on with roles that most desperately want to continue. Advocacy, carers groups, financial grants, and support for respite are crucial and ideally should provide carers with an easily accessed and coherent network of support. In the context of the Care Programme Approach, all carers have an entitlement to their own assessment and care plan. In our organization, this assessment can be offered either by the patient's care coordinator or perhaps more appropriately by an independent assessor. Various interventions may be offered to the family and carers, but the rehabilitation team should be involved at an early stage and particularly to identify if specialist input such as family therapy is needed. At present, we cannot routinely offer ward-based family therapy but we have been able to access treatment on a case-by-case basis.

The evidence base for inpatient psychiatric rehabilitation

How do we demonstrate that a service provides a good outcome: what is the evidence for this? Large-scale studies looking at models of service for these very disabled patients are thin on the ground but in the last 10 years or so there has been an increase in research looking in this area.

There is evidence that with appropriate psychiatric rehabilitation services patients with even the most enduring complex psychosis can progress to supported community living within 5 years, and of these some will progress to independent living. A large-scale cohort study in Ireland produced outcomes that supported further development of rehabilitation services: those patients who actively received rehabilitation service were eight times more likely than those on the waiting list for the service to achieve and sustain successful community living (12).

In 2013, a paper was published looking at the quality of service and clinical outcomes of rehabilitation units: the Rehabilitation Effectiveness for Activities for Life (REAL) study. It employed the QuIRC instrument. Different domains of care were initially rated by service managers and then assessed by service users' interviews. The authors found that units with a higher proportion of older, male, and detained patients were of poorer quality. However, there were strong indications that the quality of care, effectiveness, and safety were positively associated with service user's autonomy, experiences of care, and perception of their therapeutic environment (13).

Challenges for psychiatric rehabilitation inpatient care

In our experience, practice in general adult inpatient psychiatry in England is dominated by pressure to discharge patients rapidly. This is due to the need to prioritize scarce inpatient resources to those with the highest need for admission. Risk rather than degree of disability therefore becomes the dominant issue. As rehabilitation psychiatrists, we believe this can lead to difficulties as we try to focus both on risk reduction and enhancing and sustaining recovery.

Tom Edwards in 2016 (14) described how we need to recognize the developing and increasingly complex mixed economy in the UK for the community services for people with severe mental illness.

There has been a very substantial reduction in psychiatric beds in the UK since the 1960s, and a range of philosophies and practices have appeared influencing how services should be provided. Rehabilitation services have often lost out as medium- to long-term treatment has not been acknowledged as a need. The focus has been on acute/short-term management of high-risk individuals. The focus on the latter group has led to an increase in forensic psychiatric provision.

Increased numbers of private sector inpatient beds are occupied by patients paid for by NHS services which do not have adequate rehabilitation provision. In some areas, rehabilitation provision has been partially and positively reprovided by specialist community assertive outreach teams but these are now declining in number.

The growth in non-statutory housing provision is potentially positive but can be highly variable in quality and quantity. Designated 'registered' homes are subject to more scrutiny than 'supported independent living', but supported independent living is increasingly commissioned due to a simpler funding stream.

The interface between conventional adult rehabilitation wards and low secure forensic wards can also be a problematic area with some patients not 'fitting' clearly into one or the other and at times we can lose sight of their needs. This has been widely acknowledged and work is being undertaken within the faculties of the Royal College of Psychiatrists to produce joint recommendations on service development and commissioning.

We remain concerned that the needs of this highly disabled patient group are not coherently or strategically addressed (15). People who in the past have been looked after on 'back wards' in the large old hospitals can now be living in various places. Some, unfortunately, live on the street or in a range of supported community living, general adult psychiatric services, and forensic services. We believe, however, that there remains a role for designated specialist inpatient rehabilitation services for those patients who need time to attain their best possible mental health, and to help them develop the necessary skills to maintain health in the community.

On a more positive note, we have seen the development of partnerships between housing providers, health providers, and teams of individuals with specialist skills. There have been recent local developments in our area with two projects which provide accommodation for a small group of men with mental illness and ASD, and vulnerable women with psychosis. We believe that these projects could provide a future model of partnership working and that experienced rehabilitation practitioners are best placed to be involved at all stages from planning through to follow-up care of patients.

In conclusion, there is evidence to support a role for specialized inpatient psychiatric rehabilitation care. This delivers a specialist biopsychosocial approach to assessment and treatment for a small group of individuals who have severe and enduring mental health problems, often with significant comorbidity. Without such services, alternative provision of care is unlikely to meet their needs with negative outcomes including inadequate housing, homelessness, or offending with consequent need for care though the forensic pathway. Rehabilitation services have developed from the continuing care approach of the old style 'back wards' of psychiatric hospitals to dynamic, specialized, recovery-based units with future partnership with specialized community living projects for individuals with highly complex needs.

Acknowledgments

We would like to thank our colleagues in the Multidisciplinary team on our ward for their contributions, and our colleagues at the Royal College of Psychiatrists Rehabilitation Faculty for their expertise, evidence and encouragement.

REFERENCES

1. Leff J, Trieman N, Knapp M, Hallam A. The TAPS Project: a report on 13 years of research, 1985–1998. *BJPsych Bulletin* 2000;24:165–168.

2. Repper J, Perkins R. *Social Inclusion and Recovery*. London: Baillière Tindall; 2003.

3. Davies S, Killaspy H. Rehabilitation in hospital settings. In: Holloway F, Kalidindi S, Killaspy H, Roberts G (eds), *Enabling Recovery: The Principles and Practice of Rehabilitation Psychiatry*, 2nd edition, pp. 268–269. London: RCPsych Publications; 2015.

4. Poole R, Pearsall A, Ryan T. Delayed discharges in an urban in-patient mental health service in England. *Psychiatr Bull* 2014; 38:66–70.

5. Dauncey K, Patterson J. Pathways for people with severe and enduring mental illness and complex needs: a needs assessment. Unpublished local report.

6. Rodell H, Raza K (eds). *AIMS Rehab: Quality Network for rehabilitation Psychiatric Services Annual Report*. London: Royal College of Psychiatrists; 2016. http://www.rcpsych.ac.uk/pdf/Rehab%20Annual%20Report%202016%20final.pdf

7. MacKeith J, Burns S. *Mental Health Recovery Star Organisation Guide*. London: Mental Health Providers Forum; 2008.

8. Wellness Recovery Action Plan. Homepage. http://www.mentalhealthrecovery.com

9. Parkinson S, Forsyth K, Kielhofner G. *Users Guide for the Model of Human Occupation Screening Tool (MOHOST)*. Chicago, IL: University of Illinois at Chicago; 2004.

10. Killaspy H, White S, Wright C, et al. The development of the Quality Indicator for Rehabilitative Care (QuIRC): a measure of best practice for facilities for people with longer term mental health problems. *BMC Psychiatry* 2011;11:35.

11. Wolfson P, Edwards T, Killaspy H. *A Guide to Good Practice in the Use of Out of Areas Placements*. Royal College of Psychiatrists Rehabilitation and Social Faculty Report FR/RS 06. London: Royal College of Psychiatrists; 2012.

12. Lavelle E, Ijaz A, Killaspy H, et al. Mental health rehabilitation and recovery services in Ireland: a multicentre study of current service provision, characteristics of service users and outcomes for those with and without access to these services. Final report for the Mental Health Commission of Ireland. 2011. https://www.mhcirl.ie/File/Dr_Ena_Lavelle.pdf

13. Killaspy H, Davies S. Expanding the evidence base. In: Holloway F, Kalidindi S, Killaspy H, Roberts G (eds), *Enabling Recovery: The Principles and Practice of Rehabilitation Psychiatry*, pp. 436–48. London: RCPsych Publications; 2015.

14. Edwards T, Macpherson R, Commander M, et al. Services for people with complex psychosis: towards a new understanding. *BJPysch Bulletin* 2016;40:156–161.

15. Holloway F. The forgotten need for rehabilitation in contemporary mental health services. A position statement from the Executive Committee of the Faculty of Rehabilitation and Social Psychiatry, Royal College of Psychiatrists, London. 2005. https://www.rcpsych.ac.uk/pdf/frankholloway_oct05.pdf

20

Clinical pharmacy: safe prescribing and monitoring

Sandeep Bhatti, Rachel Brown, Orla Macdonald, and Dan White

Ensuring safe and evidence-based supply of medicines

In 2013, the Royal Pharmaceutical Society published a new guideline entitled *Medicines Optimisation: Helping Patients Make the Most of Medicines* (1). The aim of the publication was to support and enhance the medicines optimization agenda and improve patient outcomes. To achieve this, it suggested four principles:

1. Aim to understand the patient's experience.
2. Evidence-based choice of medicines.
3. Ensure medicines use is as safe as possible.
4. Make medicines optimization part of routine practice.

In response, NHS England launched the Medicines Optimisation Dashboard (2014) which assists Clinical Commissioning Groups (CCGs) and trusts to monitor and respond to how well their patients' medicines use is supported and how they are demonstrating optimized medicines use. Shortly afterward, the National Institute for Health and Care Excellence (NICE) produced their guideline on medicines optimization (2).

These two publications provide key guiding principles for pharmacy teams in mental health settings and build upon other central publications.

In 2001, the Audit Commission's report *A Spoonful of Sugar: Medicines Management in NHS Hospitals* (3) recommended a number of specific pharmacy initiatives to help improve aspects of the provision of medicines, the monitoring of medicines, and improving the safety of medicines. These initiatives included medicines reconciliation, the use of a patient's own drugs, individualizing supplies, medicines education, medicines review, and enhancing clinical pharmacy.

These findings were further supported in 2007 by the Healthcare Commission in a publication entitled *Talking about Medicines: The Management of Medicines in Trusts Providing Mental Health Services* (4). This report emphasized the need to manage medicines safely, effectively, and efficiently in order to generate quality, value for money, and care which is patient-centred and based upon improving patient outcomes. It made a number of recommendations to mental health

trusts. These pivotal papers have shaped the services that pharmacy departments deliver to psychiatric inpatients. The following sections describe the routine activities, typical make-up, and qualifications of pharmacy teams for psychiatric settings.

Medicines reconciliation

Medicines reconciliation is not a pharmacy-only function and the first stages are often carried out by nurses and doctors; however, invariably it is the staff from the pharmacy department that oversee and complete medicines reconciliation. Indeed, this is encouraged and recommended by NICE (2).

A systematic review of the effectiveness and cost-effectiveness of interventions aimed at preventing medication error (medicines reconciliation) at hospital admission, carried out at the University of Sheffield, School of Health and Related Research, reports that medication errors most frequently occur during interfaces of healthcare and that admission to hospital was a particularly high-risk interface (5). This report cites two other reviews that found that the variation between the medications patients were taking prior to admission and their prescriptions on admission ranged from 30% to 70%.

The National Patient Safety Agency collated the number of medication errors during admission and discharge in the UK from November 2003 to March 2007. They found 7070 medications errors, with two fatalities and 30 that caused severe harm (6).

Medicines reconciliation is defined by the Institute for Healthcare Improvement as the process of obtaining an up-to-date and accurate medication list that has been compared to the most recently available information and has documented any discrepancies, changes, deletions, and additions resulting in a complete list of medications, accurately communicated (2).

The National Prescribing Centre described a two stage process for medicines reconciliation (7):

Basic reconciliation (stage 1): basic medicines reconciliation involves the collection and accurate identification of a patient's current list of medicines. An example of basic medicines reconciliation would include medication history taking in secondary care, where a complete and accurate list of a patient's current medication regimen would be documented within 24 hours of admission.

Full reconciliation (stage 2): full medicines reconciliation builds on stage 1 of the process and involves taking the basic reconciliation information, and comparing it to the list of medicines that was most recently available for that patient (from at least one other source). In addition, it involves identifying any discrepancies between the two lists and then acting on that information accordingly. In other words, interpreting the outcome of the basic reconciliation in light of a patient's ongoing care plan, resolving any discrepancies, and accurately recording the outcome.

Patient's own medication

The ward clinical pharmacy team will often facilitate the use of patient's own medication (POM) schemes, a scheme recommended in the 2001 Audit Commission report (3). POM schemes make use of medications that patients have received while in their previous care setting and which, after assessment and review, may continue to be used within the hospital, thus ensuring continuity and avoiding interruptions. All hospitals need to ensure POM policies are in place and that they safeguard patient safety. The benefits of a POM scheme were systematically reviewed by Lummis et al. and after reviewing 19 trials they concluded that POM schemes had a number of benefits including decreased wastage of medications, improved accuracy of medications at admission and discharge, and improved opportunities for continuity of care (10). However, they also found that the trials included in this review were of generally low quality and highlight the need for robust research to strengthen the above-mentioned claims. A review by the National Mental Health Development Unit (11) concluded that POM schemes for mental health units could improve safety and decrease cost but other practices of medicines optimizations need to also be in place.

Clozapine, lithium, and long-acting antipsychotic injections

A number of medicines used to treat mental health conditions require additional input from pharmacy staff. Examples include clozapine, lithium, and long-acting injectable (or 'depot') antipsychotic drugs.

Clozapine, originally synthesized in the late 1950s as a possible antidepressant treatment, was found to be of benefit in the treatment of schizophrenia in the late 1960s. Although antipsychotic drugs that were in use at the time were known to be associated with rarely causing agranulocytosis, a significant increase in reporting incidence was noted following the introduction of clozapine, which led to it being withdrawn worldwide in 1975 (12). In the 1990s, there was a widespread reintroduction of clozapine with mandatory monitoring of full blood counts and it remains the only antipsychotic that has a superior efficacy in the treatment of resistant schizophrenia. Due to the strict regulations controlling its use, clozapine can only be initiated by psychiatrists, and supplied only to patients who have been registered with the manufacturer's clozapine monitoring service. The majority of clozapine initiations are carried out in an inpatient setting. Its licensing restricts its use to patients with treatment-resistant schizophrenia (failure to respond or to tolerate two other antipsychotics) and to psychotic disorders in Parkinson's disease and only in those who are willing to undergo the necessary routine blood tests. The selection, registration, and

close monitoring of patients, as well as the supply logistics and limits imposed on the quantity of medication that can be issued at any one time, dictates the need for close involvement of pharmacy staff. Pharmacy staff facilitate the registration process, ensure the appropriate blood test frequency is followed, obtain blood test results, and give advice on any action necessary when blood test results are abnormal. Clozapine doses must be titrated slowly and pharmacists advise about the most suitable schedule, tailoring it to individual patients based on any pre-existing physical issues, any interacting medication, and which antipsychotic is being switched from. Adverse effects, particularly during titration, are common and pharmacists can assist in the management of these side effects by discussing options with the prescribing team and the patient as well as through the development of local guidelines.

Lithium is a narrow therapeutic index drug, which, without careful use and close monitoring, can result in patient harm. In 2009, lithium was subject to a National Patient Safety Agency alert that required all NHS healthcare organizations to ensure that patients prescribed the drug would be monitored in accordance with NICE. This includes ensuring that all blood test results would be reliably communicated between laboratories and prescribers; that patients would receive appropriate ongoing verbal and written information; that prescribers and pharmacists would check that blood tests are monitored regularly and that it is safe to prescribe and issue lithium; and that medicines that might adversely interact with lithium therapy would be identified (13). Pharmacists are ideally placed to have these detailed discussions with patients, to provide NPSA booklets, monitoring cards, and any additional supporting information as necessary, and to liaise closely with the prescribing team about the necessary monitoring. Close monitoring must continue after discharge and pharmacists have been involved in strategies such as the setting up of lithium registers (14) and lithium clinics (15).

Long-acting atypical injections and depots have often been seen as a specialist-only treatment or reserved as a last resort. They are in fact just a different method of giving a medicine; one that is of particular benefit to patients who find it hard to remember to take oral medication on a daily basis. Pharmacists are involved in the discussions with patients about various choices with medication, including how it is taken or administered. For many patients, an infrequent injection may be preferred to daily oral doses. A sound knowledge of the pharmacokinetics of these injections helps pharmacists advise prescribers on cross-titration and dosing schedules, including how to manage delayed or missed injections. Despite the oral form of these medicines being readily available in primary care, the depot or long-acting preparations are often restricted to secondary care prescribing. Pharmacists are often involved in the development of local prescribing guidelines for such drugs (see 'Formulary and prescribing guidelines: development and implementation') and they can also help facilitate a change in formulary status through involvement with Area Prescribing Committees.

Not surprisingly, medicines requiring additional specialist input are often subject to shared care arrangements between secondary and primary care. Pharmacists are involved in the development of shared care guidelines for such medicines and they can assist with transferring patients into primary care by liaising with specialists, general practitioners (GPs), community pharmacists, and patients to ensure the smooth transfer of care.

Patient communication, adherence, and medicines optimization

A key role for clinical pharmacists is ensuring medicines optimization and enhancing the likelihood of adherence to medication on discharge. Non-adherence and poor adherence to medication regimens is a common, highly complex problem that contributes to substantial worsening of disease, death, and increased healthcare costs (16, 17). Up to half of all patients do not take their medicines as recommended by the prescriber (18). A report by the York Health Economics Consortium estimated that the gross annual cost of prescription medicines wasted in the National Health Service (NHS) in England was approximately £300 million per annum (17) and the opportunity cost of the health gains foregone due to non-adherence in schizophrenia is in excess of £190 million. For people with schizophrenia, poor adherence leads to a fivefold increase in relapse rates (19). For those with bipolar disorder, suicide rates are increased by up to fivefold in non-adherent individuals (20) and it also leads to increased and prolonged hospitalizations (21). Ward pharmacists can play a key role in addressing non-adherence by providing medicines advice in line with NICE adherence guidelines (18) and through patient communication. In doing so, pharmacists follow the guiding principles of the Royal Pharmaceutical Society's *Medicines Optimisation* publication (1) such as understanding the patient's experience and facilitating choice. During a ward stay, adherence is often managed by nurse-led medication administration. However, establishing adherence barriers prior to admission and planning for them on discharge are key parts to ensuring relapse management. This is often achieved through ad hoc conversations, using patient decision aids such as http://www.choiceandmedication.org and through the use of medicine education groups (22).

Discharge planning and transfer of care

Transfer of care takes place when a patient is discharged from an inpatient mental health service setting to another inpatient service, supported accommodation, or to independent living. This process involves the multidisciplinary team across both inpatient and community mental health services, as well as liaising with the patient's GP and community pharmacy. Good communication with the patient about their medication is key; what it is for, when to take it, what to do if doses are missed, where to get further supplies from, etc. Provision of well-written information about medication can also support any discussions had verbally. Pharmacy staff are particularly involved in ensuring the transfer of care of patients taking specialist medicines, such as clozapine, lithium, or long-acting antipsychotic (depot) injections goes smoothly.

The Department of Health's 2000 report *Pharmacy in the Future – Implementing the NHS Plan. A Programme for Pharmacy in the National Health Service* (23) and the Audit Commission's 2001 report *A Spoonful of Sugar: Medicines Management in NHS*

Hospitals (3) made a number of recommendations for the involvement of pharmacy services on discharge, including the following:

- Medication is ready and available for patients on discharge
- One-stop dispensing or dispensing for discharge where medication is supplied ready labelled for discharge to cover treatment for both inpatient use and discharge.
- Pharmacists write discharge prescriptions to prevent delays in discharge.
- Giving GPs and community pharmacists detailed information about when medication was started, stopped, or changed during an inpatient stay. This also reduces the delay in transfer of medication recommendations and ensures that medication prescribed short term is not continued beyond discharge.[1]

The ward pharmacy team

Pharmacists and pharmacy technicians are registered professionals regulated by the General Pharmaceutical Council. The General Pharmaceutical Council sets standards for all pharmacists and pharmacy technicians that focus on safe and effective outcomes for patients and the public (8).

All pharmacists complete a pharmacy degree and are required to successfully demonstrate competence during 1 year of preregistration training in order to register with the General Pharmaceutical Council. Many hospital pharmacists then undertake postgraduate training courses, for example, clinical pharmacy diplomas to help further their understanding of the principles of medication use in different disease states including mental health. Pharmacists specializing in the field of mental health also undertake more specialized qualifications in psychiatric therapeutics in order to develop their clinical knowledge and skills to become highly specialist practitioners.

A ward pharmacy team is made up of clinical pharmacists and pharmacy technicians, supported by the hospital pharmacy dispensary team and other specialist services and roles within pharmacy. These colleagues work together to provide patient centred healthcare.

Pharmacy technicians have all gained a level 3 National Vocational Qualification/Scottish Vocational Qualification in pharmacy services or equivalent. Some pharmacy technicians gain a further qualification to become medicines management technicians (MMTs). They are responsible for the supply of medication and ensuring the safe and secure handling and storage of medication on the wards. MMTs play a vital role in completing medicines reconciliation when a patient is first admitted into hospital (see 'Medicines reconciliation') and they are responsible for keeping patient medication records up to date and ordering medication for discharge. MMTs spend the majority of their time on allocated inpatient wards, which allows them to be integral members of the ward based team

---

[1] Audit Commission. *A Spoonful of Sugar: Medicines Management in NHS Hospitals*. London; 2001. Contains public sector information licensed under the Open Government Licence v3.0. http://www.nationalarchives.gov.uk/doc/open-government-licence/version/3/.

and to increase one to one patient contact (9). MMTs are trained to offer patient counselling to improve adherence to medication and to provide information and instructions about how to take medication for discharge.

Ward-based clinical pharmacists play a critical role in ensuring that the right medication, at the right dose, gets to the right patient, at the right time. They work as part of the multidisciplinary team to provide evidence-based advice about the use of medication, including dosages, drug administration, pharmacokinetic information, drug interactions, and the management of side effects (adverse drug reactions). This process begins when a patient is first admitted into hospital, and continues throughout their inpatient stay, up to discharge. A key skill of a pharmacist is to perform a clinical check of the medication prescribed. This process can be complex as it needs to take account of the patient's diagnosis, any comorbidities, the indication of the medication, as well as pharmacokinetic knowledge of the drug prescribed. Using the principles of pharmacokinetics and pharmacodynamics, pharmacists are able to determine the clinical significance of potential drug interactions in order to minimize any adverse reactions. Pharmacists review all prescribed medication to ensure that it has been prescribed safely, in accordance with local and national guidelines, and meets all legal requirements.

Pharmacist input to the multidisciplinary team meeting

Pharmacists are well-respected members of the multidisciplinary team and often attend multidisciplinary team meetings, also known as ward rounds. Here, many aspects of a patient's care are discussed and ongoing care decisions are made. Pharmacists bring a unique skill set to a multidisciplinary team, adding value and optimizing patients' care by discussing, evaluating, and implementing pharmacological treatment plans. During the ward round, prescribers and pharmacists often present medicines options to the patient and their families. The pharmacist may then arrange to discuss these options in more detail with the patient at a later date. Throughout a patient's admission, pharmacists provide expert advice on prescribing to medical staff, and discuss issues around administration with nursing staff. In addition, they raise awareness of adverse effects and monitoring requirements. Not only do specialist mental health pharmacists have an in-depth knowledge of mental health medication, they are also required to have a broad knowledge about medicines used to treat various physical health disorders such as hypertension, diabetes, respiratory diseases, infections, and pain management, to name but a few. Guidance is given to psychiatrists who may be less familiar with these particular areas of medicine on what to prescribe and monitor, based upon national guidelines, such as those from NICE, as well as local guidelines, such as antibiotic policies, while at the same time ensuring that local formularies are adhered to. Pharmacists are also involved in ensuring the specific physical health monitoring, which is essential with certain medicines used in mental health, is carried out and guidance is given where necessary about how to act on any abnormal results. This is again done in accordance with national and local guidelines.

Medicines reviews

Medication plays a central role in reducing relapse rates and hospitalization in mental health disorders. For these reasons, it is important that medicines reviews take place regularly. Clinical pharmacists working on inpatient wards are best placed to offer this service, adapting the frequency of review to individual patient's needs.

Following the initiation of a new drug therapy, clinical pharmacists work with the multidisciplinary team to help determine the effectiveness and tolerability of the medication and they will advise on ways to improve tolerability or treat adverse effects if necessary.

At times, a more in-depth medicines review is required, to establish the effectiveness of treatments used in the past with the aim of informing potentially suitable treatment options in the future. This process usually involves speaking to the patient and looking through old medical notes in order to establish a timeline of therapies used, their respective effectiveness, and any tolerability issues. Tailored recommendations can then be made, taking into account current treatment guidelines, consensus statements, and the patient's views about medication.

Patient involvement is a vital part of medicines reviews, allowing the opportunity for discussion about worries or concerns related to treatment. It is also an ideal platform to establish adherence with treatment and to gain insight into a patient's ideas around the use of medication to treat their illness.

Specialist pharmacy services

Medicines information services

A fundamental part of a psychiatric pharmacy service is the provision of advice and information to other professionals about medicines in order to help improve patient care and much of this is carried out at a ward level by clinical pharmacists. However, most hospital pharmacy departments in the UK also have a medicines information (MI) service based within the pharmacy department. These MI services are regulated by a virtual body called the UKMI (http://www.ukmi.nhs.uk) that, among other things, sets standards for answering enquiries about medicines and against which MI services are regularly audited.

MI services are primarily staffed by pharmacists who have specialist skills in the identification and interpretation of information and data. Pharmacists running a specialist psychiatric MI service will also have additional qualifications and experience in this field of medicine. MI services can help with any aspect of medicines use, for example, advising on the safety of medicines in pregnancy or breastfeeding, determining if a medicine is known to cause or is causing an adverse effect, and advising about the significance of drug interactions and how to manage them. A large proportion of enquiries dealt with by a specialist psychiatric MI service are complex, requiring advice about how to treat individual cases where other, often multiple, treatments have failed, or where certain treatments may be less suitable to use for a particular reason such as comorbid illnesses (e.g. cardiac disease, epilepsy, renal failure) or because of adverse effects. This requires highly specialist knowledge, familiarity with current treatment guidelines, and an ability to search for, and interpret, primary literature in order to provide tailored advice for each individual patient. Ward-based clinical pharmacists are ideally placed to provide advice to patients and prescribers about medicines; however, there may be occasions when particularly complex situations require additional expertise. MI services can provide this additional level of support. A large proportion of enquiries to mental health MI services are from consultants, but enquiries are also received from other grades of medical staff and nursing staff. The MI service is not restricted to the inpatient setting—a significant proportion of enquiries come from outpatient teams, as well as from GPs and patients. Research has shown that clinical advice from MI services to healthcare professionals results in high levels of positive impacts on patient care, outcomes, and medicines safety (24, 25).

It is a national standard (endorsed by the Royal Pharmaceutical Society) that hospital pharmacy services provide a medicines helpline for patients and their carers to contact after discharge in case of any queries or concerns about their medicines (26). Traditionally (but not exclusively), patient helplines are delivered from within the MI service.

The role of the research pharmacist

Clinical trials

The legislation on managing medicines used in research has developed significantly since 2001. That year saw the publication of the European Union (EU) directive on clinical trials (27) which was written into UK law with the Medicines for Human Use Clinical Trials Regulations in 2004 (amended 2006) (28). An updated EU directive on clinical trials published in 2014 (29) is expected to bring further changes to our regulations.

From the outset, the EU legislation introduced a requirement that all staff who are directly involved in clinical trials must be trained in 'Good Clinical Practice' (GCP)—a standard of practice that ensures that high-quality, ethical research is being carried out. As such, a clear role for nominated clinical trials pharmacists and pharmacy technicians was born. Their remit, in the broadest sense, is to manage the medicines used in clinical trials. They are trained in GCP and they understand the various laws and guidance that dictate how clinical trials medicines, or Investigational Medicines Products as they are known, should be handled.

Research active psychiatric hospitals will often be involved in a wide range of medicines studies. There are the large pharmaceutical company-sponsored studies researching new treatments for dementia, schizophrenia, or depression, or treatments for managing side effects of psychiatric medicines, such as weight gain. Quite often, these new molecules target new receptor sites, thus expanding our knowledge of the aetiology of these illnesses. There are also the non-commercial studies which evaluate marketed medicines, for example, comparing the effectiveness of oral versus injectable antipsychotics. Throughout all of these studies the medicines being investigated must be strictly handled and accounted for according to GCP principles.

Practically this means that the pharmacy research team must be involved from the early stages of a clinical trial being introduced into an NHS trust. For an inpatient study, they will assess the feasibility of storing and handling the research medicine on the ward, ensuring that this is in keeping with the legislation and the protocol. They will then write specific procedures and guidance detailing how the medicine is to be used on that site.

As pharmacists become more experienced in managing clinical trials, their expertise is sought by investigators who are developing protocols involving medicines. Research pharmacists can give important practical advice about the feasibility and costs of using a medicine in a study and help investigators address many of the medicines-related challenges they may face.

Pharmacy practice research

While the clinical trial role is clearly related to research, it is notable that the 'clinical trials' pharmacist facilitates the delivery of research projects that are carried out by others. Yet the role of the research pharmacist can be viewed from an entirely different perspective—that is, that of a professional who embarks upon their own research. There are many pharmacists working in a variety of clinical roles who undertake research directly in their field of practice. The Royal Pharmaceutical Society is very supportive of this role and they provide expert guidance on their website about how to get involved in practice research. Indeed, the Society goes further in identifying that as healthcare professionals we have a 'duty to participate actively in the improvement of systems of care. Leading and supporting the delivery of high quality research and evaluation projects demonstrates a clear commitment to improving the quality of patient care and fulfilling this duty' (30). Within Oxford Health NHS Foundation Trust, practice-based research has been carried out by numerous pharmacists; most recently, inpatient research evaluating innovative methods of medicines communication has been conducted and published (20).

Clinical audit and POMH-UK

A key tool in ensuring high-quality care and continuous improvement is clinical audit. The national Prescribing Observatory for Mental Health (POMH-UK) provides specialist advice to mental health trusts through the provision of specific clinical audit cycles (31). The POMH-UK chooses key priorities and topics related to prescribing in mental health settings. From these it develops 'Quality Improvement Programmes' (QIPs) which consist of a clinical audit cycle, with customized change interventions, to help member organizations measure and improve quality in that area of practice. POMH-UK then analyses and disseminates the data collected.

In this way, mental health trusts and organizations are able to compare their performances to other trusts and previous audits. They can also identify areas of good practice and areas for improvement which can form the basis of improvement strategies. Often the audits are set against nationally agreed standards. The bigger the number of organizations completing the QIP programmes, the richer the data becomes.

The POMH-UK selects the topics for their chosen QIPs following recommendations made by member organizations. The following are the criteria for adopting a topic:

- Relevant to the implementation of particular NICE guideline(s).
- High-cost, high-volume, or high-risk treatment.
- Seen as a clinical priority for trusts nationally by clinicians.
- Seen as a clinical priority for trusts nationally by service users.

- Change in practice that achieves the standards is likely to have a positive impact on clinical care and outcomes.
- Likely variation in practice across trusts.
- Clear standards can be formulated that relate to prescribing practice.
- It would be practical and feasible to collect the relevant audit data.

Audit in practice: a case study

In Oxford Health NHS Foundation Trust, the use of POMH-UK audits has resulted in significant prescribing improvements. The first audit carried out by POMH-UK investigated the use of high-dose antipsychotics. During this 5-year audit cycle, high-dose prescribing of antipsychotics within the inpatient setting for the trust dropped from 26% of prescriptions audited to 11% (a relative decrease of 60%). These improvements were achieved through implementing a number of strategies ultimately resulting in changing prescribing behaviour, these included prescribing changes (introducing new requirements for prescriptions), better documentation (recording clinical rationale, proposed length of high-dose treatment, and expected benefits), and promoting safety by standardizing the documentation and monitoring requirements for high-dose antipsychotic use.

Non-medical prescribers: pharmacist supplementary and independent prescribers

As part of the government's modernization agenda, pharmacists are entitled to become non-medical prescribers (NMPs). In April 2003, changes to legislation came into force allowing pharmacists to become supplementary prescribers (32, 33). Supplementary prescribers are authorized to prescribe certain medication for patients with specific conditions, in partnership with an independent prescriber (a doctor or dentist) with the agreement of the patient. Supplementary prescribers are required to work within an agreed Clinical Management Plan approved by the independent prescriber and patient. Further changes to legislation in May 2006 allowed pharmacists to extend their role and become independent prescribers (34). Pharmacist independent prescribers are able to prescribe any licensed medicine, including some controlled drugs, for any medical condition within their competency and scope of practice. At the beginning of 2015, there were 3845 NMP pharmacists in England (35). An evaluation carried out between 2008 and 2010 found that 71% were currently using their qualification and that the majority of NMP pharmacists were working in primary care (36). This evaluation also found that prescribing by NMPs is safe, clinically appropriate, viewed positively by other healthcare professionals, and had high levels of patient acceptability (36). It has also been shown to have a positive financial impact on the health service (35). There are a growing number of pharmacist NMPs working in mental health settings. On wards, they support other prescribers and review and rewrite drug charts; however, it is in the secondary care outpatient setting that NMP pharmacists have a more substantial role. While specific published examples are limited, there are NMP pharmacists running clinics in many areas of mental health, including dementia services, post-traumatic stress disorder clinics, child and adolescent mental health services, in addition to specific clinics for specialist medicines such as clozapine, lithium, and long-acting injectable antipsychotics (depots).

Formulary and prescribing guidelines: development and implementation

The medicines available to prescribe within a hospital are governed by local trust medicines committees, often called Drugs and Therapeutics Committees (DTCs) or Medicines Advisory Committees. These committees develop a trust's medicine formulary and prescribing guidelines and the formulary will complement local arrangements with CCGs. These committees are responsible for ensuring the safe, effective, efficient, and cost-effective use of medicines and they will set out the organization's strategy for medicines management. Membership is designed to ensure a spread of representation from all clinical specialties and all localities that are served by an organization, together with key stakeholders. Committees are therefore usually made up of pharmacists, prescribers, heads of nursing, hospital managers, clinical governance leads, medicines safety officers, and representation from local CCGs.

It is one of the roles of the committee to ensure that positive NICE Technology Appraisal recommendations are adopted into the formulary within the required 3-month time frame, to horizon scan for new medicines and indications, to assess new medicines from a clinical effectiveness and financial perspective, and to make recommendations about their place within the local formulary, taking into account national guidelines such as NICE and published consensus statements (e.g. British Association for Psychopharmacology guidelines).

A DTC should provide clear guidance in the form of policies and procedures to all staff on all aspects of medicines selection and use. The aim is to reduce the occurrence of poor medicines selection that could result in negative impacts on patient safety. Providing evaluations of new medicines and devising prescribing guidelines require significant expertise and a thorough transparent approach. Some hospitals employ a formulary pharmacist specifically for this role, while others use the expertise of a medicines information pharmacist.

Examples of guidance produced by or reviewed by DTCs includes the publication of a formulary list, policies for non-formulary and unlicensed medicines use and for therapeutic substitution, and prescribing guidelines for specific clinical areas (e.g. guidelines for high-dose monitoring, rapid tranquilization, antipsychotic-induced hyperprolactinaemia, and psychotropic monitoring, and local guidelines for treating specific conditions such as generalized anxiety disorder, schizophrenia, bipolar disorder, depression, etc.), and the development of shared care protocols for medicines that require ongoing input from secondary care.

Hospital trusts are required to make their formularies available in the public domain (37). Many trusts make use of software specifically designed for this purpose, which also allows the inclusion of prescribing guidelines and other prescribing support material. Platforms such as these can be used to effectively communicate formulary and prescribing decisions to staff and offer easily accessible information to help improve the safe, effective, and consistent use of medication within an organization, as well as making formulary decisions transparent to patients and the public.

Medication Safety Officer

The Medication Safety Officer (MSO) role was nationally created in March 2014, following an NHS Patient Safety Alert to improve medication error incident reporting and learning (38). A patient safety incident has been defined as 'any unintended or unexpected incident, which could have or did lead to harm for one or more patients receiving NHS care' (38). A medication error specifically relates to an error that has occurred at any point in the medicines use process that results in a patient safety incident (e.g. errors in prescribing, dispensing, administering, and monitoring). MSOs expertly promote and assure the safe use of medications within a hospital trust with the overarching objective of minimizing harm to patients. The MSO will support the development and implementation of medicines management procedures that enhance safety in practice. They are often a first point of contact for Medicines and Healthcare products Regulatory Agency (MHRA) medicines alerts into the trust and will oversee an appropriate response to these alerts. They are also responsible for reviewing and collating the trust's medicines incidents and errors, in order to support and direct appropriate preventative actions, including staff learning, when such issues arise. A variety of professionals, including nurses and pharmacists, have been designated as MSOs. To ensure that medication safety is on everyone's agenda, the MSO is also expected to lead a multidisciplinary medicines safety group.

The education and training of MSOs is facilitated by a National Medication Safety Network. This network also allows contact between MSOs, the MHRA, and NHS England so that any new risks can be disseminated in a timely manner, as well as the sharing of other information such as areas of good practice. Collaborating with MSOs from other trusts is an essential part of the role, as sharing key results and learning objectives can improve learning from incidents at a national as well as a local level.[2]

College of Mental Health Pharmacy

All pharmacists and pharmacy technicians working within the field of mental health are encouraged to become members of the College of Mental Health Pharmacy (CMHP). The CMHP is a charitable organization that aims to ensure that patients with mental health needs receive the best medicines treatment possible. Providing education and research in the practice of mental health pharmacy is a central feature of the work delivered by the college to meet this aim. The CMHP encourages the sharing of good practice through its network of members and it provides learning and development opportunities by running introductory and more specialist psychiatric pharmacy courses as well as holding an annual international conference. Specialist mental health pharmacists can gain full credentialed membership of the college by demonstrating their expertise and knowledge in a wide range of competencies, which are assessed through the presentation of a portfolio of activity and by performance at a viva voce. The CMHP works in partnership with other key bodies such as the Royal Pharmaceutical Society to ensure pharmacy is high on the health agenda. Additionally, the college and its credentialed members provide expert input to national guidelines and health policy for medicines in mental health. Research in medicines in mental health is facilitated by the college through small research bursaries, mentorship of researchers, and active dissemination of new research findings.

[2] With thanks to Maleeha Bari, Medicines Management Lead Pharmacist, and Medication Safety Officer, Oxford Health NHS Foundation Trust, for her contribution to this section.

Summary

This chapter has explored the roles of the clinical pharmacists and medicines management technicians within the inpatient psychiatric setting. In the modern inpatient setting, the clinical pharmacy team consists of highly trained specialists whose skills can, and should, be applied to a diverse number of tasks in order to enhance the optimum use of medicines. The topics described in this chapter, while covering only a small part of the whole pharmacy department, illustrate the variety and utility of the clinical pharmacy service and the involving roles that they carry out. The clinical pharmacy team is integral to improving quality of care, preventing harm, and ensuring value for money all within a patient-centred philosophy, wherever medicines are being used.

REFERENCES

1. Picton C, Wright H. *Medicines Optimisation: Helping Patients to Make the Most of Medicines.* London: Royal Pharmaceutical Society; 2013.
2. National Institute for Health and Care Excellence. Medicines optimisation: the safe and effective use of medicines to enable the best possible outcomes. NICE guideline [NG5]. 2015. https://www.nice.org.uk/guidance/ng5
3. Audit Commission. *A Spoonful of Sugar: Medicines Management in NHS Hospitals.* London: Audit Commission; 2001.
4. Healthcare Commission. *Talking about Medicines: The Management of Medicines in Trusts Providing Mental Health Services.* London: Healthcare Commission; 2007.
5. Campbell F, Karnon J, Czoski-Murray C, Jones R. A systematic review of the effectiveness and cost-effectiveness of interventions aimed at preventing medication error (medicines reconciliation) at hospital admission. 2009. http://www.eprescribingtoolkit.com/wp-content/uploads/2013/11/PatientSafetyMedsSystematicReview.pdf
6. National Patient Safety Agency. NICE/NPSA issues its first patient safety solution guidance to improve medicines reconciliation at hospital admission. 2007. http://www.npsa.nhs.uk/corporate/news/guidance-to-improve-medicines-reconciliation/?locale=en
7. National Prescribing Centre. Medicines reconciliation: a guide to implementation. 2008. https://www.nicpld.org/courses/fp/assets/MM/NPCMedicinesRecGuideImplementation.pdf
8. General Pharmaceutical Council. Standards. 2016. https://www.pharmacyregulation.org/standards
9. Faulkner B, Bateman S, Marven M, Harrison I. Medicines management technicians in mental health. *Hosp Pharm* 2006;13:58–60. http://www.pharmaceutical-journal.com/libres/pdf/hp/200602/hp_200602_technicians.pdf
10. Lummis H, Sketris I, Veldhuyzen van Zanten S. Systematic review of the use of patients' own medications in acute care institutions. *J Clin Pharm Ther* 2006;31:541–563.
11. Riley C, Branford D. Getting the medicines right: medicines management in adult and older adult acute mental health words. National Mental Health Development Unit. 2009. http://www.cmhp.org.uk/wp-content/uploads/2013/02/getting-the-medicines-right-jul-2009.pdf
12. Bleakley S, Taylor D. *Clozapine Handbook.* Stratford Upon Avon: Lloyd-Reinhold Communications LLP; 2013.
13. National Patient Safety Agency. Safer lithium therapy. NPSA/2009/PSA005. 2009. http://www.nrls.npsa.nhs.uk/resources/?EntryId45=65426

14. Kirkham E, Bazire S, Anderson T, Wood J, Grassby P, Desborough JA. Impact of active monitoring on lithium management in Norfolk. *Ther Adv Psychopharmacol* 2013;3:260–265.

15. Jordan S. How a local lithium clinic performs in comparison with national data. *Clin Pharm* 2014;6:47.

16. Simpson SH, Eurich DT, Majumdar SR, et al. A meta-analysis of the association between adherence to drug therapy and mortality. *BMJ* 2006;333:15.

17. Trueman P, Lowson K, Blighe A, et al. *Evaluation of the Scale, Causes and Costs of Waste Medicines: Final Report.* York and London: School of Pharmacy, University of London, York Health Economics Consortium; 2010.

18. National Institute for Health and Care Excellence. Medicines adherence: involving patients in decisions about prescribed medicines and supporting adherence. Clinical guideline [CG76]. 2009. https://www.nice.org.uk/Guidance/CG76

19. Velligan DI, Weiden PJ, Sajatovic M, et al. The expert consensus guideline series: adherence problems in patients with serious and persistent mental illness. *J Clin Psychiatry* 2009;70(Suppl 4):1–46.

20. Gonzalez-Pinto A, Gonzalez C, Enjuto S, et al. Psychoeducation and cognitive-behavioral therapy in bipolar disorder: an update. *Acta Psychiatr Scand* 2004;109:83–90.

21. Scott J, Pope M. Nonadherence with mood stabilizers: prevalence and predictors. *J Clin Psychiatry* 2002;63:384–390.

22. White D, Wright M, Baber B, Barrera A. A pilot study evaluating the effectiveness of a medicines education group in a mental health inpatient setting: a UK perspective. *Ment Health Clin* 2018;7:116–123.

23. Department of Health. *Pharmacy in the Future – Implementing the NHS Plan. A Programme for Pharmacy in the National Health Service.* London: The Department of Health; 2000. http://webarchive.nationalarchives.gov.uk/20130107105354/http:/www.dh.gov.uk/prod_consum_dh/groups/dh_digitalassets/@dh/@en/documents/digitalasset/dh_4068204.pdf

24. Innes AJ, Bramley DM, Wills S. The impact of UK Medicines Information services on patient care, clinical outcomes and medicines safety: an evaluation of healthcare professionals' opinions. *Eur J Hosp Pharm* 2014;21:222–228.

25. Bramley DM1, Innes AJ, Duggan C, Oborne CA. The impact of medicines information enquiry answering on patient care and outcomes. *Int J Pharm Pract* 2013;21:393–404.

26. UK Medicines Information. Medicines helpline for hospital patients: national standard. 2014. http://www.ukmi.nhs.uk/filestore/ukmiacg/MedicinesHelplineStandardsvn3_2.pdf

27. European Parliament. Directive 2001/20/EC of the European Parliament and of the council of 4 April 2001 on the approximation of the laws, regulations and administrative provisions of the Member States relating to the implementation of good clinical practice in the conduct of clinical trials on medicinal products for human use. 2001. https://ec.europa.eu/health/sites/health/files/files/eudralex/vol-1/dir_2001_20/dir_2001_20_en.pdf

28. Legislation.gov.uk. The Medicines for Human Use (Clinical Trials) Regulations no. 1031. 2004. http://www.legislation.gov.uk/uksi/2004/1031/contents/made

29. European Parliament. Regulation (EU) No 536/2014 of the European Parliament and of the Council of 16 April 2014 on clinical trials on medicinal products for human use, and repealing Directive 2001/20/EC. 2014. https://ec.europa.eu/health/sites/health/files/files/eudralex/vol-1/reg_2014_536/reg_2014_536_en.pdf

30. Royal Pharmaceutical Society of Great Britain. An introduction to research and evaluation. 2016. http://www.rpharms.com/science-and-research/research-and-evaluation-hub.asp

31. Royal College of Psychiatrists. Prescribing Observatory for Mental Health-UK (POMH-UK). 2016. http://www.rcpsych.ac.uk/quality/quality,accreditationaudit/prescribingobservatorypomh/templatehomepage.aspx

32. Department of Health. *Supplementary Prescribing by Nurses and Pharmacists within the NHS in England.* London: Department of Health; 2003.

33. Department of Health. *The Prescription Only Medicines (Human Use) Amendment Order 2003.* London: Department of Health; 2013.

34. Department of Health. *The Medicines for Human Use (Prescribing) (Miscellaneous Amendments) Order 2006.* London: Department of Health; 2006.

35. Department of Health. Evaluation of nurse and pharmacist independent prescribing. University of Southampton and Keele University; 2011. https://www.gov.uk/government/publications/evaluation-of-nurse-and-pharmacist-independent-prescribing-in-england-key-findings-and-executive-summary

36. i5 Health. Non-medical prescribing (NMP): an economic evaluation. Health Education North West; 2015. http://i5health.com/NMP/NMPEconomicEvaluation.pdf

37. National Institute for Health and Care Excellence. Developing and updating local formularies. Medicines practice guideline [MPG1]. 2014 (last updated October 2015). https://www.nice.org.uk/guidance/mpg1

38. NHS England. MHRA Patient Safety Alert. Stage three: directive. Improving medication error incident reporting and learning – supporting information. NHS/PSA/D/2014/005. 2014. https://www.england.nhs.uk/wp-content/uploads/2014/03/psa-sup-info-med-error.pdf

SECTION 4

Nursing aspects

21

Daily ward process in inpatient mental health care

Katalin Walsby and Caroline Attard

Introduction

Mental health services have gone through significant change in the last 30 years, more than any other area of the health service in England (1). This has also involved changes in how mental health inpatient wards are organized and deliver care. Trusts have established governance processes covering all areas of clinical practice, including mental health inpatient units. These governance processes and structures ensure that the quality of patient care is not only maintained but also that continuous efforts are made to improve it. It is important to acknowledge that inpatient services have significantly transformed compared to even 10 years ago. As a result, overall standards of service delivery have improved and there is a range of support available for patients and staff. In addition, inpatient services continue to focus on improving the quality of the care they provide. Change and improvement are likely to meet with some level of resistance or apprehension among staff, either due to lack of understanding, resistance to work differently, or concerns that the proposed change will add to an already heavy workload. Hopefully, there are always ways to navigate this sense of uncertainty and win over the sceptics (2).

Clinical governance structures

At national level, the work of inpatient services is guided and monitored by several organizations such as the Care Quality Commissioners, the Department of Health, the Royal College of Psychiatrists' Accreditation for Inpatient Mental Health Services (AIMS), and the National Institute for Health and Care Excellence (NICE). Importantly, reports from inquiries into service failures that led to damage to patient also influence how inpatient services are organized and how care is delivered (3). At regional and county level, the relevant Clinical Commissioning Group provides the local framework for mental health services for a determined period. Crucially, clinical governance structures within the trusts themselves will promote that services not only learn the relevant lessons from mistakes and near misses but also develop an organizational memory (4). The sources of information crucial for maintaining and improving quality include learning from incidents and complaints, getting and reflecting on patients' and carers' feedback, and audits and inspections both internal as well as from external bodies. Compliance with guidelines as well as the team's performance are monitored at the ward level by a structure that includes from the trust's chief executive, to the director of services and inpatient services, to service managers, senior matrons, nurse consultants, clinical lead specialists, clinical governance leads, as well as ward matrons, ward managers, and deputy ward managers. Importantly, the roles of modern matron, ward manager, and consultant nurse are discussed in Chapter 7.

The charge nurse

In terms of shift work, charge nurses have a very important role, providing at the coalface a leadership and supervisory role, ensuring that nursing standards are maintained by providing teaching of clinical practice and procedures as well as role modelling good professional practice, overseeing the ward environment, and assuming high visibility as the leader on the ward (5).

Charge nurses also have an important role in implementing the changes required by the clinical governance structures described previously. To fulfil this role, nurses need to feel supported and empowered, experiences that have been linked to organizational commitment, autonomy, and job satisfaction (2, 5, 6). While change is taking place, it is important to maintain safety and effectiveness of care and nurses are ideally placed to drive the safety and quality agenda within health care (7); in fact, nursing leadership, collaboration, and empowerment have a demonstrable impact on patient safety (8) and a transformational style of leadership also has encouraging effects on retention of staff as well as a decrease in staff burnout (9, 10).

The allocated nurse

When patients are admitted, they are allocated a nurse who will provide an overall point of contact throughout their inpatient stay.

The allocated nurse will work with the patient to establish a therapeutic relationship, providing psychological therapeutic support, supporting problem-solving, promoting self-care and autonomy, providing psychoeducation in relation to the patient's mental health condition, and medication, including medication's side effects. The allocated nurse also will also attend the ward reviews of their patient as well as multiprofessional meetings where their patients are discussed; they will also prepare the nursing report for the Mental Health Review Tribunals or manager meetings when patients have appealed their detention under a particular Section of the Mental Health Act 1983.

While patients ideally should have contact with their allocated nurse throughout their hospital admission, there are obstacles conspiring against achieving this. Factors such as annual leave, sickness, and shift work have an impact on the consistency of the contact. While the allocation of an associate staff member to a patient may help to mitigate this problem, the associate staff member may be unqualified, leading to gaps in the some of the roles of the allocated nurse. Importantly, the associate staff member will still be able to signpost patients to the appropriate professionals, such as the ward pharmacist, social worker, occupational therapist, psychiatrist, or the nurse in charge for further support. In any case, given the pressures resulting from shift work, leave, and sickness, good team communication with high-quality team handovers will be crucial to provide continuity of care as well as to maintain consistent and safe care (11).

Health care assistants

Health care assistants are the team members who spend the greater part of their shift with the patients on the ward, therefore their knowledge of patients is exceptional. They are a main source of information for the qualified nurses when it comes to patients' presentation, changes in their mental state and behaviour, and a whole range of needs. Health care assistants support patients' physical and dietary needs and also support patients to have safe time off the ward. Crucially, they communicate patients' needs to the qualified nurses. Given their different set of skills to that of qualified nurses, team collaborative working is fundamental to maintain a high level of care for patients as well as a safe and structured environment for staff. Without health care assistants, the qualified nurses would have a difficult task in providing good patient care; health care assistants' needs must be considered and the development of their skills will contribute to a higher standard of care.

Ward administrative support

This is an essential role for the functioning of the ward itself. Ward administrative staff carry out and support a significant part of the written and telephone communication of the ward with other teams, the wider trust, and other local agencies. The ward administrator also helps to arrange and coordinate professional meetings, ward reviews, and discharge meetings, liaising with other agencies, both statutory as well as non-statutory. They take minutes during the above-mentioned meetings and make sure the minutes are distributed to the relevant attendees. They also have an important role in relation to ordering ward stock, such as stationery, medical equipment, and related items. While the nurse in charge and the ward manager are responsible for maintaining a safe nursing level and an appropriate ward skill mix, the ward administrator also contributes to this by monitoring these issues and dealing with the administrative aspects of requesting additional staff when appropriate.

Housekeeping

The physical environment of wards is fundamental if it is going to provide a therapeutic service. The environment should not only be friendly but also clean, safe, and free from potentially harmful equipment (12). Failure to maintain a clean environment can lead to infection control issues, including outbreaks of norovirus ('diarrhoea and vomiting') as well as flu.

Daily clinical processes

A range of activities and procedures of the utmost importance will not be discussed in this chapter, as they have been addressed elsewhere, such as nursing observations (Chapter 22), serious incidents (Chapter 25), and working with relatives and friends (Chapter 26). Next, we outline the basic activities that form the backbone of a well-functioning inpatient ward, the quality and consistency of which is likely to determine the quality and safety of the care provided. These activities are handovers, shift planning, admission of new patients, therapeutic one-to-one time, and contact with carers and relatives.

Handover

The day starts with the handover of the patients first thing in the morning. This is a very important process of the day, as without a handover of good quality the ward cannot function safely. The handover should provide an accurate account of patients, their diagnosis, risk, treatment, and therapy requirements for the day. It provides the opportunity to plan suitable activities, focusing on patient recovery and moving towards discharge. More specifically, the handover should be carried out using a standardized document to avoid omissions that may end up leading to mistakes or gaps in care.

The information handed over should include the patients' personal details, their legal status and if applicable their Section's expiry date, current level of nursing observations, diagnosis, reason for admission, presentation on admission, current presentation, as well as historical and current risks. Physical health issues must also be included if relevant. Medication, its side effects, and adherence are also important. Finally, any action required on the shift must be handed over, for example, the need to contact a relative or plans to escort a patient to a clinical appointment; any missing information will impair the quality of the care provided and, at worst, the safety of patients as well as staff.

Since handovers are a crucial part of the communication in the multidisciplinary team, it is important that all relevant team members attend; the expectation is that there is attendance by all nurses on shift, consultant psychiatrist, junior doctors, clinical psychologist, ward managers, occupational therapist, and the students on placements.

Shift planning

After the handover, the nurse in charge will allocate certain patients to specific nurses and nurse assistants, with the aim of making possible that one-to-one therapeutic interactions between patients and nurses take place. As wards are busy and at times overwhelming for staff members, the nurse in charge needs to be mindful of staff members' skills and experience during the process of allocation.

Once the allocation has been completed, the daily tasks also need to be distributed, including medication administration as well as supporting patients to attend hospital appointments or other meetings. Daily activities can only be pre-planned to a certain level due to the unpredictable nature of the mental health inpatient services. While daily routines such as handover, medication, and planned meetings and assessments must go ahead as planned, other activities may require adjusting to meet safety requirements. Thus, a dramatic change in a patient's mental health, or an unplanned admission, or a serious incident may all require an unexpected review of the plan for the shift. Staffing issues also can influence some of the previously planned daily activities.

Nurse admission procedure

The Royal College of Nursing has set standards for admission procedures (13). While these standards focus on patient and carer experience, local trusts have developed their own admission procedures which are focused not only on patient and carer satisfaction, but also on risk, safety, safeguarding issues, care planning, and appropriate information sharing. Thus, an admission may take a minimum of 6 hours, as it includes not only the assessment of the patient, but also the documentation in electronic records of the patient's risk assessment as well as the preparation of a care management plan. Thus, ward teams may feel under pressure when admissions are taking place.

Therapeutic one-to-one time

Therapeutic time with patients is essential to build a therapeutic relationship and contribute to a positive inpatient experience. It also allows patients' mental health to be monitored and to recognize any improvement or deterioration. It is expected that planned therapeutic sessions cover areas such as mental health, physical health, treatment and potential side effects, accommodation or financial issues, carers or family matters, leave arrangements off the ward, and discharge planning. The timing of these meetings can be either pre-planned or conducted in response to an emergency, such as during an episode of self-harming behaviour. Any delay and potential failure of the planned one-to-one therapeutic time should be explained to the patient clearly and a specific timeframe should be given of how and when the meeting will take place.

As an inpatient stay can be long, it is essential that therapeutic relationships are built not just with the patient's allocated nurses, but with the whole team so patients can feel comfortable to approach anyone on the ward, including the ward manager.

Contact with carers

While sometimes there may be barriers, contact with carers and families is crucial. This very important aspect of practice is discussed in Chapter 26. It suffices to say here that it is now a national standard that mental health services do meet expectations of listening to and involving carers.

Documenting in electronic records

There must be electronic progress notes made for each patient during each shift which must be timely, meaningful, and individualized. In other words, to be clinically informative, staff must avoid generic or uninformative statements. Thus, the electronic documentation must indicate, in a succinct way, any changes in the patient's mental health or risk, medication concordance and side effects, level of nursing observations, physical health issues including sleep and dietary intake, as well as leave arrangements, contacts with carers and relatives, and any activities the patient may have participated in during the shift.

Liaising with other teams and agencies

When relevant, ward teams may need to liaise with agencies such as the police, housing services, drug and alcohol services, and safeguarding services. Although on occasions these activities may be time-consuming, it is crucial that they are carried out in a timely and flexible way, as the well-being of patients, their relatives, or others in the community may be put at risk due to lack of timely communication. For example, inpatient staff may have learnt that an elderly dependant of a recently admitted depressed patient is at home at risk of neglect, or the ward staff need to work collaboratively with the police if a patient has absconded from the ward and is at high risk of suicide. The interface between the community mental health team and the inpatient wards is discussed in Chapter 9.

Other issues

Audit of clinical standards

Maintaining quality of care requires that basic clinical processes are competently and timely carried out. With a view to evidence that this has been the case or otherwise, services carry out regular audits on the following areas:

- Infection control: this includes hand hygiene, management of mattresses, and other clinical equipment.
- Health and safety: this includes the review of ligature points to reduce the risk of inpatient suicides.
- Admission documentation including capacity assessment, patients' demographics, ethnicity, religious beliefs, smoking status, risk of falls, sexual orientation, and preferences.
- Physical observations (including blood pressure, temperature, pulse, and oxygen saturation) as well as assessment of risk of venous thromboembolism/deep vein thrombosis, and assessment of cardiometabolic risk.
- An individualized and timely completed care plan.
- Risk assessments and management, including safeguarding issues, prevention and management of violence and aggression.
- Quality of documentation on clinical notes.

- A discharge care plan, indicating goals to achieve and by whom (patient, carers, staff, other agencies), a time frame for these, and identification of potential barriers to discharge.
- Audit of staff supervision.
- Audit of mandatory training.

Staffing levels

The main influence on the daily routine of a ward is whether the ward is fully staffed. If that is the case, staff will be able to plan activities, following ward routines without delay effectively at the expected standard of care. The new National Health Service (NHS) safe staffing framework for mental health wards published in 2015 highlighted the importance of ensuring that the right people with the right skills are recruited into inpatient mental health settings (14). NICE recommends that healthcare providers review their organizational strategy in relation to safe staffing, setting the number of registered nurses and healthcare assistants for wards and assessing whether the nursing staff available on the day meet patients' needs (15).

Nursing shortages are becoming increasingly severe. In fact, safe staffing and retention were among the global workforce issues highlighted at a meeting of international nurse leaders in Finland in 2015 (16). When facing staff shortages, inpatient wards teams find themselves in the position of having to work with nurses supplied by external agencies. These agency nurses must complete the local induction process as per the local NHS trust policy, which must be carried out by a qualified nurse. The induction focuses on the environment of the ward, an introduction to the essentials of clinical care, infection control, health and safety matters, as well as operational and human resources policies. When on a shift, a high proportion of agency staff ward teams are put under specific pressures, not least having to work with colleagues who are not familiar with the ward processes, team members, and more importantly, with patients and their carers.

Individual supervision

A crucial aspect of maintaining quality of care is ensuring that all staff on the inpatient wards have regular supervision. Arranging this can be challenging due to the workload associated with the acuity of wards, the fact that staff work on a shift rotation basis, as well as staff's annual leave and sickness. Staff supervision must be protected as it is the cornerstone of professional support and learning which enables individual staff members to develop their knowledge and competence, assume responsibility for their own practice, and enhance patients' care and safety. Local policies may vary in terms of how often supervision must take place but the key issue is that staff receive the support, training, professional development, supervision, and appraisals that are necessary for them to carry out their role and responsibilities (17). In this regard, studies have shown that nurses who take the time to reflect on their daily experiences provide improved nursing care and have a better understanding of their actions (18).

Influences on staff morale

Morale among staff on inpatient psychiatric wards is an important condition for the maintenance of therapeutic relationships and positive patient experience, and for the successful implementation of initiatives to improve care. Inpatient staff feel sustained in their roles by joint loyalty and trust within unified ward teams (19). Clear roles, supportive ward managers, and well-designed organizational procedures and structures help to maintain morale. A well-functioning senior ward team formed by the ward matron, the ward manager, charge nurses, and the consultant psychiatrist is important in providing clinical leadership. On the other hand, low staffing levels will affect staff morale, as they will feel less safe and less able to spend time with their patients. Also, a high risk of violence as well as a lack of opportunities to be heard in the wider organization are likely to impact on staff morale.

A significant demand that can affect the daily ward work is the issue of bed availability for patients in need of hospital admission. There may be many factors involved in these issues, including the closure of many inpatient beds, young adults with substance misuse leading to hospital admission (20), as well as societal and financial factors (21).

Leadership and transparency

The Francis report on the Mid Staffordshire NHS Foundation Trust failings focused on the importance of openness, transparency, and candour. Consequently, a key challenge facing all inpatient wards is to nurture a culture where all members of staff take incidents and near misses as an opportunity to be open with patients, carers, and other colleagues, and as opportunities to learn and improve.

Ensuring continuously improving quality and safe and compassionate care requires high standards of leadership, the most influential factor in shaping organizational culture (22). Some of the attributes of high-quality leadership include a clear moral background, analytical skills, being a life-long learner, being able to influence and motivate others, creativity, an ability to effectively delegate, and knowing when and how to ask for help (23).

Student placements

Inpatient services accommodate nurse students of a range of experience. It is essential that students not only achieve their learning outcomes but that they also have a positive experience within the ward environment (17). Unsurprisingly, qualified nurses are a key factor in the achievement of such outcomes (19). Each student has a mentor and ideally a co-mentor who will support them, providing continuity and signing them off at the end of their placement (24). All mentors within the NHS would have completed a certified mentorship training delivered by the local university.

Without an appropriate learning environment, students will not have the opportunity to develop and achieve their set learning objectives so planning and structuring learning for students is a key aim of the daily ward work.

Conclusion

We have provided an outline of some of the basic nursing processes that make it possible for a ward to be able to provide care that is safe, effective, compassionate, and patient centred. There is an emphasis on providing patients with structure and predictability, as these features will help patients, carers, and staff to work together towards achieving recovery.

REFERENCES

1. Gilburt H, Peck E. Service transformation: lessons from mental health. King's Fund. 2014. https://www.kingsfund.org.uk/sites/files/kf/field/field_publication_file/service-transformation-lessons-mental-health-4-feb-2014.pdf

2. Wright S. Dealing with resistance. *Nurs Stand* 2010;24:18–24.

3. Francis R. *Report of the Mid Staffordshire NHS Foundation Trust Public Inquiry*. London: The Stationery Office; 2013.

4. Department of Health. *An Organisation with a Memory: Report of an Expert Group on Learning from Adverse Events in the NHS. Chaired by the Chief Medical Officer*. London: The Stationery Office; 2000.

5. Royal College of Nursing. *Breaking Down Barriers, Driving up Standards: The Role of the Ward Sister and Charge Nurse*. London: Royal College of Nursing; 2009.

6. Cicolini G, Comparcini D, Simonetti V. Workplace empowerment and nurses' job satisfaction: a systematic literature review. *J Nurs Manage* 2014;22:855–871.

7. Iles V, Sutherland K. *Managing Change in the NHS: Organizational Change. A Review for Healthcare Managers, Professionals and Researchers*. London: NCCSDO; 2001.

8. Richardson A, Storr J. Patient safety: a literature review on the impact of nursing empowerment, leadership and collaboration. *Int Nurs Rev* 2010;57:12–21.

9. Weberg D. Transformational leadership and staff retention: an evidence review with implications for healthcare systems. *Nurs Adm Q* 2010;34:246–258.

10. Barr J, Dowding L. *Leadership in Healthcare*, 2nd edition. London: Sage; 2012.

11. Kanerva A, Kivinen T, Lammintakanen J. Communication elements supporting patient safety in psychiatric inpatient care. *J Psychiatr Ment Health Nurs* 2015;22:298–305.

12. Jackson C, Hill K. *Mental Health Today: A Handbook*. Brighton: City & Guilds; 2006.

13. Centre for Quality Improvement. *Standards for Acute Inpatient Services Working-Age Adults (AIMS-WA) – 6th Edition*. London: Royal College of Psychiatrists; 2017. http://www.rcpsych.ac.uk/workinpsychiatry/qualityimprovement/ccqiprojects/working-agewards/standards.aspx

14. NHS England. Mental health staffing framework. 2015. https://www.england.nhs.uk/6cs/wp-content/uploads/sites/25/2015/06/mh-staffing-v4.pdf

15. National Institute for Health and Care Excellence. Safe staffing for nursing in adult inpatient wards in acute hospitals. Safe staffing guideline [SG1]. 2014. https://www.nice.org.uk/guidance/sg1

16. NHS England. New NHS safe staffing framework for mental health wards published. 2015. https://www.england.nhs.uk/2015/06/mh-safe-staffing/

17. Nursing and Midwifery Council. Standards to support learning and assessment in practice NMC standards for mentors, practice teachers and teachers. 2008. https://www.nmc.org.uk/globalassets/sitedocuments/standards/nmc-standards-to-support-learning-assessment.pdf

18. Quinn F, Hughes S. *Quinn's Principles and Practice of Nurse Education*, 6th edition. London: Cengage Learning; 2013.

19. Totman T, Hundt GL, Wearn E, Paul M, Johnson S. Factors affecting staff morale on inpatient mental health wards in England: a qualitative investigation, *BMC Psychiatry* 2011;11:68.

20. Bacon L, Bourne R, Oakley C, Humphreys M. Immigration policy: implications for mental health services. *Adv Psychiatric Treat* 2010;16:124–132.

21. Gunnell D, Donovan J, Barnes M, et al. The 2008 global financial crisis: effects on mental health and suicide. Bristol Policy; 2015. http://www.bris.ac.uk/media-library/sites/policybristol/documents/PolicyReport-3-Suicide-recession.pdf

22. West M, Armit A, Loewenthal L, Eckert R, West T, Lee A. Leadership and leadership development in health care: the evidence base. The King's Fund; 2015. https://www.kingsfund.org.uk/sites/files/kf/field/field_publication_file/leadership-leadership-development-health-care-feb-2015.pdf

23. Ledlow G, Coppola N. *Leadership for Health Professionals: Theory, Skills and Applications*. Burlington, MA: Jones and Bartlett Publishers, Inc.; 2014.

24. Elcock K, Sharples K. *A Nurse's Survival Guide to Mentoring*. London: Churchill Livingstone; 2011.

22

Nursing observations of patients on inpatient wards

Rose Warne

Introduction

This chapter refers to nursing observations and discusses the actions of nurses carrying them out; however, it is understood that other professionals or disciplines may carry out these observations at times. Nursing observations on inpatient acute admission wards are central activities carried out by staff on a daily basis and provide challenges and opportunities for the whole multidisciplinary team but especially for the staff who perform them.

The Royal College of Psychiatrists (available from (1)) describes four levels of observations and although levels and descriptions of observations vary nationally and internationally, they seem to follow a similar range from close to intermittent to general as follows:

- Low-level intermittent observation: the baseline level of observation in a specified psychiatric setting. The frequency of observation is once every 30–60 minutes.
- High-level intermittent observation: usually used if a service user is at risk of becoming violent or aggressive but does not represent an immediate risk. The frequency of observation is once every 15–30 minutes.
- Continuous observation: usually used when a service user presents an immediate threat and needs to be kept within eyesight or at arm's length of a designated one-to-one nurse, with immediate access to other members of staff if needed.
- Multiprofessional continuous observation: usually used when a service user is at the highest risk of harming themselves or others and needs to be kept within eyesight of 2 or 3 staff members and at arm's length of at least 1 staff member.[1]

The practice of observations may raise a conflict in the staff undertaking them, between needing to watch the person and keep them safe while allowing them some space, privacy, and dignity. The activity of observation has the potential to increase frustration in the patient and so increase risk and provides a challenge to the nurse of how to make them a therapeutic experience. Some studies question the effectiveness of observations in the light of the number of suicides that have occurred while patients were under observations (2, 3). The National Confidential Inquiry into Suicide and Homicide (4) reported that 9% of all suicides in mental health patients happen on inpatient wards and of these 22% are while the person is under observations, 3% being constant observations. This highlights the challenge of how best to keep patients safe on in-patient wards and raises the question of how this is possible.

Challenges of providing nursing observations

The demands on nursing staff working on inpatient wards are significant and multifaceted, so factors such as staff shortages, demands of the ward, distractions from other patients and incidents, as well as interruptions with telephone calls, visitors to the ward, and requests for information from other staff/professions can all have an impact on the efficacy and safety of the observations being undertaken. In addition, there are factors in relation to the nurse's level of knowledge, skill, and experience, for example, whether they understand the local policy in relation to observations and the therapeutic relationship they have with the patient. Often the least qualified member of staff or agency nurse will be allocated to carry out observations. This, coupled with the potential for the staff member to be carrying out observations multiple times in a shift has the potential to result in them being less vigilant and making assumptions about the safety of the patient.

Nursing observations are, as the name suggests, a nursing intervention and this can cause conflict within a team as often the decision for a patient to be placed on observation or come off observation will fall to the medical staff. Aidroos (5) identified that nursing staff often made their own judgement and decision about what level of observation a service user required irrespective of what was thought appropriate by medical staff. Nielson and Brennan (6) suggest that

---

[1] Reproduced from Royal College of Psychiatrists, 'Violence and Aggression: Short-term management in mental health, health and community settings' (2015).

the application or removal of observations should be a dynamic and responsive process based on clinical need but that the need for a medical review can at times impede this process. These factors demonstrate the importance of a multidisciplinary team approach in relation to observations. This will ensure that nursing staff are not only involved but have significant responsibility in this decision process and are able to provide a clinical rationale for their actions but also that there are also professionals more removed from the staffing pressures involved so that a decision can be based on clinical need rather than be resource driven (Figure 22.1).

It is rarely recognized that carrying out nursing observations, particularly close or one-to-one observations, can be highly stressful for the nurse in question. The nurse can feel very isolated when the patient is chaotic, agitated, intrusive, aggressive, or experiencing psychotic symptoms. It can be difficult to appreciate how it can feel for the nurse and the anxiety it can create as to how to handle these situations. This, coupled with the patient's own discomfort at being observed and having someone with them the whole time or being routinely checked, may well go towards explaining why many nurses are keen not to disturb the patient too much and to let them sleep or avoid engagement with them.

Hagen et al. (7) point out the need for nurses to balance emotional involvement (caring) and professional distance in mental health environments, which is not an easy task. In their study, they found that nurses often attempt to manage their emotions in relation to patients who are suicidal as they more often generate feelings of frustration, anger, and fear. This emotional disharmony can cause the nurse to become exhausted and depersonalized (i.e. displaying a detached attitude towards others). This may also be a factor in explaining why the nurse may not take more advantage of the opportunity to engage with a patient in a one-to-one observation situation. In addition to this, inpatient environments have become more stressful places to work with ever-greater demands and ever-reducing resources, with greater expectations being placed on the nurses providing care. All these demands may limit the amount of emotional labour (8) that nurses feel able to provide.

The practice of observation has been used for many years (2) but its effectiveness is called into question in terms of whether a purely 'surveillance'-type intervention is sufficient to safeguard patients on an inpatient unit. Jones et al. (9) reported that subjects in their study found the experience of being observed as negative since it was perceived as intrusive and often they were not spoken to during the episode of observation. Bowles and Dodds (10) found that moving towards a more 'care' approach such as spending time with the service user during the shift and offering therapeutic interventions resulted in reduced incidents of self-harm, violence and aggression, and absconding as well as staff sickness. Cox et al.

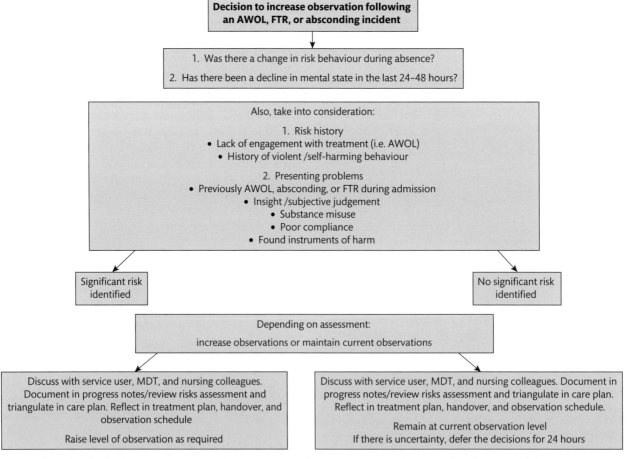

Figure 22.1 Flow chart for the decision to increase or decrease nursing observations. AWOL, absence without leave; FTR, failure to return; MDT, multidisciplinary team.

(11) carried out a literature review of alternatives to enhanced observations and concluded that while there are important insights and ideas to change clinical practice, there is no evidence that enhanced observations can be replaced. They pointed out that that a more therapeutic way of working may help to reduce the requirement for them.

Again, Martin (12) indicated that nursing observation tended to be considered a more custodial activity. A move to a more therapeutic use of time spent carrying out observations has been reflected in many hospital policies both within the UK and internationally. However, further clarity is required for nurses as to what this means and who should carry it out. The current situation on many wards is that junior and agency staff are often allocated to carry out observations, leaving more senior and regular clinicians to run the ward. It would be unrealistic to expect that observations were always carried out by qualified nurses. However, it does require time, training, and commitment to ensure that those carrying them out can do so in a safe, supportive, and patient-centred way. It requires nurses to understand that their attitude, demeanour, and approach communicate a wide range of messages to the service user and how they feel about themselves (2).

Increased observations of a patient are usually considered when there is evidence or a concern about the person's risk to themselves or others, or because the person's behaviour is chaotic, or they are at risk of absconding. However, Nielson and Brennan (6) identified that nurses often felt frustrated that observations were routinely imposed upon a patient rather than when clinically indicated. They went on to suggest that this could be due to medical staff feeling uncomfortable with the responsibility of not placing someone on observations particularly if they were not known to the clinical team. Thus, medical and nursing staff should identify a rationale for the observation level required as well as a review point, considering risk and what the patient feels they need and will be able to tolerate. Involving the patient at this point provides an opportunity to work collaboratively, moving away from a paternalistic approach to one where independence and involvement in care is maintained as much as is possible and practical. Clear communication to the patient and carer about the reasons for the level of observation and how and when it will be reviewed provides the service user with clear parameters of the care they are receiving.

Therapeutic observations

Cutliffe and Stevenson (13) provide a thoughtful template of three phases to support a suicidal patient 'back to humanity', this could be useful in thinking about how to manage other acute mental health problems:

1. Reflecting humanity, demonstrating genuineness, concern, and worth. This can help to start challenging thoughts and feelings of worthlessness. This does not require a high level of skill or expertise but rather an empathic attitude, as well as the ability to demonstrate warmth and concern and a desire to understand what the person is going through at that moment. The training of nursing staff requires that they feel able to ask difficult questions regarding risk and are able to cope with the answer, understanding how to feed/report this back.

2. Guiding the person back to humanity, where the nurse and the person work in a collaborative way, gently helping them to think about alternative views in relation to how they feel or think. This may be a point where the reduction of observations could be discussed with the patient, helping them to consider what this means as well as thinking together about what might help to replace observations. This may require some more training and support and may be utilized more by the allocated nurse rather than by every staff member carrying out observations.

3. Learning to live, where the nurse helps the person to work out what they need to do to reconnect with the world, and their life. This could involve looking towards increased independence and starting to have leave from the ward. The nurse could use this phase to reflect how far the service user has progressed and provide hope for the future. This may also involve helping the person to reconnect with their family and helping them to talk to family members and explain to family/carers what has been going on for them to re-establish their support network.

Cutliffe and Stevenson's (13) three phases offer a way of thinking that can be applied to the practice of nursing observation as an opportunity to maximize therapeutic time with the person.

Psychosocial interventions

The use of psychosocial interventions is widely recognized (14) as a beneficial approach for people with psychosis but is also of benefit to service users with a range of mental health problems. It is extremely adaptable and flexible in its application and does not require a format of formal sessions. Unfortunately, it has been identified that nursing staff trained in psychosocial interventions often underutilize these interventions, possibly due to a lack of time or difficulty in engaging unwell patients in the process. Thus, the observation periods can be seen as underused opportunities for such interventions and practices. It may be unrealistic for each hour of observation in a 12- or 24-hour period to be used in such a way. However, if some of this time could be used to provide such a psychosocial approach it would allow nurses and patients to value this enforced time together.

As with any intervention, the first step needs to be engagement and being on observations with the service user provides an invaluable opportunity to start this process. This process may involve the first phase described by Cutliffe and Stevenson (13) or it may involve finding out about the person, their circumstance, life and interests, etc. In fact, there is no reason why a thorough assessment process cannot take place during the time spent on observation, developing a shared understanding of the problem from the service user's perspective and focusing on what they would like to work on. This gives the individual some sense of control in an otherwise enforced situation. Thus, the message from the nurse to the service user is 'We need to be with you on close observations all the time, but we can use it to think about what areas you would like to work on' be it either managing difficult emotions, how to make a cup of tea or take a bath, or financial concerns. This work may also involve working towards a reduction in observations and what progress the person needs to demonstrate for this to happen. It is important to recognize that some service users will be far too unwell to engage in this process in any depth but the nurse can adapt it to the stage the person is at. However, the degree or type of illness should not prevent the nurse from suggesting using the time in a positive way and asking the person what their immediate concerns are and establishing their understanding of why they are in hospital, even if this conflicts with staff views. The nurse can then take the time to identify what the problem is, creating a problem statement and then thinking about goal setting to achieve some progress. This is also an ideal opportunity to discuss the mental disorder, diagnosis, or problem and offer some psychoeducation around it. The stress vulnerability model (15) is an ideal place to start helping people to understand how they became unwell or in hospital.

Wards can develop written resources to support staff with this work. Importantly, this should not replace the discussion as talking through aspects of a disorder is helpful in developing a shared understanding, building rapport and an atmosphere where challenge and support work together to help develop insight and awareness. The conversation may be more about what the patient does that causes them to come into hospital as opposed to talking about an illness or a diagnosis. For example, the patient may not feel that stopping medication makes them unwell but linking it with their recent admission is a starting point to thinking about its consequences and what they do that leads to others being concerned.

Observations periods are also an opportunity to discuss medication and find out about any side effects the person is experiencing, and then work with them using motivational interviewing techniques to think about what medication does to help and what it does not help. The nurse can then link the work conducted on observations with family work and utilize time on observations to offer education to the family when they visit, helping the person to start reconnecting with their family. The nurse can work with the patient to involve the family members in certain aspects of discussions, for example, helping the patient to think if any information they have gained might help certain family members. Similarly, the nurse can provide psychoeducation to the family to help them to consider whether aspects of what they do may help or hinder recovery.

All this work can then contribute to and inform a relapse prevention or safety plan. This will help both the patient and staff to feel more reassured when reducing the levels of observations, providing early warning signs for all to be aware of as well as a clear process of who will do what if they are identified. This plan can then be adapted at each stage of the patient's stay in hospital and eventual discharge home. This work must also inform the multidisciplinary discussions in relation to the decision about maintaining, reducing, or increasing observations. As previously mentioned, these can be complex and difficult decisions and it can often be left for the medical staff to take the lead. However, if nursing staff utilize observation time more effectively they will be empowered in these discussions and decisions so will have more influence in the multidisciplinary discussion about an intervention that is, mostly, a nursing role.

Documentation and communication

An important but easily overlooked aspect of providing safe and supportive observations is documentation. Triangulation of information between the care plan, risk assessment, and progress notes is essential to the provision of a consistent approach. Thomas (16) reported that observation duties are often assigned to unqualified, inexperienced qualified, or junior staff as well as agency staff. This has not changed for many inpatient units where staffing levels are a constant challenge and the use of agency staff is a daily occurrence. The use of agency, junior, or inexperienced staff to carry out observations may reduce its use as a therapeutic intervention and could lead to reduced consistency and a sense of insecurity for the patient (16). However, it is unlikely that wards are going to be able to always assign their more senior and experienced staff to this intervention. Therefore, the role of documentation along with a clear handover becomes even more crucial, allowing staff to be able to have a good understanding of the risks and rationale for the level of observations as well as the management plan for the person while on observation.

Handover between staff is essential to ensuring observations are effective and safe. The nurse handing over observations at the end of the allotted period should communicate to the nurse starting observations any risk factors and concerns, what the service user has been doing, any requests from the service user in relation to activities or how they wish to spend their time, and any other salient information. The service user should be involved in this handover as much as possible which allows the handover itself to become a therapeutic tool and offers an opportunity to summarize any discussions that have taken place, to demonstrate to the service user active listening and empathy, and to work collaboratively and develop understanding about concerns from staff and reasons for observations.

Finally, service users may often display challenging or chaotic behaviours which can be stressful for the assigned nurse to manage. Indeed, a nurse when on observations may feel very lonely as there may be unspoken expectations that they should manage any behaviour or problems the person is presenting with. Importantly, documentation and handover along with appropriate supervision can support the assigned nurse in providing guidance and a clear plan as to how to manage the person while on observations.

Culture and gender

When observations have been identified as necessary, it can be easy for ward staff to instigate them with little thought for how it may feel for the service user. For example, aspects such as gender and culture may get overlooked. In line with making this intervention therapeutic and working collaboratively with the person, it is important that the observation intervention is introduced to the service user and that explanations and rationales are given. It would be ideal if the nurse could discuss any concerns about the gender of the staff member the service user may have so that this can be addressed as much as possible. It may be impossible to assign just one gender of staff to the person but there may be certain times where this is agreed or a full explanation at this stage may be sufficient.

Cultural sensitivity should always be something that ward staff must consider in relation to the care they provide. Undoubtedly, working with the service user on the impact of observations on them is a helpful start to engagement and building of rapport. A service user's ethnicity and cultural needs should be documented as part of their care plan as a matter of routine (17). If there are specific issues in relation to the implementation of observations, they should be recorded within the care plan.

Supervision

Skills for Care (18) defines supervision as 'an accountable process which supports, assures and develops the knowledge skills and values of an individual group or team'. The Care Quality Commission (19) states that the purpose of supervision is to offer a safe and confidential opportunity for staff to reflect on the work that they do and how they respond both personally and professionally to this work. This would seem to be a crucial aspect of establishing a therapeutic approach to observations. Supervision can both support staff as regards the impact on themselves of carrying out these observations and provide a learning environment where practice and alternatives can be reflected upon. Individual and group/peer supervision can be used to help reduce the sense of isolation staff may feel in carrying out observations, particularly where staff are finding it more difficult; for example, when the service user is self-harming to an intense degree or they are aggressive or hostile. Peer supervision can give staff the opportunity to discuss these issues in a safe place as well as to think about how they can manage the observations differently both as a team and as individuals. Supervision used in this way can help foster the culture of valuing observations as a central part of a therapeutic care plan and encourage staff to further develop their skills in this intervention

Clinical vignette

David is a 20-year-old young man who was admitted to the ward 4 days ago, under Section 2 of the Mental Health Act 1983, due to a first presentation of psychotic symptoms. He lives at home with his elderly father who has been trying to cope with David's increasingly odd behaviour over the past month. David had become very suspicious of his father who reports that David had been smoking more and more cannabis recently and he was not sure how David got the money to obtain it having recently lost his bar job.

Due to David's high risk of absconding from the ward and chaotic behaviour he was placed on close observations. His allocated/primary nurse will explain to David that he is going to be placed on close observations and what this means, giving him the opportunity to understand why this intervention is going to be used, what it will involve, and how it will be reviewed. This needs to be an honest conversation with the nurse addressing the reasons clearly. An example might be: 'David, the team are aware that you don't want to be in

hospital and understand that this makes it very difficult for you. However, we are also very concerned about you and have a responsibility to keep you safe. We are worried that you may try to leave and so we are going to have a member of staff with you at all times who will be within arm's length. We will review this with you and your psychiatrist on a daily basis.' Questions to ask may be:

- Do you have any concerns or worries about this?
- Is there anything that might make this easier for you?
- Is there anything you would find helpful from the nurses when allocated to you?

The answers should be recorded as part of David's care plan with his views documented. Each member of staff allocated to David must read his care plan and be aware of his views.

At the beginning of each period of observation, the member of staff should take a handover from the previous staff member about what the immediate/ongoing risks are, how David has been up to that point, and anything significant he has said or done. If helpful, David can be included in this handover. For example, 'David, this is Helen who is going to be taking over your observations. I am going to explain to her some of the things we have discussed. If I get anything wrong, please let me know. Helen, David has explained to me that he still is very keen to get out of hospital and although is starting to accept he has to be here for now, he thinks he still would try to leave if he saw an opportunity. So he is aware that we need to keep him on close observations at present. He has said that he finds it helpful to spend some time talking in general with whoever is on observations but prefers to talk in more depth with either his psychiatrist or his named nurse. We have spent the past hour talking about some of the problems he has been having in getting a job and then playing pool.'

Over the next few days, David struggles with being on close observations but each member of staff introduces themselves to him at the beginning of the allocated period and asks if there is anything he wants to do or talk about during their time with him. The staff then try to engage with David, getting to know what he usually enjoys and what his interests are. Each day his allocated nurse spends an hour with him talking gradually more and more about the experiences he has been having.

David's allocated nurse spends time getting to know him and there is a very tentative trust between them. The allocated nurse starts to develop a shared understanding of the problem, tries to introduce small pieces of psychoeducation that fit with David's experience, and starts working with the stress vulnerability model. It is explained to David that people can have a vulnerability to becoming unwell, or if he is unable to accept the notion of being unwell then it might be helpful to focus initially on the stress rather than the vulnerability. With David, the stress may be problems in his relationship with his father, the loss of jobs, or having no money. Then the allocated nurse can point out that his cannabis use along with these issues may have resulted in him needing to be admitted to hospital.

A plan can be made with David about what information he would find helpful, with a possible option including information about psychosis, or cannabis use and its effect on mental health. Again, discussions can revolve around whether David recognizes any of this in his own experience. Similarly, information about medication may help to identify side effects and what is helpful and what is not.

The named nurse can then work with David on what he thinks his problems are, what he would like help with, and setting out some goals to try and address these. For example, thinking about how he spends his time at home and reconnecting with his friends and family.

At the point where the reduction of observations is to be considered, David's views are sought and his allocated nurse starts introducing the idea of a relapse prevention and crisis or safety plan. This is initially focused on him being in hospital and so he and the team identify signs that would suggest he is feeling unsafe or at risk of absconding. For example, David identified that if he is refused time off the ward he is more likely to be at a greater risk of absconding. Staff have agreed that if, for whatever reason, time off the ward is refused, a clear explanation will be given and a timeframe for reviewing this will be agreed with David. David agreed that if he is refused time off the ward he will await the explanation before reacting and discuss it with his allocated nurse. This plan is reviewed and applied to each change of his care while on the ward and subsequently adapted to his discharge and use with community team.

David's allocated nurse also spends some time with David's father when he visits. He has been discussing with David what information can be given to his father. David initially refused for any information about him to be shared. Therefore, the allocated nurse spent time listening to David's father about his concerns and difficulties when caring for his son; the nurse puts David's father in touch with carer support groups and offering him an assessment of his own needs. The allocated nurse continues over time to show David how some of the psychoeducation that he has been receiving might also be useful for his father.

Conclusion

Nursing observations pose many challenges and it is well recognized that they cause stress both for the nursing staff carrying them out as well as for the service user experiencing them. Although there is a strong move within healthcare trusts to try to ensure a more therapeutic approach to observations, there is little guidance on how to go about this. The National Institute for Health and Care Excellence (20) recommends as a quality standard that service users in adult mental health see a mental health care professional who is known to them on a one-to-one basis every day for at least an hour. This chapter has attempted to suggest how this might be achieved. It is possible to envisage the positive effect for each patient on close observations of having 1–2 hours a day of this type of therapeutic work woven into their observation periods. It would also undoubtedly impact nurses' levels of job satisfaction, the sharing of skills among staff, and result in a culture shift in relation to nursing observations where they become skilled and valued activities for patients, staff, and other disciplines in the multidisciplinary team.

REFERENCES

1. National Institute for Health and Care Excellence. *Violence: the Short Term Management of Disturbed/Violent Behaviour in In-Patient Psychiatric Settings and Emergency Departments*. London: Department of Health; 2005.
2. Cutcliffe JR, Barker P. Considering the care of the suicidal client and the case for 'engagement and inspiring hope' or 'observations'. *J Psychiatr Ment Health Nurs* 2002;9:611–621.
3. Cutliffe JR, Stevenson C. Feeling our way in the dark: the psychiatric nursing care of a suicidal patient – a literature review. *Int J Nurs Stud* 2008;45:942–953.
4. Healthcare Quality Improvement Partnership. *Confidential Inquiry into Suicide and Homicide by People with Mental Illness*. London: Healthcare Quality Improvement Partnership; 2016.
5. Aidroos N. Nurses' responses to doctors' orders for close observations. *Can J Psychiatry* 1986;31:831–833.
6. Nielson P, Brennan W. The use of special observation: an audit within a psychiatric unit. *J Psychiatr Ment Health Nurs* 2001;8:147–155.
7. Hagen J, Knizek BL, Hjelmeland H. Mental health nurses' experiences of caring for suicidal patients in psychiatric wards: an emotional endeavor. *Arch Psychiatr Nurs* 2017;31:31–37.
8. Hochschild AR. *The Managed Heart. The Managed Heart: Commercialization of Human Feeling*. Los Angeles, CA: University of California Press; 2003. (Original work published 1983.)
9. Jones J, Ward M, Wellman N, Hall J, Lowe T. Psychiatric inpatients' experience of nursing observation. *J Psychosoc Nurs Ment Health Serv* 2000;38:10–20.
10. Bowles N, Dodds P, Hackney D, Sunderland C, Thomas, P. Formal observations and engagement: a discussion paper. *J Psychiatr Ment Health Nurs* 2002;9:255–260.
11. Cox A, Hayter M, Ruane J. Alternative approaches to 'enhanced observations' in acute inpatient mental health care: a review of the literature. *J Psychiatr Ment Health Nurs* 2010;17:162–171.
12. Martin T. Exploring the nature of the nurse patient relationship in an acute high security forensic psychiatry unit. Doctoral thesis, LaTrobe University, Bundoora, Melbourne, 2003, unpublished. Cited in: Hamilton BE, Manias E. Rethinking nurses' observations: psychiatric nursing skills and invisibility in an acute inpatient setting. *Soc Sci Med* 2007;65:331–343.
13. Cutliffe JR, Stevenson C. *Care of the Suicidal Patient*. London: Elsevier; 2007.
14. Gamble C, Brennan G. *Working with Serious Mental Illness: A Manual for Clinical Practice*, 2nd edition. London: Elsevier; 2006.
15. Zubin J, Spring B. Vulnerability – a new view of schizophrenia. *J Abnorm Psychol* 1977;86:103–126.
16. Thomas B. Supervising suicidal patients within a hospital setting. *Br J Nurs* 1995;4:212–215.
17. Department of Health. Delivering race equality in mental health care; an action plan for reform inside and outside services and the government's response to the independent inquiry into the death of David Bennett. 2005. http://webarchive.nationalarchives.gov.uk/20130123204153/http://www.dh.gov.uk/en/Publicationsandstatistics/Publications/PublicationsPolicyAndGuidance/DH_4100773

18. Skills for Care. Providing effective supervision: a workforce development tool, including a unit of competence and supporting guidance. Skills for Care and the Children's Workforce Development Council. 2007. https://www.skillsforcare.org.uk/Document-library/Finding-and-keeping-workers/Supervision/Providing-Effective-Supervision.pdf

19. Care Quality Commission. *Supporting Information and Guidance: Supporting Effective Clinical Supervision*. London: Care Quality Commission; 2013.

20. National Institute for Health and Care Excellence. Service user experience in adult mental health services. Quality standard [QS12]. 2011. https://www.nice.org.uk/guidance/qs14

23

Assessment and management of the risk of suicide

Sue McLaughlin, Gwen Bonner, and Caroline Attard

Introduction

The assessment and management of risk of harm to self, to others, and from others remains a core task for the multidisciplinary team within the inpatient setting as this is a time of increased risk (1). However, it can also be one of the most stressful tasks for clinicians, especially the assessment of suicide risk. Multiple risk factors, warning signs, and protective factors associated with risk will present different challenges for the staff carrying out the assessment which depend upon the therapeutic relationship with the service user, personal and clinical experience of the assessor, team/service risk culture in the ward and team attitudes (2), and the ward atmosphere; resource issues also play a part (3). It can be very difficult to recognize all of the factors that influence our decision-making at any given point in time about risk, particularly in the inpatient ward due to the demands in this pressured environment. Staff often report they don't have enough time and they feel blamed when things do not go as expected; in addition, the documentation process is often seen as a hindrance and it can sometimes fall short of expectations.

We have found that providing staff with a semi-structured process along with opportunities for reflective peer review both on an individual and a team level can provide a valuable aid and learning experience for the clinician, service user, and carer. It can also improve the risk assessment and the effectiveness of the management plan as well as supporting staff to examine interventions and consider alternatives (4). We have seen a positive outcome in relation to the linking of the risk documentation (risk assessment linked to risk management plan and commentary in progress notes reflecting the interventions outlined in the plan) when using this process. This chapter will focus on the important elements of suicide risk assessment and management in the inpatient ward, and anonymous case vignettes will illustrate the skills and structures required for effective risk assessment, management, and documentation. A process for supporting staff (reflective peer review) which is an area that is sometimes missed from the risk assessment and management system will also be illustrated. Barriers to implementation and recommendations for future practice will be included.

Suicide risk assessment and management

There are several policies and guidelines, practice manuals, and research papers setting out the process of suicide risk assessment and management. It is well documented that the key variables of suicidal ideation, previous attempts, and well-formed plans are the best predictors of suicide (5–8) and the approach to gaining an understanding of this should consist of the following:

1. Collecting information related to risk factors (historical, clinical, situational), protective factors, and warning signs/triggers for suicide (Box 23.1).
2. Collecting information related to suicidal ideation, planning, behaviours, desire, and intentions (Box 23.2).
3. Making a clinical formulation of risk based on points 1 and 2.
4. Intervening to mitigate the risk.
5. Gaining collateral information where possible from family and friends.

However, this process is not always straight forward, service users may withhold intent and it is important to have an open discussion about this, but this can only be achieved through a process of authentically engaging in a compassionate and curious conversation. Service users will quickly distinguish genuine warmth, interest, and a desire to help from 'insincere professional warmth' (9). The key to engagement is listening; validation of the person's feelings and persevering with questioning in an empathetic way to build a connection. It is important to communicate verbally and non-verbally the desire to help as well as considering issues of difference and cultural safety (10). This discussion will enable the completion of the risk assessment collaboratively; steps should be taken to corroborate if possible. The assessor must also look for evidence of incongruence, hopelessness, well-formed plans to harm self, and access to lethal means. While access to certain means can be controlled while the person is on the ward, it is only possible to know the means the person is considering if an open discussion and exploration of these thoughts has taken place; it should not be assumed that a previous method will be the same in subsequent attempts. For example, a person may have taken an overdose of prescribed medication prior to admission; once

Box 23.1 Practice points: collecting information about risk factors

Historical factors are risks that have occurred previously (e.g. previous overdose). *Static risk factors* are features of the person's history that predict relapse of the risk or place them in a high-risk group but are not amenable to deliberate intervention.

Clinical factors are illness or presentations that increase risk, for example, depression, personality disorder, etc.

Situational factors are the things going on at the moment that are known to increase risk, for example, housing or financial worries, bereavement, physical illness, relationship breakup, substance misuse, anger, humiliation, court appearance, etc. The level of distress/psychosocial need, the meaning of behaviours, how and when these might be repeated, as well as other factors likely to have a bearing on risk at this point in time.

Triggers are the things known to precipitate the risk (alcohol, arguments, anger, let down, etc.); what increases or decreases the risk and under what circumstances?

Protective factors are the things that help to keep the person safe or are important to them and prevent them from acting (different for each of us).

Practice example

Historical factors: Varinia is a 30-year-old, single, unemployed woman; she has many creative skills but finds it difficult to acknowledge these at the moment. She has had no contact with her family for many years and refuses to discuss this in detail but she has disclosed a history of childhood physical abuse. She lives alone and states she has 'no real friends'. She has had previous contact with services following self-harm (overdoses of analgesia bought over the counter in 2001 and 2010). She required a period in an intensive care unit for 2 weeks following her last overdose in 2010.

Clinical factors: Varinia is currently experiencing biological symptoms of depression including loss of energy, reduced appetite, and severe insomnia, and is managing to sleep for no more than 2–3 hours before waking very early in the morning. She is exhausted on waking due to confusing and disturbing dreams.

Situational factors: ward staff have noticed a deterioration in her self-care and grooming (this is very out of character) and a reluctance to engage in ward activities; when asked about her feelings she described hopelessness, sadness, and stated she is angry with herself for 'wasting her life', she can't be bothered to carry on. She feels tired and overwhelmed and can't see a way forward.

Varinia has thoughts every day of ending her life; she wants to take a lethal overdose but does not have access to means. She has been researching methods on the Internet. She has periods of distress and tearfulness, especially in the morning and late evening—she describes these as her 'worst times'.

Protective factors: her only protective factor was her mother who died recently.

Triggers for suicidal thoughts: feeling a burden on others, loneliness, anger, and shame.

Department of Health (2007) Best Practices in Managing: Principles and Evidence for Best Practice in the Assessment and Management of Risk to Self and Others in Mental Health Services.

www.gov.uk/government/uploads/system/uploads/attachment_data/file/478595/best-practice-managing-risk-cover-webtagged.pdf. Contains public sector information licensed under the Open Government Licence v3.0.

Box 23.2 Practice points: uncovering suicidal ideation

Relationship/rapport first

Henden (9) suggests:

Pay attention to your own non-verbal communication (eye contact, gestures, facial expressions).

Unconditional positive regard (show compassion, genuine concern, and desire to understand).

Accurate empathy (fully understanding how it must feel to be the service user—in their shoes).

Questions (Do not ask in a check list/robotic style but weave into a compassionate conversation)

Have you wished you were dead or wished you could go to sleep and not wake up?

Practice example: sometimes when people are feeling this overwhelmed they wish they were dead or have thoughts of ending their life—has this ever happened to you?

Have you actually had any thoughts of killing yourself?

Practice example: when people feel in this much pain they can have thoughts of killing themselves, have you?

If the answer is *yes* it is important to follow this up:

Have you been thinking about how you might do this now?

When you have these thoughts have you had any intention of acting on them?

Have you started to work out the details of how you would kill yourself?

Do you intend to carry out this plan?

Practice examples (it is crucial that these questions are part of a conversation and not a checklist):

How often do you think about cutting your throat (every day, every hour)? How long do these thoughts last (2–3 minutes, 10 minutes, hours)?

Are you able to control these thoughts (with distraction or other techniques)?

When are you thinking of doing this?

Have you given thought to where you will do this?

Have you gone as far as thinking about what with (have you bought the knife etc.)?

Have you made any arrangements for funeral or tidied up your affairs?

Have you made a will or taken out insurance?

Protective factors

Practice example: are there things—anyone or anything (e.g., family, religion, pain of death)—that stop you from wanting to die or acting on thoughts of suicide?

Reasons for ideation

Was it to end the pain, or stop the way you were feeling (in other words you couldn't go on living with this pain or how you were feeling) or was it to get something else—to get someone to attend to you, revenge or a reaction from others? Or both?

Take extra care when there is a sudden unexpected improvement in symptoms

This may indicate a relief and a sense of peace now a decision has been made to die.

Be alert for any incongruence (discrepancy between what is said and other information/non-verbal communication).

Practice example: I'm really glad to hear you are feeling better about your situation; can you help me to understand what has changed to make you feel this way?

Source data from: Shea, S.C. (2009) Suicide assessment: part 1: uncovering suicidal intent, a sophisticated art. *Psychiatric Times*. 2009; 26 (12):17–19; and Henden, J. (2017) *Prevention Suicide: The Solution Focused Approach* (2nd Ed) Wiley.

admitted, the person no longer has access to medications on the ward but suicidal intent may have changed. The person may now be having thoughts of an alternative means and unless we ask specifically, this may not be divulged and opportunities for intervention will be lost. If the person has suicidal ideation or has attempted suicide, key questions to help understand intent are required (Box 23.2). A sensitive approach is crucial, and rapport must be established promptly—going through a rigid list of closed questions will suffice in getting the paperwork completed but it will not provide an accurate description of the distress and risk the person presents with and is highly likely to hinder a rapport being established. From the authors' reviews of risk assessments, we have found that the seriousness of suicide risk was not recognized in a high number of situations and that within peer reviews, service users' views of their risk differed from that of professionals—this was often due to the lack of exploration of intent or recognition of incongruent statements. This conversation cannot be rushed and it is preferable if it can take place in a private place on the ward (11). When attempting to uncover intent, any objective evidence of depression which is more difficult for the service user to conceal will add to the weighting of risk significantly (poor self-care, low energy, slowed responses).

Following this process, the development of a collaborative risk management plan and service user safety plan aimed at understanding suicidal ideation and behaviour, reducing the distress associated with this, and promoting the safety of the service users and others is required (Box 23.3). This plan must focus on the approach and interventions and be easily accessible and understandable for all staff including agency workers. Service users (even within the inpatient ward) can and should be involved fully in this process. There is increasing consensus that inpatient care needs to move away from custodial approaches to managing safety through observation and restrictions alone to a more interpersonal approach that focuses on connecting with the service user, 'being with' rather than 'doing to' and creating a sense of safety through a genuine caring relationship (12). The pain associated with suicidal ideation is likely to result in a number of side effects which will also need to be addressed in the risk management plan; these will be unique to the individual.

Box 23.3 Risk management and service user safety plan

1 Varinia has developed a safety plan (see later in box).
2 Varinia has identified times where an increase in contact with staff is required (waking and prior to going to bed). Varinia feels a structure is useful but struggles to get this in place without support—a short session with staff is helpful to achieve this every morning.
3 Peter Smith will be Varinia's key worker. He will focus on connecting with Varinia to understand her suicidal thoughts, validating her experiences and thoughts; this work will focus on reconnecting and strengthening her pre-suicidal self, gently encouraging Varinia to consider alternative approaches/explanations to her difficulties and interpretations.
4 All staff: focus on the rapport development and creating a relaxing non-judgemental environment. For Varinia, this entails listening carefully, responding in a timely way, or explaining when this is not possible. Help her with a structure to her day, encourage her to keep to her plan, and provide positive feedback on small accomplishments. The focus in interactions will also be on reassurance that feelings can be overcome and there is hope for the future as well as any practical support required each shift.
5 Varinia is aware of the rationale for level 3 observations—review these with her during each shift (see Chapter 22 on observations).
6 Varinia has completed the 'Recovery Star' (13): Varinia scores lowest on identity and self-esteem; information has been provided on coping with low self-esteem; Varinia will complete the first exercise—strengths and needs—with the help from staff.
7 Varinia acknowledges she has symptoms of depression and has agreed to discuss medication options with Dr Blythe and the ward pharmacist.
8 Varinia will work on the sleep hygiene programme—night staff to evaluate this with her.
9 Varinia and staff will utilize the 'Safewards' (14) interventions (calm down and soft words) at times of distress.

Safety Plan
(This is required even when the person is in an acute phase of crisis and may find such planning difficult as it can provide a useful framework for identifying coping in the next 24–48 hours rather than over a longer period.)

My current problems/risks
I think I would be better off dead, I feel I am worthless, trivial, I have poor sleep, can't see my strengths. I feel so lonely and alone. I feel a burden on the ward. I want these feelings to end.

What I can do to manage (ensure the removal of access to means is covered here) my own risks/problems on a day-to-day basis (or even hour by hour)
  Make a structure at the start of the day (shift) so I have a plan.
  Talking with my friend—Katie.
  Use the calm down box (essential oil pillow, iPod, stress tool).
  Talk to the staff and other service users, join in the ward groups especially the reading group and yoga.
  Use the breathe and relax app.

  Be honest so that staff can remove access to the means for self harming - sharp objects and tablets.

What I want from the care team to help me to get/stay safe and well
Listening not judging, help me on practical issues and with my plan. I also need help with care plan, sleep problems, my concentration is poor so reminders of groups and routines help, reviews of medication and information on other therapies have been helpful.

  When I'm on the ward I feel frightened if there is shouting—help me to move away from noise and arguments.

  I sometimes get involved in other people's problems on the ward—help me to identify when this is happening and to take steps to avoid it.

What warning signs may mean I'm becoming unwell? What triggers my problems/risk or crisis?
Distant in a world of my own, I cry. Go quiet, can't answer or put on a mask that everything is ok.

  I stop taking part in groups, I stay in bed. Isolate myself on the ward.

What have I done in the past that helps me to cope and stay safe and well?
I like photography and I make my own clothes but I haven't done this for 2 years.

What will I do to help calm and soothe myself? What will I tell myself?
Don't buy tablets, you can get through this. Remember my strengths (kind, I know myself, helpful, decent cook, good at sewing and photography). Talk to the staff—they are here to help.

What would I say to a close friend who was feeling this way?
You are going to be ok, I know it's hard I have also been through this.
  Don't agree with the solution but acknowledge the problem: 'That makes sense'; 'I would want that pain to stop'.

What could others do that would help? Who do I want/not want contact with in a crisis?
Smile at me, spend some time with me, listen, remind me I will feel better.
  Explain the ward routine and what groups are happening.
  I can't talk over the phone. I don't like being ignored or nagged. I hate queuing for my medication.
  I get worried about the observation levels—I want to reduce them as soon as possible.

Who can I call on for help (ensure contacts are clearly recorded)?
My allocated nurse on the ward.
Katrina: 97867908592.
Bart: 97867908592.
Samaritans: 090056777.
Papyrus: 08000684141.

A safe place I can go to is:
My room, the therapy room—be around others on the ward.

If I still feel I'm in a crisis or at risk to myself or others I will:
Tell the staff or Katie.

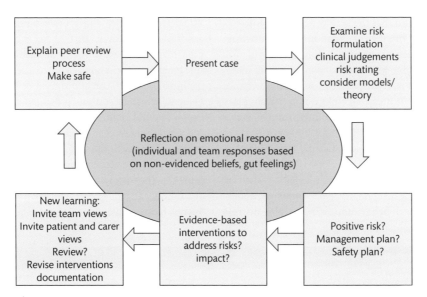

Figure 23.1 Reflective peer review process.
Adapted with permission from McLaughlin S et al. (2014), Improving confidence in suicide risk assessment. *Nursing Times* 110: 27, 16–18.

For suicide risk assessment and management to be effective, mental health inpatient staff need to feel comfortable and confident talking about death and suicide. They need to work from a compassionate stance, 'talk to listen', and feel able to move away from check lists and a surveillance approach to risk management (15, 16). However, working in this way requires training, protected time, support for staff, and a just culture that avoids criticism and blame. A commitment from the organization to create this culture is required. Significant work has been undertaken in relation to creating a positive culture and ensuring there is good morale in the ward environment through the 'Safewards' programme (17–19); this work can be usefully implemented as part of the overall risk management process. In addition, attention must also be paid to all of the factors that combine to influence the decision-making in relation to suicide risk assessment and management planning. This is important as it can have a direct impact on the risk/needs assessment/risk rating and thus the allocation of resources. A range of models and tools are available to assist clinicians in the decision-making process but it is accepted that clinical judgement in the context of a caring, genuine relationship is the overriding factor determining the level of risk the person poses and what actions will assist them during this painful time (20–24).

The individual factors affecting clinical judgement, engagement, and decision-making

All staff on the inpatient ward will vary in their level of skill and ability at any given time in carrying out these tasks. It is important to note that this is influenced by numerous factors as mentioned earlier and it is not simply level of expertise, training, grade, or profession (25). For example, the experience of having a service user in your care die by suicide and how this was subsequently managed can have an impact on risk assessment (26–29), confidence in one's own ability, and difficulties during the assessment (thoughts and feelings, transference, and counter transference). The personal situation of ward staff can also have an influence on their risk assessment. To

begin to address this, we have developed and implemented a reflective peer review process (Figure 23.1).

The peer review process by 'critical friends' is utilized in the teaching and business fields and is seen as a way to 'reinvigorate' staff as well as being beneficial to skill acquisition and competence (30). Benefits have been highlighted in terms of introducing a process of ongoing development through reflection; this can provide a support network and also create a cycle of continuous practice improvement. It is surprising then that within healthcare services we make limited use of the expertise of our peers in other teams or healthcare environments to facilitate this. The process outlined above aims to embrace the expertise of our peers within the multidisciplinary team, facilitate an objective clinical perspective, devise a more practically driven approach to building staff skill, competence, and confidence in relation to suicide risk assessment, risk management/interventions, and documentation. An example from practice is set out in Boxes 23.4 and 23.5. The facilitator must have skills and knowledge of group facilitation and adhere to the model. This should be an independent person from outside of the ward teams; for example, the nurse consultant or clinical specialist role can be utilized here. We have also found it useful to invite a peer review facilitator from outside of the organization and this can be a reciprocal arrangement.

The peer review process provides an opportunity for the team to have their anxieties about a case acknowledged and validated. In the example we have used, it came to light that John had reminded staff of a previous case with a poor outcome. Staff had been avoiding conversations about suicide with John and this was an area where more support was required as it was affecting the risk management. There was also an opportunity for individual staff to explain why there was a difference of opinion in relation to the rating of risk; myths were dispelled about John's openness about suicidal ideation reducing his risk. It came to light that the team were very focused on the physical security of John and less time had been spent discussing ways he can keep himself safe, triggers to his self-harm were not known, and the level of suicidal intent was not known fully. The team recognized that more information was required to inform the risk management plan and onward treatment plan for John; it

Box 23.4 Peer review stages

Throughout each phase, the facilitator is interested in emotional responses and gut feelings.

1 *Explain peer review process—make safe.* The facilitator explains the process, special attention is paid to the fact that this is not about blame or criticism, all feedback is confidential, and all viewpoints are neither wrong nor right but will be analysed in a respectful environment. This is particularly important when there are different views held within different multiprofessional groups. All participants' views will be considered. Explain and encourage thinking outside of 'the norm'.

Focus on support for staff and the creation of a safe environment.

2 Team or worker will briefly *present the case* (see example in Box 23.5) and talk about their own feelings and reactions.

3 *Formulation* to include what is going well, questions, dilemmas, and areas to focus on in the risk assessment—revisit reflections/gut feelings.

Consider models and theories at this stage.

4 Group to review formulation, risk management, and safety plan.

The focus here is on positive risk taking, triangulation with the current situation, ward incidents, and other observable behaviour. Emotional response and gut feelings?

5 Group to ensure that interventions proposed are service user focused and are known to alleviate suicidal desire/distress.

Explore what has been achieved so far during the inpatient stay.
How do staff feel when they engage?
Has rapport been established?
Consider and highlight service user strengths.
Ensure attention has been given to the pre-suicidal state of the service user.
Consider if we have marshalled all resources.
Questions to pose:
- Have we done everything we can?
- What are we doing that *is not* having a positive impact? Why?
- What can we do differently?
- How will we go about this?
- What are we doing that is working well?
- Emotional response and gut feelings?

6 Service user/carer views—in agreement? Conflicting views? Do they feel a rapport/connection with the team?

Hope for the future?
This can be obtained prior, during, or after the meeting depending upon the preference of the service user and carer.

7 Identify new learning, questions to ask:
- What factors are driving the decision-making?
- Can we revise the plan based on feedback?
- What is the learning for self, team, and what training is required?
- What resources do we need?
- What support do we need?
- What do we understand that is different from before?
- Intuition and gut feelings: what are they telling us now?

Box 23.5 Brief case example of reflective peer review: steps 2–7

Developmental history

One close friend at primary school, went to an all-boys secondary school—expelled at 16.

Difficult relationships with friends—aggression.
Bangs head to hurt himself from age 10 to 15.
Preoccupied with self-harm from age of 15, multiple injuries from cutting his arms.

Social environment when growing up

Father: solicitor; mother: accountant.

John cared for by grandfather—described him as cruel and punishing.
Trauma—physical violence at home between parents.
John played computer games from young age to block out violence in the home.

Relationships

Parents:
Doesn't feel loved by them.
Doesn't feel connected to them.
Can feel controlled by them.
Expectations: 'I need to be better than everyone to get noticed, nothing I do will be good enough, I will never get control.'

Ways of coping

Try to get control back with self-harm, dismiss views of others, be persuasive—push for a response or reaction from others; this is often through verbal abuse or hurtful remarks.

This admission was precipitated by John cutting his throat during an argument with his father; he required surgery for this. During admission, he has tied a ligature around his neck with the intention of ending his life. He is currently expressing suicidal ideation by hanging or overdose; he had researched various websites on suicide methods. Staff feel the risk of suicide is high due to previous history, suicidal ideation, and plan; he has expressed feeling angry and hopeless. He has been on level 2 observations for 8 weeks (see Chapter 22 for more information on observations). John is having periods of supervised Section 17 leave from the ward; however, medical staff have been refusing this following incidents of self-harm which has created some conflict with the team.

Things that are going well

- The ward environment seems to be containing John as the frequency of his self-harm thoughts has reduced.
- John understands that he needs to be on the ward now.
- The use of level 2 observations helps to contain John at times of increased distress and keeps him safe when he feels unable to manage.
- John has made use of group activities and was respectful of others.
- John responds to staff listening to him and explaining boundaries.
- Supervised leave for up to 2 hours has not resulted in untoward incidents.
- A rapport has been established with three male members of the team.

Questions/dilemmas/gut feelings

- Why has the severity of John's self-harm increased?
- Could it be that more responsibility has been given to John to manage his own safety? Prior to admission, his father had suggested he finds his own place and on the ward rather than having a blanket observation for the whole shift we have been trying to review on an hourly basis.
- John seems to communicate different messages with different groups of people, could he be concealing intent?
- John seems to be able to identify people's weaknesses; he can be hurtful at times in his communication, especially to his mother and female staff.
- Does John have a need to feel that he is in control? What effect does this have on his behaviour?

was acknowledged we needed a focus on his avoidance but also his strengths and managing his own safety. We acknowledged that staff were fearful of things going wrong and recognized the impact this might be having in terms of a paternalistic approach by some staff. The countertransference example of John regressing when observations were increased was explored and this highlighted a team split in relation to the value of observations, this was discussed and allowed both medical and nursing staff to resolve a difference of opinion that was hidden previously. The peer review process provided an opportunity for staff to put forward a plan focusing on John taking some responsibility for his own safety while on the

- John seems to become childlike around older female staff on the ward. What is happening at these times?
- Where does John's fixation and preoccupation with self-harm come from?
- What is the prognosis?
- Ongoing cycle of negative thoughts and self-harm renders staff powerless at times.
- Staff are very anxious about John's impulsivity.

Reflections offered during the process

- There seems to be something very important about control for John. We wondered if this is a learned behaviour from family relationships.
- It seems as though John's preoccupation/fixation with self-harm will remain because it is longstanding.
- Has John had any positive relationships in the past? It could be useful to find out about these relationships.
- It appears that John doesn't have a clear sense of identity.
- John seems to be limited in the way that he can communicate his needs.
- There was a sense that John is entering what could potentially be a dangerous phase of his life. There was a worry that John seems to lack awareness of the potential consequences of self-harm.
- How does he feel about death/suicide?
- There was a feeling that some staff are underestimating the consequences of Johns threats, beliefs, and behaviours.
- John reminded staff of a previous patient who ended his life after leaving the ward.
- Within the multidisciplinary team, we focus on diagnosis and symptoms—the family are looking for changes in medication to resolve the problems, how realistic is this?

Review of the plan

- The current risk management plan relies heavily on staff keeping John safe, observations, controlling access to means, and escorted time from the ward.
- The current plan does not address the issues of dependency versus safety on the ward.
- All the action focus on what staff will do.
- John's strengths are not tapped into within the plan.
- John agrees that his risk of self-harm is high; he wants staff to 'keep him safe'. He has refused to collaborate on a safety plan—he says it is pointless as he will be on the ward until he dies.

New learning

- We don't yet understand all of the factors and feelings beneath self-harm, and there has been an avoidance of specific discussions about death, suicide, and also strengths.
- We don't know about John's pre-suicidal thinking.
- Interventions to address previous trauma?
- Interventions aimed at developing the relationship—John is pushing everyone away.

Support for staff

- Case formulation with ward psychologist to devise risk management plan.
- Multidisciplinary team discussion around flexible observation system and how we can keep John safe.
- Additional group supervision.
- Risk panel—this facility enables staff to have their care plan endorsed by clinical directors and experts within the trust who hold a monthly risk panel meeting. It aims to provide an additional mechanism to ensure we are doing everything we can.

ward. Staff were able to explore some suggestions for responding to John when he talked about suicide.

Barriers with implementation of peer review

Individual barriers to staff taking part in the peer review process are often related to time constraints or anxiety about presenting the case. Setting up a safe space for multidisciplinary staff by providing clear information about confidentiality and ground rules and giving them permission to attend can help to overcome this.

Staff feeling excluded is also a barrier. The communication about the preference for the peer review to be multidisciplinary and getting buy-in from all disciplines enhances the process considerably as the most successful plans are those that the team all buy into. The sharing of views from a medical, psychological, social, and occupational health as well as nursing and support staff perspective is key to the process.

Organizational barriers also exist and buy-in from senior managers is required so that time can be protected for this important process for risk assessment and management. The process works best when a set time and day is agreed with a consistent facilitator from outside of the ward or another ward area.

While we have seen some positive results from the peer review process in terms of improvement in staff confidence and skills, and also the documentation and linking of risk assessment to management plans, more work is required to find out exactly what elements of the peer review process are most helpful.

When incidents occur

It is crucially important that formal support mechanisms are integrated into team structures so that if an incident does occur, staff feel supported. There is growing acknowledgement that untoward incidents can have a traumatic effect upon patients and staff, hence the need for structured support; this can sometimes vary in quality or be left to chance (26). An opportunity to think about one's own experiences in practice and how untoward events are processed can impact risk assessment and management in the future. The psychological first aid model is an evidence-based method of conducting post-incident support and the principles can be usefully adapted to provide support to staff following incidents (31).

Suggested approach for responding to staff following distressing incidents at work

Following an untoward incident, we may feel upset, even traumatized; however, these acute feelings gradually diminish. This can happen fairly quickly after a couple of hours or may take up to 4 weeks for some people. It is important to:

- respond to distress
- provide information/education

- provide comfort and support
- accelerate recovery
- promote mental health.

Facilitate access to further intervention if necessary but generally the following principles apply:

1. Shortly after a traumatic event those affected should be provided with practical, pragmatic psychological support. They should be provided with information about possible reactions they might have and what they can do to help themselves.
2. Early access to support should be based on an accurate and current assessment of need.
3. Individuals who experience continued symptoms for a month or more after the traumatic event can benefit from psychological intervention (32). It is important to develop protocols within the service as to how this can be accessed. Within the authors' trust, this is provided by the trauma service and staff can be fast tracked into treatment.
4. The approach should take explicit account of people's natural resilience, built on what might be termed psychological triage. People cope with stress in differing ways, and no formal intervention should be mandated for all those exposed to trauma. Use of trauma support should be voluntary, other than in cases where event-related impairment is a threat to an individual's own safety or the safety of others.

A six-stage approach to psychological first aid in group settings has been proposed (33) (see also Box 23.6):

1. Introduction: to the group leaders, explain purpose of the group, identify expected duration of the group, and explain ground rules.
2. Provide a review of the facts of the incident as you understand them.
3. Ask for clarification of facts as presented.
4. Teach: offer psychoeducational information that normalises responses to trauma, point out signs and symptoms that may require further attention, emphasise use of coping mechanisms and stress management.
5. Support the natural cohesion of the group.
6. Assist in connecting with informal support systems such as family and friends, as well as more formal supports if necessary.[1]

Useful lines of enquiry

1. Can you describe what happened?
2. How did you feel?
3. Was there anything you found helpful?
4. Was there anything you found unhelpful?
5. How did you feel afterwards?
6. How did you cope afterwards?
7. How are you coping now?
8. Is there anything else you would like to tell me about?

---

[1] Everly G.S., et al. (2008) A quantitative expression of resiliency in the workplace: an odds ratio analysis. *International Journal of Emergency Mental Health*. 10 (3). pp. 169–75. CC BY 4.0 https://creativecommons.org/licenses/by/4.0/.

> **Box 23.6** Example process of using the principles of a psychological first aid model
>
> - The meeting should take place soon but not immediately after the event, 5–14 days is preferable; immediately after the event, practical support should be offered to staff (opportunity to go home, speak to a colleague, cup of tea/coffee, etc.).
> - The group will be offered to the team or individuals within the team.
> - The group should take place away from the ward environment.
> - The group will be facilitated by two staff trained in providing group psychological support.
> - Purpose of the meeting should be explained.
> - Boundaries must be made explicit at the outset in relation to confidentiality, respect, purpose of the group is to listen, validate provide information, and signposting.
> - Time boundaries: the group will last for 1 hour.
> - Names of participants should be noted if they are agreeable.
> - Participants offered the chance to discuss the event in a non-threatening way.
> - Explanation offered with regard to the normal course of processing traumatic events.
> - Supplementary leaflets offered and any questions discussed.
> - Further support available can be highlighted and opportunities for further contact offered.
> - Closure of the meeting should re-emphasize the natural response that individuals may be experiencing.
> - Post-incident audit form should be completed.
> - A follow-up group may be offered.
> - Individual support must also be offered to those who do not want to attend a group.

9. Conclude by normalizing again, for example: 'You have experienced a stressful event, everyone has different ways of dealing with stress. It's perfectly normal for some people to experience strong emotional and/or physical reactions now or at a later date. These usually subside on their own but if they do not it may be helpful to have another opportunity to talk them over'.

Throughout the process, allow the affected person to maintain their privacy—do not press them. Create opportunities for the person to withdraw if you sense things are becoming too difficult for them. Support the affected person, but do not take responsibility away from them.

If you feel anyone may benefit from advice on ways to overcome stress (not everyone wants or needs this, some people just need you to listen) some suggestions for them are as follows:

- Talk to people you trust about what is affecting you and how you are feeling. If you cannot sleep or do not have anyone to talk to, try writing your thoughts down.
- Try to get back to your normal daily and weekly routines again. Familiar, day-to-day tasks help to keep you grounded. Occupy yourself with things that seem sensible to you.
- Allow yourself time to cry if you want to. It can be better to do this than to try and suppress or hide these feelings.
- Try to keep yourself physically active if you can (walking, sport). However, make sure you also give yourself enough time to relax—listen to music, watch TV, etc., whatever is right for you.
- Take care to eat a balanced diet if possible and to sleep.
- Set yourself small, achievable goals in order to overcome changes.

Post-incident support record form
  Date of request for post-incident support meeting:
  Names of facilitators:
  Date of meeting:
  Brief details of the incident (e.g. date, time, who was involved, events leading up to the incident, what happened during the incident, what happened afterwards):
  Who attended the meeting:
  Observations/notes during the session:
  Duration of the session:
  Outcome (e.g. any follow-up):

- Take things one step at a time rather than trying to do everything at once.
- It is common to have recurring thoughts and memories regarding the event. These will generally become less frequent and less intensive over time. Do not try to fight them.
- If you are still having problems a long time after the stressful event and things are not getting any easier, seek help. A follow-up appointment will be offered to see how you are getting on (Box 23.7).

Carer involvement in the risk assessment and management process

Wherever possible, it is crucial to involve the carer in the risk assessment and management process. An early discussion about consent to share information should take place within the first day of admission. At times in the inpatient setting, the patient may not consent to information sharing (Box 23.8); in these cases, the decision to share information should be reviewed on a regular basis paying attention to what, if any, information can be shared. It is also important to consider capacity and level of risk within this decision-making process and the fact that a breach of confidentiality only occurs when information is newly disclosed to the recipient. Even if consent is withheld, the carer's views can be still be heard and utilized to inform the safety plan (34).

Suicide risk and ward/area transfers

Within the inpatient setting, transfers between wards, teams, or areas can be times of increased risk and distress. It is important to ensure this period is recognized and given sufficient attention within the risk management plan. Factors that increase risk are often related to hopelessness, especially when a more secure placement has been identified. This must be clearly communicated within the team so that extra vigilance and support can be put into place while the transfer is being finalized. Often the service user will have built relationships within the current ward team and the transfer can trigger feelings of loss or burdensomeness; this combined with the stress of having to make new connections or retell difficult experiences can contribute to an escalating risk of harm to self. Interventions must

Box 23.8 Example of information sharing when consent is withheld by the service user

Arun was admitted to the ward following a car accident. This was a suspected suicide attempt as he had written a note to his parents. Arun strongly denies this, he feels ashamed about this admission and he does not want any information shared with any member of his family. His father (Amit) has called the ward (he accompanied Arun on admission and was aware of the car accident and contents of the note outlining what he intended to do) asking how Arun is feeling and what the prognosis is.
  Elisha, the ward doctor, takes the call.
Amit: I'm so worried, can you tell me how Arun is please, he is not answering his mobile or my text messages.
Elisha: Yes, this must be a really difficult time for all of you at the moment. Arun is safe on the ward. I'm sorry you have not been able to reach him on the mobile, can I pass on a message?
Amit: No, I know he doesn't want to speak to me at the moment; he blames us for showing the doctor his note. Can you tell me about his diagnosis and treatment please?
Elisha: This is a difficult position for you to be in, he did mention he does not want his family to have any information about his condition but I can share with you some general information about the ward and what happens when people come here in similar circumstances to Arun, would this be helpful?
Amit: Yes please, any information at all as we have never had anybody try to hurt themselves in my family.
Elisha: It is understandable you are worried. When people get admitted to the ward the team will spend the initial period trying to understand what brought them in. A risk assessment and management plan is drawn up and the team work with the person to decide upon the best treatment: this can be medications, talking treatments, and occupational therapy. We have a team meeting every day with the doctors, nurses, and other staff to monitor the plan.
Everyone has a key worker to help them and staff are available 24 hours a day. We also start working on the plan for discharge. It is not unusual for people to not want their family to know about things but we review this with them on a regular basis as we feel it is an important part of the treatment.

be targeted towards uncovering these feelings and taking steps to minimize the risk. A case example is provided to illustrate potential risks and suggested interventions (Box 23.9).

Conclusion

The system we have proposed for effective inpatient risk assessment and management in this chapter consists of the following:

- Engagement/rapport and compassion are the starting point; service user and carer are central to the process of risk assessment and we must focus on their strengths and resources.
- Develop and communicate safety plans (service user/carer/other agencies), discuss consent to share risk information and safety plans at the earliest opportunity, and review on a regular basis.
- Design information systems in a way that enables staff to record their assessment and management plans and share these with service users and cares in a clear and systematic way and one that is clear for all staff including agency workers to follow.

Box 23.9 Clinical vignette

Tasha is a 24-year-old single woman; she was admitted to the inpatient unit following an attempt to end her life by hanging. She was disturbed unexpectedly by a care worker who made an unannounced visit. Her suicide risk was rated high by the team as she stated she did not regret her actions, she was sorry she had survived the attempt, and continued to feel she would be better off dead. She was placed on level 2 observations.

Tasha was diagnosed with autism spectrum disorder at a late stage when she was 20. Prior to this, she had been diagnosed with 'mixed personality disorder'. Following a number of months on the ward with very little progress and serious self-harm when observations were reduced, it was decided that a specialist placement was required.

Prior to the placement move, Tasha's mood seemed to improve and staff attributed this to an increase in hope due to specialist treatment. Observation levels were reduced and self-harm decreased; this resulted in longer periods of leave. Risk was reviewed and rated low.

A transfer date was eventually set for the coming week. Tasha left the ward informing staff she was going into town to purchase some items for her transfer.

Instead of going shopping, Tasha made her way to the railway track; she had researched the details of the fast trains and planned her route. A member of station staff noticed her in an exposed area of the rail track and he took immediate action to prevent Tasha going onto the line.

Once back on the ward, staff spoke to Tasha to understand what had been happening in the last week. Tasha identified the following:

1 The news of the transfer to the out of area specialist placement was terrifying.
2 She did not know how she would feel when she got there.
3 She was fearful of what the other people (staff and service users) would be like.
4 She had no hope that treatment would help her because of her diagnosis of autism spectrum disorder.
5 She felt alone and isolated and the decision to end her life became stronger than ever before.
6 She felt a huge sense of relief and purpose from making the plans.

Staff interventions

1 The transfer to the new placement was discussed in detail, a visit was arranged to meet the team on the ward with a follow-up visit to the new placement.
2 Ward staff engaged with Tasha to help her to identify her feelings of hopelessness and the automatic thoughts precipitating this.
3 Direct questions were required to uncover the extent of hopelessness and suicidal intent.
4 A safety plan was devised with Tasha to focus on the transfer period.

- Peer review/reflection/supervision/support must be part of the multidisciplinary routine and carry equal weight as the multidisciplinary team meeting or medication round.
- There is already a significant burden felt by clinical professionals in relation to suicide and this can impact suicide risk assessment so it is crucial that systems for investigation do not inadvertently blame or criticize individuals.

Future research might further contribute to our knowledge of suicide risk assessment and management in the inpatient setting by investigating factors or events that are perceived to enhance risk assessment and management, for example, the peer review process and reflective practice.

REFERENCES

1. The National Confidential Inquiry into Suicide and Homicide by People with Mental Illness. Making mental health care safer: annual report and 20-year review. University of Manchester; 2016. http://documents.manchester.ac.uk/display.aspx?DocID=37580
2. Brunero S, Smith J, Bates E, Fairbrother G. Health professionals attitudes' towards suicide prevention initiatives. *J Psychiatr Ment Health Nurs* 2008;15:588–594.
3. Bowers L, Whittington R, Nolan P, et al. The relationship between service ecology, special observation and self-harm during acute inpatient care: the City 128 study. *Br J Psychiatry* 2008;193:395–401.
4. Rahman MS, Gupta S, While D, et al. Quality of risk assessment prior to suicide and homicide: a pilot study. 2013. http://research.bmh.manchester.ac.uk/cmhs/research/centreforsuicideprevention/nci/reports/
5. Joiner TE, Conwell Y, Fitzpatrick KK, et al. Four studies on how past and current suicidality relate even when "everything but the kitchen sink" is covaried. *J Abnorm Psychol* 2005;114:291–303.
6. Jobes DA. The collaborative assessment and management of suicidality (CAMS): an evolving evidence-based clinical approach to suicidal risk. *Suicide Life Threat Behav* 2012;42:640–653.
7. Department of Health. Best practices in managing: principles and evidence for best practice in the assessment and management of risk to self and others in mental health services. 2007. https://assets.publishing.service.gov.uk/government/uploads/system/uploads/attachment_data/file/478595/best-practice-managing-risk-cover-webtagged.pdf
8. Shea SC. Suicide assessment: part 1: uncovering suicidal intent, a sophisticated art. *Psychiatr Times* 2009;26:17–19.
9. Henden J. *Prevention Suicide: The Solution Focused Approach*, 2nd edition. Chichester: Wiley; 2017.
10. Cutcliffe J, Stevenson C. *Care of the Suicidal Person*. London: Churchill Livingstone; 2007.
11. Cutcliffe J, Stevenson C. Never the twain? Reconciling national suicide prevention strategies with the practice, educational, and policy needs of mental health nurses (part one and two). *Int J Ment Health Nurs* 2008;17:341–362.
12. Chen S, Krupa T, Lysaght R, McCay E, Piat M. The development of recovery competencies for in-patient mental health providers working with people with serious mental illness. *Adm Policy Ment Health* 2013;40:96–116.
13. Outcomes Star. Recovery Star: the Outcomes Star for adults managing their mental health. http://www.outcomesstar.org.uk/mental-health/
14. Safewards. Homepage. http://www.safewards.net
15. Cummins A. The road to hell is paved with good intentions: quality assurance as a social defence against anxiety. *Organ Soc Dyn* 2002;2:99e119.
16. Cole-King A, Green G, Gask L, Hines K, Platt S. Suicide mitigation: a compassionate approach to suicide prevention. *Adv Psychiatr Treat* 2013;19:276–283.
17. Bowers L, Allan T, Simpson A, Jones J, Whittington R. Morale is high in acute inpatient psychiatry. *Soc Psychiatry Psychiatr Epidemiol* 2009;44:39–46.
18. Bowers L, Chaplin R, Quirk A, Lelliott P. A conceptual model of the aims and functions of acute inpatient psychiatry. *J Ment Health* 2009;18:316–325.
19. Bowers L. Safewards: a new model of conflict and containment on psychiatric wards. *J Psychiatr Ment Health Nurs* 2014;21:499–508.

20. Hawton K, Bergen H, Cooper J, et al. Suicide following self-harm: findings from the multicentre study of self-harm in England, 2000-2012. *J Affect Disord* 2015;175:147–151.

21. Joiner TE. *Why People Die by Suicide*. Cambridge, MA: Harvard University Press; 2005.

22. Shea SC. Innovations in eliciting suicidal ideation: the Chronological Assessment of Suicide Events (CASE Approach). Presented at the Annual Meetings of the American Association of Suicidology from 1999 through 2009.

23. Delgadillo J, Moreea O, Outhwaite-Luke H, et al. Confidence in the face of risk: the Risk Assessment and Management Self-Efficacy Study (RAMSES). *Psychiatr Bull* 2014;38:58–65.

24. Vatne M, Nåden D. Patients' experiences in the aftermath of suicidal crises. *Nurs Ethics* 2014;21:163–175.

25. Boardman J, Roberts G., Risk, safety and recovery. Centre for Mental Health and Mental Health Network, NHS Confederation; 2014. https://www.centreformentalhealth.org.uk/risk-and-recovery

26. Bohan F, Doyle L. Nurses' experiences of patient suicide and suicide attempts in an acute unit. *Ment Health Pract* 2008:11:12–16.

27. Collins JM. Impact of patient suicide on clinicians. *J Am Psychiatr Nurses Assoc* 2003;9:159–162.

28. Dewar I, Eagles J, Klein S, Gray N, Alexander DA. Psychiatric trainees' experiences of, and reactions to, patient suicide. *Psychiatr Bull* 2000;24:20–23.

29. Fareberow NL. The mental health professional as suicide survivor. *Clin Neuropsychiatry* 2005;2:13–20.

30. Baskerville D, Goldblatt H. Learning to be a critical friend: from professional indifference through challenge to unguarded conversations. *Camb J Educ* 2009;39:205–221.

31. Rose S, Bisson J, Wessley S. A systematic review of single psychological interventions ('debriefing') following trauma – updating the Cochrane review and implications for good practice. In: Orner RJ, Schnyder U (eds), *Reconstructing Early Intervention after Trauma Innovations in the Care of Survivors*, pp. 24–29. Oxford: Oxford University Press; 2003.

32. Bisson J, Ehlers A, Matthews R, Pilling S, Richards D, Turner S. Psychological treatments for chronic post-traumatic stress disorder: systematic review and meta-analysis. *Br J Psychiatry* 2007;190:97–104.

33. Everly GS Jr, Sherman MF, Nucifora F Jr, Langlieb A, Kaminsky MJ, Links JM. A quantitative expression of resiliency in the workplace: an odds ratio analysis. *Int J Emerg Ment Health* 2008;10:169–175.

34. Department of Health. Information: to share to not to share. The information governance review. Department of Health; 2013. https://assets.publishing.service.gov.uk/government/uploads/system/uploads/attachment_data/file/192572/2900774_InfoGovernance_accv2.pdf

24

Implementation of the Safewards model on inpatient wards

Caroline Attard

Introduction

Aggression on inpatient mental health wards is frequent, problematic, and a major challenge for nurses and mental health services more generally. An important protective factor that can limit the likelihood of aggression is the strength of the therapeutic relationship between patients and nursing staff. The continuing need to focus on good communication and teamwork are also integral to ongoing management of aggressive behaviour (1). The Safewards programme was designed and developed by Professor Len Bowers following an extensive 16-year research programme and good evidence from a randomized control trial. Safewards offers the opportunity to reduce the frequency of these risky and harmful events, resulting in keeping patients and staff safer (2).

Background

The Safewards initiative is a multicomponent, evidence-based conflict and containment reduction intervention that has demonstrated effectiveness in general acute mental health settings (3). Bowers defines two important concepts for the model, namely conflict 'as events that threaten staff or patient safety such as verbal abuse, physical aggression to others, self-harm, suicide and absconding'; he also defines containment as 'measures taken to reduce the likelihood of these events occurring, such as: required medication, physical restraint, constant or intermittent observations, seclusion and rapid tranquilisation' (3). Safewards has a strong evidence base on its effectiveness generated by a large randomized control trial within general acute mental health wards. The results of this trial were important and reported a 15% reduction in conflict and a 25% reduction in containment (2).

A common assumption made by many organizations nationally and internationally is that two psychiatric wards in the same hospital should run similarly, following the same hospital policies, with the same numbers of staff, admitting the same client group. However, in practice they can be extremely different and safety can vary significantly from one ward to another (2). Many different factors and variables can affect safety on a ward, such as leadership, patient group, and staffing shortages among others. Attempts have been made to try to understand what makes one ward so different from another (2, 3). However, there is little evidence available as to what definitive interventions or safeguards are required to facilitate a safe ward, despite many policies and guidelines, both nationally and internationally, attempting to do so (3, 4–7). One of the main challenges is that inpatient mental health is not an easy area to research due to there being many variables and an ever-changing, complex environment. However, the Safewards initiative has clarified some aspects of the inpatient environment which are helpful for improvement purposes (2). It indicates that restrictive interventions of all types seem to have similar themes.

Safewards model

The Safewards model works with the assumption that patients that are subject to one restrictive intervention are more likely to be subject to others. The model collectively calls them *containment*, and has accumulated evidence that they are all driven by similar factors. Similar distinctions are made about behaviours of patients who threaten their own safety and that of others. Therefore, using the same thinking from the Safewards initiative, wards that have high levels of self-harm, absconding, or medication refusal also have high levels of aggression. The Safewards model describes these behaviours collectively as *conflict*, and believe they have common causes (2, 3).

The model describes six characteristics of the way that inpatient mental health wards work that have the potential to influence rates of conflict and containment (3):

- How patients relate to one another in the ward community.
- Static features such as age and gender.
- Regulatory frameworks from the Mental Health Act through to hospital policies
- Structured environment for patients.
- Staff group, and how they work together (team work) to provide a physical environment of the ward.
- Contact with friends and relatives, influences from outside the hospital and into the outside world.[1]

[1] Bowers L (2014). Safewards: A New Model of Conflict and Containment on Psychiatric Wards. *Journal of Psychiatric and Mental Health Nursing* 21:499–508. CC BY-NC-ND 4.0.

Table 24.1 Factors influencing conflict and containment

Staff modifiers	Features of the staff as individuals or teams, or ways in which the staff act in managing patients or their environment, initiating or responding to interactions with patients that have the capacity to influence the frequency of conflict and/or containment
Patient modifiers	Ways in which patients respond and behave towards each other that have the capacity to influence the frequency of conflict and/or containment, and which are susceptible to staff influence
Flashpoints	Social and psychological situations arising out of features of the originating domains, signalling and preceding imminent conflict behaviour
Conflict	'Conflict' refers to all those patient behaviours that threaten their safety or the safety of others (violence, suicide, self-harm, absconding, etc.).
Containment	'Containment' refers to all the actions staff take to prevent conflict events from occurring or seek to minimize the harmful outcomes (e.g. PRN medication, special observation, seclusion, etc.).

Each of these characteristics can increase what the Safewards model describes as 'flashpoints'. These flashpoints are particular psychological or social situations which may then trigger conflict by patients or containment by the staff. The main benefit of the model is that it allows staff and organizations to identify many 'staff modifiers', in other words, things that staff can do to prevent the flashpoints from happening, or reduce conflict or containment. Knowledge of these modifiers allows staff to develop interventions that will promote or enhance techniques and those interventions are therefore likely to reduce rates of conflict and containment (2, 3).

The most basic form of the Safewards model is summarized in Table 24.1. The table lists factors influencing rates of conflict and containment on inpatient wards, and explains why some wards have much more conflict and containment than others.

Safewards' ten interventions

Bowers designed Safewards for use on adult acute mental health inpatient units offering ten interventions (2, 3) which work together to improve the culture of the ward and improve relationships between patients and staff. However, since its launch it has been adapted for use in many different environments. Safewards was launched locally in Berkshire across four adult acute wards, one psychiatric intensive care unit, and two older adult wards. The following sections explain the ten interventions and how these were then implemented on Rowan ward, an inpatient ward for older adults with functional mental health conditions. Typical types of conditions are depression, schizophrenia, psychosis, anxiety, and personality disorder as well as people with early stages of dementia.

Intervention 1: clear mutual expectations

Bowers explains that some of the difficult and challenging behaviours exhibited by patients are due in part to a lack of clarity about how they are expected to behave, or lack of consistency between the ward staff about what those expectations are. This is particularly problematic for patients who:

- have difficulty interpreting the verbal and non-verbal communications of others
- are distracted by psychotic thinking and preoccupations
- find it hard to concentrate
- cannot think clearly
- are undergoing extreme emotional states and moods that bias their perception and interpretation of what is going on around them
- have a distorted view of the world and others, particularly those in positions of authority, possibly due to past experiences and upbringing (2, 3).

Just as the staff have expectations of patients, patients have expectations of the staff. The Safewards model allows improved communication between the two, and provides clarity in the social environment helping patients to experience less irritation and frustration. This lowered stress and anxiety can help to reduce symptoms and supports patients' recovery. Terms such as expectations, guidelines, or standards are used rather than rules, as this can have negative connotations.

On Rowan ward (Figure 24.1), mutual expectations were discussed and decided upon within staff meetings and patient community meetings. A poster highlighting these expectations was displayed in the staff room and within the ward for patients to see.

A leaflet with the mutual expectations and other ward information was produced to be given to patients and carers on admission to the ward.

Intervention 2: soft words

When a person is unwell, a nurse's role is varied and often conflicting. The nurse will need to ensure that they support the person to get sufficient sleep, get up in the morning, wash and attend to personal grooming, wear appropriate clothes, eat and drink sufficiently, etc. In addition, attempts must be made to build a relationship with the person, foster social contact between patients, and engage them in organized activities on the ward. On the other hand, nurses will also have to ensure that the patient takes their prescribed medication, does not leave the ward without permission, sees various professionals such as psychiatrists, avert or diffuse arguments between patients, and prevent them from harming themselves. Often this is in the context of patients being formally detained in hospital under the Mental Health Act 1983.

Safewards advocates reducing confrontations due to the above-mentioned stressors and promotes working more collaboratively with patients, using appropriate language and communication skills, encouraging staff to be always carefully polite and respectful—for example, saying please and thank you as any perceived lack of respect can lead from a flashpoint to a crisis. It is important not to assume that collaborative working happens already and Safewards encourages the following ways to make sure the soft words intervention is maintained by:

- a 'message of the day' poster displaying 'soft words' tips, to be placed in the ward office and regularly changed, preferably daily (Figure 24.2)
- postcards with special hints and messages in an interesting format as a booster.

Implementation on Rowan ward included leaving helpful tips and guidance notes on using the soft words approach to patients

Rowan Ward Mutual Expectations

1. **Everyone** (staff and patients) will **RESPECT** each other and **TAKE TIME to listen** to each other's opinions.

2. Staff are **OPEN AND WILLING** to hear suggestions from patients and carers/relatives.
   A 1:1 session will be held every Thursday morning to discuss any issues with the ward and listen to suggestions.

3. A Carer's Group will be held monthly at various times, to **SUPPORT** carers and relatives and give them a chance to meet others in similar circumstances.

4. The nursing staff will deal with patients' and carers' requests in a **timely** and **efficient way,** reporting back to them on progress.

5. Access to the garden will be **restricted** in extreme weather conditions for safety.

6. Patients **ONLY** are allowed to smoke in the designated garden area, visitors **MUST GO OUTSIDE** the hospital grounds.

7. Everyone will be informed about the activities and therapies available to them, and will be **encouraged to attend** them.
   Please make a REAL EFFORT to engage in activities as this is part of your treatment while on the ward.

8. Everybody should try to look after themselves, and keep themselves clean and appropriately dressed.
   Staff will assist anyone who is unable to do so.

9. Everybody should assist in keeping the ward **clean and tidy**, reporting any issues to staff. Please **do not** allow food to spoil in bedrooms. Staff will assist patients in keeping bedrooms tidy for those who are unable to do so.

10. Patients are asked **NOT** to go in other patients' rooms or **REMOVE their property.**

11. **VIOLENCE OF ANY KIND** including **threatening others, swearing** or **aggressive language, hitting** or **throwing** things **WILL NOT** be tolerated.
    If you are feeling angry, politely ask to be left alone or walk away from the situation. But **DO** try to provide an explanation when you feel calmer.

12. It may be necessary to do a ward search (including patient's bedrooms) for contraband items.
    This is for the health and safety of everybody and according to Trust policy.

13. Staff to put on a film in the cinema every afternoon and evening, they should let patients know what film is on and **encourage patients to attend.**

14. If someone wants to watch something particular on TV, politely ask others if they mind changing the channel.

15. Please be **respectful of groups** that are taking place in the activity room, TV lounge, dining room and garden room.
    Also that patients are **NOT** disturbed by visitors or ward staff when the groups are in session **unless** absolutely necessary.

16. Relatives can use all communal areas on the ward. However we politely ask that the TV lounge is for **patients ONLY,** unless invited in by staff for meetings.

17. Relatives should **inform staff** if they give food to patients as this may **affect the patients appetites.**

Figure 24.1 Some of the difficult and challenging behaviours exhibited by patients are due in part to lack of clarity about how they are expected to behave, or lack of consistency between the ward staff about what those expectations are.
© Berkshire Health Care Foundation Trust.

in the handover room. There was a ward lead in charge of changing and displaying these twice weekly. Staff decided to display the posters on the back of the staff room door instead of the office as there was a lot more space. The staff made a feature of it with 'soft words' written in big bright letters to draw focus and create an impact. The soft words poster was surrounded by flowers and leaves, decorated with glitter. Staff members commented on how much focus was drawn to the words and how bright and colourful the poster was. One staff member stated that 'it brightens my day to look at that'.

Intervention 3: talk down techniques

When patients become agitated, angry, or upset, and a crisis arises where it seems likely they might become more violent or harm themselves, it is often possible to talk to help them calm down. That process is usually called de-escalation or diffusion. Most staff have some instruction in these skills as part of prevention and management of violence training, but the coverage is not always thorough or at an advanced level. This is because no one has previously pulled all the different techniques together, or assembled them into a meaningful picture.

A poster summarizing basic to advanced de-escalation techniques is placed in an area frequented by staff, preferably the nursing office, for the duration of the intervention. On Rowan

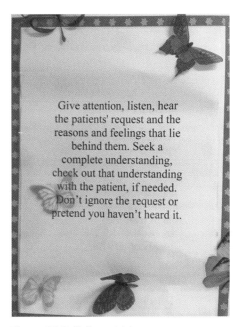

Give attention, listen, hear the patients' request and the reasons and feelings that lie behind them. Seek a complete understanding, check out that understanding with the patient, if needed. Don't ignore the request or pretend you haven't heard it.

Figure 24.2 'Soft words' tips.
© Berkshire Health Care Foundation Trust.

ward, posters were displayed in the office and staff room highlighting tips on how to use talk down techniques when communicating with patients. Training was delivered to staff to improve skills in this area and highlighted simple things such as using the patient's name, staff controlling their own emotions and responses, and offering choices to the patient to help them feel they still have some control.

Intervention 4: positive wards

Handovers are virtually the only place where the nursing team get together and discuss each patient. This has an important organizational function, making sure that the oncoming shift of nurses knows what has been happening, what the main risks are, what new patients have been admitted, and what should or must happen in the following shift. However, in their report of what has happened during the shift, they will often focus on exceptional behaviour. That is, the behaviour of patients which is difficult to manage or which presents risks to the patient or others. As such, they may promote a negative perception of patients. To balance this natural tendency, Safewards suggest that something positive must be said about each patient at the handover and that when difficult behaviour is described, potential psychological explanations are also offered, promoting a positive appreciation of patients and reducing the likelihood of further conflict.

When implementing this intervention staff were encouraged to give positive feedback as well as problematic or challenging behaviour about patients during handovers. This has mitigated the negative feelings and thoughts that staff can sometimes feel towards certain patients and behaviours so that more understanding of what might be causing those behaviours and being more thoughtful about the person as an individual is encouraged.

Intervention 5: bad news mitigation

In Safewards, it was found that some patients leave impulsively and in anger following unwelcome news. About one in four absconders leave in anger at their treatment. Some of these had long-term dissatisfactions with psychiatry, but others leave impulsively following unwelcome events, such as refused requests for leave, discharge, or negative outcomes of Mental Health Review Tribunal hearings.

Bad news from home can also precipitate conflict for patients. Severe examples would be a death in the family, or the termination of a relationship with an intimate partner. Things like the loss of tenancy, a burglary, and illness in the family, or childcare issues, can all represent blows to patients. The resulting stress and distress can then be acted out on the ward with increased irritability, aggression, violent incidents, and absconding. Safewards helps to notice these moments rapidly, and acts fast to mobilize psychological and social support for the patient, before the distress turns into a conflict incident.

When implementing this, staff were encouraged to consider what was bad news beforehand for each individual patient and discuss a plan of action of how to manage and approach a patient before they receive bad news. This helped the team to think about how the patient may take the news so that the staff members approached them in a more supportive manner and, importantly, information was not imparted in an off-hand way.

Intervention 6: know each other

It is a well-known fact that the cornerstone of mental health nursing is the formation of good therapeutic relationships with patients. However, putting it into practice with patients on an acute ward can be difficult. There are many factors that can get in the way of this such as the shift system, the turnover of patients, the pace of admissions and discharges, the amount of routine work to do, the filling out of forms, the phone calls, the ward rounds, etc. When staff do have time to spend with patients it is helpful to know about their background and interests as these provide conversation topics that can be raised. Also, when staff find out about a patient's interests, this information is often passed around the team so that everyone can use it to engage with the patient.

However, the same process can work in reverse. If the patients are given a little more information about staff, they can find areas of common interest and conversational topics. The mutual familiarity and knowledge gleaned can help speed up the forming of relationships and those relationships can help staff to orientate patients, enhance their coping skills, ameliorate their more difficult behaviour, and make them feel more comfortable and reassured during their admission.

Rowan ward staff members were asked to complete a questionnaire which gave details of topics such as their hobbies and roles, which were then typed up, laminated, and displayed in a folder. The aim was for patients to get to know staff better and to increase rapport. The key factor in implementing this was to ensure the folder was bright and colourful and in large print. The same photos as shown on the staff photo identification board were used to aid patient memory. Different fonts, borders, and pictures helped to personalize each person's profile and make it interesting to look at. The folder is left in the patient's main TV lounge for easy accessibility (Box 24.1).

On Rowan ward, patients have been responsive to the folder. For example, a patient stated that they had used the folder and had remembered what one of the nurses had stated about their values. This had initiated the client talking about this in conversation with the nurse which eased rapport.

Intervention 7: mutual help meeting

The ward as a social community is a perspective that should not be ignored, as this is a powerful engine to help patients, shape their behaviour, and progress them towards discharge. The help and assistance that patients give each other is highly valued by them. Moreover, the giving of help, even in the most minor of respects between patients, offers the giver a socially valued role, the chance to make a meaningful contribution and the potential to increase their self-esteem. Furthermore, about half of all patient violence arises from patient behaviour and/or patient–patient interaction. If we can teach patients to positively appreciate each other, contain their own emotional reactions to each other's behaviour, and uphold behavioural expectations, then this will equally contribute to reduced levels of conflict.

On Rowan ward, meetings were held twice a week and aimed to give patients an opportunity to thank others for things they had done or give suggestions for making the ward a better place to be. Patients were reminded throughout the week what had been suggested. Facilitation of the meeting was consistent and attendance was generally good.

Box 24.1 Orchid Ward mutual expectations

1 Everyone (staff and patients) will *respect* each other and *take time* to listen to each other's opinions.
2 Staff are *open and willing* to hear suggestions from patients and carers/relatives.
3 A community meeting will be held every Wednesday morning to discuss any issues with the ward and listen to suggestions.
4 A carer's group will be held monthly at various times, to *support* carers and relatives and give them a chance to meet others in similar circumstances.
5 The nursing staff will deal with patients' and carers' requests in a *timely* and *efficient* way, reporting back to them on progress.
6 Access to certain areas will be *restricted* in relation to risks identified on a health and safety basis.
7 Smoking *is not* allowed anywhere within Prospect Park hospital grounds. Nicotine replacement therapy will be provided for patients during their inpatient stay.
8 Everyone will be informed about the activities and therapies available to them, and will be encouraged to attend them.
9 Please make a *real effort* to engage in activities as this is part of your treatment while on the ward.
10 Everybody should try to look after themselves: *keeping clean* and *appropriately dressed*. Staff will assist anyone unable to do so.
11 Everybody should assist in *keeping the ward clean* and *tidy*, reporting any issues to staff. Please *do not* allow food to spoil in bedrooms. Staff will assist patients in keeping bedrooms tidy for those unable to do so.
12 Patients are asked *not to go* in other patients' rooms or *remove their property*.
13 *Violence* of any kind including *threatening others, hurting others, swearing, aggression, or destroying property* will not be tolerated. If you are feeling *angry*, politely ask if you could be left alone or walk away from the situation. But *do* try to provide an explanation when you feel calmer so we can learn how to prevent this occurring again.
14 It may be necessary to conduct *random ward searches* (including patients' bedrooms) for contraband items. This is for the health and safety of everybody and according to trust policy.
15 If someone wants something particular on TV, *politely ask* others if they mind changing the channel.
16 Please be respectful of *groups* that are taking place in the activity room, TV lounge, dining room, and garden room.
17 Visitors are requested *not to disturb* any groups *unless* absolutely necessary.
18 Relatives can use all communal areas on the ward; however, we politely ask that the TV lounge is for *patients only* unless invited in by staff for meetings.

Intervention 8: calm down methods

Sometimes it is possible to anticipate when something is brewing for a patient. It might be their facial expression, tone of voice, abrupt response to a normal reminder, restlessness, breathing pattern, body language, eye contact, movement around the ward, and other cues. Although 'as needed' (PRN) medication may be an effective strategy, it is perhaps reached for too easily and quickly on occasions and even considered to be the answer to everything. In fact, it might be better sometimes to use the patient's own strengths and usual coping mechanisms to help them calm down. This intervention suggests a range of alternatives and provides the means to make them available to patients where possible.

On Rowan ward, a calm down box was developed and kept in the staff office to prompt and encourage staff to think about using alternatives to medication in an incident where clients are agitated. There was a poster advertising the box on the back of the office door which stated that staff should think about alternatives before using any PRN medication. Contents included a breathing cat and dog teddy, CD players, relaxation CDs, mood lighting, reflexology stress balls, colourful Japanese fans for hot and bothered patients, a soft snuggly blanket to keep the cold at bay, a book of best loved poems, and stress balls.

Intervention 9: reassurance

Patients can react with fear or anger after events or episodes. Events such as violence, absconding, the admission of disturbed patients, arguments, and containment measures such as manual restraint or coerced intramuscular medication can all have an impact on everyone on the ward. Night-time may be particularly frightening for patients, particularly if they are not used to sharing a sleeping area with other people that they do not know and their illness may make them particularly vulnerable to additional stress. Patients may wake to the sound of shouting in the middle of the night, and lie awake fearfully imagining what might be going on. These reactions partly explain why one event triggers another as if there is one significant incident on the ward, a second is more likely to occur. Reassurance seeks to reduce the risk of 'contagion' between patients by allaying the anxieties that occur in these circumstances.

Rowan ward staff developed helpful tips and guidance notes which were left in the handover room for reassurance for staff to access. This was being highlighted and advertised to staff in the weekly staff meetings for staff to become more aware of accessing and using them to guide interventions.

Intervention 10: discharge messages

Many patients are admitted in a state of depression and hopelessness, even if that is masked sometimes with anger and resentment towards the staff and the hospital. There are many ways of assisting patients to regain hope, and get a sense of purpose about what their admission is for, for example, expressing care and concern for them as well as attending and listening to their concerns. This intervention attempts to provide a further method to imbue hope and convey authoritative messages about the purpose and benefit of an admission left by patients at the point of discharge.

On Rowan ward, patients that were nearing discharge from the ward were encouraged to write a message either about their experience or tips for coping on a ward to others. These messages were then displayed on the ward 'discharge tree' (Figure 24.3). Staff decided that the best place for the tree would be somewhere highly visible, so it was put opposite the patients' main TV lounge. Patients were asked to draw designs of how the tree should look in the ward art groups. All patients involved drew a scene and in response to that the tree had a sky-blue background and green grass. A wall art sticker of a magnolia tree with birds and butterflies was added which brightened it up. There were not many patient discharges initially and so motivational quotes were added on some of the leaves. Patients have suggested that the tree is seasonal, such

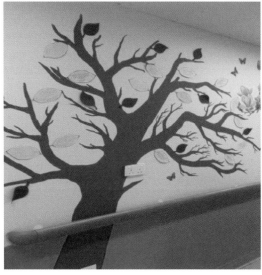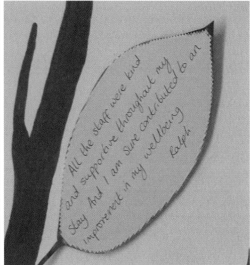

Figure 24.3 The discharge tree.
© Berkshire Health Care Foundation Trust.

as adding autumnal colour leaves, and bunnies on the grass for Easter!

Other positive effects

Results were also positive on other wards. Safewards was successfully implemented on all acute wards at Prospect Park hospital and achieved an increase in duration between conflict incidents by 16% in 2015/2016 compared to 2014/2015. There was also a 15% increase in patients reporting feeling safe on the ward, through patient feedback.

Feedback from staff on the ten interventions

There was the perception from staff that low staffing levels made interventions that required engagement with patients, such as the calm down box and mutual help meetings, difficult to implement; however, when they did implement them, they made a big difference to the level of incidents on the ward. Staff said that the handover-based interventions, such as positive words and bad news mitigation, had benefited from role modelling by the nurse consultant and other senior staff by clarifying what was expected of them. Following feedback from staff, the interventions were added to the handover template to make sure they were completed.

The 'reassurance' intervention was one of the most well received, and many staff recommended adding a tick box to the hospital's incident forms to ensure it had taken place as routine practice.

There was evidence of rather superficial understanding of a number of the interventions. A number of staff felt that the 'positive words' intervention was perceived to have improved team's cohesion enabling some wards to deal with perceived attempts from a given patient to create splits in the ward team. The 'calm down box' was reported to be of value in helping to reduce anxiety and agitation and, importantly, it communicated to patients that staff cared about them.

Challenges

The main challenge for all the Safewards interventions was to embed them into the practice and culture of the wards and ward staff routines, so that, for example, staff read the posters and used the tips and information available around the ward. It was also important for staff to make patients aware of information such as the 'know each other folder' and to remember to obtain messages for the discharge tree before the patient left the ward. To address these challenges some interventions were highlighted in regular staff meetings or documented on an interventions checklist. Another challenge was to motivate patients to attend the mutual help meeting. If there were mobility issues for individuals making it difficult for them to attend, patients were met with on a one-to-one basis to update and encourage them to use the approach.

Training method

A train-the-trainer model was adopted as recommended by the Safewards model, which consisted of an afternoon's training for the ward managers and team leaders in all wards. The training consisted of the following:

- An in-depth discussion of the Safewards model including originating domains of conflict in inpatient settings, and the patient and staff-level modifiers of conflict.
- A discussion of the process through which this evidence was used to develop the ten conflict reduction interventions.
- In-depth training in the use of the ten interventions.
- Factors increasing the likelihood of successful adoption, such as the importance of appointing 'intervention champions' to promote and take ownership of their implementation on each ward.
- Staff on wards were trained in the week before the first 10-week period of Safewards implementation.

- All wards were provided with a folder with the intervention descriptions, and web links to the training videos were emailed to every staff member.
- The physical materials required to implement the interventions were also provided in the training session.

These methods were supplemented by follow-up visits to the wards by the senior team for further discussion of the interventions and to train staff in the completion of the outcome measures. The inpatient nurse consultant visited each ward on a weekly basis to provide support and supervision of the clinical leads for each of the project wards.

Embedding 'talk down' skills into prevention and management of violence and aggression training

Despite the training that was provided for all staff on all participating wards, staff indicated that there was still a lack of confidence in utilizing talk down skills in conflict situations. Therefore, a practical, robust way of embedding the skill was developed, using technology, role play, and peer review to build, consolidate, and test knowledge and skills in a safe environment, thus improving confidence and competence.

Overall, this innovative training strategy was well evaluated by staff and student nurses. Staff engaged well with the opportunity to consolidate the talk down skills in training, despite some early trepidation. There appeared to be increased confidence in using talk down skills and increased confidence utilizing skills in the ward setting as evidenced by the change in use of prevention and management of violence and aggression and from the results of a self-assessment.

Conclusion

Listening to patients' points of view, negotiating with them, being generous, and showing flexibility and willingness to compromise unsurprisingly seem to contribute to reducing conflict and containment. The Safewards model talks about balancing restrictions by giving autonomy to patients in other areas that might compensate for the restrictions necessary for detention (2, 3). This might mean giving a voice and allowing choices on the ward activities, meals, snacks, furnishings, and timings, all of which might address detained patients' needs for respect and freedom. Staff may also intervene to address hopelessness and self-stigmatization due to hospitalization in a variety of both informal and organized ways.

The Safewards model also brings significant new considerations to the fore. For the first time, patient–patient interactions are seriously considered and included in explanations for rates of conflict and containment (3, 8). While patient characteristics and symptoms have been widely reported as causes of conflict and containment, the Safewards model identifies treatments as an effective safety-producing strategy, and identifies that the way staff respond to patients' characteristics can significantly impact on the occurrence of actual conflict or containment events (9, 10). The results described in this chapter show that Safewards is effective at increasing safety as well as increasing the perception of safety among patients. Importantly, the Safewards model incorporates influences on patients' behaviour from outside hospital, providing new understandings and therefore new ways to intervene (2, 3).

REFERENCES

1. Emmerson E, Einfield SL. *Challenging Behaviour*. Cambridge: Cambridge University Press; 2011.
2. Bowers L. The Safewards model. 2015. http://www.safewards.net./easy
3. Bowers L. Safewards: a new model of conflict and containment on psychiatric wards. *J Psychiatr Ment Health Nurs* 2014;21:499–508.
4. Centre for Quality Improvement. *Accreditation for Inpatient Mental Health Services (AIMS). Standards for Inpatient Wards – Working Age Adults*, 4th edition. London: Royal College of Psychiatrists; 2010.
5. National Institute for Health and Care Excellence. *Core Interventions in the Treatment and Management of Schizophrenia in Primary and Secondary Care*. Clinical Guideline [CG82]. London: National Institute for Health and Care Excellence; 2009.
6. Royal College of Psychiatrists. *Looking Ahead—Future Development of UK Mental Health Services: Recommendations from a Royal College of Psychiatrists' Enquiry*. Occasional Paper OP75. London: Royal College of Psychiatrists; 2010.
7. Care Quality Commission. *Monitoring the Use of the Mental Health Act in 2009/10: The Care Quality Commission's First Report on the Exercise of Its Functions in Keeping under Review the Operation of the Mental Health Act 1983*. London: Care Quality Commission; 2010.
8. Bowers L, James K, Quirk A, et al. Reducing conflict and containment rates on acute psychiatric wards: the Safewards cluster randomised controlled trial. *Int J Nurs Stud* 2015;52:1412–1422.
9. Dickens G, Piccirillo M, Alderman N. Causes and management of aggression and violence in a forensic mental health service: perspectives of nurses and patients. *Int J Ment Health Nurs* 2013;22 532–544.
10. Duxbury J, Whittington R. Causes and management of patient aggression and violence: staff and patient perspectives. *J Adv Nurs* 2005;50:469–478.

25

Post-incident debriefing, team formulation and staff support

Claudia Kustner

Closeness, chaos, crisis, and control—describing acute adult inpatient mental health wards: case notes

Clinical vignette

In the weekly staff support group, staff members are encouraged by the consultant nurse to reflect on how the week has been on the ward. Lydia, an experienced staff nurse, comments that she is too scared to say the 'q' word, in fear that the quietness of the ward will soon be disrupted. As if on cue, the loud, piercing sounds of an emergency pit alarm fills the room. Staff members rush out to find a heated altercation between Theo, an experienced, middle-aged support worker and Joe, a 25-year-old service user, who was recently admitted, involuntarily, on Section 2 of the Mental Health Act 1983. Joe is adamant and furious that he should be allowed to go out for a smoke break despite not having been assessed by the consultant yet. Joe picks up a chair from the communal sitting area and attempts to throw it at Theo, who is trying to de-escalate the situation. Szymon, another young service user on the ward, has, over the 3 months of being on the ward, developed a close, respectful relationship with support worker Theo. In an attempt to protect Theo, he rushes towards Joe and is knocked out by the chair. Staff members have to restrain Joe while Theo calls an ambulance for Szymon, who appears to be dazed and injured.

Discussion

Acute adult inpatient mental health wards have been observed by researchers to encapsulate the following factors—closeness, chaos, crisis, and control (1, 2). In a milieu characterized by high bed occupancy, quick staff turnover rates, acutely unwell service users, and unpredictable interactions and incidents, the environment can often feel chaotic, critical, and uncontained.

The National Health Service (NHS) community-based mental health care has also increased the threshold for admission to inpatient wards, with more service users detained under the Mental Health Act 1983. Service users are thus often dependent on staff for their care and freedom to leave the ward, which can leave them feeling disempowered and wanting to be heard. Due to staff often being in this position of control, volatile behavioural patterns and symmetrical struggles may emerge in the dynamics between staff and service users. An intolerable and restrictive environment can often create a culture where aggressive acts may be seen as justified among service users who are attempting to feel self-empowered.

With high levels of stress, low support, and lack of psychological knowledge, staff may often respond to service users punitively (3), increasing the use of restraints and reducing caring behaviour, which could then reinforce negative patterns of interactions and negatively affect relationships between management, staff, service users, and carers (3).

Studies of serious untoward incidents (suicide, absconding, homicide, suicide attempt, serious assault) and restrictive practices (physical restraints, seclusion) on acute inpatient mental health wards have highlighted an urgent need for improved post-incident support for both service users and staff (4, 5). Service users often report feeling ashamed, helpless, re-traumatized, and uncontained after a serious incident on the ward (1, 6). Staff, in turn, also report feeling traumatized, guilty, fearful, and hopeless (1, 2, 7). But while these studies provide valuable information on the experiences of staff and service users, they provide limited guidance on the process and content of psychologically focused debriefing frameworks.

Despite their acuity and unpredictability, inpatient mental health wards are also locked wards and safe spaces, which can often nurture a familiar closeness between staff and service users (8). On the wards where the author currently works, service users have often commented that they feel the 'ward is like their home and staff members are like family'. This was echoed in a study by Beech and Norman (9) where service users commented that quality psychiatric nursing care included a warm, safe, and homely environment.

Studies of acute inpatient mental health units show that highly developed communication and personal skills are key for staff who work with service users in this challenging 'home away from home' environment (10). The quality of ward staff and service user relationships has also been shown to be a key determinant of outcomes, including severity of symptoms and level of social functioning among service users, and frequency of violence and aggression on the ward (11).

In addition, factors associated with incidents on the wards often correlate with the interactions and relationship dynamics between service users and staff (12). From a service user's perspective, the theme of powerlessness is predominant. Morrison (13) highlights the latter, in confirming that aggressive and violent behaviour on a ward could often be predicted by a coercive, rigid, and controlling style by staff, as opposed to an accommodating and empathetic interpersonal style. Hence, collaborative partnership approaches to care have been associated with a reduction in incidents and violence (12).

It is thus evident that the overall well-being of staff working on these wards is critical to the care they provide to service users. Staff members who have a holistic and trauma-informed understanding of service users, as well as a common, systemic understanding of the role and purpose of interactions and incidents on the ward, are more likely to be understanding of and attuned to service users' needs and behaviours. To wit, research shows that ward environments that create regular spaces and processes for staff to talk to one another, debrief, learn, and review incidents and interactions are more likely to be peaceful and offer good-quality, restorative care (12).

It has thus been advocated that further research should focus on the specific conditions and processes that enable the development of therapeutic interactional skills among staff, and encourage the practice of these skills within the nuanced context of a mental health inpatient ward (10). In addition, when conditions for effective team working are instilled, there is also evidence that that service delivery improves and health care organisations operate more effectively (14). West and Spendlove (15) also reiterated that in the UK there is a strong need for psychological interventions that improve interprofessional team working, as weak processes appear to have potentially detrimental effects on organizational productivity, as well as the well-being of staff and service users.

Today's dynamic NHS environment is characterized by high levels of work demands and rapidly changing structures and culture. In a time when time is limited, it is integral to create psychologically minded spaces for teams to reflect upon their joint functioning, their wider work systems, and the service users who they care for. This chapter argues that the creation of facilitated talking spaces for teams to reflect with each other is integral for both staff and service user well-being on acute inpatient mental health wards. It also advocates for and explores the client-centred philosophy and principles of trauma-informed care whereby service users' strengths are highlighted over pathology and skills building over symptom reduction (16). A systemic team formulation model is proposed as a useful, trauma-informed, staff supervision intervention that could be used on the wards, as it offers numerous intra- and interpersonal benefits for teams that engage in the process of shared formulations. A case example illustrating the methodology of systemic team formulation will be explored. Towards the end of the chapter, post-incident debriefing will be discussed as a necessary form of staff support after serious untoward incidents and restrictive practices.

Trauma-informed care

Clinical vignette

Helen is a feisty, impulsive, 20-year-old woman with a childhood history of being looked after in various foster care homes. She has been calm and stable on the acute inpatient mental health ward after a crisis admission 3 weeks ago, but is fearful of living on her own. She was admitted following a break-up with her boyfriend and an attempted overdose. In a Care Programme Approach (CPA) (see Chapters 5 and 9) meeting with Helen present, the multidisciplinary team (MDT) suggest that she is ready to be discharged from the ward. Helen feels upset that her care coordinator could not make the CPA meeting time arranged by the ward to attend, but she reluctantly agrees with the discharge plans and denies having any suicidal ideation or intent. Her discharge summary is prepared, medication is organized for her, and transport is arranged. That afternoon after coming back from her usual leave time off the ward, Helen collapses on the floor and reports to staff that she has taken a big overdose of painkiller pills. She has to be rushed to hospital where she remains in a critical condition for a few days but manages to recover.

In the regular staff reflective practice support group at the end of the week, staff members share their feelings of anger, confusion, disappointment, and concern about Helen's behaviour, and are unsure about how to proceed further with her care. The ward psychologist helps the team formulate about the link between Helen's past traumas of abandonment and her current destructive and deliberate self-harming behaviour. The team explores the importance of creating a care plan that is informed by her past trauma around being abandoned, and its impact on her current functioning. They identify that establishing stable sources of support for Helen is going to be crucial for a safe and successful discharge.

Discussion

The link between childhood exposure to trauma and long-term mental health outcomes is irrefutable (16–19). These studies indicate that up to 90% of individuals diagnosed with serious and enduring mental illnesses, personality disorders, substance abuse, and those in contact with criminal justice systems, were exposed to significant emotional, physical, and or sexual abuse in childhood.

Childhood trauma is not a distinct, isolated event that occurs to an individual in time and space, but rather a defining experience that deeply influences the core of an individual's identity. An individual's early childhood experiences shape their expectations of relationships and the way they learn to deal with intense feelings, such as fear, loss, distress, and threat. Reflecting on these attachment narratives is key to understanding how individuals respond when hurt and how they cope (17, 20). Attachment theory is fundamentally a theory of emotional regulation (17). When a child is distressed and agitated, they seek comfort and protection from their parents. How this reassurance is offered provides a sense of safety for the child and shapes how s/he learns how to regulate their feelings.

Violence, abuse, and neglect in early childhood can negatively disrupt and compromise an individual's attachment narrative and their internal working model (how an individual sees themselves, others, and their relationships) (17). This then may have cognitive, emotional, relational, and physical ramifications in later life. Individuals may then develop maladaptive and destructive methods of getting their needs met. Traumatic experiences can also inhibit new learning and influence an individual's response to future stressors (19).

There is thus a convincing and emerging evidence base for inpatient mental health staff to become trauma informed and to employ the principles of trauma-informed care in their everyday practice (18, 19). Trauma-informed care is a client-centred philosophy and model of care service delivery that acknowledges the role of early trauma on behaviour across the lifespan (21). Trauma-informed organizations are also those that recognize that their services can re-traumatize admitted service users with significant trauma histories through the undiscerning and coercive practices of physical restraint and loss of autonomy. Admission to, and like in the case example of Helen described earlier, discharge from mental health services, the onset of destabilizing symptoms, and dislocation from normal support networks and family can all be sources that could trigger re-trauma for service users (21).

The nature of nurse–service user relationships is crucial to service users' perceptions of quality and effectiveness of care on inpatient wards. Service users with a history of trauma, abandonment, and/or poor attachment in childhood may be highly sensitive to suboptimal care from staff, that is, perceiving staff to be disinterested, disrespectful, or disempowering towards them, which then may reinforce negative thoughts of inferiority and rejection leading to feelings of being re-victimized (19).

The following key principles of trauma-informed care can be applied on an inpatient mental health ward to avoid re-traumatization and to promote emotionally corrective experiences for service users who have experienced trauma in the past (16, 18, 21):

1. Service users should feel connected to and valued by staff as fellow human beings, and not just service users. They should be informed in a timely and emotionally supportive manner about care plans and treatment options to encourage feelings of hope and safety around recovery. Service users and their family members should be actively included and participate in all care provision decisions.

2. Staff should attempt to model collaborative and respectful communication to avoid reinforcing and repeating the very types of disempowering, traumatic relational patterns they seek to treat.

3. Staff should try to work mindfully and in empowering ways with service users, carers, and other social services agencies to promote and protect the autonomy of the individual.

4. When appropriate and relevant, psychologists and psychiatrists can incorporate the principles of trauma-informed care in their therapeutic work with inpatient service users, by exploring and raising awareness of relational themes and maladaptive coping patterns that developed as a result of traumatic relationships and events in a service user's life. Service users should be encouraged to recognize recurring relational patterns in the therapeutic setting when they occur, rehearse new skills, and adopt healthier, non-destructive strategies for coping with trauma triggers and meeting emotional needs.

5. Staff members should be aware of and understand possible connections between childhood trauma and adult psychopathology, and the ways they can be played out in patterns of behaviour on the ward. Regular and consistent staff group meetings should be offered, where staff can reflect, formulate, and debrief as a team. These meetings should be facilitated by health care professionals capable of containing and listening to staff in a non-judgemental and objective manner.

In order to develop a culture and belief in the value and benefits of trauma-informed care, staff should develop knowledge and skills of the recurring impact of past traumas on service users and understand their responsibilities in preventing possible re-traumatization (16).

A systemic approach understands the importance of context in shaping behaviour and considers patterns of interaction that may follow exposure to traumatic events (22). Understanding the connections between current 'symptomatic' behaviours and past traumatic events are integral to understanding the current situation and to develop ideas on how to change it. Smith (22, p. 56) also notes that:

> unacknowledged trauma has a way of reasserting its shaping influence on our lives through 'inexplicable' episodes of anxiety and distress, both physical and emotional.

In line with the principles of trauma-informed care, systemic team formulation sessions can provide staff with an opportunity to holistically discuss the possible meanings service users attach to their early relationships and traumatic events. In these discussions, staff can then explore how maladaptive and unhealthy coping mechanisms and behaviours (aggression, self-harm, irrational thoughts, avoidance), may have once been adaptive, interpersonal behaviours in the abusive childhood contexts of service users. Thus, as opposed to seeing service users' actions as being challenging, 'behavioural', and 'acting out', staff are encouraged to reframe an individual's attempts to cope as survival skills and communication attempts that were once important, but now interfere with the establishment of healthy interpersonal relationships and boundaries (18).

Within these formulation meetings, staff members should be given an opportunity to self reflect, debrief and regain empathy for service users' concerns and communication attempts. Staff members that have a psychological perspective on challenging behaviours on the ward are more likely to create a safe and caring environment where choice, collaboration, and empowerment are emphasized (16). Staff can also then explore caring interventions that may serve as corrective emotional experiences. These care planning points on how to engage and interact more effectively with service users may help them move forward from the iterative, generational cycle of trauma and victimization, and ensure that abusive relationships are not unknowingly replicated in the helping relationship (18). A more detailed discussion of systemic team formulation follows.

Systemic team formulation

Clinical vignette

Jimmy is a 63-year-old, white man from Scotland who was admitted to the ward after assaulting a black policeman. He is a man of small stature, generally well groomed, but presents with a flat affect and pressured speech. He has a long-standing diagnosis of bipolar mood disorder with psychotic symptoms. He presents with very limited insight into his mental state and need for admission, and often expresses delusional ideas that he is a secret agent of MI5. On the ward, he presents as verbally hostile towards staff and other service users. At times, he is physically aggressive and makes derogatory racist comments, particularly towards staff members of a different race and culture. There have been numerous incidents, some serious, involving him on the ward. He has unpredictably attacked two black staff members, by kicking them in the shins and spitting at them, requiring physical restraint. Jimmy has put in an official complaint to the ward manager, that he feels a black staff member injured him during a restraint. He frequently gets overinvolved in other service users' care, often provoking conflict between staff and service users. He has been on the ward for 3 months, as he is currently homeless and he has made limited progress in his clinical presentation. Staff requested that a team formulation be done to discuss Jimmy, as they are concerned for the well-being and morale of fellow black staff members on the ward. They also feel they are losing their patience with Jimmy and feel increasingly unable to empathize with his concerns.

Discussion

Dallos and Vetere (17) stated that change happens by assisting people to see that problems do not only lie essentially with the individual, but are also created and maintained relationally. Emotions and attachment-related feelings are also at the centre of relational dynamics (23). Having a reflective space to explore and formulate the links between individual experiences and relational processes can often help ward staff better understand challenging behaviours that could, and do, lead up to conflict and incidents on the ward. In psychology practice, a working hypothesis or summary of a client's difficulties and relational processes, based on psychological theory, and informing the intervention is known as a formulation. Team formulation is thus the use of formulation in teams to develop a shared understanding of the client's difficulties (24). While formulation is a key competence area for psychology practice (25), team formulation is a more recent and specialized development in the field, with a growing literature base (24–28).

Despite recent guidelines by the British Psychological Society (14) recommending the applied psychology intervention of team formulation as 'an effective use of a psychologist's limited time' and 'a powerful way of shifting cultures towards more psychosocial perspectives' (24, 26), very little has been written about the actual contribution formulation can make within an acute adult inpatient mental health setting.

Systemic team formulation is an area that is yet to be researched. Systemic theory provides a unique lens to make hypotheses about the reasons for people's difficulties, in light of their relationships and interactional patterns.

The objective of team formulation meetings is to facilitate a supervision process among staff of formulating a shared team understanding of a service user that can then be used in interventions and collaborative care plans with the service user, their support teams, and carers. Team formulation can be done from various psychological perspectives. An integrative model of team formulation, such as the one proposed by Lake (28), provides a useful structure for the adult inpatient environment, as it encourages a holistic, open-ended, participatory discussion about a service user's history, and highlights any gaps in the history that still needs to be explored.

Drawing from the latter model, systemic team formulation, in the context of my ward practice, is a staff-focused, psychological, group supervision intervention that encourages the ward team to develop a shared understanding of a patient's difficulties and behaviours, from a systemic psychology perspective. A systemic perspective involves viewing individuals' concerns and problems as happening *between* people rather than just *within* people (24). It involves thinking about wider contexts and agencies, families and relationships, beliefs and discourses, lifespan development and trauma, and power and culture. The focus of systemic team formulation, in contrast to other team formulation models, is that its main focus is relational.

In systemic team formulation supervision sessions, team members are encouraged to self-reflect on and share their own feelings, beliefs, and responses towards a patient, and to identify how this may affect how the patient may feel and respond back to staff members.

A discussion is held about possible circular patterns of interaction that may occur between staff and patients, and how these interactions may mirror interactions that patients may have with their families and support systems. Hypotheses are then explored about different ways in which staff could interact with patients more effectively on the ward. The theoretical approach underlying this model of team formulation will be discussed further in this chapter.

Essentially, there are three aspects that are usually covered in the systemic team formulation supervision meetings that the author of this chapter usually facilitates on the wards (28):

1. There is a biopsychosocial discussion about a service user's history and relationships, including an exploration of possible traumas that the individual has endured, which ensures that all disciplines are able to contribute their viewpoints and historical accounts of the service user and their relationships:
   • Genogram.
   • Temperament.
   • Developmental, school, and work history.
   • Social environment while growing up.
   • Trauma.
   • Cultural context.
   • Relationship history.

With regard to the case study of Jimmy, staff members contributed important historical information about him in the team formulation session held, listed in Table 25.1. After this discussion, some staff reported that they were unaware that Jimmy came from a 'broken home' (words used by staff members) and that he had limited schooling and a past history of being assaulted and restrained on the ward. Staff felt that knowing this information helped them feel more empathic towards him and understanding of his antisocial behaviours. Staff members also reflected that they didn't know much about Jimmy's cultural and developmental background, as they were so focused on his disruptive behaviour.

2. There is then a hypothetical discussion about the systemic pattern of interaction that could be occurring between the service user and staff (Figure 25.1). In Figure 25.1, the term 'client system' is used, indicating that systemic formulation is not only about the service user but also the system around them, which staff may or may not have contact with, but should be considered in the formulation (family, carers, friends, services, agencies).

With regard to the case study of Jimmy, staff reflected that due to his poor insight and unpredictability in interactions they were divided in their feelings towards him. Some felt fond of him while others felt very angry and uncomfortable around him. This led to staff responding to him in different ways. Some attempted to reprimand him and remove him away from triggers, while others tried distracting him and validating his concerns. Staff hypothesized that due to this split in staff responses, as well as his traumatic developmental history, Jimmy's core beliefs could be that 'some people can't be trusted'. His coping strategies were then to get overinvolved when he felt he couldn't 'trust' some staff and that he then tried to make himself more 'powerful' among some staff, which then resulted in him verbally and physically assaulting some staff and service users. Staff also noticed that Jimmy had no support sources in his system, and that ward and staff had 'become Jimmy's world'.

Table 25.1 Discussion points brought up by staff regarding what they knew of *Jimmy

Developmental history	Relationship history	School and work history
• He lost contact with his mum when he was aged 3 • His father worked for the RAF and was absent from his life • He was married 10 years ago, but is now divorced. He has two children	• Appears to be estranged and isolated from his family • He does not appear to have contact with his children	• Left school when he was 13 • He describes himself as a musician and song writer • He is currently unemployed
Trauma	**Temperament**	**Culture**
• He has had multiple admissions into acute services in the last 3 years • He has been assaulted by peers on the ward before • He has also attacked a nurse and members of the police which has led to him being restrained numerous times • (Possible childhood trauma due to lack of supportive home environment?)	• Generally pleasant • He has a good sense of humour • He does not like being challenged • He can be stubborn and non-compliant • He often uses racist language and can be hostile to people of different cultures	• Was born in London but grew up in Scotland • He grew up in the 1950s

3. Based on the team formulation points from 1 and 2 above, there is then a brief discussion about care planning points that could be useful and effective in future interactions with the service user. This discussion involves staff engaging in a process of relational reflexivity, that is, they are taking a 'bird's eye view' of their own interactional patterns. They are observing and reflecting on the way in which they relate with others, and the circular impact that may have in interactions with clients, their families, agencies, and other staff. With regard to the case of Jimmy, staff reflected that it was useful for them to distinguish the different viewpoints of staff members in relation to Jimmy, and that they had a better systemic understanding of the possible pattern of behaviour in Jimmy's life and on the ward. They identified the split in staff behaviour as being part of the problem-maintaining feedback loop in Jimmy's behaviour as well as Jimmy's social isolation, and they formulated care planning points to work as a team in supporting Jimmy to feel safer on the ward, in an attempt to prevent further antisocial behaviour on his part. Staff reflected that they were now curious about Jimmy's cultural and developmental background, and would ask him to share information on this, to get to know him better. They also agreed on the importance of exploring possible community support resources for Jimmy. The key nurse would take these care planning points back to Jimmy to get his perspective on them, and for him to contribute his perspective of what could be helpful for him on the ward.

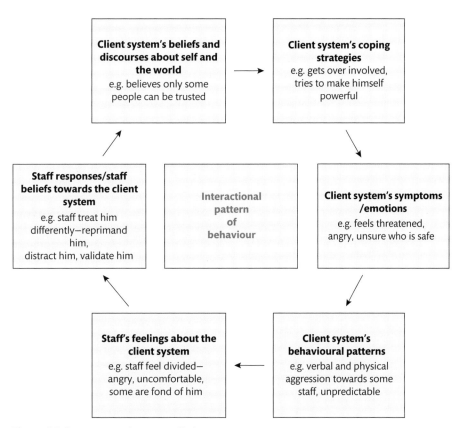

Figure 25.1 Interactional pattern of behaviour.

Team formulation has been recommended as being particularly useful with complex clients, such as Jimmy, who have long histories with mental health services, where 'transference and countertransference issues are likely played out in relation to the whole team' (14, p. 22). System team formulation allows for 'symptoms' and 'challenging behaviours' to be seen as problems in interactions and communication between people, rather than residing within individuals (24).

Some have even argued strongly that team formulation should be seen as a radical alternative to psychiatric diagnosis (24), a powerful instrument for culture change, and a much-needed space for busy teams to think, process, and understand intrapersonal and interpersonal feelings and behaviours.

Team formulation meetings as discussed in the context of this chapter is a form of supervision, consultation, or group therapy (27), whereby team members, who are in effect the client, approach the facilitator of team formulation, usually a psychologist, with a presenting complaint of feeling confused, stuck, and angry in their interactions with certain service users in their care. The team formulation meetings, much like group therapy sessions, often need to be facilitated with careful, psychotherapeutic skills of containing, reflecting, and reframing, as feelings of anger, frustration, stuckness, or sadness are often expressed. Disagreements, splits and conflict within the team are also often discussed. These moments in team formulation are often significant reflections of the service user's own conflicts, dilemmas (24), and relational narratives. These need careful handling, as do the splits and disagreements that sometimes arise within the team, reflecting the service user's own conflicts and dilemmas. This is crucial information that can be used to enhance our understanding of the service user rather than, as so often happens, simply being acted out through disintegrated, contradictory, and sometimes punitive interventions, based on primitive formulations such as 'he's just doing it for attention'.

The team formulation approach is ideally implemented by trained psychologists through meetings that are a standard part of the weekly timetable, attended by all professionals. Essentially, the aim is to facilitate a process of developing a formulation with the whole team, resulting in a shared team understanding that can be used as the basis for intervention and collaborative work with the service user and, as appropriate, their carers. A typical format for the meeting is to summarize the background information; identify the main current concerns or 'stuck points'; develop the formulation in discussion with the team; outline possible ways forward based on the formulation; write up and circulate the formulation and intervention plan to all staff; and re-visit the formulation and the plan as necessary.

It should be noted that in the proposed version of systemic formulation practice, the main client is, in effect, the team, whose feelings of stuckness, hopelessness, anger, or despair are likely to have prompted the request for a discussion (24). In effect, a team formulation meeting is a type of supervision or consultation, and in the same way as with those activities, it may not always be appropriate or helpful to share the aspects that deal with strong staff reactions directly with the service user.

The involvement of service users in discussing and contributing to care planning points drawn from the team formulation sessions, has been found to be useful for both staff and service users. In some cases on the ward, it has been useful to share and discuss team formulation discussions with service users, but this often depends on the service user's mental state and stage of recovery.

Systemic team formulation, based on systemic family theory, is a co-constructional process which, in itself, is an intervention to perturb and change the team system. Thus, the process of how the formulation takes place, the questions asked, when and how they are asked, and by whom, all have the potential to create a change in the system (24). An acute inpatient psychiatric ward offers a unique opportunity to 'map the family dance' between inpatients and ward staff (i.e. to observe interactions between staff and inpatients that could mirror interactional patterns between inpatients and their families), thereby raising awareness that problems service users face in their respective systems are often mimicked and maintained through circular processes in their daily interactions with ward staff too. Systemic team formulation, as a psychotherapeutic intervention, thus provides a reflective space for the ward team to explore these interactional dynamics and to think strategically about addressing these patterns, and to use the language of relationships to describe and understand behaviour, beliefs, and feelings.

An individual's presenting problem and distress is a multifaceted, iterative process that should be understood 'in terms of relational dynamics at many levels of contextual understanding' (29). Based on systemic formulation for individuals, a systemic team formulation would include the following elements: context (current, historical, developmental, social, cultural); a genogram indicating family relationships and dynamics; traumas, transitions, and attachments; and support sources, coping strategies, and protective factors. In addition, examining the circular and recursive patterns of behaviours, beliefs, and feelings between staff and service user is key, as the inpatient ward environment often becomes a microcosm of the service user's familial system. Examining circular systems of causation was a key proponent of Gregory Bateson's cybernetic epistemology. Bateson, an anthropologist, social scientist, and cyberneticist, is often credited with providing the epistemological foundation and language for systemic theories. Cause and effect are thus circular in nature, whereby problems are maintained through iterative cycles of unhelpful feedback (24).

Systemic team formulation also provides a necessary space for ward staff to become aware of their own thoughts, feelings, and reactions towards service users in crisis, and towards each other in the team. They can reflect on their positioning, with regard to professional status, gender, class, ethnicity, age, etc., and how these may impact the care they deliver to inpatients, especially as the work context is often highly emotive. It provides a space where intense feelings between staff and service users are acknowledged, shared, and normalized. It also creates a shared formulation space whereby staff can take a higher perspective (a meta-perspective) on the relationships and dynamics between staff members within the team, and with the wider hospital and mental health system. Thus, systemic team formulation changes the lens on the 'problematic patient' to the problems being a product of the interactional dynamics in the ward community, including staff, service users, and the wider mental health system (24).

The team formulation thus becomes a systemic intervention, in and of itself. Johnston (27) proposes that:

> constructing a team formulation of a complex client can itself be enough to facilitate change by enabling the staff to share and process their emotions, put their feelings and views about a service user in a theoretical context, and view a service user with new insight, compassion and hope.

Post-incident debriefing and staff support

A controversial Cochrane meta-analysis of research conducted across a variety of settings (including studies with staff working in high trauma-risk occupations) (30) concluded that single-session psychological debriefing had little to no effect on the psychological distress of individuals and failed to prevent post-traumatic stress disorder, thereby claiming that debriefing was ineffective. In this section, it will be argued that creating *regular* spaces for staff to meet, talk, and debrief are crucial in maintaining staff well-being and in mitigating the negative, short- and long-term psychological impact of working in a space where serious untoward incidents often occur and where physical restraint of service users is often required.

Psychological debriefing is defined as an early intervention technique for staff exposed to a stressful event that carries the risk of psychological trauma (4). The intervention model that is most commonly used is the critical incident stress debriefing model, which encourages the expression of emotions and allows individuals to talk about and process the traumatic incident without judgement or criticism (4). In mental health care, the addition of reflective practice principles in debriefing sessions, such as the critical analysis of clinical practices, the exploration of the suitability of the therapeutic skills used, and the promotion of safe practices, has increased the efficacy and value of debriefing sessions in this emotionally intense context (4).

Acute inpatient mental health wards are often unpredictable and volatile environments (8) where staff often remain wary of quiet periods on the ward, and anticipate the next inevitable incident. Strong working relations in the staff team is often the anchor in maintaining stability on the ward, and a team approach to care assists in making the ward feel less unpredictable and chaotic. Due to high staff turnover, absenteeism, and lack of permanent nursing staff on wards, this anchoring stability is, however, often threatened (8). The influx of agency or temporary workers on the wards, who do not really know the service users or the system, contribute to ward instability. In a setting where there is a hugely varying patient group, chaotic interactions and socially disagreeable behaviour can often occur. Acutely ill service users are often on the ward with less ill service users awaiting social support. Some service users can be demanding treatment, while others may reject it and be legally compelled to take it (8). All of these factors could increase the likelihood and incidence of serious incidents occurring on the ward, which may require physical restraint.

Incidents can include serious, antisocial, or violent and aggressive untoward events between service users and/or staff and others. Sometimes these events require the use of restraint by staff on service users, which is an incident on its own. Restraint can be defined as any incident where staff have to physically lay hands on a service user in the course of managing an untoward incident (12).

Serious incidents are defined by NHS policy (31) as:

events in health care where the potential for learning is so great, or the consequences to service users, families and carers, staff or organisations are so significant, that they warrant using additional resources to mount a comprehensive response. Serious incidents can extend beyond incidents which affect service users directly and include incidents which may indirectly impact service user safety or an organisation's ability to deliver on-going healthcare.[1]

These events can be isolated, single events or multiple, linked or unlinked events. There is no definite list of what constitutes a serious incident, but it includes unexpected or avoidable death (e.g. suicide or homicide); unexpected or avoidable injury that has resulted in serious harm or requires further treatment; actual or alleged abuse (sexual, physical, psychological, acts of omission that results in neglect, exploitation, etc.); and an incident (or series of incidents) that prevents, or threatens to prevent, an organization's ability to continue to deliver an acceptable quality of health care services (e.g. property damage, security breach, and inappropriate enforcement/care under the Mental Health Act 1983 and the Mental Capacity Act 2005, including Mental Capacity Act, Deprivation of Liberty Safeguards (31)) (see Chapter 2).

The NHS serious incident framework policy (31) recognizes that serious incidents can be impactful on staff who were involved, or who may have witnessed an incident. Staff members, much like victims and carers, often want information on how and why the incident occurred, as well as on the outcomes of the incident. Staff may thus experience an array of feelings as a result of it, especially if they are aware that an investigation around the incident will be taking place. To allay anxiety, staff should be provided with information about the stages of the investigation and how they will be expected to contribute to the process.

The following factors influence the emotional impact of serious incidents on staff: severity and outcome of the incident; the closeness of the relationship with the service user involved; the perception of whether the incident may have been prevented; support and response from management; and importantly, the availability of external support and psychological aftercare after the incident (1).

Staff working in inpatient acute settings express that they are often affected by feelings at work which cause personal discomfort (8). This is often mirrored from the agitation and distress felt by their service users which can reach intensely intolerable levels. Thus, a circular tension may develop, where service users attempt to communicate their pain, anguish, confusion, and fear, and staff put up barriers to protect against these intense emotions. The latter is characterized by complaining about the piles of paperwork, avoidance and retreating to the office, insensitivity towards agitated service users, rapid turnover, rigidity in care planning, and being over-concerned with risk assessments (32). To cope with this inevitable pattern, staff members need regular, consistent, and supportive safe spaces to think and 'share the weight of projections, anger, and anxieties that they are asked to carry' (32, p. 197).

Multidisciplinary conflict may also emerge when relations with a particular service user brings feelings to the surface and creates a split in the team. This can be reinforced by the, at times, hierarchical individual silos that professions within a MDT find themselves operating within.

Thinking and working towards a superordinate goal minimizes the splits and often highlights the complementary skills that are often mutually inclusive. A collaborative approach to care is created in the form of MDT handovers, CPA meetings, staff support meetings, and post-incident reviews, where staff can meet to integrate different perspectives, to review lessons learned, and to create shared formulations (32). Teams are then able to take corporate responsibility and professional accountability for the services they provide.

The serious incidents framework policy (31) also promotes that staff should be offered counselling, occupational health services, and

---

[1] NHS. *Serious Incident Framework: supporting learning to prevent recurrence.* NHS England. 2015. Contains public sector information licensed under the Open Government Licence v3.0.

access to professional advice from a union or relevant professional body in the aftermath of serious incidents and restraints conducted (31). Regular Staff support groups are thus an invaluable source of support for staff to reflect on difficult feelings, to prevent a destructive reactive response, to curtail early dissatisfaction, and to mitigate burnout (4, 33).

However, due to the propulsive power and pace of the ward routine, changes in shift patterns and unpredictability of service user demands and needs, staff are often prevented from having a regular and consistent reflective space to discuss and review incidents. The context of acute mental health in the UK makes the post-incident support actions recommended earlier difficult to follow. Occupancy and throughput of service users are high, as well as staff vacancy rates (12). On the wards where the author works, the hiring of supernumerary staff during staff group times has been invaluable, as it allows ward staff to attend the group, ensuring safe staffing numbers.

Studies have shown that a high frequency of violence, aggression, and incidents on the ward undermine the quality of therapeutic services provided (34), affect the morale of staff, and can lead staff to feelings of depression and being burnt out (1). In addition, failure to deal with feelings elicited by incidents hinders the ability to learn from the event, and to critically reflect on it (12). Regular and safe spaces for ward staff to talk, reflect, and debrief are thus crucial.

Despite the results of the Cochrane meta-analysis (30), mentioned at the beginning of this section, Richards (35) and Nurmi (36) identified beneficial outcomes following psychological debriefing, but recommended that a single, isolated intervention appeared to be of little benefit. Matthews (37) found lower levels of stress among workers in areas where post-incident debriefing was available for staff who wanted to access it. In addition to lowering levels of stress among staff, debriefing was also found to foster reflective practice (38). Thus, creating and sustaining regular spaces for mental health staff to meet and talk and receive support is crucial in maintaining a healthy workforce, healthy service users, and a healthy ward. It is also crucial for ward management to consider staffing numbers during staff group times, to ensure regular staff can attend.

REFERENCES

1. Bowers L, Simpson A, Eyres S, et al. Serious untoward incidents and their aftermath in acute inpatient psychiatry: the Tompkins Acute Ward Study. *Int J Ment Health Nurs* 2006;15:226–234.

2. Johansson IM, Skärsäter I, Danielson E. The health-care environment on a locked psychiatric ward: an ethnographic study. *Int J Ment Health Nurs* 2006;15:242–250.

3. Daffern M, Howells K, Ogloff J. What's the point? Towards a methodology for assessing the function of psychiatric inpatient aggression. *Behav Res Ther* 2007;45:101–111.

4. Goulet MH, Larue C. Post-seclusion and/or restraint review in psychiatry: a scoping review. *Arch Psychiatr Nurs* 2016;30:120–128.

5. Ryan R, Happell B. Learning from experience: using action research to discover consumer needs in post-seclusion debriefing. *Int J Ment Health Nurs* 2009;18:100–107.

6. Kontio R, Joffe G, Putkonen H, et al. Seclusion and restraint in psychiatry: patients' experiences and practical suggestions on how to improve practices and use alternatives. *Perspect Psychiatr Care* 2012;48:16–24.

7. Sequeira H, Halstead S. The psychological effects on nursing staff of administering physical restraint in a secure psychiatric hospital: 'When I go home, it's then that I think about it'. *Br J Forensic Pract* 2004;6:3–15.

8. Bowers L, Chaplin R, Quirk A, Lelliott P. A conceptual model of the aims and functions of acute inpatient psychiatry. *J Mental Health* 2009;18:316–325.

9. Beech P, Norman IJ. Patients' perceptions of the quality of psychiatric nursing care: findings from a small-scale descriptive study. *J Clin Nurs* 1995;4:117–123.

10. Cleary M. The realities of mental health nursing in acute inpatient environments. *Int J Ment Health Nurs* 2004;13:53–60.

11. Berry K, Barrowclough C, Haddock G. The role of expressed emotion in relationships between psychiatric staff and people with a diagnosis of psychosis: a review of the literature. *Schizophr Bull* 2011;37:958–972.

12. Secker J, Benson A, Balfe E, Lipsedge M, Robinson S, Walker J. Understanding the social context of violent and aggressive incidents on an inpatient unit. *J Psychiatr Ment Health Nurs* 2004;11:172–178.

13. Morrison EF. The tradition of toughness: a study of nonprofessional nursing care in psychiatric settings. *J Nurs Scholarsh* 1990;22:32–38.

14. Onyett S. *Working Psychologically in Teams*. Leicester: British Psychological Society; 2007.

15. West M, Spendlove M. The impact of culture and climate in healthcare organisations. In: Cox J, King J, Hutchinson A, McAvoy P (eds), *Understanding Doctors' Performance*, pp. 91–105. Oxford: Radcliffe Publishing; 2006.

16. Elliott DE, Bjelajac P, Fallot RD, Markoff LS, Reed BG. Trauma-informed or trauma-denied: principles and implementation of trauma-informed services for women. *J Community Psychol* 2005;33:461–477.

17. Dallos R, Vetere A. *Systemic Therapy and Attachment Narratives: Applications in a Range of Clinical Settings*. London: Routledge; 2009.

18. Harris ME, Fallot RD. *Using Trauma Theory to Design Service Systems*. San Francisco, CA: Jossey-Bass; 2001.

19. Muskett C. Trauma-informed care in inpatient mental health settings: a review of the literature. *Int J Ment Health Nurs* 2014;23:51–59.

20. Fonagy P. Thinking about thinking: some clinical and theoretical considerations in the treatment of a borderline patient. *Int J Psychoanal* 1991;72:639–656.

21. Hodas GR. *Responding to Childhood Trauma: The Promise and Practice of Trauma Informed Care*. Harrisburg, PA: Pennsylvania Office of Mental Health and Substance Abuse Services; 2006.

22. Smith G. *Working with Trauma: Systemic Approaches*. London: Palgrave Macmillan; 2012.

23. Dallos R, Vetere A. Systemic therapy and attachment narratives: attachment narrative therapy. *Clin Child Psychol Psychiatry* 2014;19:494–502.

24. Johnstone L, Dallos R. *Formulation in Psychology and Psychotherapy: Making Sense of People's Problems*. London: Routledge; 2013.

25. Johnstone L, Whomsley S, Cole S, Oliver N. *Good Practice Guidelines on the Use of Psychological Formulation*. Leicester: British Psychological Society; 2011.

26. Christofides S, Johnstone L, Musa M. 'Chipping in': clinical psychologists' descriptions of their use of formulation in multidisciplinary team working. *Psychol Psychother* 2012;85:424–435.

27. Johnstone L. *Using Formulation in Teams. Formulation in Psychology and Psychotherapy: Making Sense of People's Problems*. Hove: Routledge; 2013.

28. Lake N. Developing skills in consultation. 2: a team formulation approach. *Clin Psychol Forum* 2008;186:18–24.

29. Vetere A, Dallos R. *Working Systemically with Families: Formulation, Intervention and Evaluation*. London: Karnac Books; 2003.

30. Rose SC, Bisson J, Churchill R, Wessely S. Psychological debriefing for preventing post traumatic stress disorder (PTSD). *Cochrane Database Syst Rev* 2002;2:CD000560.

31. NHS England. *Serious Incident Framework: Supporting Learning to Prevent Recurrence*. London: NHS England; 2015.

32. Hardcastle M, Kennard D. *Experiences of Mental Health In-Patient Care: Narratives from Service Users, Carers and Professionals*. London: Routledge; 2007.

33. Hinshelwood RD. *Suffering Insanity: Psychoanalytic Essays on Psychosis*. New York: Psychology Press; 2004.

34. Whittington R, Wykes T. An observational study of associations between nurse behaviour and violence in psychiatric hospitals. *J Psychiatr Ment Health Nurs* 1994;1:85–92.

35. Richards D. A field study of critical incident stress debriefing versus critical incident stress management. *J Ment Health* 2001;10:351–362.

36. Nurmi LA. The sinking of the Estonia: the effects of critical incident stress debriefing (CISD) on rescuers. *Int J Emerg Ment Health* 1999;1:23–31.

37. Matthews LR. Effect of staff debriefing on posttraumatic stress symptoms after assaults by community housing residents. *Psychiatr Serv* 2006;49:207–212.

38. Bell JL. Traumatic event debriefing: service delivery designs and the role of social work. *Soc Work* 1995;40:36–43.

Working with relatives and friends

Nicki Moone

Introduction

The term 'carers' will be used throughout this chapter to outline approaches and considerations when working with relatives and significant others of service users on the inpatient ward. However, it should be made clear that not all individuals may see themselves as 'carers' so mental health practitioners need to be mindful of this when working with a service user's family and friends (1).

The UK has seen in the last few decades a significant shift in the way that mental health services are delivered (2–4). A move towards community-based care, except in periods of high distress and acute illness, has meant that the role of relatives and carers of those with mental health difficulties has likewise changed (5, 6). Service users are likely to have been in the community in the weeks preceding admission to an inpatient ward and are likely to have received informal care from those close to them (7). There has been increasing recognition of the role that informal carers play and that they should be considered as partners in the process (8). Government policies have introduced strategies to highlight and support the role that carers play and ensure their needs are addressed (9).

Within mental health services, the 'Triangle of Care' provides specific guidance to support carers, acknowledging the vital role they play in the service user's journey towards recovery (10). Central to this triangle is the intention to promote collaboration and develop responsive services that provide both information and support. The six standards that underpin the 'Triangle of Care' provide a benchmark against which services can measure their performance (Figure 26.1).

Mental health services must be well rehearsed in best practice to promote carer involvement (11, 12). In adapting and adopting a carer-inclusive approach, services must aim at meeting the demands of carer involvement at all stages of the service user's journey toward recovery (13). Significantly, the Care Act 2014 has ensured that carers are given equivalent entitlement to support as those that they care for, giving the caring role the recognition it merits (14) by ensuring support for carers in their role and maintaining their well-being. This includes an obligation on the part of mental health services to involve carers in developing the service user's support plan (15).

Understanding the experiences of relatives and carers

The experiences of carers in the events leading up to hospital admission need to be understood to help develop a service that is responsive and sensitive to their needs. Their expectations can provide some suggestions of how services need to evolve to develop an all-inclusive approach to meet with the guiding principles of best practice initiatives (16). Often overlooked, the skills that are necessary to work effectively with carers require exploration and may be best enhanced by understanding the carer perspective and experience (17).

Carers can experience a range of emotions at the point at which they come into contact with mental health services. This is particularly so when it is their first contact and therefore most likely within an acute care setting or inpatient ward. The ward may be an unfamiliar place and the language used and the way mental health services work may seem confusing. Admission to hospital may have been traumatic, precipitated by difficult events that have included involvement of agencies such as police and social services. Carers can often be physically exhausted due to lack of sleep, worry, disruptions at home, and changes in usual daily routines as the service user has become increasingly unwell. Consideration therefore needs to be given to the following:

- Relatives and carers may have been coping with stressful situations 24 hours a day in the days and weeks leading up to the admission.
- Events leading up to admission may have been traumatic.
- They may have been struggling to manage difficult behaviours with little or no support or advice.
- They have a strong emotional connection to the person who has been admitted, it is natural for them to want to be involved.
- They will be exhausted, fearful, and may have feelings of guilt that they should have done more. There may also be a sense of relief that they will now get the support that they need.
- The impact of someone becoming mentally unwell can lead to other difficulties, ranging from financial concerns through to becoming isolated from other support networks.

To understand these experiences in more detail and their potential effect upon carers, further consideration should be given to stress and well-being as well as emotional and practical impact.

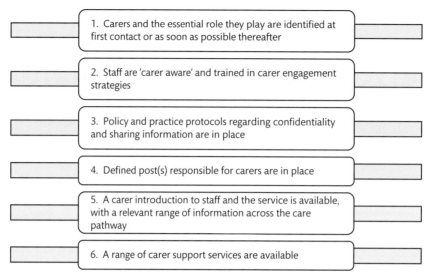

Figure 26.1 The key six standards of the 'Triangle of Care'.

1. Carers and the essential role they play are identified at first contact or as soon as possible thereafter

2. Staff are 'carer aware' and trained in carer engagement strategies

3. Policy and practice protocols regarding confidentiality and sharing information are in place

4. Defined post(s) responsible for carers are in place

5. A carer introduction to staff and the service is available, with a relevant range of information across the care pathway

6. A range of carer support services are available

Stress and well-being

General levels of stress, widely acknowledged as a major factor in reduced well-being, can be high when support is being provided to someone with mental health difficulties (18). Considering the range of emotional experiences and managing significant changes in their lives, carers and relatives can be prone to developing physical or mental health difficulties themselves (19). At times, relationships within the family or social network can become strained as each person tries to adapt to what has been happening. It can be particularly difficult for children to understand what is happening to their relative. Changes in the family routine can be unsettling and this can be evident occasionally by changes in children's behaviour at home or at school. It is therefore unsurprising that a high proportion of carers report difficulties in physical and mental well-being (19, 20). Carers can also neglect their health needs (21). They also report that a significant contributing factor to increased levels of stress can be a lack of support from services, and thus not getting the help that they need, further compounding stress.

Regarding the health needs of carers, it can be easily understood that they might neglect their own health when prioritizing supporting someone who is acutely unwell (21). The reasons for this can be varied and may be practical in nature, for example, relating to not having the time while trying to support the service user. Equally, being distracted by the competing demands of the caring role alongside usual everyday life may result in the carer overlooking their own health needs. There are other potential reasons why carers may not look after their health or seek out help and this relates to how this would impact the pivotal role that they play and the fear that they may not be able to continue with their caring role. It is therefore imperative that mental health practitioners take time to consider the well-being of carers and ascertain whether they have any difficulties. This can provide a sense that services care and acknowledge the impact that caring can have on health and well-being. As indicated earlier, carers report that a significant contributing factor to increased levels of stress can be the lack of support from services.

Emotional impact of caring

The experiences of carers supporting a service user before admission to hospital can be emotionally exhausting. When a carer is supporting a service user in acute mental distress, the feelings experienced can be varied and the impact wide ranging (22). In particular, if this is the first experience of contact with mental health services there can be a sense of being overwhelmed and confused by the way services operate and the terms and language used, leading to feelings of loss, fear, and frustration. The parents of a service user may have thoughts about the possible causes of the service user's mental health issues as well as a sense of isolation and stigma (23). Although these feelings can be experienced at the point of admission, practitioners should keep in mind that similar feelings can occur at any stage throughout the service user's journey towards recovery.

Services must capture and use the wealth of knowledge that the carer has of the service user's life before admission as this can greatly inform the recovery process (24). The carer may be aware of the aspirations that the service user has and adjusting to changes in their general functioning can be difficult for the carer to come to terms with. Evidence suggests that approximately 40% of carers experience distress and depression (25). Of relevance to mental health carers, it appears that dealing with behavioural problems is associated with the highest levels of distress (26). Significantly, the evidence suggests that distress is most notable in those new to their caring role (27).

Practical impact of caring

A range of areas can be impacted by the caring role, including from financial concerns through to isolation from friends and family. The following list highlights areas that mental health practitioners should consider when meeting with carers in the ward environment:

- *Financial implications*: supporting a service user can come at considerable financial cost. Providing additional support to ensure adequate dietary intake alongside attendance at appointments can lead to extra expense. If the carer is working, the disruption caused by the caring role can lead to further financial repercussions, which in turn can add to the stress experienced.

- *Disturbance of daily routines*: in the weeks leading up to admission the carer may have been involved in many activities to support the service user ranging from seeking help and support through to ensuring medication concordance. Thus, the routines of both the carer and the wider family may have been disrupted, which can be disconcerting and lead to feelings of stress and not being able to manage competing demands.
- *The consuming nature of caring*: the caring role can become the focus in a carer's life. The demands of supporting someone who is experiencing mental distress can be overwhelming and the carer may have dedicated all their time to keeping the service user emotionally and physically safe before admission. Taking on responsibility and then relinquishing it upon admission to hospital can be a difficult period of adjustment.
- *Social isolation*: many carers can become isolated from family and friends as they have increasingly focused on their caring role, adding to the emotional impact of the situation.
- *Difficulties at work*: although there is recognition of the need to support those in a caring role in the workplace, the reality may be different. Needing to take time out of work to support the service user can lead to difficulties, further compounding the stress experienced by the carer.

What do relatives and carers expect from acute inpatient services?

Mental health practitioners must meet the needs of carers and families and involve them in all aspects of care delivery (28, 29). In simple terms, carers want to be involved in decisions that have a direct impact on the service user as well as to receive timely information to support their carer role (30). Carers want to be acknowledged for the role that they play in the service user's life and, crucially, be listened to by professionals (31).

Sharing information with carers

Issues around sharing information or not with carers remains a complex issue for mental health practitioners. National Health Service (NHS) trusts have local guidelines that support staff in making decisions about how best to share information with a service user's carer. However, there are several factors that need to be considered. On the one hand, services must keep in mind the impact that not sharing information can have on both an emotional and practical level for both the service user and the carer. On the other hand, seeking consent from a service user to share information with their carer at a time of acute mental distress can be problematic (32). Similarly, while mental health professionals are bound by professional, legal, and ethical obligations, there are also codes of professional conduct and law protecting the service user's right to confidentiality. Similarly, professionals should also respect the carer's right to confidentiality. The following key themes should be considered:

- Carers should be given sufficient information to support them in their role.

- Consent to share information should be sought early in the admission from the service user and clearly recorded.
- Consent should be revisited throughout the admission with the service user as appropriate.
- Explore what exactly the service user is willing to share.
- Work with both the service user and the carer throughout the care pathway to ensure commitment to good practice guidelines.
- Discuss and seek clarification on any potential challenges to sharing information.

Receiving information from carers

Carers can also expect respect to be afforded to their privacy and right to confidentiality, the exception being if someone is felt to be at risk or harm if the information was not shared. It is not always easy to share information with professionals about a loved one and this warrants consideration. If the carer has concerns about the service user's presentation or aspects of their behaviour, it can be difficult to discuss this openly and the carer should be afforded an opportunity to do so. The carer may be reluctant to share information which may upset the service user and therefore should be assured a right to privacy. Ideally, the goal will be that all information is shared openly between carers, professionals, and the service user and this can be done over time as the service user moves towards recovery.

Adopting a carer-inclusive approach

Working with relatives and carers in an inpatient setting requires a collaborative relationship and that consideration is given to the expertise in supporting the service user that the carer has shown in the build up to the hospital admission. It is crucial to be empathic and understand the carer's perspective. The carer will have been acting with the best intention often in very difficult circumstances to support the service user. Each carer has a unique set of experiences and skills, and help, support, and advice during a crisis are often well received and can offer much-needed reassurance. In light of national policy and guidelines, acute inpatient services should consider the following carer-valued expectations:

- The opportunity to talk to someone on the ward.
- To be included throughout the admission process.
- Opportunities to be involved in all stages of treatment through to recovery and discharge unless deemed otherwise (issues of consent and right to information need to be considered).
- To be given information that is both written and verbal about treatment, diagnosis, and follow-up care.
- To be given advice on how to manage difficult behaviour and self-harm.
- To be offered an assessment of their needs.
- To be signposted to additional practical and emotional support.

The opportunity to talk to someone

As previously indicated, prior to the admission to the inpatient ward, carers will have been coping with a range of difficult experiences that may have had a considerable impact on their well-being. Giving them the opportunity to talk to staff shows recognition of their valuable role. In fact, offering time to a carer can begin a process of reducing the emotional impact that caring may have and be the first step in developing a working partnership. Initial conversations will enable practitioners to ascertain whether the carer needs help and support and to advise on the options available. This may be the first time that someone has afforded the carer the opportunity to share their experiences. Indeed, sharing experiences with a professional can be reassuring. Importantly, the communication should be a two-way process throughout the duration of the admission to hospital. Taking time to listen will help staff to have a clear picture of events leading up to admission and to identify specific issues that may warrant further consideration. The carer may have questions about the service user's recent experiences so the type of information that is shared and how this is done should be in line with policies and procedures for sharing information.

Being included

The opportunity for the carer to be included throughout the service user's journey through mental health services is essential unless deemed otherwise in light of confidentiality issues or risks to the service user and/or carer. The carer's knowledge of the service user can prove invaluable when planning care and the recovery journey. Upon discharge, it can often be carers who will assume some responsibility for the care plan implementation and this reinforces the importance of cooperation and partnership. Listening to the views of carers and involving them in the decision-making process can ensure better concordance with the treatment plan and therefore better outcomes for the service user. The following questions warrant consideration by the ward team when working with carers:

- Are carers able to be present when decisions are made?
- Are there opportunities for carers to meet with professionals regularly throughout the service user's time on the ward?
- Is information sharing with the carer regularly reviewed with the service user?
- Are carers routinely asked about concerns or difficulties that they may have?
- Are carers asked about the best course of action in light of their experience with the service user?
- Are carers asked to provide feedback on difficulties encountered with the treatment plan?
- Do all team members view carers as experts in their own right?
- Is feedback on the service provided regularly sought from carers and suggestions acted upon?

To be given information

Inpatient services must offer a range of information to support the carer in their role. Attempts to share and provide information need to be explored throughout the admission and not be seen as a one-off event at the time of admission. At times of crisis, the ability to retain information may be reduced which is why it is essential that providing information is regularly attempted throughout the admission (13). In the first instance, the primary worker should take responsibility for sharing basic information, including arrangements to meet with the wider ward team to discuss concerns in more detail. Regarding written information, it goes without saying that it should be clear, concise, and regularly reviewed by the ward team to ensure ongoing relevance.

The information to be shared should include key themes regarding mental health, treatment, and information sharing, alongside an overview of the team as shown in Figure 26.2.

To be given specific advice about managing difficult behaviours

It is likely that leading up to admission to hospital the carer may have been involved in handling and coping with difficult and stressful behaviours. It is therefore important to offer clear and concise information about such behaviours; some suggestions follow.

Self-harm

Supporting someone who self-harms can provoke strong feelings in the carer and this needs time to be explored (33). The carer may require advice on how to manage these feelings and how to respond to the service user's behaviour, including information on how to look after themselves at times of such stressful situations. It is important to acknowledge feelings of fear and anger and suggest strategies to help manage feelings of responsibility and blame. Having resources such a list of useful websites may help the practitioner to signpost the carer towards appropriate ongoing support.

Difficult behaviours

Several behaviours can be exhibited because of being acutely unwell or in extreme distress. Interacting with the person they care for may have become increasingly difficult, leading to feelings of frustration and fear. Difficult behaviours that include aggressive behaviour can be particularly distressing for the carer so they need advice and reassurance on how they have managed it. It is useful to offer information and advice on possible reasons for the behaviour as well as how the behaviour will be managed in the hospital setting. Again, it is important to signpost the carer to additional support and to provide useful contacts such as local carer support groups.

To be offered a carer assessment

When someone provides a regular or substantial amount of care to a family member or a friend, they are entitled to support from the local council and mental health services have a duty to offer a

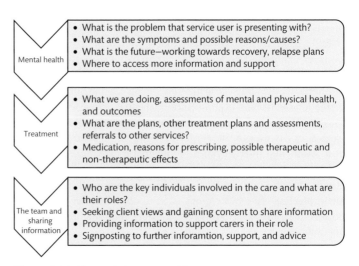

Figure 26.2 Sharing information with carers.

carer's assessment. Although there is no definition of what constitutes either regular or substantial care, if more than one relative or carer has been involved in supporting the service user then each is entitled to a carer assessment in their own right (29). The purpose of the carer assessment is to explore the impact that the caring role is having on their life and well-being and its outcome should be a plan that will support the carer in their role. This plan can include additional support that the carer can access alongside practical support that may be needed. The practice of conducting a carer assessment provides the carer with the opportunity to be listened to and to receive recognition of their role. Importantly, if the ward does not routinely offer carers assessments then the ward staff need to be aware of who is best placed to complete them and how to refer the carer to them.

To be signposted to support

The expectation here is that the team will be able to signpost carers to additional available support. The ward must have a list of contacts and resources that can be shared with carers, including:

- further sources of advice and information including information on carer assessments and how to access financial advice and information on benefits
- useful contacts—a list of local and national support groups, forums, and carers courses that can be accessed
- carer rights—many carers remain unaware of the rights they have so this information should be readily shared with them.

Mental health practitioner skills to support relatives and carers

It is important to consider the skills that are essential to developing a therapeutic and collaborative relationship with carers and relatives. In keeping with contemporary mental health care, there is an expectation that carers and relatives will meet mental health professionals who convey warmth, empathy, and commitment (34). Specifically, professionals need to be proactive in offering support and information which includes:

- that the expertise of the relative or carer must be acknowledged
- building an honest and respectful relationship from the start
- that a collaborative relationship needs to be maintained over time.

Skills and values needed to work with relatives and carers

Being a mental health practitioner requires considerable knowledge and interpersonal skills. Central to it are core therapeutic skills needed to ensure engagement and to develop a rapport including communication skills, active listening, using reflective statements, affirmation, and summarizing. These skills underpin developing a meaningful relationship with carers. There are also interpersonal skills and qualities on the part of the mental health practitioner that need to be demonstrated when working with carers. Conveying warmth and understanding alongside patience and attentiveness are key. In line with a focus on recovery, the mental health practitioner should display a hopeful and optimistic

outlook and be personally reflective and reflexive (35). Also, in line with contemporary professional values and effective mental health care, the values of empathy, compassion, and treating individuals with dignity and respect are critical to meeting the needs of service users and their relatives and carers. Finally, it is essential that mental health practitioners keep an open mind and avoid bias based on their own interpretation of events and are mindful of understanding the carer's perspective.

Communication skills

Working with carers and relatives who may have experienced feelings of emotional distress requires an ability to communicate effectively and without it, a collaborative partnership is unlikely to follow. Poor initial communication with a carer can greatly hinder future attempts to work as partners in care. In fact, poor communication between hospital staff and carers can lead to anguish and frustration, and is a common topic of NHS complaints (36). Taking time to consider practical ways to engage with carers and foster effective communication can improve carer experiences.

Active listening

Active listening to the experiences of carers will convey a sense of acknowledgement and validation of their recent experiences and of the difficulties they have encountered and what these have meant to them. This, in itself, can act as a source of comfort as they will sense both concern and interest on the part of the practitioner. Active listening requires verbal and non-verbal interaction skills as well as the ability to use silence when appropriate, to 'hear' what is being said. All of this is particularly relevant when working with carers who are experiencing distress and emotional upset.

Working in partnership

Mental health practitioners should consider the carer to be an expert by the very nature of their experiences. It is the carer who will have been present during a period of deterioration for the service user and will have assumed various roles during the lead up to admission to hospital, often in difficult circumstances.

The term partnership implies both parts sharing the same goal, namely working towards the recovery of the service user. However, mental health practitioners can feel unprepared to work as partners with carers (37), which requires developing a carer-inclusive approach that acknowledges their expertise as well as the sense of bewilderment and stress that are experiencing when the service user is admitted to an acute inpatient ward (38). Self-awareness on the part of the mental health practitioners and exploration of their attitudes towards carers can ensure that the partnership garners the best outcomes for the service user. In particular, understanding how to respond to criticism of mental health services in a non-defensive way can ensure the principles of carer inclusiveness are embraced (39).

Exploring attitudes and beliefs as a ward team and reflecting on how best to work in genuine partnership with carers require consideration of both personal and professional values. On a busy acute inpatient ward, it may be best to remember simple key points to support the approach to carers (Figure 26.3).

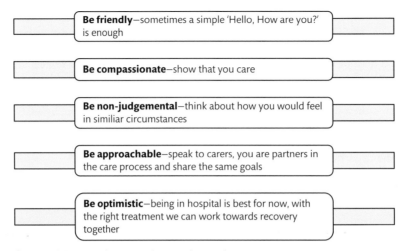

Be friendly—sometimes a simple 'Hello, How are you?' is enough

Be compassionate—show that you care

Be non-judgemental—think about how you would feel in similiar circumstances

Be approachable—speak to carers, you are partners in the care process and share the same goals

Be optimistic—being in hospital is best for now, with the right treatment we can work towards recovery together

Figure 26.3 A simple approach to working with carers.

Working with a carer on an inpatient ward: a clinical vignette

The following clinical vignette highlights how using a systematic and considered approach to meeting a carer's needs can transform and enhance their experience.

Martin is a 20-year-old service user who lives at home with his mother and sister. He first became unwell approximately 1 year ago, when he left university after just one term. His family had tried to get him to get help but he had steadfastly refused saying that they needed help, not him. He was referred to services 1 month ago, following an argument with a neighbour who Martin believed had been spying on him. Following this event, he was arrested and assessed while in custody, where it became apparent that he was very suspicious and believed that he was being monitored by government spies. Although prescribed olanzapine at the time, he refused to take it and his behaviour became increasingly worrying for his family. He was admitted to the ward a week ago, having been found in the middle of the night walking on the motorway.

Tracey, Martin's mother, has given up her job as an administrator with a local building company to care for him. She feels that since Martin became unwell their family life has been shattered and they are at the mercy of his moods and unpredictable behaviour. She is very upset and worried about her son and thus has been asked to consider taking antidepressants by her general practitioner. She is particularly worried about her daughter who is struggling to cope with the changes in her brother's behaviour. Tracey has tried to get help for Martin but felt that he had to be critically unwell before anyone listened to her. When Martin left university, she knew he was mentally unwell but he refused to get help. Tracey has seen him deteriorate over the last few months during which he has become anxious, isolative, irritable, and very suspicious.

Before Martin was admitted to the ward, Tracey felt overwhelmed. She felt that she had no support and that services were not responsive to her attempts to get urgent help for her son. She had no useful information that she could use to help her manage or cope and she felt lost and alone.

By adopting the approach outlined and working alongside Tracey, her thoughts and feelings can be transformed to provide her with a sense of optimism and confidence to manage in the future.

Someone to talk to

Tracey meets with her son's named nurse on the ward and with the wider team when she requests it. She has been given time to talk through her experiences and the impact that recent events have had on her and her family. She has been signposted to additional support and has been given a guide on useful contacts, including a local carers' course where she can meet people with similar experiences.

To be given information

Tracey has been given information that is specific to Martin. At first, he would not allow any information to be shared with her which was fully explained to her and she was given information that would help her situation. The named nurse spent time checking with Martin throughout his admission to ensure that his views were respected. Tracey also shared her thoughts and was given assurance of her right to privacy in line with protocols. Martin eventually was happy that Tracey had the information that she needed. She seems less stressed to him.

To understand rights as a carer

Tracey was given an information sheet that included information on her rights as a carer and on her right to have a carer's assessment. Tracey now has a carer plan which indicates the support that she needs.

To be a partner in the care process

Tracey was supported to feel as an important part of the care team. She was involved in decisions about Martin's discharge and felt listened to when she suggested that some of the planned interventions were not feasible given Martin's current mental health.

Improving the carer experience

Tracey feels proud of her son and feels that as a family they have grown because of their recent experiences. She feels that she has developed some useful skills to manage and is looking forward to the future; she feels positive and reassured about it.

Practical considerations for inpatient services when working with carers

- *Identification of carers.* Carers should be identified at the point of admission to hospital. It is important to consider that there may be more than one carer involved and this should be clarified early on.
- *Staff training.* All staff should receive carers training and this should not be seen as an isolated event. Staff should regularly have opportunities to explore and consider issues related to carers and the service that they are offering. The team should ensure regular informal and formal opportunities to meet as a team and with carers to review and revisit their approach to working with them.
- *Information sharing.* Alongside local policies and guidelines for best practice for sharing information, staff should endeavour to learn from their experiences and use case examples to explore lessons learnt as well as more complex issues around sharing information with carers. This will promote greater confidence and competence.
- *All staff should be carer champions.* Although it is useful to have a designated role of a 'carers' lead', all staff should take responsibility to ensure that carer needs are addressed. Each team member being responsive to carer requests and enquiries avoids delays in meeting carer needs and enhances the working relationships with them.
- *Carer information packs.* Carers should receive information that includes an overview of services and relevant information related to the specific issues of the service user. This information should be regularly reviewed and updated. Ideally, each pack should be adapted to meet the specific needs of the carer.
- *A range of options to carers* should be offered on the ward with a view to support them and promote their involvement in the care process.
- *The inpatient team* should ensure that all staff are aware of their role in supporting carers and how best to build on strengths and address needs. Support for carers should be timely, prompt, and provide an account of the nature of acute mental distress and its impact on them.
- *Working closely with other services and agencies* will ensure that relatives and carers are offered a seamless service.

Summary

Current national directives, policies, and guidelines acknowledge the role that relatives and carers play and outline how services should respond to build on carers' strengths and address their needs (40). Modernization of mental health services has had a direct impact on carers and families as the development of alternatives to admission services means that service users often stay at home longer before admission to hospital (41). An admission to an inpatient facility can be precipitated by periods of disruption to many aspects of both the service user's and the carer's day-to-day life (42). Working effectively with carers requires consideration of the impact that the caring role has had and of the ways in which the ward can facilitate an effective working relationship. Attention to best practice, guidance, and protocols go some way to addressing the need to be carer inclusive. A systematic approach to addressing the needs of carers must be adopted to improve not only the carers' experiences but also service user outcomes.

REFERENCES

1. Molyneaux V, Butchard S, Simpson J, Murray C. Reconsidering the term 'carer': a critique of the universal adoption of the term 'carer'. *Ageing Soc* 2011;31:422–437.
2. Norman IJ, Peck E. Working together in adult community mental health services: an inter-professional dialogue. *J Ment Health* 1999;8:217–230.
3. Wood VJ, Curtis SE, Gesler W, et al. Creating 'therapeutic landscapes' for mental health carers in inpatient settings: a dynamic perspective on permeability and inclusivity. *Soc Sci Med* 2013;91:122–129.
4. Curtis S. *Space, Place and Mental Health.* Geographies of Health Series. Farnham: Ashgate; 2010.
5. Milligan C. Location or dis-location? Towards a conceptualization of people and place in the care-giving experience. *Soc Cult Geogr* 2003;4:455–470.
6. Wiles J. Daily geographies of caregivers: mobility, routine, scale. *Soc Sci Med* 2003;57:1307–1325.
7. Milligan C, Atkinson S, Skinner M, Wiles J. Geographies of care: a commentary. *N Z Geog* 2007;63:135–140.
8. Department of Health. *Recognised Valued and Supported: Next Steps for the Carers Strategy.* London: Department of Health; 2010.
9. Simpson EL, House AO. User and carer involvement in mental health services: from rhetoric to science. *Br J Psychiatry* 2003;183:89–91.
10. Worthington A, Rooney P. *The Triangle of Care, Carers Included: A Guide to Best Practice in Acute Mental Health Care.* London: The Princess Royal Trust for Carers, National Mental Health Development Unit; 2010.
11. Royal College of Psychiatrists. Good psychiatric practice: confidentiality and information sharing. 2018. http://www.rcpsych.ac.uk/healthadvice/partnersincarecampaign/carersandconfidentiality.aspx
12. National Institute for Health and Care Excellence. Psychosis and schizophrenia in adults: treatment and management. Clinical guideline [CG178]. 2014. https://www.nice.org.uk/guidance/cg178
13. Crawford MJ, Rutter D, Manley C, et al. Systematic review of involving patients in the planning and development of health care. *BMJ* 2002;325:1263.
14. Department of Health & Social Care. Care Act 2014: care and support statutory guidance. 2015. https://www.gov.uk/government/publications/care-act-statutory-guidance/care-and-support-statutory-guidance
15. Cree L, Brooks HL, Berzins K, Fraser C, Lovell K, Bee P. Carers' experiences of involvement in care planning: a qualitative exploration of the facilitators and barriers to engagement with mental health services. *BMC Psychiatry* 2015;15:1.
16. Rowe J. Great expectations: a systematic review of the literature on the role of family carers in severe mental illness, and their relationships and engagement with professionals. *J Psychiatr Ment Health Nurs* 2012;19:70–82.
17. Wood VJ, Curtis SE, Gesler W, et al. Creating 'therapeutic landscapes' for mental health carers in inpatient settings: a dynamic perspective on permeability and inclusivity. *Soc Sci Med* 2013;91:122–129.
18. Oyebode J. Assessment of carers' psychological needs. *Adv Psychiatr Treat* 2003;9:45–53.
19. Cormac I, Tihanyi P. Meeting the mental and physical healthcare needs of carers. *Adv Psychiatr Treat* 2006;12:162–172.

20. Smith L, Onwumere J, Craig T, McManus S, Bebbington P, Kuipers E. Mental and physical illness in caregivers: results from an English national survey sample. *Br J Psychiatry* 2014;205:197–203.

21. Pinquart M, Sörensen S. Correlates of physical health of informal caregivers: a meta-analysis. *J Gerontol B Psychol Sci Soc Sci* 2007;62:P126–137.

22. Fadden G, Bebbington P, Kuipers L. The burden of care: the impact of functional psychiatric illness on the patient's family. *Br J Psychiatry* 1987;150:285–292.

23. Albert R, Simpson A. Double deprivation: a phenomenological study into the experience of being a carer during a mental health crisis. *J Adv Nurs* 2015;71:2753–2762.

24. Bee P, Brooks H, Fraser C, Lovell K. Professional perspectives on service user and carer involvement in mental health care planning: a qualitative study. *Int J Nurs Stud* 2015;52:1834–1845.

25. Pinquart M, Sorensen S. Associations of stressors and uplifts of caregiving with caregiver burden and depressive mood: a meta-analysis. *J Gerontol B Psychol Sci Soc Sci* 2003;58: P112–P128.

26. Ornstein K, Gaugler JE. The problem with "problem behaviors": a systematic review of the association between individual patient behavioral and psychological symptoms and caregiver depression and burden within the dementia patient–caregiver dyad. *Int Psychogeriatr* 2012;24:1536–1552.

27. Hirst M. Carer distress: a prospective population based study. *Soc Sci Med* 2005;61:697–708.

28. Department of Health. *Healthy Lives, Healthy People: Our Strategy for Public Health in England*. London: The Stationery Office; 2010.

29. Seddon D, Robinson C, Reeves C, Tommis Y, Woods B, Russell I. In their own right: translating the policy of carer assessment into practice. *Br J Soc Work* 2007;37:1335–1352.

30. Simpson EL, House AO. Involving users in the delivery and evaluation of mental health services: systematic review. *BMJ* 2002;325:1265.

31. Repper J, Breeze J. User and carer involvement in the training and education of health professionals: a review of the literature. *Int J Nurs Stud* 2007;44:511–519.

32. Slade M, Pinfold V, Rapaport J, et al. Best practice when service users do not consent to sharing information with carers. *Br J Psychiatry* 2007;190:148–155.

33. McLaughlin C, McGowan I, O'Neill S, Kernohan G. The burden of living with and caring for a suicidal family member. *J Ment Health* 2014;23:236–240.

34. Birch L. Strategies to implement the recommendations of the Francis report. *J Healthc Manag* 2015;21:558–563.

35. Scaife J. *Supervising the Reflective Practitioner: An Essential Guide to Theory and Practice*. Hove: Routledge; 2014.

36. Parliamentary and Health Service Ombudsman. Communication and complaint handling. 2011. http://www.ombudsman.org.uk/listening-and-learning-2011/case-studies2/communication-and-complaint-handling

37. Stanbridge RI, Burbach FR, Rapsey EH, Leftwich SH, McIver CC. Improving partnerships with families and carers in in-patient mental health services for older people: a staff training programme and family liaison service. *J Fam Ther* 2013;35:176–197.

38. Walker E, Jane Dewar B. How do we facilitate carers' involvement in decision making? *J Adv Nurs* 2001;34:329–337.

39. Coyle J. Understanding dissatisfied users: developing a framework for comprehending criticisms of health care work. *J Adv Nurs* 1999;30:723–731.

40. Petch A, Cook A, Miller E. Partnership working and outcomes: do health and social care partnerships deliver for users and carers? *Health Soc Care Community* 2013;21:623–633.

41. Department of Health and Social Care. *No Health Without Mental Health: A Cross-Government Mental Health Outcomes Strategy for People of all Ages*. London: Stationery Office; 2011.

42. Carers UK. In sickness and in health. 2012. https://www.carersuk.org/for-professionals/policy/policy-library/in-sickness-and-in-health

27

Accreditation of inpatient mental health services

Robert Chaplin

Introduction

This chapter outlines how a programme of accreditation can help improve the standards of care on inpatient units by describing the Accreditation for Inpatient Mental Health Services (AIMS). The development of and need for accreditation are outlined with evidence of how accreditation adds value to the process of audit. There is a discussion of how data obtained from national audits of inpatient care and accreditation have been used to describe the quality of inpatient mental health services. There follows a report of the local use of the accreditation programme for an acute mental health inpatient ward for men in Oxford. Finally, some key standards are provided in order to describe what a high-quality inpatient unit may look like.

The need for accreditation

Since the Sainsbury Centre for Mental Health (1) carried out a survey of the quality of care in acute inpatient wards, highlighting the existence of unpleasant and non-therapeutic settings, there have been persisting concerns regarding inpatient psychiatric wards (2). Policies and guidance have been introduced in an attempt to improve the quality and safety on psychiatric inpatient wards. These included the clinical guidelines for the management of disturbed behaviour on inpatient wards established by the National Institute for Health and Care Excellence (3). However, when auditing the implementation of these guidelines, the Healthcare Commission (4) funded and the Royal College of Psychiatrists managed the National Audit of Violence. This concluded that wards are often noisy, unsafe environments, providing little structure for service users. Nursing staff felt poorly trained to deal with the challenging situations that occurred on the wards.

Despite attempts to reform and modernize the National Health Service (NHS) through the vision set out in the NHS Plan (5), healthcare staff have voiced scepticism and resistance to organizational change. Perceptions regarding 'top-down approaches' originating and imposed by government or senior managers have left ordinary staff feeling unengaged with little opportunity to influence plans (6). Furthermore, simply distributing guidelines or educational material rarely changes clinical behaviour of staff (7).

In an attempt to both improve the quality of care on inpatient wards and challenge this struggle with motivation for change, the Royal College of Psychiatrists developed the AIMS programme. It was felt that there had been too much focus on problems without recognition of the excellent work that staff do under difficult circumstances and that accreditation would help recognize and reward wards that achieve high standards (8).

Accreditation

First developed in 1917 in the US, accreditation is a system of non-governmental self-regulation in which an independent agency defines and monitors standards of quality in hospitals and other health service providers participating in the scheme (9). The earliest accreditation programme in the UK was the Hospital Accreditation Scheme for non-acute community hospitals, with its standards first published in 1988. It was found that accreditation tended to encourage change through a clearer organizational focus on driving quality improvement and facilitated communication between staff, managers, and other sites (9). Indeed, the goal of AIMS is to foster those principles by supporting wards in adopting common national standards and building a culture of improvement (8).

Currently in the UK, accreditation is being developed in a variety of health care settings. These include dental services, diagnostic services (pathology and radiology), allergy and immunology endoscopy, occupational health, and anaesthetic departments.

The process of accreditation was first introduced by the Royal College of Psychiatrists' Centre for Quality Improvement as a means of improving the quality of the administration of electroconvulsive therapy. There had been three national audits during the 1980s and 1990s carried out by the Royal College of Psychiatrists into the administration of electroconvulsive therapy which had shown a failure of practice to improve against key standards of care and administration. The adoption of accreditation, which involved the awarding of a certificate to reward the meeting of these key standards, was associated with a sustained improvement in practice over the period of 2004–2011 (10).

Accreditation was hence rolled out to augment other quality improvement networks, including inpatient mental health units, to support audits which were already in the process of being carried out. Essentially, accreditation is a voluntary process, as distinct from statutory regulation by the Care Quality Commission and is self-funded by the member organizations. The AIMS process involves a period of self-review, which requires the completion of questionnaires by staff, service users, and carers and an examination of healthcare records and policies and procedures. This is followed by a peer review visit by members of other wards enrolled in the programme together with a service user or carer. On the basis of the findings of these reviews, the ward's strengths and weaknesses are identified and a recommendation is made regarding the ward's accreditation status by the AIMS Accreditation Advisory Committee, which is then ratified by the Royal College's Education, Training and Standards Committee, a process that altogether lasts at least 8 months.

AIMS requires its member wards to demonstrate adherence to a common set of national standards drawn from a number of sources including the Mental Health Policy Implementation Guide (11, 12) and the findings of the National Confidential Inquiry into Suicide and Homicide (13) as well as consultations with frontline staff, service users, and carers.

The process of accreditation

Initially, an expert advisory group with strong multidisciplinary membership was set up. This included psychiatrists, inpatient nurses, psychologists, occupational therapists, ward managers, service users, and carers. The evidence for good-quality care was reviewed and a series of standards developed which undergo 2 yearly revision. These standards are divided into three types:

1. Failure to meet these standards would result in a significant threat to patient safety, rights, or dignity and/or would breach the law.
2. Standards that an accredited ward/unit would be expected to meet.
3. Standards that an excellent ward/unit should meet or standards that are not the direct responsibility of the ward/unit.

Examples of some of the standards are shown in Table 27.1 and they are grouped here with an example of one or more key standards to reflect each theme of care. These standards have been deliberately selected to give an illustration of the breadth and comprehensiveness of the types of care assessed in AIMS from a more comprehensive list of over 100 standards. They should also give an overview of high-quality inpatient care.

Following the development of standards, a series of instruments to measure these standards were then developed. These included questionnaires to be completed by service users, staff, carers, and the ward manager, an environmental audit checklist, an audit of policies procedures and protocols, and a case notes review. Each ward then completes a self-review and submits that to the system administrators. Subsequently, there is a peer review visit to the ward comprising

a psychiatrist, a nurse, and a service user from an external service which serves to check the data from the self-review and to interview staff and provide support and suggestions for practice development. A report is presented to an independent Accreditation Committee at the Royal College of Psychiatrists' Centre for Quality Improvement which comprises multidisciplinary professional staff, service users, and carers who work in inpatient care. Accreditation can be granted for a 3-year period, deferred, or not granted. Accreditation is not granted if the service fails to meet one or more 'type 1' standards and do not show the capacity to meet these within a short time. If there is the capacity to meet these standards, then accreditation is 'deferred' until they have been met.

Standards

The standards which inpatient units are judged against are derived from a number of sources. These include the Department of Health Policy Implementation Guides, the findings of the National Confidential Inquiry into Suicide and Homicide (14), guidance from the National Institute of Health and Care Excellence, recommendations by the National Health Service Estates and the Royal College of Psychiatrists about ward design, the National Patient Safety Agency's Safer Wards for Acute Psychiatry Initiative, and recommendations arising from the National Audit of Violence (15). The standards are underpinned by a core set of values developed by expert advisory groups, and have been refined in consultation with frontline staff, patients, carers, other interested groups such as national charities, and professional bodies. The standards cover five domains:

- General standards, including policies, protocols, and staffing-related issues.
- Timely and purposeful admission.
- Safety.
- Environment and facilities.
- Therapies and activities.

The complete set of standards in 2017 is aspirational and services are not expected to meet every standard; services can still be accredited without meeting all the standards. Table 27.1 contains a sample of the standards with at least one example from every domain. Failure to meet one of these standards is likely to defer accreditation.

Results of the original pilot study of AIMS and relevance to current practice

The Accreditation of Mental Health Service Quality Network was piloted initially in 16 acute mental health wards in the UK. An evaluation in 2010 of the effectiveness of the original pilot of the AIMS project (16) reported on the extent to which the first 16 acute mental health wards met the standards required for accreditation. Four wards achieved immediate accreditation while a further 11 were subsequently accredited. The most common reasons for initial failure of accreditation were lack of psychological therapies (7 of the 11 wards), lack of an invitation to patients for one-to-one contact with each patient on daytime shifts (5/11), the presence of ligature points (4/11), and the availability of medical staff for emergencies

Table 27.1 Standards that an accredited inpatient unit would be expected to meet in 2017

Domain	Example of standard
Access and referral	Clear information is made available, in paper and/or electronic format, to patients, carers, and healthcare practitioners on: • a simple description of the ward/unit and its purpose • admission criteria • clinical pathways describing access and discharge • main interventions and treatments available • contact details for the ward/unit and hospital
Control of bed occupancy	Senior clinical staff members make decisions about patient admission or transfer. They can refuse to accept patients if they fear that the mix will compromise safety and/or therapeutic activity
First hour of admission	On admission to the ward/unit, or when the patient is well enough, staff members show the patient around
First 4 hours of admission	Patients have a comprehensive physical health review started within 4 hours of admission and is completed within 1 week, or prior to discharge. It includes: *First 4 hours*: • Details of past medical history • Current medication, including side effects and compliance (information is sought from the patient history and collateral information within the first 4 hours. Further details can be sought from medical reconciliation after this) • Physical observations including blood pressure, heart rate, and respiratory rate *First 24 hours*: • Physical examination • Height, weight • Blood tests (can use recent blood tests if appropriate) • Electrocardiogram
Completing the admission process	All patients have a documented diagnosis and a clinical formulation *Guidance: the formulation includes the presenting problem and predisposing, precipitating, perpetuating, and protective factors as appropriate*
Reviews and care planning	The practitioner develops the care plan collaboratively with the patient and their carer (with patient consent)
Leave from the ward/unit	Patients are sent on leave into the care of carers only with carer agreement and timely contact with them beforehand
Care and therapeutic activities	Activities are provided 7 days a week and out of hours
	Every patient is engaged in active conversation at least twice a day by a staff member
	Patients and carers are offered written and verbal information about the patient's mental illness
	Patients are able to leave the ward/unit to access safe outdoor space every day
	Patients have their medications reviewed at least weekly. Medication reviews include an assessment of therapeutic response, safety, side effects, and adherence to medication regimen
	The safe use of high-risk medication is audited, at least annually and at a service level
Physical health care	The team gives targeted lifestyle advice and provides health promotion activities for patients. This includes: • smoking cessation advice • healthy eating advice • physical exercise advice and opportunities to exercise Long-stay patients who are prescribed mood stabilizers or antipsychotics are reviewed at the start of treatment (baseline), at 3 months, and then annually unless a physical health abnormality arises. The clinician monitors the following information about the patient: • A personal/family history (at baseline and annual review) • Lifestyle review (at every review) • Weight (every week for the first 6 weeks) • Waist circumference (at baseline and annual review) • Blood pressure (at every review) • Fasting plasma glucose/ HbA1c (glycated haemoglobin) (at every review) • Lipid profile (at every review)
Risk and safeguarding	If a patient is identified as at risk of absconding, the team completes a crisis plan, which includes clear instructions for alerting and communicating with carers, people at risk, and the relevant authorities
Discharge planning	The team makes sure that patients who are discharged from hospital to the care of the community team have arrangements in place to be followed up within 1 week of discharge, or within 48 hours of discharge if they are at risk
Interface with other services	There are joint working protocols/care pathways in place to support patients in accessing the following services: • Accident and emergency • Social services • Local and specialist mental health services, e.g. liaison, eating disorders, rehabilitation • Secondary physical healthcare
Capacity and consent	Patients have an assessment of their capacity to consent to admission, care, and treatment within 24 hours of admission

(*continued*)

Table 27.1   Continued

Domain	Example of standard
Patient involvement	Patients and their carers are given the opportunity to feed back about their experiences of using the service, and their feedback is used to improve the service
Carer engagement and support	Carers are involved in discussions about the patient's care, treatment, and discharge planning
Compassion, dignity, and respect	Patients are treated with compassion, dignity, and respect *Guidance: this includes respect of a patient's race, age, sex, gender reassignment, marital status, sexual orientation, maternity, disability, and social background*
Information	The ward/unit has access to interpreters and the patient's relatives are not used in this role unless there are exceptional circumstances
Confidentiality	Confidentiality and its limits are explained to the patient and carer on admission, both verbally and in writing
Ward environment	Male and female patients (self-defined by the patient) have separate bedrooms, toilets, and washing facilities
	There are clear lines of sight to enable staff members to view patients. Measures are taken to address blind spots and ensure sightlines are not impeded, e.g. by using mirrors
	There is an alarm system in place (e.g. panic buttons) and this is easily accessible
Staff:	
• Leadership and culture	Staff members feel able to raise any concerns they may have about standards of care
• Team working	When the team meets for handover, adequate time is allocated to discuss patients' needs, risks, and management plans
• Staff levels and skill mix	There is an identified duty doctor available at all times to attend the ward/unit, including out of hours. The doctor can: • attend the ward/unit within 30 minutes in the event of a psychiatric emergency • attend the ward/unit within 1 hour during normal working hours • attend the ward/unit within 4 hours when out of hours
• Staff induction and retention	All newly qualified staff members are allocated a preceptor to oversee their transition onto the ward/unit
• Appraisal support and supervision	All staff members receive an annual appraisal and personal development planning (or equivalent)
• Staff well-being	Staff members are able to take breaks during their shift that comply with the European Working Time Directive
• Staff training and development	Staff receive training in the use of legal frameworks, such as the Mental Health Act 1983, Section 17 (or equivalent) and the Mental Capacity Act 2005 (or equivalent)
• General management	The team attends business meetings that are held at least monthly
Outcome measurement	Clinical outcome measurement data is collected at two time points (admission and discharge) as a minimum, and at clinical reviews where possible
Audit/service evaluation	A range of local and multicentre clinical audits is conducted which include the use of evidence-based treatments, as a minimum
Learning from complaints and incidents	Staff members share information about any serious untoward incidents involving a patient with the patient themselves and their carer, in line with the Duty of Candour agreement
Commissioning and financial management	The ward/unit is explicitly commissioned or contracted against agreed ward/unit standards. *Guidance: this is detailed in the Service Level Agreement, operational policy, or similar, and has been agreed by funders*

Source data from *Standards for Acute Inpatient Services – Working-Age Adults (AIMS-WA)*, 6th edition, Beavon M., Raphael H., Shaygan S. (eds). Royal College of Psychiatry, 2017.

within 30 minutes (2/11). Staff from these 11 wards that were later accredited were interviewed by telephone to enquire what changes had led to this achievement. They responded that the process improved communication within the multidisciplinary team, gave power to negotiate for resources needed to achieve accreditation as the managers of the services had signed up to the project, provided clear guidance how to practice, rewarded good practice, and led to additional unrelated improvements in care. The observation that these wards subsequently met 100% of these standards showed clear improvement in safety and quality although it could not be assumed that the AIMS process was the only factor driving up standards.

An unpublished review was carried out by this chapter's author in February 2016 of the current reasons for inpatient units being deferred from accreditation in order to make a rough estimate of the changing picture of the challenges for inpatient units. The meeting of the Accreditation Committee reviewed the accreditation status

of 23 wards of whom six received accreditation, three did not receive accreditation, and the remainder received deferred status in order to implement improvements that would likely result in accreditation over the ensuing 3 months. The most common reason for not initially achieving accreditation was the lack of availability of activities in the evenings and weekends (13 wards). Staffing issues, for example, inability of staff to take breaks (seven wards), cancelled staff training (seven wards), inadequate staff supervision (six wards), deficiencies in staff training (five wards), and the lack of annual assessment in competency of medicines administration (nine wards) were the next most common problems. Lack of psychological services was still a major issue, absent in eight wards, although three members of the meeting stated that their trust had achieved the appointment psychology sessions on their wards due to the AIMS process. Problems with the design and safety of wards were evident in the presence of blind spots on six wards and ligature points on four wards. The standard of the availability of doctors within 30 minutes had not improved and was noted in four wards. Overall, this snapshot of data suggested that there were some improvements, notably in provision of one-to-one therapeutic contact, provision of psychological service, and a safer environment, but the challenges facing inpatient units were largely similar 6 years later.

Local impact of the AIMS programme

The author has worked on an inpatient unit in Oxford. This ward and the other acute psychiatric admission wards were enrolled on the AIMS programme in 2015 and the wards received a peer review visit. This involved a consultant psychiatrist, a nurse, and a ward manager from other parts of the country. As well as measuring the standards, there was a face-to-face interview with myself and other members of the inpatient clinical team. They discussed how they practised in their individual units, allowing an exchange of ideas and exposure of our team to other ways of working. The unit and others in our organization were originally 'deferred' from accreditation in order to implement changes: for example, provision of ward psychological therapy input for a day per week, allowing unsupervised access to the ward garden, and permission for the use of mobile telephones by patients. The ward and the others in the organization were subsequently accredited. It is important to state though that the ward was participating in other quality improvement activities alongside the accreditation programme which may also have influenced practice.

Research arising from the national audits of inpatient care

A programme of research has been carried out at the Royal College of Psychiatrists' Centre for Quality Improvement in order to obtain a national picture of the quality of inpatient care and to compare the standards of care between the different types of inpatient units. There has been a particular focus on obtaining the opinions of service users and staff about their experiences of violence and aggression on the units. Prior to the adoption of accreditation, inpatient care was subject to two national audits focused on the clinical practice guidelines to prevent and manage violence, referred to as the 'National Audits of Violence'. In 2006, over 400 questionnaires were analysed from the service users and staff at 184 acute adult inpatient units. The study highlighted the common experiences of violence, with nurses (78%) significantly more likely to report the experience of violence than service users (37%). Drugs and alcohol were particularly seen as contributory factors. Other standards frequently not met in the 2006 National Audit of Violence included staffing levels, training, provision of activities, and ward design (17). Staff from each ward that participated attended joint sessions where they developed and discussed the implementation of local improvement plans.

Comparisons of the safety on wards for adults of working age have been made with those caring for older adults with mental health problems and with psychiatric intensive care units (PICUs). The studies highlighted that it was the nursing staff who were most likely to bear the burden of experience of violence on all types of inpatient units studied (acute working age, older adult, forensic, and PICUs),

being significantly more likely than patients to report assaults. Nurses working on acute working age wards were more likely to report violent experiences than their colleagues working on forensic wards but less likely than those working in PICUs (18). Somewhat surprisingly, nursing staff working on older adult wards were more likely to report an assault than nurses working on acute working age wards but had received less training in its management and were less likely to have access to safety alarms (19).

Further challenges for accreditation

Accreditation, by its very nature, is a complex intervention. It involves the engagement of a service and its staff in order to positively impact direct clinical care. Moreover, the services that are engaged in an accreditation process may be involved in one or more local or national quality improvement initiatives. It is therefore difficult to measure the actual impact of an accreditation programme above the confounding effects of other quality improvement activity. In particular, it is necessary to ascertain that if improvements in the quality of care have been made, were these as a direct result of the accreditation process or was change driven by other factors? To date, there has been no satisfactory answer to this question. At the Royal College of Psychiatrists' Centre for Quality Improvement, the impact of accreditation programmes has been measured by determining the adherence to evidence-based standards before and after the interventions. In the case of the evaluation previously discussed (10) on electroconvulsive therapy standards, it is possible to demonstrate serial improvements in compliance with standards over a 10-year period. However, this is not sufficient to state that it was the accreditation programme that *caused* the improvements.

A systematic review of health care accreditation programmes to measure their impact (20) concluded that programmes identified (mainly in the US and involving acute rather than mental health care) a limited level of evidence to support accreditation's effectiveness. Furthermore, accreditation programmes like any intervention may have unintended negative outcomes. This was highlighted in a study of clinical medical students in Taiwan where the hospital accreditation programme was perceived to lead to increased trivial workloads, decreased clinical learning opportunities, and violation of professional integrity (21). A further systematic review in 2015 (22) identified only one randomized controlled trial of an accreditation programme and concluded that there was no evidence to demonstrate its effectiveness in changing the quality of care. Currently, work is undergoing at the Royal College of Psychiatrists' Centre for Quality Improvement to systematically evaluate a new mental health service accreditation programme by comparing the standard adherence outcomes of services randomly allocated to immediate accreditation interventions or waiting list controls. Not only will this be important to establish whether the accreditation programme is effective, but if so, what the important components of the programme are that are effective: for example, the dissemination of evidence-based practice, the dissemination of good or innovative practice, the highlighting of poor or outdated practice, the peer review process, the process of certification, or other aspects of the programme. Further, it will help identify how the programme changes care. Currently the standards are undergoing review in order to update and reduce the number, so reducing administrative time for services and reviewers.

Conclusion

Accreditation programmes are important means by which to engage staff and collaboratively work to improve the safety and quality of inpatient care. They differ from the statutory regulator, the Care Quality Commission, as engagement with them is generally voluntary and they do not have enforcement powers. They encourage the sharing of good practice as well as the identification of poor practice in an atmosphere which is designed to be supportive and non-judgemental. For example, initial failure to gain accreditation status most usually leads to a deferred status where the ward is supported with a plan to gain accreditation, which usually they manage to achieve. Challenges for the future are to ensure that the evidence-based guidelines are frequently revised according to new research and policy initiatives and to incorporate more standards based upon patient outcomes (primarily clinical outcome, safety, and patient experience). Some key quality indicators are being introduced to further improve the standards and rigorous research evaluations are being piloted to investigate their effectiveness.

REFERENCES

1. Sainsbury Centre for Mental Health. *Acute Problems: A Survey of the Quality of Care in Acute Psychiatric Wards.* London: Sainsbury Centre for Mental Health; 1998.
2. Mental Health Act Commission. *In Place of Fear: 11th Biennial Report 2003–2005.* London: The Stationery Office; 2005.
3. National Institute for Health and Care Excellence. *Violence: The Short Term Management of Disturbed/Violent Behaviour in Inpatient Psychiatric Settings and Emergency Departments.* London: National Institute for Health and Care Excellence; 2005.
4. Healthcare Commission. *National Audit of Violence.* London: Healthcare Commission; 2005.
5. Department of Health. *The NHS Plan: A Plan for Investment, A Plan for Reform.* London: The Stationery Office; 2000.
6. Gollop R, Whitby E, Buchanan D, Ketley D. Influencing sceptical staff to become supporters of service improvement: a qualitative study of doctors' and managers' views. *Qual Saf Health Care* 2004;13:108–114.
7. Roland M. Choosing effective strategies for quality improvement. *Qual Health Care* 2001;10:66–67.
8. Lelliott P, Bennett H, McGeorge M, Turner T. Accreditation of acute inpatient mental health services. *Psychiatr Bull* 2006;30:361–363.
9. Scrivens E. *Accreditation: Protecting the Professional or the Consumer?* Buckingham: Open University Press; 1995.
10. Murphy G, Doncaster E, Chaplin R, Cresswell J, Worrall A, Three decades of quality improvement in electroconvulsive therapy: exploring the role of accreditation. *J ECT* 2013;29: 312–317.
11. Department of Health. *Mental Health Policy Implementation Guide: Acute Adult Mental Healthcare Provision.* London: The Stationary Office; 2002.
12. Department of Health. *Mental Health Policy Implementation Guide: Developing Positive Practice to Support the Safe and Therapeutic Management of Aggression and Violence in Mental Health Inpatient Settings.* London: The Stationary Office; 2004.
13. Department of Health. *Safety First: Five Year Report of the National Confidential Enquiry into Suicide and Homicide by People with Mental Illness.* London: The Stationary Office; 2001.
14. National Confidential Inquiry into Suicide and Homicide by People with Mental Illness. Annual report England, Northern Ireland, Scotland and Wales, July 2015. University of Manchester; 2015. http://documents.manchester.ac.uk/display.aspx?DocID= 37591
15. Royal College of Psychiatrists. *The National Audit of Violence (2003–2005): Final Report.* London: Royal College of Psychiatrists; 2005. http://www.rcpsych.ac.uk/PDF/Final Report shortened for website.pdf
16. Baskind R, Kordowicz M, Chaplin R. How does an accreditation programme drive improvement on acute inpatient mental health wards? An exploration of members' views. *J Ment Health* 2010;19:405–411.
17. Chaplin R, McGeorge M, Lelliott P. The National Audit of Violence: in-patient care for adults of working age. *Psychiatr Bull* 2006;30:444–446.
18. Loubser I, Chaplin R, Quirk A. Violence, alcohol and drugs: the views of nurses and patients on psychiatric intensive care units, acute adult wards and forensic wards. *J Psychiatr Intens Care* 2009;5:33–35.
19. Chaplin R, McGeorge M, Hinchcliffe G, Shinkwin L. Aggression on psychiatric inpatient units for older adults and adults of working age. *Int J Geriatr Psychiatry* 2008;23:874–876.
20. Hinchcliff R, Greenfield D, Moldovan D, et al. Narrative synthesis of health service accreditation literature. *BMJ Qual Saf* 2012;21:979–991.
21. Ho MJ, Chang HH, Chiu YT, Norris JL. Effects of hospital accreditation on medical students: a national qualitative study in Taiwan. *Acad Med* 2014;89:1533–1539.
22. Brubakk K, Vist GE, Bukholm G, Barach P, Tjomsland O. A systematic review of hospital accreditation: the challenges of measuring complex intervention effects. *BMC Health Serv Res* 2015;15:280.

SECTION 5
Psychological aspects

28

Psychological treatment on the acute ward

Ian Barkataki and Louise Ross

Introduction

Psychological approaches to the treatment of mental disorders on inpatient wards have been a relatively recent development in the UK (1). However, there has been a rising demand for psychological interventions and expertise within mental health services. This increase in demand has been supported by guidelines and policy, which have extended to acute and inpatient settings (2). The increased emphasis of psychological approaches to working within this context has resulted in the British Psychological Society developing specific guidelines around the commissioning and delivery of high-quality psychological practice in inpatient units (3). This has been subsequently incorporated into criteria and standards used to evaluate the quality of inpatient service provision.

In contrast to models of mental illness that are rooted in disease or biological cause (4, 5), psychological approaches have traditionally favoured a biopsychosocial framework to understanding mental health (6). Influenced by systemic theory, a psychological understanding takes a holistic view of a person rather than a narrow focus on illness. Individuals are situated within the context of their family, friends, and occupational and social environment, in addition to their relationship with their problem(s). In acute inpatient settings, a systemic approach also extends to the influence of fellow patients, healthcare professionals, external specialists, community teams, and the broader organizational health system where the person is located (7). Understanding this series of overlapping systems can help direct a course of clinical treatment, and lead to one that is meaningful for the individual and can be sustained on the ward and beyond.

A psychological formulation encapsulates symptoms, cognition, and observable behaviour as a means of communication and expressing personal agency, and is integral to a psychological approach. Such formulations are a conceptualization of the underlying precipitation, maintenance, and explanatory factors that underlie a problem or condition, as well as a framework of how these fit together. In contrast to discrete and static diagnostic criteria, formulations are generally considered working models predicated around testable hypotheses which are constantly refined and developed as more is learnt during the course of clinical practice. Through the lens of formulation, an individual's difficulties are seen as making sense to them and can be understood in relation to their own life history and individual context (8).

Formulation can empower service users to understand their own problems, develop insight, make sense of their current crisis, and also inform a personalized treatment plan. This can range from an intervention provided by an individual clinician, or could involve a multidisciplinary team and would be planned in collaboration with the service user. A formulation-driven intervention is expected to be subject to some form of evaluation. Whereas traditionally such an evaluation can come from psychometrically validated scales, outcome measures, or tests, this can also include externally observable behaviours, self-reported symptoms, or feedback from the clinical team (3).

Underpinning all psychological approaches is a reflective stance that seeks to understand the impact of the work on the individual service user and the care team. It questions how things may have been done differently, taking into account failures in treatment as well as successes. Under such a framework, a psychologically informed treatment is not simply a discrete piece of work conducted in isolation, or as a technical procedure applied by a member of ward staff to a service user, but is a reiterative process that informs future care for that service user and impacts the wider ward culture.

As a discipline focusing on applying psychological approaches to clinical problems, psychology is well placed to contribute to high-quality inpatient working (9). In the UK, psychologists have an extensive training that involves an undergraduate degree in psychology where academic theory and research methods are taught, a period of pre-qualified work experience in an applied setting that is usually clinical or research related, and a further doctoral programme that combines academic teaching, research, and service evaluation, as well as supervised clinical practice. In particular, clinical psychologists are required to develop competencies across the lifespan in adult mental health, child and adolescent services, older adult services, and learning difficulties services. During their training they will be expected to develop expertise in delivering evidence-based psychotherapies across multiple models and work closely with professionals from a multidisciplinary team. As a consequence, many clinical psychologists will have had exposure to inpatient wards or will have learned many of their skills in similar National Health Service environments.

Psychological working within a multidisciplinary team

In multidisciplinary working, individual clinicians and specialists bring together different skills, training, and backgrounds to work collectively as a team. On an inpatient ward, specific skills and competencies often 'belong' to particular team members who are then tasked with working in a particular capacity (e.g. prescribing medication, control and restraint) or speciality (e.g. nursing, occupational therapy, and pharmacy). While there can be such defined roles for psychologists, psychological thinking is not solely the preserve of psychologists, but is an approach that can influence a wider ward culture (3).

Instead of viewing the psychologist in a defined role as a sole provider of psychological working (in the form of assessment, therapy, etc.), it can be more beneficial to staff and patients to start with the premise that members of the whole multidisciplinary team are capable of integrating psychological thinking within their routine working practice, and for psychologists to actively develop this capability. This is not incompatible with maintaining the integrity of individual roles, as most clinical professions will already draw from psychology or psychological models during their training, or at least acknowledge there are psychological factors involved when working with patients.

Clarke (10) proposes a four-level model of competencies required to deliver high-quality inpatient care. A possible framework of how this can be translated for staff, based on job role, duties, and background training is provided in the following subsections (see Table 28.1). Under this model of working, psychologists can be deployed most effectively by distributing expertise and facilitating the development of a psychologically skilled ward workforce.

Psychology and staff well-being

Heavy demands, close proximity, severity of illness, and rapid admission/discharge of service users combined with large, rotating staff teams contribute to the intensity and difficulty of clinical work within a modern inpatient unit. This poses unique challenges to staff in the form of inconsistency, unpredictable workflow, personal risk of injury, and the powerful interpersonal dynamics that can play out among ward teams. Staff morale, cohesion, retention, and positive attitudes to service users are essential to the smooth functioning of the ward and effective clinical outcomes (11). Conversely, high turnover of personnel, high levels of stress, poor job satisfaction, and ongoing staff conflicts undermine the efficiency of the ward, and contribute to adverse ward conditions for patients (12).

Psychology can play a useful role in supporting the ward workforce. Through guidance and reflection, staff can feel valued and more effective in conducting their duties. Use of psychological frameworks can help staff teams understand group dynamics and become aware of psychological processes that may be being played out on the ward, such as in-groups, splitting, or scapegoating. They can elicit the metacognitive or systemic issues about the working context, and help process the less tangible burdens of emotional labour, such as working with ambiguity and sitting with emotional distress.

Evaluation, audit, and research

As a discipline based in applied science, psychology places as much emphasis on evaluation and measurement as on delivery of treatment. This is reflected in the expertise in research methodology required by psychologists, as well as the increasing emphasis on outcome and impact for all psychological therapies. Moreover, psychologists are expected to plan, execute, and facilitate audits, service evaluation, and practice-based research as part of their role, which extends to the inpatient environment (13). Data collected from audits and evaluations of routine ward clinical practice can be used to inform and refine treatment, as well as contribute to the continuous improvement of the ward. As the findings and recommendations are grounded in data collected from a specific service, they will have greater ecological validity than externally published evidence, which is often carried out in tightly controlled research environments. Evidence gathered on a ward is therefore more likely to have a greater impact when informing treatment or care planning. Furthermore, methodologies, findings, and recommendations from such evaluations can be disseminated more widely, replicated on other wards, or adapted for local service requirements, thus contributing to the development of good clinical practice across all inpatient settings.

Service user involvement and recovery model

Psychological practice has been heavily influenced by the service user movement, which has stimulated reciprocal demand for increased psychological input. The service user movement centres on empowering individuals to have greater involvement in their own clinical care, destigmatization of mental health conditions, recognition of expertise derived from lived experience, and establishing a more equitable balance of power between the service user and clinician. Service user views are actively elicited and care is centred on the needs and desires of the individual rather than being directed by professionals (14). In some cases, service users are involved in training healthcare professionals, providing peer support

Table 28.1 Psychological competencies according to level and specific inpatient role

Level	Requirements	Ward role	Typical competencies
1	All ward staff	Health care assistant, technical instructor	Engagement skills, active listening, use of recovery principles
2	Post registered practice	Newly qualified nurse	Problem-solving, relapse prevention, de-escalation, suicide prevention
3	Advanced practice	Occupational therapist, senior nurse	Motivational interviewing, manualized psychological treatments (e.g. anxiety management), relaxation training
4	Independent practice	Clinical psychologist, medical psychotherapist	Evidence-based psychological therapies, supervision, and training

and advocacy or otherwise actively influencing policy and service development.

In an inpatient context, a psychological approach to treatment would position the service user as a co-creator of a therapeutic plan rather than a passive recipient of care. Service users may be involved in holding ward meetings, having direct input with clinical decision-making during ward rounds, or advocating for changes on the ward. Approaching problems using the framework of psychological formulation can work against mental health stigma by individualization of care, in contrast to fitting individuals to diagnostic categories. Advantages to this approach are its broader understanding and insight of individual difficulties, reduced conflicts around diagnostic ambiguity, and potential reduction of polarization between inpatient staff ('the well') and service users ('the ill'). The aforementioned distribution of psychological expertise can empower service users to develop insight into their behaviour, peer educate around self-care, and validate each other's own expertise and experience.

Allied to service user involvement is the recovery model, an approach that emphasizes recovery as a life process or personal journey, rather than aiming for cure or alleviation of symptoms (15). There is greater emphasis on quality of life and markers of social or functional improvement. Recovery-oriented goals are developed by the service user and can guide treatment, inform clinical decision-making, and cultivate optimism in conditions that are traditionally seen as 'treatment resistant' or 'incurable'. Increased acknowledgement and dominance of this philosophy has led to the development of many 'recovery-oriented' services underpinned by standards and practices that position the service user as an expert of their recovery (16). Thus, psychological approaches in an inpatient context would focus on providing a secure and safe psychological environment, instilling hope for change, and developing personal meaning of one's illness.

Forms of psychological treatment on inpatient wards

The most straightforward view of psychological treatment on an acute ward is psychologists (and psychology-related practitioners, such as psychotherapists, arts therapists, occupational therapists, and counsellors) delivering evidence-based psychological therapies directly to individual service users. While this forms part of the remit of psychology, this can be problematic as access to psychological input on wards is generally scarce (17). Moreover, service users are often on a ward during a short period of crisis, and may not be stable or be on the ward for long enough to engage in conventional psychotherapies that can take months to complete. The dynamic nature of the ward necessitates any treatment to be delivered in conjunction with the rest of the multidisciplinary team in order to follow a coherent and consistent care plan. Effective psychological treatment on wards can be better conceptualized as a spectrum of direct or indirect working (3).

Direct psychological working

Individual

Although the inpatient environment is not the most typical setting for psychotherapy, there is still some scope for a variety of adapted therapeutic options. Psychotherapy on the ward may be suitable for service users who have attained some psychological stability and are likely to remain on the ward for some time. There are briefer, more directive adaptations of evidence-based therapies such as cognitive behavioural therapy or solution-focused therapy (9). There may also be a role for humanistic, person-centred counselling approaches that are non-directive, but offer the service user empathy, positive regard, or help make sense of their experiences (18). Psychoeducation around a condition, problem, or disorder can be useful as a means of empowering the service user, increasing confidence, and reducing distress resulting from lack of knowledge or understanding about their experience (19). It can also help combat internalized mental health stigma and facilitate service users talking about their individual story.

During the assessment phase of inpatient work, psychological expertise can bring together disparate strands of the clinical conceptualization of the presentation, the service user's subjective experience of their condition, and the role of early experiences and family background. It can also highlight precipitant and maintaining factors. A robust assessment can draw from a range of empirically validated psychometric measures, scales, or tests to look at cognition, behaviour, and symptomatology. Alternatively, it is possible to develop subjective or idiosyncratic methods of capturing specific clinical data or any other observations. Building a preliminary psychological formulation of the problem is one of the key goals of any assessment and this will be used to inform subsequent care (20).

More structured psychological work can support an individual's transition from inpatient to the community. Understanding underlying motivations, strengths, and weaknesses can contribute to prevention or crisis management, and inform the processes around inpatient discharge or transfer of care. Similarly, identifying areas of outstanding work, preventative measures, or risk is part of good care planning and post-ward care on behalf of the service, which can be shared with community teams and external agencies. While some of this work may focus on the actual content of the plan or specific elements of aftercare, underlying the psychological approach to recovery will be the cultivation of hopefulness regarding improvement, preparing service users for setbacks and relapses and developing resiliency.

Patient group

Therapeutic interventions using a group format are an established method of treatment in regular inpatient practice. These vary in content, frequency, and duration across a range of subjects such as relaxation, creative activities, and psychoeducational teaching. Many will be delivered by practitioners from a range of backgrounds, such as nursing staff, occupational therapy, and health care assistants, depending on training and therapeutic milieu. Such approaches are wholly compatible with psychology, where there are already established practices for delivering group therapy across most psychological models and therapeutic orientations (9). More recently, skills-based interventions such as mentalization-based therapy (21) and dialectical behavioural therapy (22) originally oriented towards the treatment personality disorders have been developed, modified, and applied by clinical psychologists for inpatient settings (23). Additionally, group work can be helpful to recognise interpersonal interactions, unconscious dynamics, and systemic factors that may be otherwise left unattended during treatment. While this can come directly from psychologists and psychological practitioners as facilitators of such groups, these issues can also be attended to during the psychological supervision of ward staff.

While therapeutic groups have advantages in contributing to the structure or routine of the ward, ensuring equality of provision and allowing a degree of standardization within the treatment regimen, there are other implications that need to be considered. From a managerial perspective, there can be resource costs in taking staff off general duties and finding suitable space and time. Additionally, facilitators are required to be committed to regularly running a group which may impact rotas and shift planning to accommodate this. For staff themselves, they will need a moderate level of skill in presentation, teaching, and public speaking as well as a basic understanding of how to manage groups of people. For service users, due to the varying severity and type of presentations there will need to be some form of screening regarding suitability for group treatment, and this may lead to a visible division between patients who are eligible for groups and those who are not. While none of these factors should prevent group-based activities from being conducted, they do need to be considered and appropriately accommodated.

As well as treatment and intervention, psychologically informed practice could also be used in more routine ward activities that typically adopt a group-based format. Psychological thinking is integral to debriefing and processing significant events, de-escalating emerging ward dynamics, or in other situations where formulation and systemic approaches can help shed light or address splits. Lastly, service user involvement and patient advocacy can be developed through group formats, and in some instances this has led to service user-led practices such as regular patient meetings about how the ward is run, holding peer-led hearing voices groups, and having former residents come back to the ward to give advice to current service users. All of these service user involvement advances are geared towards equalizing the balance of power between clinicians and service users.

Family and friends

The involvement of family, friends, and carers is critical to an individual's experience of an acute inpatient service. Systemic psychological approaches view the individual as inseparable from their wider context, paying particular attention to how a person is situated across social, occupational, and family contexts (8). In particular, relationships (or lack of them) are frequently a crucial element of an individual's entry into mental health services, and can heavily affect their treatment on the ward as well as their subsequent recovery. Lack of support, isolation, over-involvement, ongoing conflicts, work pressures, and social attitudes towards mental illness are all common historical experiences for many service users. While some of these may recede into the background in an inpatient setting, they will still have to be encountered when an individual leaves.

A robust psychological approach would incorporate these systemic issues into treatment and view the wider network as integral to longer-term recovery. Sometimes formal family therapy can be offered, in which significant relational ruptures and breakdowns can be addressed, and emotional support and education about disorders can be provided (24). Particularly relevant to acute inpatient settings, family sessions can focus on the challenges of discharge, identifying early warning signs, encouraging treatment compliance,

and emergency planning. This can help consolidate wider treatment plans and can potentially prevent future episodes or admissions (24). At a broader level, some of the more generic psychological communication skills such as active listening, maintaining positive regard, and validation may help when dealing with sensitive topics, complaints, or achieving compromises between different parties, including service users, family, friends, and professionals (25).

Indirect psychological working

While delivering clinical treatments and interventions directly to service users, families, and carers is the most visible form of psychological work; indirect psychological work has a potentially wider impact and can constitute a more efficient allocation of psychology resources. Indirect psychological working consists of a variety of activities across various levels of the organization, that still have a substantive effect on the running of the acute inpatient service and the service user's experience.

Ward staff

Psychological supervision is a mandatory requirement for psychotherapists. Unlike other clinical forms of oversight or management, psychological supervision has been defined as the formal provision by a senior or qualified practitioner of an intensive relational space which supports the work of clinical colleagues. This is provided in order to maintain quality and ensure competence and effective working (26). Although such a relational form of supervision is not typically offered to all ward-based staff, there are some indications that it can be helpful for staff in managing the burden of ward work and enhancing clinical effectiveness (27). While supervision is usually conducted on an individual basis, it is possible to also deliver supervision for staff groups or introduce facilitated 'reflective' practice sessions. In contrast to the task-orientated and fast-paced work on a ward, clinical supervision allows a space for thinking, validation, and the toleration of ambiguity (9).

Additionally, indirect working may include workforce development to upskill staff. This can take on the form of teaching, training, and dissemination of psychological theory, techniques, and practices. Part of this educative process may also involve activities such as helping ward staff develop formulations or introducing psychological perspectives during ward rounds, care planning meetings, or case discussions. Developing staff may also involve examining personal attitudes, acknowledging the influencing of language and understanding culture. On wards, clinical psychologists have been traditionally assigned to this function due to the role of supervision within their own training and their emphasis on reflective practice (3), but other disciplines have increasingly adopted supervision within their practices. As an added benefit, as well as helping form a more skilled, effective, and capable workforce, investment in training can help raise morale as well as fostering more inclusive and collaborative attitudes (28).

Physical environment

Inpatient wards are dynamic, intense, and constantly changing locations and good psychological practice actively engages with the surrounding physical environment. Although much consideration is already given to the environment in terms of risk, security, and safety, there is increasing awareness that the structural elements of inpatient units can have psychological effects on both service users and staff. Such psychological factors have been shown to have a bearing on the clinical activities taking place on the ward such as aggression levels and the increased use of restraint or seclusion (29). The utilization of evidence-based design for wards (30), programmes such as 'Safewards' (31), and similar initiatives aimed at enhancing aesthetics, comfort, and utility of clinical spaces all come under the auspices of environmental psychology. These factors are increasingly incorporated at the design, maintenance, and ongoing physical shaping of the inpatient environment.

Organization

Psychology's competency in evaluation of research evidence, audit, and systemic thinking makes it particularly helpful in informing leadership and service development. Often, this has been used in the implementation of protocols and guidelines that direct treatment choice, which can be helpful in preventing ineffective or potentially harmful treatments or practices. Beyond directing treatments within an individual service or organization, such expertise can also be used to inform strategic planning, resource allocation, or commissioning decisions and can even have an impact on directing good practice at the national level.

Challenges of psychological working within an acute setting

Compulsory treatment

Due to the nature of the type of work conducted on acute inpatient units, service users may be held under the Mental Health Act or otherwise undergo treatment under compulsion. Regardless, the core principles of good psychological practice remains the collaborative stance, instilling hope of improvement, and encouraging engagement in treatment under an individual's own volition. As compulsorily imposed treatment can work against these principles, it poses a significant challenge.

Professional practice guidelines and codes of ethics and conduct require practitioners to respect the service user's rights to choose to receive treatment and for this consent to be informed on the basis of the best available information. It is important that where individuals are detained under legislation, treatment has to be provided in accordance with legal requirements. Any relevant local and national policies, and the needs of individual and public safety always take precedence. However, under compulsory treatment, psychological approaches can still be conducted as long as the best interests of the service user are considered.

Any attempts to intervene against the express wishes of a client should only be done after careful deliberation and on the basis of clearly identified needs. Part of this can be addressed by breaking down the various aspects of treatment that an individual may or may not consent to (rather than seeking an all-encompassing global consent). By allowing individuals to accept or reject these individual treatment components, it can go some way towards enhancing engagement and reducing non-compliance. Timing of obtaining consent in the starting of a particular therapeutic activity within compulsory treatment should be carefully considered, as this may have an effect on engagement or an intervention's longer-term success. Clear information regarding what a given intervention involves, its benefits, risks, and the likelihood of success, needs to be provided. It is also important to be clear about the role, function, and expertise level of the clinician delivering any psychological intervention, as well as any information regarding possible alternative forms of treatment. Throughout any compulsory treatment, psychological approaches will still advocate that service users are empowered to their own choice in accepting or rejecting interventions, or being allowed to withdraw from them at a later time.

It should also be recognized that psychological treatment under such circumstances may be limited due to imbalances in power between staff and service user, and that factors relating to positive outcomes such as therapeutic rapport, intrinsic motivation to change, and openness may be affected. Under such restrictions, psychological interventions may be more focused towards skills training such as relaxation, anxiety management, or psychoeducation. The merits of refraining from intervention during the acute setting should be recognized, as an ill-timed, under-motivated, or badly delivered intervention may not only be unhelpful, but can impede openness to future psychological treatment. In such cases, maintaining clinical optimism and engendering motivation for post-ward psychological treatment can be a more effective use of resources.

Limits on healthcare/short-term working

In community settings, most psychological interventions are conducted over the space of several weeks or months. Psychotherapies or other psychological pieces of work are frequently held on a weekly basis, with independent work or homework tasks to consolidate progress carried out in between sessions. However, the concentrated timeframes involved with inpatient working require psychological interventions to be adapted and further modified, especially in the event of unexpected discharge or transfer (9). Such adaptations may be relatively straightforward, such as emphasizing treatment on more acute symptoms, arranging daily sessions instead of weekly, or taking advantage of the constant presence of staff. The ward environment may also lead to increased use of shorter, targeted group-based interventions, especially those that are open to new entrants. Other adaptations may be more complex and require careful planning, handover between staff, or subsequent involvement of other healthcare professionals, friends and family, and external agencies.

With shorter-term interventions, the focus on treatment may be geared towards reduction of distress, stabilization, and short-term management of symptoms, rather than longer-term recovery and growth. Expectations of observable change are likely be lower due to the shortened period of treatment, as well as the increased severity of presentation that would typically necessitate inpatient admission. Nonetheless, service users can be well placed in a ward context to learn tangible skills that reduce risk or help them develop insight. Therapeutic rapport, trust, and expectations around continuity of treatment are likely to be different, with the intense, close-quarter nature of the ward often expediting the formation of close relationships. Depending on the service model and resourcing, it may be possible for inpatient staff to contract to continue working with a service user after leaving the ward, especially if there are conditions around discharge or if ongoing monitoring is required to ensure their well-being (e.g. under a compulsory treatment order under the Mental Health Act). In turn, this may help with service users developing rapport, trust, and comfort with a clinician or service.

Managing demand

Unfortunately, the demand for psychological expertise often outweighs supply. Moreover, psychological interventions can have substantial time commitments, are labour intensive, and are difficult to scale up in the event of increased need without additional substantial investment of resources or personnel. Therefore, it is imperative that there is ongoing active planning and strategic management around the capacity and delivery of psychological input on the ward. Often, awareness of seasonal fluctuations in admissions, shifting profiles of those who are admitted, and routine data gathering about which interventions are most effective can help managers deploy limited psychological resources to best effect. There may be some benefits in having a psychological triage or prioritization systems around allocating input, or having a method of clear communication regarding availability of psychological personnel at a given time, which can be shared at handovers or ward rounds. Variations in demand may also involve reconsidering the use of experienced, trained clinicians as teachers and disseminators of skills, or overseeing the work of more junior members of staff rather than delivering treatment directly at busy times. In some instances, demand can also be managed by mobilizing additional psychological resources such as fostering links to clinical researchers developing inpatient treatments who need access to clinical settings, or hosting speciality trainees, students, or other types of supernumerary staff.

Maintaining a presence

One of the challenges of staff working psychologically is being visible and maintaining a presence on the ward. If this is not prioritized, there are risks that the psychological work becomes seen as obscure or an optional luxury rather than an essential part of the wider multidisciplinary team. Moreover, clinicians run the risk that they are viewed as precious and unfairly exempt from more routine duties, which can cause resentment among other staff. Therefore, it is important that psychological practitioners make a conscious effort to be present on the ward where possible, and to be approachable by actively encouraging consultation, reflection, and discussion. Although much of psychological work is intangible, taking opportunities to highlight and notify the wider team of outcomes and completed objectives, as well as highlighting when ward staff demonstrate psychological thinking and skills, can go some way to increasing visibility of psychological approaches in an inpatient setting.

REFERENCES

1. Durrant C, Clarke I, Tolland A, Wilson H. Designing a CBT service for an acute inpatient setting: a pilot evaluation study. *Clin Psychol Psychother* 2007;14:117–125.
2. Sainsbury Centre for Mental Health. *Acute Care 2004: A National Survey of Adult Psychiatric Wards in England*. London: Sainsbury Centre for Mental Health; 2005.
3. British Psychological Society. *Commissioning and Delivering Clinical Psychology in Acute Adult Mental Health Care: Guidelines for Commissioners, Service Managers, Psychology Managers and Practitioners*. London: British Psychological Society; 2012.
4. Engel G. The application of the biopsychosocial model: a challenge for biomedicine. *Science* 1977;196:129–136.
5. Deacon BJ. The biomedical model of mental disorder: a critical analysis of its validity, utility, and effects on psychotherapy research. *Clin Psychol Rev* 2013;33:846–861.
6. Butler G. Clinical formulation. In: Bellack A, Hersen M eds), *Comprehensive Clinical Psychology*, pp. 1–24. New York: Pergammon Press; 1998.
7. Jones A, Bowles N. Best practice from admission to discharge in acute inpatient care: considerations and standards from a whole system perspective. *J Psychiatr Ment Health Nurs* 2005;12:642–647.
8. Johnstone L, Dallos R. *Formulation in Psychology and Psychotherapy: Making Sense of People's Problems of Work*. Hove: Routledge; 2013.
9. Clarke I, Wilson H. *Cognitive Behaviour Therapy for Acute Inpatient Mental Health Units: Working with Clients, Staff and the Milieu of Work*. Hove: Taylor & Francis; 2009.
10. Clarke S. *Acute Inpatient Mental Health Care: Education, Training and Continuing Professional Development for All*. London: NIMHE/SCMH; 2004.
11. Lemieux-Charles L, McGuire WL. What do we know about health care team effectiveness? A review of the literature. *Med Care Res Rev* 2006;63:263–300.
12. Totman J, Hundt GL, Wearn E, Paul M, Johnson S. Factors affecting staff morale on inpatient mental health wards in England: a qualitative investigation. *BMC Psychiatry* 2011;11:68.
13. British Psychological Society. *Core Competencies: Clinical Psychology – A Guide*. London: British Psychological Society; 2006.
14. Campbell P. The history of the user movement in the United Kingdom. In: Heller T, Reynolds J, Gomm R, Muston R, Pattison S (eds), *Mental Health Matters*, pp. 218–225. Basingstoke: Macmillan; 1996.
15. Jacobson N, Greenley D. What is recovery? A conceptual model and explication. *Psychiatr Serv* 2001;52:482–485.
16. Anthony WA. A recovery-oriented service system: setting some system level standards. *Psychiatr Rehabil J* 2000;24:159–168.
17. Bowers L, Whittington R, Nolan P, et al. *The City 128 Study of Observation and Outcomes on Acute Psychiatric Wards: Research Report*. Produced for the National Co-ordinating Centre for the National Institute for Health Research Service Delivery and Organisation Programme (NCCSDO). London: City University; 2006.
18. Stickley T. Counselling and mental health nursing: a qualitative study. *J Psychiatr Ment Health Nurs* 2002;9:301–308.
19. Duman ZC, Yildirim NK, Ucok A, Er F, Kanik T. The effectiveness of a psychoeducational group program with inpatients being treated for chronic mental illness. *Soc Behav Pers* 2010;38:657–666.
20. British Psychological Society. *Good Practice Guidelines on the Use of Psychological Formulation*. Leicester: British Psychological Society; 2011.
21. Fonagy P, Gergely G, Jurist EL. *Affect Regulation, Mentalization and the Development of the Self of Work*. London: Karnac Books; 2004.
22. Linehan M. *Cognitive-Behavioral Treatment of Borderline Personality Disorder of Work*. New York: Guilford Press; 1993.
23. Dimeff LA, Koerner KE. *Dialectical Behavior Therapy in Clinical Practice: Applications across Disorders and Settings of Work*. New York: Guilford Press; 2007.
24. Carr A. The effectiveness of family therapy and systemic interventions for adult-focused problems. *J Fam Ther* 2009;31:46–74.
25. Shattell M, Hogan B. Facilitating communication: how to truly understand what patients mean. *J Psychosoc Nurs Ment Health Serv* 2005;43:29–32.

26. Milne D. An empirical definition of clinical supervision. *Br J Clin Psychol* 2007;46:437–447.

27. Dunn C, Bishop V. Clinical supervision: its implementation in one acute sector trust. In: Bishop V (ed), *Clinical Supervision in Practice*, pp. 85–108. New York: Springer; 1998.

28. Whittington R, Wykes T. An evaluation of staff training in psychological techniques for the management of patient aggression. *J Clin Nurs* 1996;5:257–261.

29. Van der Schaaf P, Dusseldorp E, Keuning F, Janssen W, Noorthoorn E. Impact of the physical environment of psychiatric wards on the use of seclusion. *Br J Psychiatry* 2013;202:142–149.

30. Huisman E, Morales E, Van Hoof J, Kort H. Healing environment: a review of the impact of physical environmental factors on users. *Build Environ* 2012;58:70–80.

31. Bowers L. Safewards: a new model of conflict and containment on psychiatric wards. *J Psychiatr Ment Health Nurs* 2014;21:499–508.

29

Interventions for specific conditions

Ian Barkataki and Louise Ross

Psychology in the inpatient context

As discussed in Chapter 28, access to psychological expertise and approaches is now considered an essential part of inpatient psychiatric treatment, with the application of these interventions in an acute setting increasingly endorsed in healthcare guidelines (1). However, due to the low amount of research activity being carried out in acute settings, the evidence base and its ecological validity has been limited. As a consequence, psychologists, therapists, and psychological practitioners working in this sector have often had to draw on the wider body of research and make pragmatic adaptations to accommodate inpatient working. Nonetheless, a combination of evidence-based practice (2) and feedback from service users (3) has informed the development of good psychological practice for inpatient working.

Adaptations and considerations

Delivery of any psychological intervention requires considerable planning and this is no different when it comes to ward work. As the primary function of a hospital admission is to stabilize mental health and reduce risk, psychological interventions are geared towards supporting that aim and avoiding any unintentional compromising of this. Furthermore, as the inpatient setting is frequently unpredictable, with decisions made on the basis of urgency and need, careful consideration regarding allocation of resources, personnel, and timing are critical. Planning for psychological work also has to take into account that individuals may be discharged or transferred at short notice in response to changes in presentation, housing, and availability of support post discharge, as well as the legalities of the Mental Health Act. Additional complications arise from the fact that treatment planning occurs at an individual level yet is subject to a myriad of external influences that ward staff often have little control over, which can have a huge impact on service user experience (4). This unpredictability means that it is not always feasible to deliver psychological interventions in a traditional format and it is difficult to standardize or establish fixed protocols that can be universally applied.

Robust psychological interventions are tailored to focus on what is most likely to alleviate distress in line with identified goals set by the patient. Due to the brevity of inpatient stays, psychological interventions need to be proportional, responsive, and timely. Input varies among individuals with differing emphasis and focus on assessment, formulation, and intervention stages depending on the needs identified. This can be guided by whether the person has previously received psychological input, their current motivation and insight, the severity and duration of illness, and their likely length of stay. To maximize effectiveness, there has to be a degree of fluidity to the approach, while also providing psychological containment for any anxieties and the maintenance of hope regarding recovery (2). As hospital admission enables a period of sustained observation, the development of a psychological formulation in collaboration with the patient is an important early step in developing insight into a given presentation, which in turn can inform into discussions around diagnosis and treatment.

Overview of psychological interventions

Although there are a multiplicity of views and approaches to a given condition, which will depend on the orientation of the individual psychological practitioner conducting the intervention, most are likely to draw upon one or more of the following psychological models. These models are generally considered to be transdiagnostic in nature and have a wide variety of applications.

Cognitive and behavioural therapies

The focus of behavioural therapies is externally observable behaviour and actions, what maintains and reinforces behaviour, and how it can be modified. Behavioural approaches are generally symptom focused and often aim to reduce or extinguish distressing or unhelpful behaviours. This is mainly achieved through action-oriented methods such as exposure to previously avoided situations, or the positive reinforcement of desired behaviours via reward strategies (5). In contrast, cognitive therapies emphasize the importance of thoughts, beliefs, and assumptions and their contributions to psychological distress. As such, cognitive techniques are geared towards identification of dysfunctional thinking and how it contributes to the view of one's self and the world (6). Cognitive behavioural therapy (CBT) integrates elements of these two approaches and furthers them by exploring the interactions between thought and behaviour, and how such experiences can be interpreted. Moreover, CBT has evolved to incorporate different philosophical approaches including mindfulness, acceptance and commitment therapy, compassion-focused therapy, and dialectic behavioural therapy, all of which are aimed at enhancing individual functioning and tolerating distress (7).

There are several factors that lend support to the delivery of CBT-based interventions within the inpatient context (2). The emphasis on observable change can engender therapeutic optimism and hope about recovery. The focus on measurement facilitates audit/research activity and growth of an evidence base specific to the ward. CBT interventions can often be adapted for short-term work or modularized to be discrete and self-contained pieces of work that can be carried out both on and off the ward. They can also potentially be supported by a range of ward professionals of varying expertise and training. However, engagement in CBT approaches can require the individual service user to have a certain degree of intellectual and literacy skills due to the frequent emphasis on recording, self-report and written work. Furthermore, it is necessary for the service user to have some insight into their difficulties and to be willing to take the personal responsibility to address them.

Psychodynamic psychotherapies

Psychodynamic therapies focus on unconscious processes and the impact of early experiences and attachments on present functioning. The goal of psychodynamic therapy is to increase an individual's awareness of these unconscious drives with particular emphasis on unresolved conflicts or underlying issues that cause distress (8). In this type of treatment, the processes enacted between the patient and therapist are as important as the content of the material discussed and can be used as a frame to understand the impact of significant past relationships. Treatment may not always be symptom or illness focused but can instead be oriented towards developing insight, enabling psychological security, and establishing self-identity.

Traditional psychodynamic therapies require a substantial time commitment, so are not generally delivered within inpatient settings, although the benefits and feasibility of group and short-term forms is debated (9, 10). However, psychodynamic frameworks have been used to good effect in assessment and formulation, guiding interventions and helping ward staff understand strong interpersonal dynamics or reactions (2). Often the work carried out under psychodynamic therapies is hard to observe and is reliant on subjective experience, so can lead to difficulties in quantifying and measuring effectiveness, with interpretations being difficult to validate or evidence. There can also be problems in terms of consistency in delivery across settings, and the need to have highly trained and supervised staff to deliver this type of treatment.

Systemic therapies

Systemic therapies situate the person within a given social context, viewing behaviours as a response to interactions within a wider system (11). This can include families, intimate relationships, workplaces, schools, hospitals, or broader societies. Under this model, mental health difficulties are viewed as an interplay between individual characteristics, distress, communication difficulties, and dysfunctional interactions between people. Systemic therapies can be useful to identify problem-maintaining behaviours, restrictive belief systems, and the impact of historical, contextual, and constitutional factors on the individual and their surrounding network (12).

Systemic approaches benefit from moving away from apportioning blame or identifying particular individuals as 'sick', to focusing on the difficulties in relationships and how people are positioned within their wider context. Moreover, systemic ideas can be used flexibly with individuals, families, and staff teams to explore different perspectives and to look at different ways of tackling problems. They also have the advantage of addressing wider societal-level issues, such as power and inequality. However, it can be hard to deliver a systemic intervention within a ward setting due to the logistics of coordinating attendance of multiple stakeholders, and the need for identified individuals to have a degree of insight, willingness, and motivation to work on the 'problem'. Furthermore, other people may not want to consider their potential role in maintaining difficulties and there may be limited scope in changing aspects of an individual's environment.

Interventions for specific conditions

Individuals are admitted to an acute inpatient setting for a range of difficulties. While this chapter cannot comprehensively account for all conditions, or the myriad of potential comorbid variables, several common presentations are discussed in greater detail in the following subsections. Although specific techniques and approaches are discussed in the context of different conditions, often as they were developed to be used, in practice they are implemented according to the formulation, needs, and preferences of patients.

Mood disorders

'Mood disorders' is an umbrella term encompassing a range of mental health conditions where there is some disturbance in an individual's affect. Mood disorders can include conditions of elevated mood, such as mania or hypomania; depressed mood, such as unipolar or major depression; and bipolar disorder, in which moods cycle between mania and depression.

Depression

From a psychological perspective, depression is an interaction of low mood, sustained negative thinking, isolative and self-neglecting behaviours that perpetuate a cycle of unhappiness. Withdrawal from other people and a gradual reduction in activities combined with persistent negative interpretations of experiences result in the individual discounting positive events and overestimating the importance of negative ones.

Depression is one of the most well-researched mental health conditions. A large body of psychological research exists which concludes that a range of different psychological interventions, including CBT, interpersonal therapy, problem-solving, and behavioural activation, can be effective in treating depression across multiple populations and settings, including those with severe or chronic depression and inpatients (13). In addition to standard practice, psychological interventions adapted for a ward environment have helped reduce symptoms of depression when delivered in individual and group formats (14, 15), although the longer-term impact on readmission and relapse rates remains unclear. Crucially, interventions can be adapted to specifically target high levels of suicidality and/or self-neglect (16), which are pertinent for this client group. Several specific psychological tools are evidence based in the treatment of depression:

Behavioural activation

This is an approach that specifically focuses on engaging with desired behaviours and eliminating avoidance. It involves scheduling of diminishing, avoided, or new activities with the aim of increasing opportunities to gain positive reinforcement from 'doing' (17). Activity diaries are used to measure baseline activity levels and then monitor the impact of increasing these on a person's mood. In particular, individuals are encouraged to record levels of achievement and satisfaction from engagement in scheduled activities. Mood diaries can be implemented independently to exclusively rate emotional states throughout the day at pre-agreed intervals. This can aid understanding of how emotions are influenced by a variety of internal and external factors, as well as identify particular periods of elevated risk. In the context of depression, given that reduced activity is considered a key maintaining factor, measurement of the impact of activity on mood is recommended.

Activity/mood diaries are relatively simple to implement. They can constitute part of more formal therapy or be used as a tool during one-to-one meetings with ward staff who can monitor and evaluate the impact of engagement in activities available during an admission, and set targets for future activity. It is crucial that such an approach is adopted by the whole ward team, as it is important that engagement in activity is consistency reinforced and opportunities for a gradual systematic introduction of additional beneficial activities are sought (18).

Positive data logging

When depressed, individuals can become prone to negative cognitive biases such as overgeneralization, all-or-nothing thinking, and selective attention. This can result in only focusing on experiences that confirm negative beliefs. The active noticing of positive events, and proactively searching and systematically recording evidence to support alternative beliefs via data logging can become very useful when tackling low mood (19). Ward staff can also use such logs to help an individual think about their progress, positive interactions with other service users, or other goals that have been attained.

Bipolar affective disorder

'Bipolar' refers to the two extremes of emotion: depression and mania. While mood naturally fluctuates across time, in bipolar disorder there can be frequent or intense changes or cycling of emotional state. Although it is recognized that extreme mood states are often associated with biological and physiological factors, a psychological perspective would emphasize the role of thought and behaviour in the initiation and perpetuation of mood instability. Development of insight and awareness following an episode is therefore central to managing the symptoms of the disorder and mitigation of relapses.

A recent comprehensive review of psychological interventions for bipolar disorder concluded that some, but not all, approaches may have a beneficial effect on relapse, readmission to hospital, and symptoms of depression (20). The strongest evidence was reported for family psychoeducation, which substantially reduced relapse rates. However, there was little evidence of reduction in symptoms of mania, which fits with the argument that engaging psychologically during an acute phase should be done sensitively and may be counterproductive (21). Given that symptoms of mania are one of the main reasons for inpatient treatment, efforts should focus on engaging with families and provision of well-planned collaborative care. Once there is a degree of mood stabilization, the techniques outlined in the following subsections can aid development of insight and mood management:

Mood monitoring

One of the main goals of any bipolar-related intervention is to increase insight into the cyclical nature of the condition. Tracking fluctuations in mood can be helpful in this regard and can serve as an early warning for particular highs and lows by rating moods across time. They can also help track the disorder across time and capture variations within and between cycles of mania and depression. Mood tracking can be carried out physically with a diary or chart, or can be conducted electronically using programmes such as 'True Colours' which prompts an individual to record and monitor symptoms using text, email, and Internet technology; promotes self-management; and enables sharing of information with friends, family, and professionals (22). The relative immediacy of staff contact while an individual is an inpatient provides the ideal environment to trial using a mood tracking system and to receive coaching and support around this.

Relapse prevention planning

Allied to mood tracking, a formal relapse plan can be useful. Such a plan would be developed collaboratively between ward staff, family and the service user, and can be idiosyncratically adapted to specific presentations. A good plan would incorporate some element of identifying early warning signs, triggers, psychoeducation about the disorder, mapping out a relapse signature along with early warning signs, and some advance planning about potential mitigating factors such as diet, drug use, exercise, and sleep. With the consent of the individual, significant people in their network should be invited to feed into the development of such a plan to draw together different perspectives. Observations of ward staff can be incorporated into this and prior to discharge, a joint meeting can be held where the relapse prevention plan can be finalized and shared with relevant professionals. As it is common for feelings of shame to emerge as insight increases in the aftermath of a manic or hypomanic episode, support and education about how to repair relationships or account for decisions made during the episode should be incorporated into this (23).

Structural limits

As there are risks around erratic or unwise decisions made during acute phases of bipolar disorder, advanced planning of physical limits can be helpful. This may include restrictions around access to finances, motor vehicles, alcohol, or other such attendant factors. It is essential that these limits are developed in collaboration with the person in advance and that the rationale is clearly explained.

Anxiety

A psychological formulation of anxiety would view it as the misinterpretation of non-threatening stimuli as threatening. This results in physiological changes (e.g. increased heart rate and laboured breathing) accompanying the activation of the body's sympathetic nervous system. Although adaptive and motivating during situations of danger, it is debilitating and counterproductive in the absence of such harm. Anxiety can self-perpetuate via a cycle of avoidance and limiting exposure to evidence that contradicts anticipated fear.

Anxiety underpins a myriad of distinct disorders, including panic disorder, obsessive–compulsive disorder, post-traumatic stress disorder, acute stress disorder, social anxiety disorder, and generalized anxiety disorder. CBT is consistently reported as an effective intervention in all of these (24). Although anxiety disorders are often not the primary diagnosis in an acute setting, there are high levels of comorbidity and admission to hospital can be anxiety provoking. There is some evidence that demonstrates ward-based transdiagnostic interventions can decrease levels of anxiety (25). There are numerous techniques that have been deployed effectively in an inpatient setting, including the following:

Thought records

Thought records are used for a number of purposes. They are structured tools designed to systematically elicit negative thoughts and to allow an individual to consider contradictory evidence and develop alternative thinking patterns (26). Thought records also collect data on specific triggers, patterns, and thinking styles. Although standard record forms exist, it is recommended that they are tailored to the individual and take into account specific areas of distress. For example, additional information can be collected on bodily sensations in panic disorder, interpretation of intrusive thoughts for obsessive–compulsive disorder, or beliefs about evaluation by others in social phobia. Once completed, thought records can be used to highlight the link between thoughts and feelings and psychoeducation can be delivered to normalize experiences and make sense of anxious thoughts.

Behavioural experiments

In order to test the veracity of anxiety related thoughts, situational exposure to feared stimuli can be conducted. Such behavioural experiments allow the individual to make a prediction, check if it comes true, and then to incorporate this evidence into future cognitions (19). Such experiments often coincide with exposure to previously avoided situations or activities, such as avoiding leaving the house due to fear of collapsing. Key cognitions such as 'I will lose control' and associated behavioural predictions can be clearly operationalized, tested without resorting to safety behaviours, and used to review beliefs. Reassurance seeking is a common way that people try to reduce the anxiety they experience. Although it may provide temporary relief, this process prevents the individual from learning to tolerate emotional discomfort and prevents opportunities to challenge beliefs and specific cognitions. Furthermore, time spent reassurance seeking does not promote alternative ways of coping, such as distraction or use of relaxation. Within a ward setting, it is important that details of behavioural experiments are clearly communicated to ward staff so that the rationale for not providing reassurance can be discussed and a consistent approach is developed in terms of how to manage this behaviour. Ward staff are well positioned to encourage and facilitate recording and rating of beliefs and predictions (before and after experiments) and exploring the meaning of data recorded.

Breathing and relaxation techniques

These techniques are an effective way to manage the physical symptoms of anxiety, as they slow breathing and intake of oxygen and are effective in reducing hyperventilation. This involves the teaching of various techniques and skills such as diaphragmatic breathing or progressive muscular relaxation. Such skills can be taught individually or within a group setting by a variety of healthcare staff, as they often follow a protocol or set of instructions.

Psychotic disorders

Psychological frameworks for understanding psychosis would focus on the interpretation and meaning behind phenomenological experiences such as hallucinations, delusions, and disorganized thinking and exploring the distressed caused by these (27). For example, if critical voices are appraised as being external and threatening, it would naturally follow that strategies such as avoidance and hypervigilance are used, and that these can be potentially changed. Furthermore, a therapeutic stance that emphasizes normalization and a shared understanding of psychosis as a part of the spectrum of human experience can help by cultivating a more positive view of the self, encouraging general functioning, and facilitating communication within relationships and reducing stigma. By actively tackling self-isolation and distress, and providing opportunities to question the validity of unusual perceptions, strongly held beliefs that accompany the disorder can often be weakened and challenged.

There is a wealth of research interest in psychological interventions for psychosis. The consensus view is that intervening early is important (28), and provision of CBT can reduce symptoms, improve medication adherence, and provide superior relapse prevention in comparison to other therapies. There is evidence from inpatient (29) and outpatient (30) settings that CBT delivered in a group format can be as effective as individual CBT sessions. Although a group format may not be appropriate for all, this format enables multiple individuals to receive psychological input and is an important consideration for the inpatient setting where time constraints and limited resources can reduce access to psychological interventions during an admission. Alternatively, some groups are run by former or current service users. The 'Hearing Voices Network' runs groups where individuals can share their experiences in a non-judgemental and supportive environment. Such groups can be particularly useful when individuals are recently discharged from hospital, as attendance can commence during an admission and continue following discharge, thus providing much-needed stability.

Validation

It is important that clinicians and ward staff do not dismiss or ignore experiences of psychosis, particularly when an individual is highly distressed by them. Direct challenging, dismissal, or trivializing of positive symptoms such as delusional beliefs or hearing voices can cause distress and increased resistance, and can contribute to worsen mistrust of others. While active collusion or agreement with the unusual experience should be avoided, validating the fact that these are experienced by the service user and are causing them distress is helpful (31). Ward staff can enhance validation through active listening, normalization, recognition of their distress, and dispelling myths about the disorder through psychoeducation.

Theory A versus theory B

This is a technique that involves evidence gathering but without the explicit aim of belief modification. It can be particularly helpful when there are conflicting views about the nature or validity of events. For example, for the delusional belief 'I am being followed by MI5', two theories would be developed: one which supports the belief and the other which refutes it. Information regarding both of these approaches would be gathered by the service user and staff and subsequently compared. These kinds of interventions in psychosis aim to increase flexibility in thinking in an open and collaborative way that does not position the service user as 'wrong' or elicit shame for being different.

Family intervention

To counter messages that recovery is the sole responsibility of the 'patient', family involvement can be useful. In addition to the involvement of family members and significant others in ward review meetings (if appropriate), family therapy sessions can focus on improving communication within the family system and are recommended alongside individual CBT sessions. Such an approach can help family members learn ways to listen to each other, openly discuss problems, and come up with potential solutions together (32). Increasing the shared understanding of psychosis, relapse signatures, and prevention is crucial and should take place irrespective of whether the individual experiencing psychosis engages so that significant others can be supported (32). Although family interventions should be readily available, individuals with 'treatment-resistant' psychosis should be prioritized due to difficulties with engagement. Family work can begin during an admission, and specific skills such as problem-solving developed to aid management of difficulties that arise following discharge from hospital, with the overall aim of reducing the likelihood of relapse.

Narrative techniques

These techniques can focus on an individual's relationship to their voices and over time work towards understanding the meaning behind voices, hallucinations, or other unusual experiences. This can help with strong emotions, such as anger or fear, that can increase the severity and frequency of psychotic experiences (33). Direct communication with voices is advocated by some researchers as a method of improving this relationship, reducing fear and hostility, and limiting the impact of experiences. This can be achieved through negotiations with voices to develop boundaries around frequency, volume, and voice-free periods (33). Although not strictly a narrative technique, recent developments in CBT also emphasize the importance of increasing a person's sense of control, particularly for persecutory delusions. Instead of challenging the content of delusions, reduction of worry is prioritized, as it is argued to play a central role in the development and maintenance of paranoia (34). Effective worry interventions have included psychoeducation about worry (e.g. positive and negative beliefs about worry), identification of worry triggers, psychological formulations that emphasize the role of thinking processes (e.g. rumination), and techniques of how to respond to worry (34).

Personality disorders

Personality disorders often relate to difficulties in self-regulation of emotion and difficulties with communication in relationships. Psychological approaches would recognize the role of invalidating experiences resulting in beliefs around worthlessness, defectiveness, or abandonment (35). Individuals with such diagnoses often have disruptions in early attachments with caregivers, so become desperate to form and maintain attachments to others but have not learnt the skills required to negotiate relationships (36). Self-harm,

suicidal intention/actions, and other destructive behaviours can be used in an attempt to gain some control over distressing feelings and under duress, risk behaviours can quickly escalate and lead to negative effects on the individual and those around them. Such emotional instability can contribute to the loss of relationships, work, or school and alienate the individual from the surrounding social environment, which in turn reinforces negative views of the self and amplifies further emotional instability.

The majority of research has focused specifically on borderline personality disorder, as often treatment programmes are designed with this client group in mind to reduce life-threatening behaviours. The challenges of working psychologically with this group are compounded by patterns of behaviour that are longstanding and unlikely to change as a result of a short-term admission (37). Moreover, due to issues related to attachment and disruption in early relationships, continuity of care and longer-term therapeutic relationships are critical. For these reasons, the main focus on psychological work on a ward is likely to be at a staff level to develop and support consistent ways of working. However, the skills training component of dialectical behaviour therapy, an evidence-based approach for this client group, has been trialled in a ward setting and there is some evidence that it can be effective in reducing self-injurious behaviours and distress (38). The following subsections will outline some of these skills. Working with personality disorders in an inpatient setting is addressed more comprehensively in Chapter 17.

Distraction

Distraction can be a useful way to direct attention away from internal distress and serve as a short-term alleviation of intense emotions. Ward staff can proactively encourage activities, teach distraction methods, or engage in general conversation in response to increased instability in mood or behaviour. Encouraging individuals to seek this out with staff and fellow service users is also a way of enhancing interpersonal effectiveness.

Mindfulness

Mindfulness involves focusing on the present in a purposeful way without judgement. This strategy can reduce the power of distressing thoughts, images, feelings, or urges, by encouraging observation without engagement or struggle (39). Ward staff are well positioned to support this by teaching methods individually or in groups, providing mindfulness scripts and audio files and encouraging repeated practice.

Distress tolerance

These techniques aim to help the individual tolerate and cope with feelings as and when they arise. These usually target the physiological side of emotional dysregulation, such as increased adrenaline, temperature, tension, and hyperventilation. Toleration strategies include diaphragmatic breathing, progressive muscle relaxation, and submergence in cold water (ice diving). Personalized coping plans can be developed based on what an individual finds effective and should be shared with community teams.

Chain analysis

Chain analysis is a detailed examination of events in the lead up to risk-related behaviour and evaluation of the consequences (40). In particular, the individual is supported to identify specific thoughts, feelings, and actions and opportunities to respond differently in the future. Consideration is also given to factors that may have made a person vulnerable to emotional distress, such as lack of sleep, which can inform relapse plans. Chain analysis should include interactions with ward staff and can sensitively feed into multidisciplinary discussions about the function of behaviours and help develop a consistent approach to behaviours such as self-harm.

Team-based psychological working

Development of a shared formulation can facilitate discussion of a patient's personal history while drawing upon relevant psychological theories to identify precipitating and maintaining factors around the patient's difficulties. Drawing on psychodynamic theory, particularly ideas of transference and countertransference (41), can be helpful in explaining difficult or uncomfortable feelings ward staff might have towards patients. Understanding self-harm or other self-destructive behaviours as maladaptive ways of coping can help both staff and patients foster compassion and shift attitudes that may be otherwise confrontational or adversarial.

REFERENCES

1. British Psychological Society. *Commissioning and Delivering Clinical Psychology in Acute Adult Mental Health Care: Guidelines for Commissioners, Service Managers, Psychology Managers and Practitioners*. London: British Psychological Society; 2012.
2. Clarke I, Wilson H. *Cognitive Behaviour Therapy for Acute Inpatient Mental Health Units: Working with Clients, Staff and the Milieu*. London: Taylor & Francis; 2009.
3. Hopkins J, Loeb S, Fick D. Beyond satisfaction, what service users expect of inpatient mental health care: a literature review. *J Psychiatr Ment Health Nurs* 2009;16:927–937.
4. Gilburt H, Rose D, Slade M. The importance of relationships in mental health care: a qualitative study of service users' experiences of psychiatric hospital admission in the UK. *BMC Health Serv Res* 2008;8:1.
5. Wolpe J, Brady JP, Serber M, Agras WS, Liberman RP. The current status of systematic densitization. *Am J Psychiatry* 1973;130:961–965.
6. Beck AT. *Cognitive Therapy and the Emotional Disorders*. New York: Penguin; 1979.
7. Hayes SC. Acceptance and commitment therapy, relational frame theory, and the third wave of behavioral and cognitive therapies. *Behav Ther* 2004;35:639–665.
8. Leichsenring F, Leibing E. Psychodynamic psychotherapy: a systematic review of techniques, indications and empirical evidence. *Psychol Psychother* 2007;80:217–228.
9. Kösters M, Burlingame GM, Nachtigall C, Strauss B. A meta-analytic review of the effectiveness of inpatient group psychotherapy. *Group Dyn* 2006;10:146–163.
10. Haase M, Frommer J, Franke G-H, et al. From symptom relief to interpersonal change: treatment outcome and effectiveness in inpatient psychotherapy. *Psychother Res* 2008;18:615–624.
11. Dallos R, Draper R. *An Introduction to Family Therapy: Systemic Theory and Practice*. Maidenhead: McGraw-Hill Education (UK); 2010.
12. Carr A. *Family Therapy: Concepts, Process and Practice*. Chichester: John Wiley & Sons; 2012.
13. Cuijpers P, Andersson G, Donker T, van Straten A. Psychological treatment of depression: results of a series of meta-analyses. *Nord J Psychiatry* 2011;65:354–364.
14. Köhler S, Hoffmann S, Unger T, Steinacher B, Dierstein N, Fydrich T. Effectiveness of cognitive–behavioural therapy plus pharmacotherapy in inpatient treatment of depressive disorders. *Clin Psychol Psychother* 2013;20:97–106.
15. Schramm E, Dietrich van Calker M, Dykierek P, et al. An intensive treatment program of interpersonal psychotherapy plus pharmacotherapy for depressed inpatients: acute and long-term results. *Am J Psychiatry* 2007;164:768–777.
16. Brown GK, Ten Have T, Henriques GR, Xie SX, Hollander JE, Beck AT. Cognitive therapy for the prevention of suicide attempts: a randomized controlled trial. *JAMA* 2005;294:563–570.
17. Veale D. Behavioural activation for depression. *Adv Psychiatr Treat* 2008;14:29–36.
18. Curran J, Lawson P, Houghton S, Gournay K. Implementing behavioural activation in inpatient psychiatric wards. *J Ment Health Train Educ Pract* 2007;2:28–35.
19. Bennett-Levy JE, Butler GE, Fennell ME, Hackman AE, Mueller ME, Westbrook DE. *Oxford Guide to Behavioural Experiments in Cognitive Therapy*. Oxford: Oxford University Press; 2004.
20. Oud M, Mayo-Wilson E, Braidwood R, et al. Psychological interventions for adults with bipolar disorder: systematic review and meta-analysis. *Br J Psychiatry* 2016;208:213–222.
21. Scott J, Colom F, Vieta E. A meta-analysis of relapse rates with adjunctive psychological therapies compared to usual psychiatric treatment for bipolar disorders. *Int J Neuropsychopharmacol* 2007;10:123–129.
22. Miklowitz DJ, Price J, Holmes EA, et al. Facilitated integrated mood management for adults with bipolar disorder. *Bipolar Disord* 2012;14:185–197.
23. Jones S. Psychotherapy of bipolar disorder: a review. *J Affect Disord* 2004;80:101–114.
24. Hofmann SG, Smits JA. Cognitive-behavioral therapy for adult anxiety disorders: a meta-analysis of randomized placebo-controlled trials. *J Clin Psychiatry* 2008;69:621–632.
25. Raune D, Daddi I. Pilot study of group cognitive behaviour therapy for heterogeneous acute psychiatric inpatients: treatment in a sole-standalone session allowing patients to choose the therapeutic target. *Behav Cogn Psychother* 2011;39:359–365.
26. Greenberger D, Padesky CA. *Mind Over Mood: Change How You Feel by Changing the Way You Think*. New York: Guilford Publications; 2015.
27. Morrison AP. The interpretation of intrusions in psychosis: an integrative cognitive approach to hallucinations and delusions. *Behav Cogn Psychother* 2001;29:257–276.
28. Birchwood M, Todd P, Jackson C. Early intervention in psychosis: the critical-period hypothesis. *Int Clin Psychopharmacol* 1998;13:S31–S40.
29. Owen M, Sellwood W, Kan S, Murray J, Sarsam M. Group CBT for psychosis: a longitudinal, controlled trial with inpatients. *Behav Res Ther* 2015;65:76–85.
30. Lecomte T, Leclerc C, Corbiere M, Wykes T, Wallace CJ, Spidel A. Group cognitive behavior therapy or social skills training for individuals with a recent onset of psychosis?: results of a randomized controlled trial. *J Nerv Ment Dis* 2008;196:866–875.
31. Pitt L, Kilbride M, Nothard S, Welford M, Morrison AP. Researching recovery from psychosis: a user-led project. *Psychiatrist* 2007;31:55–60.
32. Garety PA, Fowler DG, Freeman D, Bebbington P, Dunn G, Kuipers E. Cognitive–behavioural therapy and family intervention for relapse prevention and symptom reduction in psychosis: randomised controlled trial. *Br J Psychiatry* 2008;192:412–423.

33. Corstens D, Longden E, May R. Talking with voices: exploring what is expressed by the voices people hear. *Psychosis* 2012;4:95–104.

34. Freeman D, Dunn G, Startup H, et al. Effects of cognitive behaviour therapy for worry on persecutory delusions in patients with psychosis (WIT): a parallel, single-blind, randomised controlled trial with a mediation analysis. *Lancet Psychiatry* 2015;2:305–313.

35. Young JE. *Cognitive Therapy for Personality Disorders: A Schema-Focused Approach*. Sarasota, FL: Professional Resource Press; 1994.

36. Fonagy P, Target M, Gergely G. Attachment and borderline personality disorder: a theory and some evidence. *Psychiatr Clin North Am* 2000;23:103–122.

37. Paris J. Is hospitalization useful for suicidal patients with borderline personality disorder? *J Person Disord* 2004;18(3: special issue):240–247.

38. Bohus M, Haaf B, Simms T, et al. Effectiveness of inpatient dialectical behavioral therapy for borderline personality disorder: a controlled trial. *Behav Res Ther* 2004;42:487–499.

39. Allen NB, Chambers R, Knight W, Melbourne Academic Mindfulness Interest Group. Mindfulness-based psychotherapies: a review of conceptual foundations, empirical evidence and practical considerations. *Aust N Z J Psychiatry* 2006;40:285–294.

40. Linehan M. *Cognitive-Behavioral Treatment of Borderline Personality Disorder*. New York: Guilford Press; 1993.

41. Leiper R. Psychodynamic formulation: looking beneath the surface. In: Johnstone L, Dallos R (eds), *Formulation in Psychology and Psychotherapy: Making Sense of People's Problems*, pp. 45–66. New York: Routledge; 2014.

Diversity, advocacy, staffing issues

30

Diversity in inpatient care

Michelle Mbayiwa

Introduction

The National Health Service (NHS) is a unique and comprehensive service that is available for everyone regardless of their income, employment status, race, disability, gender reassignment, age, religion or belief, sex, sexual orientation, and marriage and civil partnership status. The service is bound by the core values and principles of the 'NHS Constitution' (1) and has a duty of care to respect the human rights of whom they provide a service to. The Department of Health is committed to ensuring that equality and human rights are at the heart of policy and that this is based on the best available evidence. The NHS has a social responsibility to promote equality through the services it provides and to particularly acknowledge groups where improvements in health and life expectancy are not aligned to the changes observed in the general population. This chapter will highlight the issues around diversity within inpatient care in relation to each of the protected characteristics, the effect diversity has on patient care, the importance of challenging and addressing these issues, and suggest some points of best practice. As some diversity issues are addressed, it will be apparent that they affect both patients as well as staff providing care.

What is diversity?

When we talk about diversity we mean respecting and valuing all forms of difference in individuals. People differ in all sorts of ways which may not always be obvious or visible. These differences might include race and ethnicity, culture and belief, gender and sexuality, age and social status, ability, and use of health and social care services (2). Diversity means understanding that everyone is unique, and recognizing our individual differences, practising mutual respect of those unique experiences and qualities so we can all collaboratively endeavour to eradicate all forms of discrimination. The Equality Act 2010 was introduced to replace legislations such as the Race Relations Act 1976 and the Disability Discrimination Act 1995, making any form of discrimination illegal. It contains all of the UK's legal requirements on equality, protecting people from discrimination based on certain explicitly protected characteristics. Whether at work as an employee or when using the service, the purpose of the Equality Act is to ensure that everyone has the right to be treated fairly. The following characteristics are defined as protected: race, disability, gender reassignment, age, religion or belief, sex, sexual orientation, and marriage and civil partnership. This chapter will outline the first six of these characteristics.

Race

Race as a protected characteristic refers to a group of people defined by their race, colour, and nationality (including citizenship), and ethnic or national origins (3). Black and minority ethnic (BME) communities have significantly poorer mental health outcomes and poorer experiences of services (4). Patients from ethnic minorities with severe mental illness have been reported to be at greater disadvantage and inequality with respect to service needs and provision (5–7). Thus, tackling race diversity is a challenge for mental health services and professionals. In this connection, a study in the US found that aligning patients with a clinician from the same ethnic background decreased the use and need for emergency services and increased the use of community services (8). Another study in Australia confirmed this finding, with a reduction in inpatient admissions for some ethnic groups and a low level of crisis intervention required. The picture seems more complex as in England some patients were not keen to work with staff from their own community (4). There are several factors that fall within the race category that need to be taken into consideration to address diversity and equality, for example, language, cultural factors, and diet.

Language barriers

There has been an increase in the number of patients from different ethnic and language backgrounds in contact with mental health services so provisions to meet this demand need to be made available. Several documents set out principles that ensure a safe, high-quality interpreting and translation service is provided (e.g. 'Working with an interpreter' (9)). NHS guidance states that professional interpreters should be provided for clinically significant events such as care planning. For example, mental health wards in the Berkshire Healthcare NHS Foundation Trust have multilingual DVDs providing information on patients' rights and they also have a range of different types of translation, including face to face, telephone, and British Sign Language. Not infrequently, however, ward staff often do not have the skills to work with interpreters or the latter are not readily available. Therefore, staff members who speak the same language of a given patient may occasionally aid as an unofficial interpreter during the assessments process (10), facilitating the assessment as well as reducing the risk of incidents due to potential misunderstandings. Even after language barriers are dealt with, professionals may not yet be equipped with the skills to assess and manage mental distress in patients from different cultural groups, with lack of knowledge about cultural issues, difficulties in communication, and stereotyping cited as the main areas of concern (11–14).

Dietary needs

Inpatient services have sought to establish flexibility around patients' dietary needs providing a variety of choices (halal meals, vegetarian meals, etc.). It is recognized that having this option contributes to the patient's recovery, reducing the risk of patients' malnutrition (14). Since 1990, a variety of documents have provided guidance and opinion on food service in UK hospitals and institutions (15–19).

Developing culturally sensitive care plans

Mental health professionals conducting assessments of and developing care plans with patients should be mindful of the potentially relevant cultural differences and be alert to the possibility that an individual's ethnic heritage may affect the clinical team's ability to identify and meet those needs. For example, patients of African heritage may be less likely to be aware of, or report, their needs, making it more difficult for the clinical teams to meet them (20). The independent inquiry into inequalities in health (21) keenly proposed for 'cultural competency' to be developed and embedded in staff's everyday practice at work. Staff are required to acquire the skills to understand and be sensitive to cultural differences in illness and treatment as well as to address issues of institutional racism, which occur when organizational structure, policies, processes, and practices result in minority ethnic groups being treated unfairly and less equally, often without intent or knowledge.

Race from the staff's perspective

Abuse toward staff sometimes is racially motivated and it can sadly be accompanied by violence and aggression. NHS trusts have been working towards a zero-tolerance policy of abuse to staff, for example, by publicly displaying posters to demonstrate their support to them. At a practical level, although staff have been encouraged to report this type of behaviour to the police, they often feel there is no point on doing that as their perception is that it is unlikely that anything will be done. However, work continues with staff to emphasize that it must not be seen as a lost cause and that organizations must continue to strive for zero tolerance of violence and aggression from patients in any form, verbal or physical. Daily, staff members are encouraged to report any such abuse via incident reporting systems (many of them electronic forms which are easy to complete) as well as to the police. A local trust works closely with security management services when staff have been assaulted with a view to press charges on the perpetrator as well as supporting and guiding staff through the process.

Recruitment and selection

Recent research indicates that there has been very little progress in the past 20 years in terms of addressing discrimination against BME staff in the NHS (22). In this regard, the NHS Workforce Race Equality Standards (WRES) is a compilation of nine indicators which have been made available to the NHS since 2015 to be used as a tool to improve workplace experiences and representation at all levels for BME staff. The WRES focuses on equality and on the BME workforce in relation to their experiences and treatment, as NHS England and its partners are committed to tackling race discrimination and to create an environment where the talents of all staff are valued and developed (23). All this is important, not least because research shows that discrimination increases sickness and absence, with staff leaving organizations, an outcome that is both clinically and financially costly (24).

Disability

A person has a disability if she or he has a physical or mental impairment which has a substantial and long-term adverse effect on that person's ability to carry their normal day-to-day activities (4), including people with cancer or HIV.

Clinical vignette

Camila is an 18-year-old female with features of emotionally unstable personality disorder as well as a history of a depressive episode with anxiety who was taken to the accident and emergency (A&E) department by her school following thoughts to harm herself; she was subsequently admitted to hospital informally. She was known to the child and adolescent mental health services and was profoundly deaf, which made it difficult for the team to assess her; the team had to rely on the information provided by the school and by her mother. None of the A&E professionals were trained to use sign language making the assessment process difficult. Similarly, none of the inpatient ward staff had that training either. Ward staff decided to use picture messages to communicate with her regarding her basic needs, which was helpful at the time. However, it took a few days to access British Sign Language translation. Had the latter been timely available, the whole process would have been much less distressing, and from the onset would have improved the level of care provided.

Impact of the physical environment

Mental health inpatient units have over the years made considerable changes to their physical environments to ensure they can look after patients with physical disabilities who utilize wheelchairs by installing ramps leading into open courtyards to enable access to fresh air; this also been accompanied by the provision of bathroom facilities for the disabled.

Support for staff with disabilities

Staff with disabilities report high levels of discrimination (22). A crucial role of a ward manager is to be able to get their staff to speak openly about any disabilities they may have and how they can be supported. For example, a staff member with hearing difficulties should be included in deciding what supportive measures would assist them to do their job efficiently and as to how they wanted the rest of the team members to be informed of their disability and by whom. Staff at all levels need training on how to maintain this level of support once a staff member's disability is acknowledged.

Gender reassignment

If the person is proposing to undergo, is undergoing, or has undergone a process (or part of a process) for sex reassignment then they have a protected characteristic (3). Guidance, information, policies, and education about gender reassignment must be shared with staff to build their confidence in caring for patients. More recently, there has been a national drive for single-sex inpatient units, which is now implemented across most mental health wards, to promote patients' privacy and dignity as well as to reduce the risk of sexual incidents and to protect vulnerable patients. Those hospitals which still have mixed-sex wards essentially make provisions, particularly sleeping arrangements, by cordoning off part of the ward so that patients from the opposite sex do not have access to the other side of the ward. Not much research exists on which is the better option for patients and staff but the risk of sexual vulnerability has been reduced and many patients now have en-suite rooms. There remain other challenges in need of addressing. For instance, for a same-sex ward, the question would be the male to female staffing ratio, an issue to be taken into consideration when, for example, putting together a ward's duty roster.

Age

In 2015, there were nearly 9.4 million workers over 50 years old in the UK, with 1.17 million of them aged 65 or over, a number that is set to increase. It is predicted that older people will make up 32% of the workforce by 2020, because of the increase in the state pension age and longer life expectancy. This demographic change will put increasing pressure on mental health inpatient services. The key issue here is that care is provided based on the patient's needs (e.g. mobility, frailty, and vulnerability to exploitation and neglect) and not merely and exclusively based on the person's age (25).

Religion or belief

Religion as a protected characteristic refers to any religion, and also includes having no religion. A religion must have a clear structure and belief system while belief means any religious or philosophical belief or no belief. To be protected, a belief must satisfy various criteria, including that it is a weighty and substantial aspect of human life and behaviour. Denominations or sects within a religion can be considered a protected religion or religious belief (4). People from all religions report experiencing discrimination on the basis of their faith, the highest reporting being by Muslims (22.2%) (22).

Every ward should have a specified system for assessing spirituality needs, incorporating them into care planning and making links with relevant community services (26). The admitting nurse should record the patient's religion so the care plans integrate spiritual care for the duration of the patient's admission (26). Also, spiritual care resources boxes must be available on all inpatient wards to give patients the opportunity to practise their religion should they wish to do so. These boxes contain religious resources (e.g. prayer mat, holy books from the main faiths, prayer/meditation beads, and leaflets of comforting quotes). It is also essential for hospitals to have faith rooms for patients (26) and professionals need to make sure these services are accessible to patients. For example, Berkshire Healthcare NHS Foundation Trust (27) has a sanctuary multifaith space, which contains facilities for those who wash before prayers. Patients are given a choice in advance of what they would like to happen at the multifaith service which is held on a Sunday. This can vary according to who is at the service. The trust's chaplain acts as a link to several faiths and can access information, for example, about the respective leaders in local churches who can work with the hospital to cater for patients' needs. The chaplain also provides one-to-one support for patients. The faith visitors are a group of people who visit hospitals monthly, representing the main religions such as Buddhism, Judaism, Islam, and Sikhism. Monthly cultural and religious briefings are distributed to staff containing information on what faith visitors will be able to offer at upcoming religious festivals. Finally, with a view to provide information to the wider staff, the Berkshire Healthcare NHS Foundation Trust website contains information produced by faith visitors about typical attitudes around social issues including sexuality, gender, and ageing which staff can access. These resources help staff to understand cultural features, pressures, or stigma the patient may be experiencing around their diagnosis or current experiences.

Sex

The NHS needs to improve its data collection of the sexual orientation of people with mental illness to comply with the Equality Act. However, this is just part of a far bigger issue as most mental health nurses remain reluctant to assess the sexuality and sexual health needs of their patients (28) even though they are critical aspects of who we are as individuals and of how we view ourselves. Sexuality is a topic that can potentially arouse discomfort (29) but ignoring it will leave an important aspect of patients' lives in the dark, potentially affecting areas such as relationships and engagement with medication and support. Clearly, a therapeutic relationship between the mental health nurse and the patient is an opportunity to take a sexual history, promote safe sexual practices, and discuss sexual health issues.

Avoiding discrimination against staff and supporting staff

The NHS must avoid discrimination against its staff, especially of job applicants with issues that correspond to any of the protected characteristics. The NHS undertook a review of how potential candidates were recruited. For example, standardized online application forms used by all NHS trusts are processed according to guidance provided by the Department of Health, the Data Protection Act 2018, and the Equality Act. All this was done with a view to reducing the possibility of discrimination, be it because of sex, sexual orientation, marital status, or any other protected characteristic.

The National Institute for Health and Care Excellence guidelines on workplace management point out that the role and leadership style of line managers is particularly important when supporting staff in the workplace (30). It is important to challenge stereotypes and to not make assumptions that, for example, an older employee may find learning new tasks difficult or that a younger employee might be less dependable. Reflective practice and commitment to the understanding of everyone as a person and considering and respecting cultural diversity will enable mental health staff to work with service users to establish supportive care strategies and achieve good and valid outcomes (31).

Conclusion

Services and professionals must continue working towards inclusivity and promotion of diversity. Evidence shows that BME communities have poorer experiences of services and significantly poorer mental health outcomes, although several programmes have been developed to address these inequalities (3). As the UK's population becomes more diverse, it is imperative that improvements occur in this area.

REFERENCES

1. Department of Health and Social Care. The NHS constitution: the NHS belongs to us all. 2015. https://www.gov.uk/government/uploads/system/uploads/attachment_data/file/480482/NHS_Constitution_WEB.pdf

2. Simons L, INVOLVE Coordinating Centre. Diversity and inclusion: what's it about and why is it important for public involvement in research? INVOLVE, National Institute for Health Research. 2012. http://www.invo.org.uk/posttypepublication/diversity-and-inclusion-what%E2%80%99s-it-about-and-why-is-it-important-for-public-involvement-in-research

3. Legislation.gov.uk. Equality Act 2010. 2010. https://www.legislation.gov.uk/ukpga/2010/15/contents

4. Mental Health Providers Forum, Race Equality Foundation. Better practice in mental health for black and minority ethnic communities. 2015. http://raceequalityfoundation.org.uk/wp-content/uploads/2018/10/Better-practice-in-mental-health.pdf

5. Keating F, Robertson D, McCulloch A. *Breaking Circles of Fear*. London: Sainsbury Centre for Mental Health; 2002.

6. Ndegwa D. *Social Division and Difference: Black and Ethnic Minorities*. London: NHS National Programme on Forensic Mental Health Research and Development; 2003.

7. Bennet J, Keating F. Training to redress racial disadvantage in mental health care: race equality or cultural competence? *Ethn Inequal Health Soc Care* 2008;1:52–59.

8. Ziguras S, Klimidis S, Lewis J, Stuart G. Ethnic matching of clients and clinicians and use of mental health services by ethnic minority clients. 2003. http://psychservices.psychiatryonline.org

9. Working with an interpreter: toolkit – for practitioners and interpreters. Improving communication for people who use mental health and learning disability services in Scotland. Mental Welfare Commission for Scotland; 2013. http://www.mwcscot.org.uk/media/127976/interpreter_toolkit_for_practitioners_and_interpreters_march_2013.pdf

10. Murphy K, Maclead Clark J. Nurses' experiences of caring for ethnic minority clients. *J Adv Nurs* 1993;18:442–450.

11. Bhugra D, Bhui, K. *Cross-Cultural Psychiatry: A Practical Guide*. London: Arnold; 2001.

12. Dobson SM. Bringing culture into care. *Nurs Times* 1983;79:464–466.

13. Jones DC, Van Amelsvoort Jones GM. Communication patterns between nursing staff and the ethnic elderly in long term facility. *J Adv Nurs* 1986;11:265–272.

14. Royal College of Psychiatrists. Improving in-patient mental health services for black and minority ethnic patients: recommendations to inform accreditation standards. Occasional paper OP71. 2009. https://www.rcpsych.ac.uk/usefulresources/publications/collegereports/op/op71.aspx

15. Department of Health. *Equity and Excellence: Liberating the NHS*. London: Department of Health; 2010.

16. McWhirter J, Pennington CR. Incidence and recognition of malnutrition in hospital. *BMJ* 1994;308:945–948.

17. Centre for Health Services Research. *Eating Matters*. London: University of Newcastle upon Tyne; 1997.

18. Association of Community Health Councils for England and Wales. *Hungry in Hospital?* London: ACH-CEW; 1997.

19. British Association of Enteral and Parenteral Nutrition. *Hospital Food as Treatment*. Maidenhead: BA-PEN; 1999.

20. Bruce M, Gwaspari M, Cobb D, Nedgwa D. Ethnic differences in reported unmet needs among male inpatients with severe mental illness. *J Psychiatr Ment Health Nurs* 2011;19:830–838.

21. Acheson D. *Independent Inquiry into Inequalities in Health*. London: HMSO; 1998.

22. The Kings Fund. Making the difference: diversity and inclusion in the NHS. 2015. https://www.kingsfund.org.uk/sites/files/kf/field/field_publication_file/Making-the-difference-summary-Kings-Fund-Dec-2015.pdf

23. NHS England. Technical guidance for the NHS Workforce Race Equality Standard (WRES). 2016. https://www.england.nhs.uk/wp-content/uploads/2014/10/wres-technical-guidance-april-16.pdf

24. NHS England. Briefing for NHS Boards on the NHS workforce race equality: NHS workforce race equality delivers better care, outcomes and performance. 2015. https://www.england.nhs.uk/wp-content/uploads/2015/10/wres-nhs-board-bulletin.pdf

25. Audit Commission. *Forget Me Not 2002: Developing Mental Health Services for Older People in England*. London: Audit Commission Publications; 2002.

26. Royal College of Psychiatrists. Accreditation for Inpatient Mental Health Services (AIMS). Standards for inpatient wards –working-age adults. 2010. https://www.rcpsych.ac.uk/pdf/Standards%20for%20Inpatient%20Wards%20-%20Working%20Age%20Adults%-%20Fourth%20Edition.pdf

27. Berkshire Healthcare NHS Foundation Trust. Chaplaincy. https://www.berkshirehealthcare.nhs.uk/our-services/other-services/chaplaincy/

28. Woolf L, Jackson B. Coffee and condoms: the implementation of a sexual health programme in acute psychiatry in an inner city area. *J Adv Nurs* 1996;23:299–304.

29. Higgins A, Barker P, Begley CM. 'Veiling sexualities': a grounded theory of mental health nurses responses to issues of sexuality. *J Adv Nurs* 2008;62:307–317.

30. National Institute for Health and Care Excellence. Workplace health: management practices. NICE guideline [NG13]. 2016. https://www.nice.org.uk/guidance/ng13

31. Bradley P, DeSouza R. Mental health and illness in Australia and New Zealand. In Elder R, Evans K, Nizette D (eds), *Practical Perspectives in Psychiatric and Mental Health Nursing*, 3rd edition, pp. 87–108. New South Wales: Mosby, Elsevier Australia; 2012.

31

Advocacy

Georga Godwin

Introduction

This chapter is not a comprehensive examination on the avenues open to patients to advocate for their rights, it would be impossible to cover in detail all aspects of this. This chapter therefore outlines the principles and signposts where further information can be obtained.

The tension between psychiatry and law

Inpatient psychiatry is the practice of treating patients with mental health conditions in a hospital setting. However, many of those patients do not agree that they have a mental disorder, they disagree that they need treatment, and that they need to be in hospital. These patients require detention and compulsion to receive the treatment their psychiatrists consider necessary. The Mental Health Act 1983 as amended by the Mental Health Act 2007 ('MHA') (1) gives psychiatrists the power to do this. Although, the decision to detain is taken by psychiatrists and AMHPs, detention is technically by a 'detaining authority', or 'responsible authority', usually the local mental health National Health Service (NHS) trust.

Some psychiatric inpatients, like patients admitted to general hospitals, are 'informal' rather than detained (although this too is covered by the MHA, in Section (S.) 131 MHA). Such patients are allowed to come and go off a ward as they choose, and cannot be medicated against their will. Unfortunately, in the author's experience it is not uncommon to find informal patients denied time off the ward, and therefore de facto detained. For example, it is unlawful to write in an informal patient's notes that they are not allowed to leave the ward as denying leave off the ward would amount to detention.

The issue for inpatient psychiatry is how to provide treatment to a patient who disagrees that they need that treatment. Historically, patients with mental disorders were detained against their will with little recourse to the law, or thought given to how that felt for them, indeed it seems that having a mental disorder precluded a patient from having any legal rights (2). This is now not the case, but there remains a tension between the objectives of inpatient psychiatry and the law.

Psychiatrists are trained to provide treatment that they consider is in a patient's best interests. But if a patient is detained against their will, they will want to leave hospital before they are as well as the

psychiatrist would like. So, on the one hand, there are psychiatrists who wish to do the best for their patients; and on the other, there are patients who are detained against their will. Holding the balance between these two is the law. And it is the same law that allows psychiatrists to detain that protects the rights of the patients.

The law agrees with the aim of inpatient psychiatry, if not to cure, at least to alleviate symptoms[1] but a patient can only be detained if the treatment is necessary.[2] What is necessary is different from what is in the patient's best interests. The tension therefore extends to the focus of psychiatrists and lawyers.

Mental health law is complicated and evolving, such that in order to practise in this area lawyers must be accredited on The Law Society's Mental Health Accreditation Scheme. While psychiatrists have some training and understanding of the MHA,[3] they are not lawyers so do not have the training to interpret and apply legal principles. However, psychiatrists do not do deal with the law alone and each NHS trust employs Mental Health Act Administrators (MHAAs), also not legally trained, whose job it is to ensure compliance with the law, and who themselves have access to legal advice.

The MHA gives psychiatrists the power to detain patients[4] and enforce medication when less restrictive care has failed or is inappropriate, and allows patients to seek to be discharged from detention. However, once discharged, if the patient stops medication psychiatrists will re-detain and enforce medication because they believe there is a need for treatment. Thus, in the doctor–patient relationship, psychiatrists have the power.

The legal framework

Mental health law is today encapsulated in the MHA (1) and a body of extensive case law. Like most human rights law, it arose out of the aftermath of World War II. The Universal Declaration of Human

---

[1] S. 145(4) MHA.

[2] S. 72 MHA.

[3] A 2-day course with 1-day yearly refresher for S. 12(2) MHA-approved clinician, whereas an Approved Mental Health Practitioner (AMHP) must complete a 6-month university course.

[4] It takes two doctors, one must be S. 12(2) MHA approved, and an AMHP to detain.

Rights. Article 9 states, 'no one shall be subjected to arbitrary arrest, detention or exile'. This is also codified in in Article 5 of the European Convention on Human Rights (ECHR) (3). In the UK, the ECHR is enacted by the Human Rights Act 1998, and Article 5 of the ECHR is enshrined in the MHA.

The MHA gives a detained patient the right to a court hearing to seek discharge via the First-tier Tribunal Mental Health ('Tribunal'), and the right to a lawyer to represent them both at those hearings and generally because they are detained.

Lawyers are not free, and it is seen as only right that someone who is detained and is seeking discharge from that detention should have their legal representation paid for by the state. All patients who apply for a Tribunal hearing therefore qualify for legal aid. Patients who require legal advice other than for a Tribunal hearing also qualify for legal aid but this is means-tested.

Good practice under the MHA is outlined in the Code of Practice ('the Code') published by the Department of Health in 2015 (4). The Code outlines the responsibilities of the detaining authority, and the professionals, regarding how to protect the patient's rights and how care, support, and treatment should be delivered.

Patients/clients

In legal terms, there are two types of detained patients:

- Those whose discharge is controlled by clinical teams (civil patients).[5]
- Those detained under Part III of the MHA (restricted/forensic patients).[6, 7]

The difference between them is that restricted patients may have been sent to psychiatric hospital for assessment while awaiting trial, or their detention has been ordered in lieu of a sentence of imprisonment. They are subject to restrictions overseen by the Ministry of Justice.

Capacity

Difficulties for the mental health lawyer arise when their client does not have the capacity to give instructions. Some clients can give basic instructions, 'I want to go home', but are unable to provide details; and some clients give instructions that are not based in reality. Guidance is provided only in the case of clients who have applied for a Tribunal (5).

Recent jurisprudence (6) held that there is a different level of capacity for applying for a Tribunal and withdrawing that application. That said, a mental health lawyer will act on instructions at a far lower threshold than would be acceptable in any other area of law.

If a patient does not have capacity to instruct then a lawyer may be appointed for them under Rule 11 of The Tribunal Procedure (First-tier Tribunal) (Health, Education and Social Care Chamber, Rules 2008 ('Tribunal Rules') (7). Once appointed, the lawyer must act in the client's best interests rather than follow incapacitous

instructions, although they must make the patient's wishes known to the Tribunal (5).

There is no guidance on how to represent a client who lacks capacity outside the Tribunal procedure. In these cases, the client could be referred for a Tribunal and Rule 11 will then apply. Otherwise, the lawyer must follow instructions from someone acting as litigation friend.

Information

There is a duty on the detaining authority to provide information to the patient regarding their detention as soon as practicable after the patient has been detained. Information given includes details of the Section the patient is detained under, how to apply for a Tribunal, other means of securing discharge,[8] that medication can be enforced, that there is a Code of Practice for the MHA, and that their post may be withheld.[9]

Information is often provided when the patient is first admitted and not able to understand, and often patients remain confused and distressed. In order to help tackle this issue, the author of this chapter launched a website to help: https://www.mentalhealthsolicitor.co.uk/services-for-you.html.

Solicitors

It would be unfair for a mentally disordered patient to advocate for themselves. Given the complexity of the law, it is difficult for lay people to pick their way through the legal morass. Therefore, there is a need for specialist lawyers. The lawyer's role is to help the client understand the law that is being applied to them, and to use that law to further their rights.

Relationships between psychiatrists and patients continue after detention has ended, therefore a lawyer should help their client to find common ground so they can work together. But while solicitors must provide realistic advice, clients may choose not to take that advice and solicitors must act on the instructions given regardless. Clients' instructions can be changeable, so what might appear straightforward to a psychiatrist can change drastically and therefore be understandable only within the privileged relationship. Because of legal privilege, psychiatrists do not know the instructions or to what extent the solicitor is acting contrary to their legal advice. Further, a client may tell their psychiatrist one thing but instruct their lawyer quite differently.

For the lawyer, it is hard to understand why some psychiatrists give legal advice when they do not fully understand the law and are not privy to the instructions. This is especially true when a client is deciding whether to apply for a Tribunal. The decision process that a client and solicitor go through is more complex than whether the psychiatrist agrees that their patient is ready for discharge. A psychiatrist will base their advice on their medical opinion; a lawyer will base their legal advice on a longer-term and wider view of the issues.

---

[5] SS. 2, 3, 7 (Guardianship), 17A to 17G (Community Treatment Orders), 37, notional 37 MHA.

[6] S. 79 MHA.

[7] SS. 35, 36, 37/41, 42 (Conditional Discharge), 45A, 47/49, 48 MHA.

[8] By the consultant psychiatrist, the hospital managers, or the patient's nearest relative.

[9] S. 132 MHA.

Choosing a lawyer

Lists of solicitors' firms that provide mental health legal services are kept by the detaining authority, but there is no guide as to how competent each lawyer is. Only recently the law changed so that only people (they need not be qualified lawyers) who are accredited on the Mental Health Accreditation Scheme of The Law Society can represent at Tribunals.

For some patients trust is a real issue. They find themselves detained against their will, forced to take medication, and they believe no one is on their side. These patients can be desperate because they genuinely believe that they should not be in hospital and not be receiving treatment. In mental health law, where most of the legal advice given is negative, for example, that medication can be enforced despite protestations that the patient does not need it, trust is vital to help the client come to terms with their situation. The relationship therefore between a mental health lawyer and their client requires time and patience to build. It is impossible to understand how a client feels being detained against their will but trying to get small concessions into the amount of freedom they have certainly helps.

Ensuring good practice

In England and Wales, all qualified lawyers are regulated by the Legal Services Board. Each type of lawyer has its own secondary regulator, with solicitors regulated by the Solicitors Regulation Authority. The Solicitors Regulation Authority sets principles and codes of conduct to ensure that solicitors operate independently, with integrity, and in the interests of clients and the public (5).

The Law Society issued a practice note entitled 'Representation Before Mental Health Tribunals' (8), which sets out good practice within the Tribunal procedure. The Law Society also has a Mental Health Accreditation Scheme, to which all representatives that appear before the Tribunal must belong. Accreditation is only gained after proving competency, and also has a Code of Practice (9).

Mental health lawyers may also become a member of the Mental Health Lawyers Association (10). This has its own Code of Conduct (11), which stresses the need for the highest ethical and professional standards when dealing with clients and other patients.

Funding for mental health representatives is by the state via the Legal Aid Agency, which uses peer review (12) to ensure best practice and good quality of work.

First-tier Tribunal Mental Health

Composition of the Tribunal

The court that has jurisdiction for the MHA is the First-tier Tribunal Mental Health ('Tribunal').[10] The Tribunal is administered by the Tribunal Service Mental Health ('TSMH') (13).

A Tribunal is made up of a panel of three experts: a medical member (a consultant psychiatrist), a Tribunal Judge (often a full-time Salaried Tribunal Judge), and a specialist lay member (a social worker or other mental health professional). It is independent of the detaining authority and must have no conflict of interest or bias in the proceedings.

The Tribunal is a check to the power of the detaining authorities (14) in that it ensures that psychiatrists can only detain and enforce treatment if the law agrees. If the Tribunal finds that detention is not necessary, then it will discharge the patient regardless of the medical opinion.

Application and reference periods

When a patient can apply for a Tribunal depends on which Section they are detained under. Generally, an application can be made once in every period of time that the Section lasts for, therefore a renewal of a Section starts a new application period. However, this varies depending on the Section (15).

A lawyer will advise their client when to apply based on the merits of their case, but patients often apply when they are at their most desperate to go home. Patients have the right to withdraw their application at any stage prior to the Tribunal's decision.

Some patients rarely exercise their right to apply, which can prolong detention. If a psychiatrist thinks that is the case, they should recommend that the patient instructs a lawyer, in the same way that lawyers should recommend their client get a doctor rather than give medical advice.

The process for listing a Tribunal hearing date is problematic because the patient, their representative, the psychiatrist, care coordinator, and a nurse must all attend. Finding a convenient date can be difficult. In Oxford, the parties give their availability to the MHAA, who sends time slots to the TSMH. However, problems occur when a date is agreed before a lawyer has been instructed, or a hearing is listed on a date that none can do. Relisting can cause long delays, which can prolong detention.

Procedural rules

There are rules that govern the Tribunal, the Tribunal Procedure (First-tier Tribunal) (Health, Education and Social Care Chamber) Rules 2008 ('Tribunal Rules') (7). These rules have an overriding objective to deal with the case 'fairly and justly',[11] which governs how Tribunal procedure is to be carried out.

Powers of the Tribunal

The powers of the Tribunal differ according to the section under which the patient is detained. For civil patients, the Tribunal can discharge (now or on a later date) either because the legal criteria are not made out or it exercises its discretion.[12] Tribunals have no power, however, to make any judgment on the original sectioning of a patient (16).

Discretion to discharge is used where the Tribunal is satisfied that sufficient treatment and risk management is available outside of hospital, it is therefore used only in 'exceptional circumstances' (17).

The Tribunal can recommend that the consultant psychiatrist considers whether to place the patient on a community treatment order,[13] which allows for enforced medication to enable the patient to remain out of hospital.[14] Also 'with a view to facilitating discharge on a future date', it has the power to recommend leave or transfer to

---

[10] Also known as the Mental Health Tribunal, previously the Mental Health Review Tribunal.

[11] Rule 2 of the Tribunal Rules.
[12] S. 72(1) MHA.
[13] S. 72 (3A) MHA.
[14] SS. 17A to 17G MHA.

another hospital.[15] Using these recommendations, a mental health lawyer can help their client to get appropriate treatment in hospital and aftercare in the community.

For forensic patients, the Tribunal can grant an absolute discharge (18),[16] discharge with conditions on the day (conditional discharge),[17] or defer a conditional discharge for arrangements to be made.[18] Here, the Tribunal has no statutory power to make recommendations, but it can on a non-statutory basis (19), although case law suggests that the Tribunal can decide not to hear any submissions on this point (20).

A Tribunal does examine whether a psychiatrist's treatment plan is appropriate. Thus, some issues before the Tribunal are medical, and that a member of the Tribunal is a psychiatrist allows the Tribunal to exercise its own expertise (21). Further, it is for the Tribunal to decide what evidence it accepts (22).

Legal criteria

To make a decision, the Tribunal applies a legal test based on *Winterwerp* v *Netherlands* [1979] ECHR 4. The basic legal criteria for all sections are the existence of a mental disorder, nature, degree, own health, own safety, protection of others, and available treatment. The legal tests for discharge are found in S. 72 MHA. The test to decide whether to absolutely or conditionally discharge a forensic patient is found at S. 73 MHA.

The criteria differ slightly depending on the Section the patient is detained under, but is the same as those used when a person is originally detained (23).

The criteria are applied on the day of the hearing, so any disorder or symptoms not suffered from on that day cannot necessitate detention. Thus, psychiatrists who do not see their patients often can find themselves unable to make out the legal criteria.

Mental disorder

According to Article 5 of the ECHR, a person can be detained if they are of 'unsound mind'.[19] Today the term used is mental disorder. This is defined in the MHA,[20] and includes learning disability, which is also defined.[21] Unless under S. 2 MHA, to be detained a person with a learning disability must exhibit 'abnormally aggressive or seriously irresponsible conduct'.[22]

Article 5 ECHR states that a person can be detained if they are an alcoholic or drug addict.[23] This is not reflected in the MHA where a person cannot be detained just for those reasons.[24]

The law is clear that to be detained, a patient must be suffering from a disorder but psychiatry is not an exact science. Psychiatrists will sometimes argue that a patient's personality traits are a reason to detain; however, *personality traits* are not a disorder. The law always requires clarity.

[15] S. 72 (3) MHA.
[16] S. 73 (1) MHA/S. 75(3) MHA.
[17] S. 73 (2) MHA.
[18] S. 73 (7) MHA.
[19] Article 5 (1)(e) of the ECHR.
[20] S. 1(2) MHA.
[21] S. 1 (4) MHA.
[22] S. 1(2A) MHA.
[23] Art. 5(1)(e) ECHR.
[24] S. 1(3) MHA.

Nature

The 'nature' criterion covers the long-term prognosis of the mental disorder, the response to medication, other treatment, and any stress factors, including how likely a disorder is to relapse in the community (24).

The law accepts that 'nature' is difficult to quantify and while the term is defined in *ex parte Smith* [1998] by Popplewell J, it is also accepted that it is so interlinked with degree that the issues dealt with under one criterion can also be dealt with under the other. However, in a hearing the psychiatrist must be clear what evidence they have for each criteria.

Degree

'Degree' refers to the current manifestation of the patient's disorder' (23), i.e. the symptoms that are exhibited on the day of the hearing.

There are patients with residual symptoms who function adequately in the community, and it is arguable therefore that there is a threshold that should be applied here. Some such patients can be discharged, while some still require inpatient treatment. It is the effect of those symptoms on functioning and distress that necessitates inpatient care.

Own health

The own health criterion is the ability of a patient to care for their own physical and mental health and accept support to do so (4).

The patient probably needs to understand that they have a mental disorder in order to guard against risks of relapse therefore 'insight' comes under this criterion. However, some patients accept treatment because they trust medical advice, or because they know that if they refuse they may be readmitted.

Own safety

The own safety criterion (4) covers self-harm, suicidal ideation, self-neglect, and behaviour that makes the patient vulnerable, including financial and other forms of exploitation. A patient's ability to accept support to look after their own safety is paramount when considering this criterion.

Occasionally, psychiatrists argue that female patients are vulnerable to sexual exploitation; however, consideration must be given to whether a female patient consents to sexual relations (25) before citing this. A bad decision is not necessarily an incapacitous decision.

Protection of others

The protection of others[25] is simply any risk the patient may cause to others as a result of their mental disorder. Any violent behaviour that is not connected to a mental disorder is irrelevant to the Tribunal (26).

It is for the psychiatrist to provide evidence as to risk, usually past incidents, which the Tribunal will use to form their own judgment, it does not assess risk itself (27).

Some patients are violent only when unwell and when well there is no such risk; the question is how well is that patient on the day of the hearing.

[25] Code of Practice paragraph 14.10.

The availability of appropriate treatment

Treatment must be available to the patient at the hospital where the patient is detained (28), it must be appropriate,[26] and be provided to alleviate or prevent deterioration of the disorder.[27]

Treatment is defined in the MHA,[28] and the Code of Practice 2015 states that it can be simply detention in hospital under the supervision of a psychiatrist and nursing staff (4).

Best interests

Psychiatrists are trained to act in a patient's best interests but the MHA requires a higher threshold (29):

> Suffering from mental disorder … which **warrants** his detention in a hospital.[29]
>
> Detention as aforesaid is **justified**.[30]
>
> Mental disorder … which makes it **appropriate** for him to be liable to be detained.[31]
>
> That it is **necessary**.[32]

According to the *Oxford English Dictionary*, 'warrant' means to 'justify or necessitate', and 'appropriate' means 'suitable or proper in the circumstances'. None of these words mean best interests.

ECHR legal concepts

Other legal concepts have been incorporated from the European Court of Human Rights jurisprudence:

- Detention must be a necessary and proportionate response (30).
- Detention must be the least restrictive measure: less restrictive measures must be insufficient to safeguard, therefore detention is the only option (31).

What these concepts mean is that there is a threshold for meeting the criteria: if the patient could manage the disorder and risks accruing in the community with sufficient support then the Tribunal should discharge them. It is good practice for the psychiatrist to grant leave and provide medication prior to the hearing to allow the Tribunal to assess the proportionality of continued detention.

Evidence

Tribunal hearings are inquisitorial and not adversarial but the clinical witnesses will be arguing for continued detention and the patient for discharge. As one side is trying to make a case, to ensure fairness, rules of evidence apply.

In a Tribunal, all evidence is admissible, even hearsay, but there is a burden of proof and standard of proof.

Burden of proof

Burden of proof places the onus on one side to prove their case. For example, in a criminal court the onus is on the prosecution to prove that the defendant is guilty.

Until the case of *R (H) v London North and East Region Mental Health Review Tribunal (Secretary of State for Health intervening)* [2001] 3 WLR 512 (CA), the burden of proof had been on the patient to prove they did not suffer from a mental disorder. This was held to be incompatible with Article 5 ECHR, so the wording of the MHA was changed (32), and now it is for the detaining authority to prove that the patient has a disorder and should be detained.

The detaining authority makes out its case through the evidence provided by the clinical witnesses. This means that if the psychiatrist does not provide evidence for their medical opinion, the legal criteria is not made out and the patient will be discharged.

Standard of proof

According to the *Oxford Dictionary of Law*, standard of proof is defined as 'the degree of proof required for any fact in issue in litigation, which is established by assessing the evidence relevant to it'.

In English law, there are two standards of proof: the civil standard, which is on the balance of probabilities, and the criminal standard, which is beyond reasonable doubt.

In the case of *Reid v Secretary of State for Scotland* [1998] UKHL 43, it was confirmed that the standard of proof in a Tribunal is the civil standard. What this means is: 'If the evidence is such that the tribunal can say "we think it more probable than not" the burden is discharged, but if the probabilities are equal it is not' (33).

In percentage terms, a Tribunal starts without bias at a balance of 50%. If on the evidence the balance is not moved to 51% in favour of detention, the patient will be discharged. Because the burden of proof lies with the detaining authority, the psychiatrist must prove the extra 1%. All the patient's legal representative has to do is suggest that this extra 1% is not made out.

Hearsay and weight

A witness who is giving evidence that is not their direct knowledge is giving hearsay evidence. In a Tribunal, most of the evidence would constitute hearsay because it is taken from medical notes written by a group of people.

In *R (on the application of DJ) v MHRT; R (on the application of AN) v MHT* [2005] EWHC 587 (Admin), Munby J stated that the Tribunal:

> must take into account that it is hearsay and must take into account … institutional folklore with no secure foundation in either recorded or provable fact. The Tribunal must guard against too quickly jumping to conclusions adverse to the patient.

Munby J acknowledged a problem with psychiatric evidence, that as a patient gains a longer history with psychiatric services, more medical notes and reports are generated and some incidents that were insignificant get blown out of proportion in later reports. The effect of the ruling in this case is that the more damming the hearsay evidence, the more verification the Tribunal will require, and without that verification less weight will be given to it.

It is vital that psychiatrists check their evidence against contemporaneous notes and do not simply take the last report at face value. Relying on evidence that is not correct could cost credibility and make it harder to make out their case. For example, one sexually inappropriate comment made by a patient 10 years prior to a Tribunal appeared in evidence as a sexual assault. Luckily for the patient, the legal representative checked in the medical notes and was able to produce the correct evidence for the Tribunal.

[26] S. 3 (4) MHA.
[27] S. 145 (4) MHA.
[28] S. 145 (1) MHA.
[29] S. 72 (1)(a)(i) MHA.
[30] S. 72 (1)(a)(ii) MHA.
[31] S. 72 (1)(b)(i) MHA.
[32] S. 72 (1)(b)(ii) MHA.

Further, psychiatrists must provide evidence, not simply opinions or assertions, especially when discussing potential future risks to the patient or to others. A concern that something may happen is not proof.

Statutory reports

The following reports must be submitted in evidence (34):

- Statement of Information by the responsible authority/detaining authority that sets out who has legal responsibility for the patient.
- Psychiatric report by the responsible clinician (psychiatrist).
- Social circumstances report by the care coordinator/social worker.

Other papers are also submitted:

- Nursing report for inpatients.
- The section papers for patients under S. 2 MHA.
- Statement by the Secretary of State for Justice for forensic patients.
- A victim statement for forensic patients[33].

Reports are to be submitted 3 weeks after the TSMH has received the application or referral.[34] If the case is S. 2 MHA, whatever information is available must be provided in the time available,[35] For restricted patients, reports must also be sent to the Ministry of Justice.[36]

Content

Two guidance documents set out what each report should contain: 'First-tier Tribunal Health Education and Social Care Chamber: Statements and Reports in Mental Health Cases', 28 October 2013 (34), and Guidance Booklet T124, 'Reports for Mental Health Tribunals' (HMCTS, April 2012) (35), but the focus is to make a clear argument for detention using the legal criteria.

Reports are usually based on the patient's medical records, which are contemporaneous to any incidents. However, occasionally mistakes are made in the records so it is important to check that the records are not contaminated with those of another patient because if so, this contamination will appear in the reports. Further, any inaccuracies will cast doubt on the integrity of the evidence as a whole. It is therefore vital that the patient's social and psychiatric history not be misrepresented.

Not for disclosure

The report authors may consider some information to be detrimental to the patient and/or others so wish that to be withheld. This is possible under Rule 14 of the Tribunal Rules. Information will be disclosed to the patient unless the Tribunal is satisfied:

- that disclosure would be likely to cause the patient or others serious harm; and
- it is proportionate and in the interests of justice not to disclose.

This is a high threshold so it is rare that such information is not disclosed.

---

[33] If the Domestic Violence, Crime and Victims Act 2004 applies.
[34] Rule 32(6) of the Tribunal Rules.
[35] Rule 32(5) of the Tribunal Rules.
[36] Rule 32(7) of the Tribunal Rules.

The Tribunal hearing

Preliminary medical examination

Prior to the hearing, the patient can have an interview with the medical member if they request one.[37] The detaining authority must ensure that this is facilitated, and that the medical member can read the patient's medical notes. It is not good practice to deny access to the patient's notes, indeed denying access to the patient or their notes to a person authorized under the MHA is a criminal act of obstruction and can result in up to 3 months in prison.[38]

Procedure

The procedure followed in a Tribunal hearing is flexible to ensure that the patient can participate in the proceedings.

The decision of the Tribunal is usually given on the day of the hearing,[39] with written reasons to follow.

Legal issues

During the hearing, the legal representative may meet in private with the Tribunal to make legal submissions.[40] It is impossible to know what legel issues will arise so one learns to expect the unexpected.

Witnesses

The Tribunal has the powers to exclude witnesses if they consider that their presence will prevent another person from providing their evidence freely.[41] Likewise, the Tribunal has the power to direct for further witnesses to appear before it.[42]

Public hearings

Rule 38 also gives the Tribunal the power to direct that the hearing be held in public if it considers it would be in the interests of justice to do so. This was famously done recently in the Brady case (36).

Adjournment

If any issues cannot be resolved on the day, the Tribunal can adjourn.[43] This is usually due to insufficient evidence such that a decision cannot be reached. If the Tribunal has heard some evidence then the hearing is part-heard and the relisted hearing will be before the same panel, otherwise the matter can be relisted before any panel. The Tribunal can also make directions to ensure there is then sufficient evidence to proceed.[44]

Oral evidence

Oral evidence is usually given by the authors of the reports. Witnesses are questioned by the Tribunal and cross-examined by the patient's representative.

---

[37] Rule 34 of the Tribunal Rules.
[38] S. 129 MHA.
[39] Rule 41 of the Tribunal Rules.
[40] Rule 5(3)(e) of the Tribunal Rules.
[41] Rule 38(4) of the Tribunal Rules.
[42] Rules 5 and 15 of the Tribunal Rules.
[43] Rule 5(3)(h) of the Tribunal Rules.
[44] Rule 5(3)(d) of the Tribunal Rules.

There must be very little new evidence submitted orally at the hearing, as the patient's representative has to prepare a case. Given the expense and time it takes to list a Tribunal, as well as any distress to the patient caused by adjourning it, not putting full evidence in the reports is to be avoided.

Occasionally, psychiatrists will be asked if they are representing the detaining authority. Such decisions are usually up to the management of the detaining authority, and will have been decided prior to the hearing. A psychiatrist who decides to represent the detaining authority has the right to cross-examine all the witnesses, including the patient. Cross-examining the patient will necessitate asking them distressing questions and will mar the therapeutic relationship. If not representing the detaining authority, the psychiatrist is there as a professional witness only and therefore is emotionally detached from the proceedings. Thus, if the patient remains detained, the patient knows that the psychiatrist was just presenting their opinion and the decision was made by the Tribunal.

Writing a report and attending a Tribunal adds to the psychiatrist's workload, often leading to reports submitted late.

Psychiatrists also ask to leave hearings early, usually before the patient has given their evidence. Given that the outcome of most Tribunals is that the patient remains detained, the focus for the patient is that the psychiatrist gets to hear their side uninterrupted. Staying to hear is good practice, and can be a therapeutic tool and help foster a better relationship.

The lawyer at the Tribunal

A legal representative's role is to follow the client's instructions but also to aid the Tribunal, and ensure that the Tribunal gets all the evidence it needs. However, for the client who is detained and medicated against their will it is vital that their representative makes sure that the Tribunal is conducted so that they feel that their evidence has been considered.

Unlike ward rounds, Tribunal hearings are structured so that each person has their say without interruption from others. Even if not discharged, a Tribunal can be a catalyst towards discharge because the psychiatrist has heard the patient's point of view and changes in care and treatment are made in light of that.

A question often put to a mental health lawyer is: 'What is it like to represent people who should not be discharged?' The answer, like that given by criminal law specialists, is that one does one's best without making a judgement. It is for the Tribunal to make the decision based on all the evidence. Problems occur when psychiatrists are not sufficiently experienced or trained to put their case forward. There are occasions therefore when patients are discharged because the evidence for maintaining detention is not put forward.

The patient at the Tribunal

After the evidence has been given, the Tribunal will tell the patient whether they are discharged. Those who are not discharged may feel disheartened. But even so, the patient should feel comfortable with the clinical witnesses so they can continue to work with the psychiatrist to progress towards discharge. They therefore need to understand that the evidence given was based on facts that are a true representation of their histories, and that none of the evidence was spurious.

Appeals

The Tribunal will provide written reasons outlining how they came to their decision. These are open to appeal but only for an error of law.[45] There is no appeal on the basis that the Tribunal made the wrong decision (37).

In some instances, rather than allow an appeal to the Upper Tribunal, the First-tier Tribunal will review its own decision,[46] quash that decision, and list a hearing under a newly constituted Tribunal.[47]

An appeal of a decision of the Upper Tribunal would be to the Court of Appeal and thence to the Supreme Court, but only if the appeal raises an important principle of law.[48]

Judicial review

Other rights of challenge for a patient when the detaining authority acts unlawfully is by a judicial review (38).

Because the Upper Tribunal has no jurisdiction to hear an appeal against the decision of a hospital managers' hearing (see below), any appeal would be via a judicial review (39).

Issues outside the remit of the Tribunal

Often achieving a desirable outcome for a client occurs outside of the Tribunal process by negotiating with the clinical team. While a lawyer is focused on legal aspects of detention, their experience of the psychiatric system provides them with the knowledge of a wide range of services to which a client could be referred.

Leave MHA conditions

Leave under Section 17 off the ward is subject to conditions that are set by the psychiatrist[49] for civil patients, with conditions to protect the patient or others.[50]

For restricted patients, the psychiatrist must ask the Ministry of Justice to grant leave, and it is they who set the conditions.[51] Guidance for granting leave is set out in the National Offender Management Service's 'Mental Health Casework Section: Section 17 – Leave of Absence' (40). Conditions include exclusion zones set due to risk to the public and the views of the victims (41), which must be proportionate, lawful, and necessary (42). These are within the remit of the law so any issues can be raised by the patient's legal representative. It is important therefore that the clinical team keep the patient's legal representative up to date so they can ensure that the patient's rights are respected by other agencies.

Specialist treatment needs

Some patients require specialist treatment that cannot be provided on general psychiatric wards. This is especially the case for those with

---

[45] S. 11 Tribunals, Courts and Enforcement Act.
[46] Rule 49 of the Tribunal Rules.
[47] S. 9 Tribunals, Courts and Enforcement Act; Rule 45 of the Tribunal Rules.
[48] Appeals from the Up Tribunal to the Court of Appeal Order 2008, SI 2008/2834.
[49] Schedule 1, part 2, paragraph 2 MHA.
[50] S. 17(1) MHA.
[51] S. 41(3)(c) MHA.

an autism spectrum disorder who struggle with the chaotic environment of an acute psychiatric ward. However, specialist provision is scarce and expensive, and often it is only through the intervention of a mental health lawyer that appropriate provision is provided.

After-care

S. 117 MHA places a duty on health and local authorities to provide aftercare services[52] to meet the needs of a patient that arise because of their mental disorder to minimize the chances of readmission.[53]

For patients with complex needs, aftercare services are not always provided as a matter of course, hence the need for legal intervention. By pointing out the legal responsibilities to the relevant authorities, funding can be secured and arrangements expedited so patients can return to the community.

Many professionals who work within inpatient psychiatric services are unaware that mental health lawyers can secure appropriate aftercare, and this remains an underused avenue for many patients.

Hospital managers

Under the MHA, hospital managers are not people who manage the hospitals but are independent individuals whose role is to oversee admissions and transfers, and to ensure that the rights of patients are protected.

Hospital managers' hearings

Hospital managers' hearings are held to renew or discharge a patient's detention.[54] A patient can apply for a hospital managers' hearing every 28 days.

They are quasi-judicial and bound by the rules of natural justice. Rather than use legal criteria, hospital managers' hearings have questions set out in the Code of Practice 2015 that are similar.[55]

They are independent of the Tribunal and a public body and therefore open to judicial review (43).

Habeas corpus

A patient can seek a writ of habeas corpus in the High Court if they think their original detention was unlawful. It is for the detaining authority to prove that there was lawful justification for the detention, otherwise the patient will be released (44).

Independent advocates

Each detaining authority is obliged to provide Independent Mental Health Advocates (IMHAs) for those detained under the MHA, and Independent Mental Capacity Advocates (IMCAs) for those held under the Mental Capacity Act 2005.

Independent Mental Health Advocates

IMHAs are not legal representatives, they advocate for the patient in a non-legal way to help patients obtain information regarding their detention and their medical treatment. They also help patients to complain and deal with other non-legal issues. Their functions are set out in the MHA[56] and the Code of Practice.[57] Who can be an IMHA is regulated (45).

IMHAs may attend Tribunals and hospital managers' hearings, but their role in Tribunals is set out in a TSMH Practice Note, 'Role of the Independent Mental Health Advocate (IMHA) in First-tier Tribunal (Mental Health) Hearings' (46), attending only to offer support to the patient.

Because of legal aid constraints, the majority of hospital managers' hearings are not attended by mental health lawyers. In such hearings, therefore, IMHAs help the patient to represent themselves.

Independent Mental Capacity Advocates

IMCAs are independent advocates for people held under the Mental Capacity Act 2005 (MCA).

The MCA, applies only to those lack capacity, and is rarely used in general adult psychiatry, where patients are detained under the MHA, although it is occasionally used for older adult inpatients.

IMCAs are generally appointed when an application for a Deprivation of Liberty Safeguard authorization is made in a hospital setting.[58] IMCAs can also help with decisions regarding serious medical treatment, long-term NHS residential accommodation,[59] and can challenge those decisions in the Court of Protection (47).

Nearest relatives

A patient's 'nearest relative' (NR) is not a 'next of kin'. The NR is defined by law in S. 26 MHA, but they can be displaced in County Court proceedings if that person is unsuitable.[60]

The NR can ask the detaining authority to discharge the patient.[61] However, if the psychiatrist considers that the patient would be likely to act in a manner dangerous to themselves or others then a barring notice under S. 25 MHA can be issued, which automatically refers the case for a hospital managers' hearing. The NR can also apply for a Tribunal.

Information about the patient should be shared with the NR.[62] The Code of Practice states that the patient should be asked at the earliest time what information they are happy to share.[63]

The psychiatrist can disclose information even if the patient has refused,[64] providing doing so would not put the patient at risk of harm or have any other detrimental effect. Disclosure should only be made against the patient's wishes if the advantages outweigh the

---

[52] S. 117 MHA.
[53] S. 117 (6) MHA.
[54] Code of Practice, Chapter 38.
[55] See Code of Practice 38.15–38.18.

[56] S. 130A, S. 130B, S. 130C, S. 130D MHA.
[57] Code of Practice, Chapter 6.
[58] SS. 39A, 39B, 40(1) MCA.
[59] MCA Code of Practice paragraph 6.45, SS. 35 to 41 MCA.
[60] SS. 29, 30, 31 MHA.
[61] S. 23 MHA.
[62] S. 132 (4) MHA.
[63] Code of Practice paragraph 4.32.
[64] Code of Practice paragraph 4.36.

disadvantages to the patient. However, jurisprudence states that providing information to an NR when a patient has requested not to is a breach of their rights under Article 8 ECHR (48).

Conclusion

The MHA introduces legal aspects into a clinical environment. It exists both to enable a detaining authority to act within a proper legal framework and patients to challenge what is being done. Mental health jurisprudence does not exist to question clinical decisions, it exists to question legal decisions made by detaining authorities and the clinicians who work for them. It is designed therefore for the benefit of both psychiatrists and patients. The role of the lawyer is to provide parity within that legal framework.

REFERENCES

1. Legislation.gov.uk. Mental Health Act 1983. 1983. http://www.legislation.gov.uk/ukpga/1983/20/contents

2. Porter R. Gods and demons. In: *Madness: A Brief History*, pp. 10–33. New York: Oxford University Press; 2002.

3. Council of Europe. European Convention on Human Rights. 2013. http://www.echr.coe.int/Documents/Convention_ENG.pdf

4. Department of Health. *Mental Health Act 1983: Code of Practice*. London: The Stationery Office; 2015. https://www.gov.uk/government/uploads/system/uploads/attachment_data/file/435512/MHA_Code_of_Practice.PDF

5. Solicitors Regulation Authority. SRA Handbook. 2018. https://www.sra.org.uk/solicitors/handbook/welcome.page

6. *AMA v Greater Manchester West Mental Health NHS Foundation Trust & Others* [2015] UKUT 0036 (AAC).

7. Legislation.gov.uk. The Tribunal Procedure (First-tier Tribunal) (Health, Education and Social Care Chamber) Rules. 2008. http://www.legislation.gov.uk/uksi/2008/2699/contents/made

8. The Law Society. Representation before mental health tribunals. 2016. http://www.lawsociety.org.uk/support-services/advice/practice-notes/representation-before-mental-health-tribunals/

9. The Law Society. Mental health accreditation. http://www.lawsociety.org.uk/support-services/accreditation/mental-health/

10. Mental Health Lawyers Association. The MHLA. 2018. http://www.mhla.co.uk/about/about-the-mhla/

11. Mental Health Lawyers Association. Code of Conduct. 2013. http://www.mhla.co.uk/about/code-of-conduct/

12. Legal Aid Agency. Improving your quality in mental health: a guide to common issues identified through peer review. 2016. https://www.gov.uk/government/uploads/system/uploads/attachment_data/file/556275/improving-your-quality-guide-mental-health.pdf

13. Gov.uk. First-tier Tribunal (Mental Health). https://www.gov.uk/courts-tribunals/first-tier-tribunal-mental-health

14. *Winterwerp v The Netherlands* [1979] ECHR 4.

15. Mental Health Law Online. Eligibility periods. http://www.mentalhealthlaw.co.uk/Eligibility_periods

16. *R v East London and The City Mental Health Trust Ex parte Brandenburg* [2003] UKHL 58.

17. *GA v Betsi Cadwaladr University LHB* [2013] 0280 (AAC).

18. *R (on the application of SC) v Mental Health Review Tribunal and the Secretary of State for Health* [2005] EWHC 17 (Admin).

19. *Hansard* HC Deb., vol. 121, col. 261 (28 October 1987).

20. *EC v Birmingham and Solihull Mental Health NHS Trust* [2013] EWCA Civ 701.

21. *K v The Mental Health Tribunal for Scotland* [2015] S. L. T. (Sh Ct) 197.

22. *WH v Partnerships in Care* [2015] UKUT 695 (AAC).

23. *Reid v Secretary of State for Scotland* [1999] 1 All ER 481.

24. *R v Mental Health Review Tribunal for the South Thames Region Ex parte Smith* [1998] EWHC 832.

25. *The London Borough of Southwark v KA, MA, RN "Capacity to Marry"* [2016] EWCOP 20.

26. *R (on the application of Li) v Mental Health Review Tribunal* [2004] EWHC 51 (Admin).

27. *R (on the application of N) the Mental Health Review Tribunal* [2001] EWHC 1133 (Admin).

28. *WH v Partnerships in Care* [2015] UKUT 695 (AAC)

29. *R v Hallstrom (ex parte W) (No.2)* [1986] 2 All ER 306.

30. *Winterwerp v Netherlands* [1979] ECHR 4.

31. *Witold Litwa v Poland* [2001] ECHR 2000-III.

32. Mental Health Act 1983 (Remedial) Order 2001. SI 2001/3712. 2001. https://www.legislation.gov.uk/uksi/2001/3712/contents/made

33. *Miller v Minister of Pensions* [1947] 2 All ER 372, as per Denning J.

34. Courts and Tribunals Judiciary. Practice direction: First-tier Tribunal Health Education and Social Care Chamber: statements and reports in mental health cases. 2013. https://www.judiciary.gov.uk/publications/practice-direction-first-tier-tribunal-health-education-and-social-care-chamber-statements-and-reports-in-mental-health-cases/

35. Mental Health Law Online. Guidance booklet: reports for mental health tribunals. 2012. http://www.mentalhealthlaw.co.uk/Guidance_Booklet:_Reports_for_Mental_Health_Tribunals

36. Courts and Tribunals Judiciary. In the matter of Ian Brady. 2014. https://www.judiciary.uk/judgments/ian-brady-mh-tribunal-240114/

37. *JLG v Managers of Llanarth Court* [2011] UKUT 62 (AAC).

38. Legislation.gov.uk. Judicial review. Tribunals, Courts and Enforcement Act 2007. http://www.legislation.gov.uk/ukpga/2007/15/part/1/chapter/2/crossheading/judicial-review

39. *South Staffordshire and Shropshire Healthcare NHSFT v Hospital Managers of St George's Hospital* [2016] EWHC 1196 (Admin).

40. National Offender Management Service. Mental Health Casework Section: section 17 – leave of absence. 2017. https://assets.publishing.service.gov.uk/government/uploads/system/uploads/attachment_data/file/595085/mhcs-guidance-s17-leave_.pdf

41. *X v Secretary of State for Justice* [2009] EWHC 2465 (Admin).

42. *Craven v Secretary of State for the Home Department* [2001] EWHC Admin 850.

43. *South Staffordshire and Shropshire Healthcare NHSFT v Hospital Managers of St George's Hospital* [2016] EWHC 1196 (Admin).

44. *R v Secretary of State for the Home Department Ex parte Cheblak* [1991] 2 All ER 319.

45. Legislation.gov.uk. Mental Health Act 1983 (Independent Mental Health Advocates) (England) Regulations 2008 (SI 2008/3166). 2008. http://www.legislation.gov.uk/uksi/2008/3166/made

46. Mental Health Law Online. Practice Note: Role of the Independent Mental Health Advocate in First-tier Tribunal (Mental Health) Hearings. 2011. http://www.mentalhealthlaw.co.uk/Practice_Note:_Role_of_the_Independent_Mental_Health_Advocate_in_First-tier_Tribunal_(Mental_Health)_Hearings

47. Legislation.gov.uk. The Mental Capacity Act 2005 (Independent Mental Capacity Advocates) (General) Regulations. SI 2006/1832, paragraphs 6 and 7. 2005. http://www.legislation.gov.uk/uksi/2006/1832/regulation/7/made

48. *R (on the application of E) v Bristol City Council* [2005] EWHC 74 (Admin).

32

Staff burnout and staff turnover on inpatient wards

Helen Robson and Caroline Attard

The context

Mental health services are under increasingly huge pressure as funding for the sector has been reduced (1). These funding cuts occur in the context of sweeping implementation of transformational change to services involving both the workforce and the infrastructure. The impact of these changes has been to reduce costs and has allowed many mental health providers to balance the books. Despite this, The King's Fund (1) found that 40% of mental health trusts had experienced reductions in their income across the financial years 2013/2014 and 2014/2015.

There has been a 9% reduction in overall inpatient mental health bed numbers in England from 2011 to 2013 (2). Three-quarters of the bed closures are reported to be within acute adult services, older peoples' mental health services, and psychiatric intensive care units. However, there has been no reduction in the demand for inpatient beds and the numbers of detentions under the Mental Health Act 1983 have risen (1). There has been an increase in bed occupancy rates, with large numbers of trusts running at 100% occupancy, which is well above the 85% occupancy rate recommended by the Royal College of Psychiatrists (3). Such increases in the bed occupancy rates impact negatively on the quality of care offered by inpatient services and on the number of violent incidents experienced on mental health wards (4).

The reduction in beds is occurring at the same time as an increasing demand for mental health services partly due to the reduction in social services funding and the general economic situation which has a negative impact on the overall health of the population (1). Despite the claims made about 'Parity of Esteem' for mental and physical health (5), the gap appears to be widening, with 92% of people with physical health problems reporting that they have received the care they need, compared with only 36% of people with mental health problems (6).

The impact on patients of these changes in services has been well documented (1, 7). There are examples of patients being held in police cells for unacceptably long periods of time while a bed is sought, people being turned away from accident and emergency departments, and community services being told that unless a patient is detained under the Mental Health Act, there is little or no hope of a bed being found in the near future (8). Where a person is detained, the lack of beds has resulted in severely distressed patients having to be transferred miles away from their homes and support networks, as there are no free beds in their local area (8). Again, these 'out of area' placements not only have a negative impact on the patient's experience of services but have also been found to increase the risk of suicide within inpatient services (9).

Mental health services have also seen a change in the shape of the workforce and in the skill mix. Between 2003 and 2013, there was an increase of 41% in the full-time equivalent numbers of consultant psychiatrists, as well as an increase of 33% in the number of clinical psychologists (1). In contrast, there has been an overall reduction of 2% in the number of full-time equivalent mental health nurses, with some trusts having reduced their numbers by 10% across the same timeframe (10). In addition, there is evidence that this decrease in numbers includes a disproportionately high number of experienced nurses whose roles have been cut from services, and an increase in junior nurses, peer support workers, assistant practitioners, and volunteers (1). Staff shortages, lack of experienced and consistent staff on wards, and the current high turnover of staff have all been implicated in the inquiries into inpatient deaths on wards (9).

What is stress and burnout?

Stress is the feeling of being under too much mental or emotional pressure and this can have an impact on how individuals think, behave, and feel as well as manifesting itself in both physical and mental health conditions (11). Hoff indicated that 'stress is the discomfort, pain or troubled feeling arising from emotional, social or physical sources and resulting in the need to relax, be treated or otherwise seek relief' (12, p. 42). Occupational stress is that distressing, uncomfortable feeling which is directly related to paid employment and it is known to diminish productivity in nurses, increase absenteeism, illness, poor morale, and human error, and have a detrimental impact on staff turnover (13). Each of these issues further compounds the experience of stress within the workforce (13). Galvin et al. (14)

report that in the 2013 National Health Service (NHS) staff survey, 39% of respondents reported feeling ill due to work-related stress, however, 46% of mental health nurses reported work-related stress, higher than any other branch of nursing. Work-related chronic stress conditions are a major risk factor in developing 'burnout' in employees.

Burnout has been defined as 'a popular term for the condition of having mental or physical energy depletion after a period of chronic unrelieved job related stress characterized sometimes by physical illness. The person suffering from burnout may lose concern or respect for other people and often has cynical, dehumanized perceptions of people, labelling them in a derogatory manner' (15). The concept of burnout has been attributed to Fredeunberger, who in 1974 identified this pattern in occupations where the individuals work directly with people (16). It has been stated that there are serious consequences for the person who has 'burnout' as well as the population that they serve. Examples of effects of burnout include the person leaving the profession, job dissatisfaction, marital and personal disharmony, social isolation, fatigue, loss of self-esteem and self-confidence, poor concentration, reduced libido, sleep disorders and drug and alcohol problems, gastrointestinal upset, headaches, and colds (16). These characteristics reflect the symptoms attributed to stress-related conditions. Maslach and Jackson (17) studied the concept of burnout in detail, dividing the concept into three categories, namely emotional exhaustion, depersonalization, and lack of personal accomplishment. They described emotional exhaustion as resulting from a decrease or loss of self-confidence and interest in the chosen profession, alongside feelings of weakness and fatigue. Depersonalization was described by them as the person behaving towards the recipients of their care without emotion, treating the person as if they were not a unique and individual. Personal accomplishment was described as the feelings of productivity, coping, and adequacy. These three categories of the effects of burnout are still routinely used to study the phenomenon today. Nursing is commonly held to be a profession which is heavily laden with an emotional burden and therefore those who enter the profession are at great risk of burnout (18). Studies suggest that a perceived lack of organization, order, and structure within the workplace also add to the risk of burnout within the staff group (19).

Causes of stress in inpatient services

Recruitment and retention of staff

There are higher rates of stress-related sickness within health professionals, in particular within the population of mental health nurses (20), and stress is consistently identified as a major cause of low productivity, high absenteeism, bad judgement, misallocation of resources, and poor morale (21). Acute mental inpatient facilities are extremely busy environments which are generally understaffed and under-resourced (22). The recruitment and retention of staff within inpatient services is a continual concern for the profession, with many of the staff within these highly stressful environments being unqualified frontline staff and the most newly qualified and inexperienced nurses within the workforce. Recent data details an international shortage of registered nurses choosing to work in this speciality due to low morale and the consistent workforce pressures

inherent in the day-to-day work (23, 24). Retaining staff is equally challenging, as nurses are choosing to take advantage of the early retirement clauses in the NHS pension scheme, or taking positions working within community services, where the pressures are less critical and the hours of working are more regular in many cases.

The deficit in the available qualified nursing workforce required to provide mental health services is currently felt to be reaching a crisis point, with mental health trusts across the UK currently unable to recruit into their vacant posts (25). Buckland (26) reported that more than 1260 mental health nurses had left the NHS in the 12 months prior to his article. He stated that vacancy levels were averaging 10% across the UK with a shortfall of 25,000 posts. Within those figures, there are areas where the vacancies of band 5 posts, the posts which newly qualified nurses would be applying for, were tipping 50%, particularly in the South of England and the areas of the country where there is a very high cost of living. The Royal College of Nursing reported that over 4500 mental health nurses' posts had been lost up to October 2015. The decision to withdraw the offer of NHS bursaries for students undertaking nurse training from September 2017 is anticipated to further compound the deficit, as students will be required to pay their fees as well as losing their subsistence allowance. This decision will have the biggest impact on the mature student group, who may have families to support, and consequently nurse training will not be a financially viable option open to them. Mature students are often particularly sought-after candidates for mental health nursing programmes as they can bring the required life experience and maturity to deal with the specific demands and challenges that caring for people with mental health problems can bring.

Working conditions

Over recent years, various reports have criticized mental health inpatient units for failing to provide a safe and therapeutic environment (27, 28). However, as has already been outlined, mental health nurses are working in an environment with increasingly limited resources alongside escalating workloads and increasing public expectations. Inpatient wards are fraught with ever-increasing pressure and a chaotic atmosphere, within which nurses are dealing with acutely unwell patients with very complex health and social needs, involuntary admissions, frequent crises, and the additional rise in the number of aggressive behaviours seen in inpatient settings over recent years (13). Inpatient services have for a long time practised in a traditional, biomedical model of mental health care, whereby the focus is on the management of illness and biological pathology. The consultant psychiatrist was appointed as the lead for the multidisciplinary team, and the term 'Responsible Clinician', used within the Mental Health Act reinforces the paternalistic and powerful position traditionally held by medics (29).

It could be argued that there exists a tension between old and new approaches to mental health practice. Current approaches to mental health care advocate a recovery focus, in which partnership working with the client to identify his or her goals and interventions to support a person's progress towards those goals is viewed as the gold standard of nursing practice. These ideologies have been fundamental to mental health nurse training curriculums over recent years, and form the basis of a plethora of recent publications around service provision and mental health nursing practice (30–33). Nurses within inpatient settings are often working in a situation where there is a clash of cultures, and the fundamental principles of recovery may be compromised by the pervading biomedical approach (29). The fundamental principle of personal choice within the recovery model, which includes treatment choices, is particularly difficult to negotiate, as patients often have a loss of capacity affecting their decision-making at these times. However, recovery requires workers to maximize choice regardless of the situation and within the constraints and not to hold on to power when a person does have capacity. How often is the personal choice of patients restricted by inpatient services that suspend leave, restrict visits, or delay a discharge plan because a patient is not adhering to the rules? This conflict of ideologies and nurses compromising their values to meet those of their teams, creates a thorny dilemma for those working most closely with patients, and can lead to a dysfunctional culture within the team, thus increasing stress on individual nurses working within this conflicting culture. It may also have a detrimental impact on the advancement of nursing practice as a profession as the culture of consultant psychiatrists determining treatment methods restricts the role and range of interventions utilized by nurses with patients, which further increases their risk of stress and burnout. Doyle et al. (34) established a direct link between training nursing staff to integrate psychosocial interventions in their practice, and reduced levels of burnout. However, if the culture of the environment prevents nurses utilizing newly acquired psychosocial skills it may simply have the adverse effect of decreasing personal accomplishment levels and therefore increasing levels and rates of burnout.

Lifestyle factors/shift working

Zhao and Turner (35) published a literature review relating to the health behaviours and health impact of people who routinely work shifts. The findings of this review established that shift work had a negative impact on diet, nutritional status, and more generally on the quality of life of those studied. The findings suggested that there was an increased incidence in the carbohydrate intake of those working shifts and that they tended to eat more frequently, or snack, rather than eat a full meal, compared to other groups. This may be perceived to be unsurprising given the experience of a lack of 'regular' routine experienced by shift workers, and the more limited availability of a cooked meal being provided in a workplace at irregular hours of the day and night. These adverse health impacts were associated with high body mass index scores and an increased risk of smoking in shift workers, which were found to be more prevalent in those routinely working night shifts. The studies relating to increased alcohol intake were too few for them to conclude a direct correlation; however, each of these lifestyle factors studied would independently and collectively explain the increased risk of coronary heart disease and peptic ulcer disease which has been associated with shift working. Also, working night shift has been found to be a specific risk factor in developing burnout in nurses (16). This can be partially explained by the argument that nurses working night shifts are not able to maintain adequate quality or quantity of sleep due to their irregular hours of working, and the frequent transition between their work pattern of sleep and their 'normal' routines. In addition to this, nurses working nights work for longer hours, and routinely work with reduced ratios of staff to patients. The experience of fatigue due to working night shifts may also adversely affect physical activity and motivation, which could also increase the risk

of burnout, increase their sickness rates, and consequently adversely affect the stress and burnout rates of their colleagues, as they are left working with a depleted or unfamiliar team.

Temporary staffing

Shortfalls in recruited, 'regular staff' within inpatient services are routinely filled by casual bank staff or agency staff who are paid to work on a shift-to-shift basis. The difficulties experienced by the patients, carers, multidisciplinary teams, and regular nursing staff in this situation are extremely complex and significant in the overall experiences of stress in this setting. Patients report feelings of being unsafe due to a constant change in nursing staff personnel, and the inability to develop any consistent and supportive relationships with staff who are looking after them. The regular staff are in a position of not having a sense of being part of a team of people who consistently work together, know each other's strengths and weaknesses, and develop good working relationships whereby they feel secure within their team, where everyone knows their roles and ward routines, are familiar with the specific risks and care needs of patients, and feel able to rely on each other for support and cohesion in this highly pressured environment. The team members and carers report a lack of consistent and clear communication between nurses and between different shifts leading to poor understanding of the individual patient's needs, relapse signatures, and triggers in relation to risk factors. This situation increases not only the risks of aggression and threatening behaviours as patients become frustrated and angry, but it also increases the risk of self-harming behaviours and suicide risk, as staff do not necessarily know the patients they are caring for.

There are other potential negative effects. Discharge planning becomes more problematic, the relationships between the community staff and the inpatient ward team become less consistent, and miscommunications may occur, leading to delays in discharge or more risky transfers of care from one service to another. On a shift-to-shift basis, bank and agency staff, who are unfamiliar with the ward routines, policies and procedures, and the patient population require an in-depth handover and orientation to the ward environment. They require far more supervision and support from the regular staff and do not have access to the patients' online electronic record systems, which places them in a position of having limited information available to them, and equally places additional pressure on regular staff as they have the burden of inputting and updating all the information for each of the patients on the ward. This creates a situation whereby much of the information entered onto the electronic records is second-hand and its recording is undertaken in a hurried manner, which detracts from the quality and any truly analytical thought about the information being written.

Increased acuity on inpatient wards

The described reduction in inpatient beds, increased rates of detained patients, and the constant pressure to discharge patients early to manage demand have created a situation where the acuity of the patients within any inpatient setting has increased. Dealing with patients who are acutely unwell and often unhappy to be admitted to hospital is inherently stressful and challenging to staff who are on the 'frontline'. Studies have shown that higher levels of depersonalization exist where large numbers of patients are acutely unwell (36). Feelings of depersonalization, and a lack of perceived control over work events, due to the acuity of the patient group, diminishes nurses' perceived levels of personal accomplishment, which in turn, increases the risks of burnout over time. Currid (36) identified that nurses reported having been motivated to work in mental health settings on the basis of high levels of patient contact, and the use of skills supporting the development of a therapeutic relationship. However, the same nurses reported in their practice a lack of opportunity to undertake direct clinical positive engagement with patients, and an overemphasis on administrative work.

The fundamental aspect of care in inpatient settings is that of maintaining a safe and supportive environment for patients, visitors, and staff and this represents a constant challenge. Patients are admitted to hospital when the community services are unable to minimize the person's risks to either themselves or to others and the person cannot therefore be safely managed at home. The patient's risks may include harming themselves, self-mutilating, and attempts at suicide, all of which are distressing and testing of the staff trying to care for that person. In addition, there is a need to manage patients who may wish to abscond from the ward or may be irritable and abusive or violent towards others or who simply refuse to comply with any of the treatment being offered. The underlying pressure on staff of attempting to regulate another person's behaviours, against that person's will, is stressful and not without limitation, and staff can become demotivated by the experience of the same clients rotating in and out of services, which may erodes nurses' feelings of personal accomplishment. The impact of this is frequently noted in the reported experience of the clinical care for patients; they have been found to report lower levels of satisfaction with the services provided alongside perceived lower thresholds for the use of sedation, and seclusion by staff (37).

Nursing observations

The emotional pressure of being on an enhanced observation with a patient who is either actively suicidal or self-harming is very difficult for frontline staff to cope with. Hearing distressing details of historical abuse or traumatic life events which the patient may wish to disclose in these moments of close interaction has an emotional impact on the nurse hearing them. This situation happens in the context of the previously identified increased acuity of inpatients, which in itself increases the number of enhanced observations within a ward population. This, it is easy to see that frontline staff can find themselves in a position of having to manage these inherent risks and the emotional distress of patients on enhanced observations for large proportions of their working shifts. This experience is difficult and emotionally draining in itself, but the complexities and anxieties are further increased where the patient is non-compliant with the treatment plan and therefore refuses to work with the nursing staff to keep themselves safer from self-injury or suicidal behaviour. The emotional strain on nurses required to work with people who are actively working against their care team in their efforts to maintain their safety and manage their risks is huge. The care team take on the responsibility for another person's safety against the will of that person, and this can create a situation where the two are at odds with each other, in a continual game of 'cat and mouse', where the patient is trying to create a situation whereby he or she can carry out an act of self-harm or suicide, while the caregiver is continually trying to prevent that from happening.

Mentorship and supervision as a source of stress

Addition pressures are reported by nurses when they act as mentors or preceptors for nursing students or newly qualified staff. The Nursing and Midwifery Council (NMC) requires nurses to support and develop others within the profession and the importance placed on this role is evident throughout the NHS, as nursing staff are frequently required to undertake a mentorship course as a prerequisite to further training or promotion. This supervisory role requires the nurse to have dedicated time to spend in direct contact with the person they are tasked to mentor, and demands that the nurse emotionally invests in this work, so that the person feels supported and valued in their development. When this requirement is placed upon an individual already working on a pressured, under-resourced inpatient clinical setting, the teaching and supportive role, which would have been otherwise embraced, can engender negative feelings and become a burden to the nurse, thus increasing their experience of stress. These issues are evident in the reported experience of nursing students, who often express feelings of being unwelcome in placement areas and symptoms of burnout in their mentors (14). The opportunities to work in direct and supervisory contact with their mentors are frequently reported as being minimal, which would inevitably impact the assessment process offered to students, and newly qualified staff. A lack of robust assessment and detailed direct feedback may lead on to competency issues not being identified or addressed. The impact on the student or new nurse is that they might feel undervalued, eroding their motivation to develop their skills and perform well. Over time, this may erode their levels of confidence, increase their fear of making mistakes, and cause them to avoid responsibilities around problem-solving, engaging with clients and other team members, and diminishing their personal development. The downward trajectory that this situation may create leads to further levels of stress in the workforce over time, as newly qualified staff and nursing students are the future of the profession.

Interventions to support a reduction of stress and burnout

Teamwork

The experience of working within a cohesive, consistent team with clear leadership and structures has been found to have a protective influence in reducing rates of stress experienced by mental health inpatient staff, and therefore in reducing the rates of burnout for individuals (38). Where there exists a team of staff who know each other and are able to anticipate each other's strengths and deficits as well as understanding individual member's personal traits, who work with clarity among themselves, and have an understanding of the ward structures, this not only reduces exhaustion but also sustains the camaraderie of staff in the face of challenges (38). Leadership within teams occurs across a range of individuals within the multidisciplinary team and those at more senior levels, each of whom needs to offer a sense of containment, support, and motivation to those around them. Communication across inpatient teams is fraught with difficulty as due to the nature of the shift work, teams never get an opportunity to meet to discuss the challenges of developing new ways of working, as well as handing over the pertinent and comprehensive information of the day-to-day clinical work. The result of teams handing over three (or more) times within each 24-hour period is frequently a loss of essential pieces of detailed information over time, leading to a lack of clarity and consistency. In addition, the communication from senior levels and the ward manager into their teams can also become fractured. It is therefore essential that lines of communication are multifaceted, to ensure that structure, organization, and teamwork are consistently promoted. Interventions to support this culture might include leadership training for ward managers and deputy ward managers to develop their own skills in this area as well as teambuilding interventions for the whole team (39). Supporting the team to get to know each other and to communicate in an honest and open manner serves to enhance team working and clarity across shifts, offering containment and a sense of security within the team as well as the patient population (39).

Hill et al. (40) argue that a team approach to training can be an ideal opportunity to enhance teamwork as well as to support the need for leadership, structure, and communication among team members. They argue that this provides the right set of circumstances to affect whole team cultures and to embed interventions aimed at reducing levels of stress. As mentioned earlier, there are challenges to creating a situation whereby a whole inpatient team can come together; however, it may be argued that making this happen is worth the time and investment of resources for this opportunity to be created, in order for teams to develop a positive culture as well as to convey the message that the team members are valued and respected. Teams can benefit from these events in several ways, for instance, boosting communication, creating a sense of team, skills training, and enhancing relationships and trust. Access to opportunities to enable nurses to learn and grow professionally have been found to be very important to nurses' job satisfaction rates, alongside their perceived autonomy and control over their practice and decision-making processes (41). Whole team training would enhance nurses' sense of empowerment, and would reduce staff frustration, stress, and burnout and therefore reduce staff turnover. Lautizi et al. (41) also argue that another benefit is the satisfaction reported through team advancement, progress, and growth alongside the rapport established with colleagues.

Personal attributes as a protective factor

Chang and Chan (18) carried out a large study of general nurses in Taiwan to examine the impact of proactive coping and optimism in relation to the experience of burnout. They hypothesized that individuals who utilize proactive coping skills or personal motivational strategies to overcome difficulties and achieve their desired outcomes, were able to increase their own, personal resources to enable them to respond to work pressure and demands. They identified a sense of personal optimism in order to drive a person's proactive coping strategies. They argued that people who have a sense of optimism when faced with challenges display a better ability to adjust and work flexibly, affording them greater strength for overcoming difficulties, and they therefore experience less stress. Optimists are more likely to seek out resources to manage stress and to then appropriately utilize those resources when facing a challenge. They thought in a more positive way when faced with obstacles and possessed greater flexibility to adapt and resolve problems, rather than giving in to negative thoughts and moods which would leave a person vulnerable to stress and burnout (18).

From personal experience of working in inpatient services over many years, it is evident that there are wide variations in the coping styles and strategies of staff facing the same sorts of problems and demands, and on how those individual styles affect the team functioning. In this sense, it might be beneficial for inpatient services to undertake psychometric tests on applicants prior to recruitment to establish whether they would be at a risk of burnout within this healthcare setting. In fact, Gustafsson et al. (42) identified specific personality traits which they linked to a reduced risk of burnout in their small-scale Swedish study. Those traits included higher rates of emotional stability, liveliness, and an enhanced sense of personal privacy. These individuals were able to manage everyday life and its challenges in a more balanced, adaptable, and flexible way with openness and spontaneity when dealing with other people without feeling overwhelmed or overly sentimental. The group less likely to experience burnout demonstrated a healthy barrier in terms of their expression of empathy to avoid being burdened with other people's problems. Gustafsson et al. (42) argue that to prevent burnout the person must find the right balance between hardiness and sensitivity and that the ability to stay healthy within caring work is based upon the person having an outlook on life that is realistic in terms of expectations and understanding of what is within that person's control.

In 2014, NHS England published a 'Values Based Framework' for recruitment which sets out to attract students and employees on the basis that their individual values and behaviours align with the values of the NHS Constitution (43). The initiative was partly in response to the concerns on compassion and care raised within the Francis report (44) and was intended to help ensure that the NHS has a workforce not only with the right skills and in the right numbers, but with the right values to support effective team working in delivering excellent patient care and experience. If this recruitment strategy does achieve what it sets out to do, it could have a potentially beneficial impact on reducing the rates of burnout within the workforce in the long term. If the future workforce has a commonly held set of values which genuinely support teamwork, then this would move towards a mutual commitment to NHS employees caring about each other, recognizing and responding to colleagues' work pressures and stress, and empowering staff to value and engage with support strategies to maintain the health and well-being of the workforce.

Clinical supervision

Clinical supervision is one of the cornerstones of good professional practice and is viewed as a professional requirement by each of the members of the multidisciplinary team. It is inconceivable, for example, that a psychologist or psychology assistant would not receive supervision on a routine basis. Within nursing, regular clinical supervision is also a fundamental requirement for supporting good standards of care and affording the nurse the opportunity to learn from their more experienced supervisor. The NMC sets out the expectations for their profession to share skills knowledge and experience with colleagues, within clause 9 of the NMC Code (45). Clinical supervision is the formal structure in which this requirement can be achieved. It supports staff to spend time thinking through clinical experiences, focusing on difficult or challenging situations, with the supervisor offering different ways of approaching those difficulties, or thinking with the person about what was challenging about the situation and how it might have been approached in a different way, to improve the experience for both the nurse and other people involved. In this way, the supervisee is encouraged to examine their own practice, with a critical eye, and learn from experience, supported by a more experienced and skilled colleague.

The opportunity to talk through frustrations, distressing situations, and adverse outcomes, as well as expressing a sense of pride and achievement where things have gone well, has a cathartic effect and leads to developing in knowledge, skills, and experience. Thus, the supervisee should feel unburdened by the process and restored in a personal sense. Clinical supervision also demonstrates in a tangible way that the person is valued by their employer and that they are being invested in by having this regular time out of clinical practice with someone who can offer support and guidance. However, it is interesting to note that there are several examples of negative results being found where staff support systems are put in place within NHS inpatient settings. Further analysis of these negative results ironically demonstrates that the systems have often failed due to lack of managerial support in their implementation (20). Interested staff have been unable to access these support systems due to lack of protected time being allocated, with the converse effect on staff morale. The important issue is that nurses must be empowered to place similar importance on their personal supervision as their fellow professionals within the multidisciplinary team. It is precisely these supportive structures that will sustain individuals to continue to deliver good clinical care when circumstances are challenging and there is increasing pressure on services.

Supervision should be broadly focused on the aspects of their work that the supervisee finds rewarding and therefore promotes the nurse's development on those aspects. Ward (46) undertook a small-scale study on 13 female mental health nurses in Australia, focusing on their practice, stress management, and professional well-being. She identified that the common theme among the participants was their dedication to their role and the immense job satisfaction they received from working with clients. They viewed their roles as important as they were with patients at the most critical time in their life. Although they found these experiences emotionally distressing and stressful, they expressed a sense of privilege to be sharing that moment in the client's life. They chose to look at the positive aspects of the job role rather than its frustrations and challenges, and highlighted satisfaction in perceived small achievements rather than the larger context. The role of advocating for patients when those people may have no one else, and the sense of belonging that it engendered, helped the participants to maintain a sense of balance and reduced the experience of stress. Working through the difficult and challenging aspects of a nurse's role to focus on these clinical and positive features requires great skill and investment in the supervisee by the supervisor, but the rewards are significant for everyone involved.

Supervision can be offered in a variety of different ways and at different times of the day, depending upon the needs of the service and staff. One-to-one supervision is widely regarded as the gold standard, however, group supervision to staff who may be part of the same ward team, or staff who are linked by their role, for example, ward managers, support workers, band 5 or band 6 nurses is also possible. Any opportunity for teams to spend time communicating about issues affecting their practice should be beneficial to patient care and teamwork. If the focus of this time together extends beyond factual clinical 'handover' information into the expression of thoughts and emotions, the effect on the team is that of a cathartic

experience which can be beneficial, reducing stress levels and sustaining individual and collective well-being.

Creating a situation whereby role-specific staff from a variety of different teams can spend similarly focused time together, talking through some of the difficult situations and experiences they have faced at work, affords those staff members not just the chance to air their frustrations and concerns, but also to learn from the experiences of others who might have a different perspective or the benefit of more knowledge or skill relating to the situation described. Learning from each other and hearing direct from colleagues about difficulties and anxieties also encourages a greater understanding of colleagues from other areas and how different wards might work slightly differently to each other. The sharing of experiences might lead to positive change across a diverse range of services and influence more cohesive and consistent working practices between them.

Preceptorship

Preceptorship refers to the enhanced support and supervision afforded to newly qualified nurses and allied health professionals. It varies greatly from one employer to another, but the framework is based on best practice guidance issued by the Department of Health in 2010 (47) and it is defined as:

A period of structured transition for the newly registered practitioner during which he or she will be supported by a preceptor, to develop their confidence as an autonomous professional, refine skills, values and behaviours and to continue their journey of lifelong learning. (47, p. 11)

The longer-term benefits of having this period of enhanced support for newly qualified practitioners has been reported to be improved retention of recruited staff, as well as enhanced recruitment results, reduced sickness in staff, and increased confidence and competence for the new professional (48). Preceptorship has also been found to be of benefit to the preceptor in terms of enhancing supporting skills, mentoring, and supervisory and appraisal skills (48). Employers who invest time and resources in developing robust preceptorship programmes for their new registrants set the tone for nurses and other professions to expect and to value the benefits of professional supervision and review throughout their career, which further supports their lifelong development of essential clinical skills and coping mechanisms (48). The advantage of specific employers designing and delivering their own preceptorship programme is that it allows for it to be tailored to local processes and procedures as well as training and coaching being tailored to the services that preceptees are working within and addressing the specific issues and needs of the individual new registrants.

Mindfulness training

Whereas the causes and negative consequences of stress among nurses are well documented, there is less written about effective ways to reduce or prevent the problem. There is some evidence that mindfulness-based stress reduction programmes may provide one effective way of reducing stress and improving health within clinicians. One such study included a brief 4-week mindfulness intervention for nurses and support workers (49). The study found that the mindfulness intervention group experienced significant improvements in burnout symptoms, relaxation, and life satisfaction, compared with a control group. The results suggest that mindfulness training may provide a relatively inexpensive and brief intervention approach, which is in keeping with the clinical interventions they would routinely recommend for patients, to help those in the nursing profession manage their work-related and home life stress. Another potentially beneficial intervention has been proposed by Kravits et al. (50). They applied a psychoeducational approach to proactively teach nurses techniques to identify and subsequently manage their stress levels. Techniques such as self-care, stress, and responses were taught, as well as supporting nurses to create their own wellness plans, identifying their own coping strategies and options, and subsequently evaluating their wellness planning intervention. The findings demonstrated that those nurses who actively participated in the psychoeducation programme showed fewer symptoms of burnout and reported greater psychological resources to enhance their own personal well-being (50).

These techniques can all be taught in group settings and self-administered as required, in the same way as other brief psychological interventions can be, for example, cognitive behavioural therapy. The person can learn the techniques and utilize them as they experience their own symptoms of increased levels of stress individually as required. In addition to this, work places can offer group sessions for staff, in the lunchtime period, or just prior to or following a shift, to encourage employees to effectively manage stress levels, demonstrating a respect for employees as well as an appreciation of the potential negative effects that their work may place upon them alongside a commitment to support employees. This is a promissory area of research which needs to be developed as the effect may demonstrate a fall in sickness rates, reduced turnover of staff in the workplace, and increased retention of staff. The overall value of this small investment in staff could also be reflected in improved patient satisfaction and safer services being provided.

Conclusion

The pressures on staff in mental health inpatient services are significant and increasing and there appears to be no resolution to them on the horizon. Patient acuity and the proportion of patients detained in hospital are both increasing in a context where staffing resources, bed numbers, and community and social care resources are already putting pressure on the system. The impact of these pressures on inpatient staff is an increased level of workload, decreased financial reward and working flexibility, and increasing stress. The long-term impact of high levels of stress on staff are multifarious and potentially affect a range of aspects, including their mental and physical health, social well-being, and their ability to provide a compassionate, holistic, and high standard of care. It is not difficult to envisage the cycle of stress as self-perpetuating, with staff going off work sick, leading to further pressure on their colleagues, with a detrimental effect on the quality of the experience for patients in their care, thus increasing risks of violence, absconsion, poor engagement with treatment, and more complaints and investigations, which all add to workloads and diminish staff morale. Recruitment to inpatient services also brings many challenges partly due to the unavoidable need for unsociable shift working practices, which can make this speciality less attractive when compared to services provided between 9 a.m. and 5 p.m., which are generally far more conducive to family life. In addition, patients are more unwell and challenging than those in the community, bringing additional stress to the role.

This chapter has reviewed some of the strategies available to address these issues. An increasing focus on team working, within individual teams and across teams, needs to be fostered. Incorporating a 'values-based' recruitment process or even psychometric testing to support the recruitment of individuals with the appropriate personal attributes was also discussed. Trusts need to demonstrate their commitment and the value that they place upon their staff. In particular, robust processes for clinical support and supervision alongside opportunities for improving the health and well-being of staff through interventions such as mindfulness are important. These activities should be viewed by trusts as one of their priorities and as a means by which staff can be invested in, developed, and valued. These approaches can support staff in managing workloads, reducing levels of stress, and avoiding burnout, which would ultimately increase patient satisfaction and the quality of care.

REFERENCES

1. The King's Fund. Mental health under pressure. 2016. https://www.kingsfund.org.uk/publications/mental-health-under-pressure
2. Buchanan M. England's mental health services in crisis. BBC News. 2013. http://www.bbc.co.uk/news/health-24537304
3. Royal College of Psychiatrists. Do the right thing: how to judge a good ward: ten standards for adult inpatient mental healthcare. 2011. http://www.rcpsych.ac.uk/pdf/OP79_forweb.pdf
4. Virtanen M, Vahtera J, Batty GB, et al. Overcrowding in psychiatric wards and physical assaults on staff: data linked longitudinal study. *Br J Psychiatry* 2011;198:149–155.
5. Department of Health. Achieving parity of esteem between mental and physical health. 2013. https://www.gov.uk/government/speeches/achieving-parity-of-esteem-between-mental-and-physical-health.
6. Cooper B. The headlines about 'parity of esteem' between mental and physical health remain just that. *NewStatesman*, 28 August 2015. http://www.newstatesman.com/politics/health/2015/08/british-mental-health-crisis
7. Hutchinson S. Mental health budgets 'still being cut despite pledge'. 2016. http://www.bbc.co.uk/news/health-37657954
8. McNicoll A. More mental health patients sent hundreds of miles for care due to local bed shortages. 2016. http://www.communitycare.co.uk/2016/05/20/mental-health-beds-crisis-thousands-acutely-ill-patients-sent-area-care/
9. National Confidential Inquiry into Suicide and Homicide by People with Mental Illness. *Annual Report: England, Northern Ireland, Scotland and Wales, July 2015*. Manchester: University of Manchester; 2015.
10. Royal College of Nursing. *Frontline First: Turning Back the Clock? Mental Health Services in the UK*. London: Royal College of Nursing; 2014.
11. NHS Choices. Struggling with stress? 2016. http://www.nhs.uk/Conditions/stress-anxiety-depression/Pages/understanding-stress.aspx
12. Hoff L. *People in Crisis: Clinical and Public Health Perspectives*. San Francisco, CA: Josey-Bass; 2001.
13. McTiernan K, McDonald N. Occupational stressors, burnout and coping strategies between hospital and community psychiatric nurses in a Dublin region. *J Psychiatr Ment Health Nurs* 2015;22:208–218
14. Galvin J, Suominen E, Morgan C, O'Connell EJ, Smith AP. Mental health nursing students' experiences of stress during training: a thematic analysis of qualitative interviews. *J Psychiatr Ment Health Nurs* 2015;22:773–783.

15. Anderson KN, Anderson LE, Glanze WD. *Mosby's Medical, Nursing and Allied Health Dictionary*, 5th edition. St. Louis, MO: Mosby; 1998.

16. Demir A, Ulusoy M, Ulusoy MF. Investigation of factors influencing burnout levels in the professional and private lives of nurses. *Int J Nurs Stud* 2003;40:807–827.

17. Maslach C, Jackson SE. Burnout in organisational settings. *Appl Soc Psychol Annu* 1984;5:133–135.

18. Chang Y, Chan H. Optimism and proactive coping in relation to burnout amongst nurses. *J Nurs Manag* 2015;23:401–408.

19. Bowers L, Allan T, Simpson A, Jones J, Whittington R. Morale is high in acute inpatient psychiatry. *Soc Psychiatry Psychiatr Epidemiol* 2009;44:39–46.

20. Gibb J, Cameron IM, Hamilton R, Murphy E, Naji S. Mental health nurses and allied health professionals' perceptions of the role of the occupational health service in the management of work related stress: how do they self care? *J Psychiatr Ment Health Nurs* 2010;17:838–845.

21. Hill RG, Rinaldi M, Gilleard C, Babbs M. Connecting the individual to the organisation: employers response to stress in the workplace. *Int J Ment Health Promot* 2003;5:23–30.

22. Brennan G, Flood C, Bowers L. Constraints and blocks to change and improvement on acute psychiatric ward; lessons from the city nurse project. *J Psychiatr Ment Health Nurs* 2006;13:475–482.

23. Happell B. Appreciating history: the Australian experience of direct entry mental health nursing education in universities. *Int J Ment Health Nurs* 2009;18:35–41

24. Happell B. Exploring workforce issues in mental health nursing. *Contemp Nurse* 2008;29:43–51

25. Royal College of Nursing. Urgent action needed to combat major UK nursing shortage. 2016. https://www.rcn.org.uk/news-and-events/news/urgent-action-needed-to-combat-major-uk-nursing-shortage-warns-rcn

26. Buckland D. Staff crisis as nurses quit NHS. *The Express*, 20 March 2016. http://www.express.co.uk/life-style/health/653954/Staffing-crisis-nurses-quit-NHS-health-Britain-mental-health

27. Mind. *Environmentally Friendly? Patient's Views on Conditions in Psychiatric Wards*. London: Mind; 2003.

28. Sainsbury Centre for Mental Health. *Acute Care: A National Survey of Adult Psychiatric Wards in England*. London: Sainsbury Centre Publications; 2004.

29. Robson H, Gomme S, Thompson F. Supporting recovery. In: Trenoweth S (ed), *Promoting Recovery in Mental Health Nursing*, pp. 31–48. London: Sage; 2016.

30. Repper J, Perkins J. *Social Inclusion and Recovery: A Model for Mental Health Practice*. London: Elsevier; 2003.

31. Shepherd G, Boardman J, Slade M. *Making Recovery a Reality*. London: Sainsbury Centre for Mental Health; 2008.

32. Slade M. *Personal Recovery and Mental Illness: A Guide for Mental Health Professionals*. Cambridge: Cambridge University Press; 2009.

33. Department of Health. Positive and proactive care: reducing the need for restrictive interventions. 2014. https://www.gov.uk/government/publications/positive-and-proactive

34. Doyle M, Kelly D, Clarke S, Braynion P. Burnout: the impact of psychosocial interventions training. *Ment Health Pract* 2007;10:16–19.

35. Zhao I, Turner C. The impact of shift work on people's daily health habits and adverse health outcomes. *Aust J Adv Nurs* 2007;25:8–22.

36. Currid TJ. The lived experience and meaning of stress in acute mental health nurses. *Br J Nurs* 2008;17:880–884.

37. Happell B, Koehn S. Seclusion as a necessary intervention: the relationship between burnout, job satisfaction and therapeutic optimism and justification for the use of seclusion. *J Adv Nurs* 2011;67:1222–1231.

38. Cordwell J, Bradley L. Enhancing effective multidisciplinary teamworking: a psychoeducational approach. In: Lynch JE, Trenoweth S (eds), *Contemporary Issues in Mental Health Nursing*, pp. 169–179. Chichester: John Wiley and Sons; 2008.

39. Bowers L, Nijam H, Simpson A, Jones J. The relationship between leadership, teamwork, structure, burnout and attitude to patients on acute psychiatric wards. *Soc Psychiatry Psychiatr Epidemiol* 2011;46:143–148.

40. Hill RG, Atnas CI, Ryan P, Ashby K, Winnington J. Whole team training to reduce burnout amongst staff on an inpatient alcohol ward. *J Subst Use* 2010;15:42–50.

41. Lautizi M, Laschinger HKS, Ravazzolo S. Workplace empowerment, job satisfaction and job stress among Italian mental health nurses: an exploratory study. *J Nurs Manag* 2009;17:446–452.

42. Gustafsson G, Persson B, Eriksson S, Norberg A, Strandberg G. Personality traits among burn out and non-burn out health care personnel at the same workplaces: a pilot study. *Int J Ment Health Nurs* 2009;18:336–348.

43. NHS England. Values based recruitment. 2014. https://www.hee.nhs.uk/our-work/attracting-recruiting/values-based-recruitment

44. Francis RF. Report of the Mid Staffordshire NHS Foundation Trust Public Inquiry. 2013. http://webarchive.nationalarchives.gov.uk/20150407084003/http://www.midstaffspublicinquiry.com/sites/default/files/report/executive%20summary.pdf

45. Nursing and Midwifery Council. The code: professional standards of practice and behaviour for nurses and midwives. 2015. https://www.nmc.org.uk/standards/code/read-the-code-online/

46. Ward L. Mental health nursing and stress: maintaining balance. *Int J Ment Health Nurs* 2011;20:77–85.

47. Department of Health. Preceptorship framework for newly registered nurses, midwives and allied health professionals. 2010. http://webarchive.nationalarchives.gov.uk/20130107105354/http://www.dh.gov.uk/prod_consum_dh/groups/dh_digitalassets/@dh/@en/@abous/documents/digitalasset/dh_114116.pdf

48. Sharples K, Elcock K. *Preceptorship for Newly Registered Nurses*. Exeter: Learning Matters Ltd.

49. Mackenzie CS, Poulin, PA, Seidman-Carlson R. A brief mindfulness based stress reduction intervention for nurses and nurse aides. *Appl Nurs Res* 2006;19:105–109.

50. Kravits K, McAllister-Black R, Grant M, Kirk C. Self-care strategies for nurses: a psychoeducational intervention of stress reduction and the prevention of burnout. *Appl Nurs Res* 2010;23:130–138.

SECTION 7

Specialist services across the life span

33

Acute inpatient care for children and adolescents

Anthony James

Admissions to an inpatient unit

There has been a change in the type of adolescent admissions to hospitals over the last several years. There are a number of factors behind this:

1. Increasing levels of self-harm and suicide attempts leading to requests for emergency admissions. Suicide is one of the leading causes of deaths in adolescents, and such deaths following self-harm have been underestimated, and have increased in the twenty-first century (1).
2. The rates of emotional disorders including depression have increased (2).
3. In recent years, there has been an increase in the admission rates for anorexia nervosa: not only have admission rates increased but so too have multiple admissions per person with anorexia nervosa. The increase in admission rates might reflect an increase in prevalence rates of anorexia nervosa in the general population, but other explanations, including lower clinical thresholds for admission, are possible (3).
4. The prevalence of autism and autistic spectrum disorder (ASD) appears to be increasing (4), with an estimated prevalence of ASD in the US of 14.6 per 1000 (one in 68) children aged 8 years, many of who display self-harming behaviours.
5. Therapeutic developments—early intervention psychosis services and community dialectic behavioural therapy for severe and persistent self-harm have led to a reduction in certain admissions.

Characteristics of who is admitted

Admission practices vary between countries, and in England the admission rate is low (2.2/1000 population at age 19 years), with schizophrenia, affective disorders, neurotic disorders, and eating disorders being the most frequent diagnoses (5). Eating disorders represent a major use of bed days as the length of stay is longer (see Chapter 36).

There have been significant changes in admissions to inpatient services: in the US, psychiatric discharges increased for children from 155 per 100,000 children in 1996 to 283 per 100,000 in 2007; for adolescents, from 683 to 969 per 100,000; and for adults, only slightly from 921 to 995 per 100,000 (6).

Involuntary admissions vary across countries, with a rate of 29.5% or prevalence rate of 2.5 per 10,000/12–17-year-olds in a national Finnish survey (7). In one study (8), psychotic disorders, violent and hostile behaviours, and suicidal ideation and talk were linked to involuntary admission, but not family adversities (e.g. family violence, divorce or separation, severe financial difficulties, and unemployment) except for parental substance use problems. The risk for being admitted when presenting with aggressive behaviours was greater in girls, which may be linked to the finding that admissions are often associated with childhood adversities, including abuse (9).

Besides psychiatric illness however, in practice it is clear that social factors play a significant role in who is admitted (10). Children in the welfare system are overrepresented in the child and adolescent psychiatric units (11), reflecting the high rates of psychiatric morbidity in this population (12). Indeed, alongside any principal psychiatric problem, adolescent inpatients suffer a multitude of difficulties including educational and social difficulties (13). A high level of family dysfunction is common, and many but not all studies report parental personality or psychological disturbance (13). Not surprisingly then, given the multiple problems that adolescent inpatients suffer, treatment that focuses on only some of these factors is likely to have limited effectiveness.

Assessment

Unfortunately, even in inpatient services standardized assessments of psychopathology are not routinely undertaken. This has led to the systematic under-reporting and, therefore, treatment of various disorders such as post-traumatic stress disorder (PTSD) (14). In one study, the introduction of standardized semi-structured instruments such as the Kiddie-Schedule for Affective Disorders and Schizophrenia (K-SADS) (15) led to the increasing recognition of several main diagnostic categories (depressive, anxiety, bipolar, and disruptive disorders), suggesting that those disorders were likely underreported.

International comparisons of admission rates

Comparisons of health care provisions, including admission rates, is fraught with methodological problems; however, a striking difference has been noted for paediatric bipolar disorder, where in the US the admission rate, especially for those under 13 years of age, is particularly high (16). For those aged under 20 years, the discharge rates for paediatric bipolar disorder per 100,000 population are as follows: the US 95.6, Australia 11.7, New Zealand 6.3, Germany 1.5, and England 0.9. The most marked divergence in discharge rates is in 5–9-year-olds: the US 27, New Zealand 0.22, Australia 0.14, Germany 0.03, and England 0.00. The disparity between the US and other discharge rates for paediatric bipolar disorder is markedly greater than the variation for child psychiatric discharge rates overall, and for adult rates of bipolar disorder, suggesting this may be due to differing diagnostic practices for paediatric bipolar disorder in the US. However, there may be a possible under-recognition of paediatric bipolar disorder in England.

Types of unit

Units are divided as general or specialized by function, and usually by age of the children and adolescents.

Age-based units

The major division of inpatient psychiatric services for children and adolescents is based upon age, with the differing developmental needs, particularly those between prepubertal and postpubertal children and adolescents. Child units often have a greater involvement of parents and family, including in some cases the provision to stay, which reflects the finding that compared to adolescents, younger children tend to come from more problematic families (17). Adolescence marks a transition for the individual and socially, with the greater influence of peers, and change in schooling and the possibility of leaving home. Such a large transitional period means in practice that general adolescent units often have an informal distinction between the older adolescents (>16 years) and younger adolescents.

In some countries, particularly those in Scandinavia and Northern Europe, child psychiatric units with an emphasis upon family and parental involvement continue to flourish. Recent surveys in the US (6) point to a substantial increase in the use of child psychiatric beds, while in the UK, the number of child psychiatric units has decreased substantially (18). The latter may reflect not only the increased provision of community child and adolescent mental health services (CAMHS), but also a reluctance to separate children from families.

Specialized units

There are specialized inpatient services for eating disorders. The need for this specialized service may reflect parental or indeed adolescent demands. However, while there is accumulating evidence for better outcomes for eating disorders with specialized community eating disorder services (19), there is no such evidence for an advantage for dedicated adolescent eating disorder inpatient units.

In England, adolescent intensive care units for violent, and/or persistently disruptive behaviours, as well as serious self-harming behaviours and persistent suicide attempts, are organized on a supra-regional level. While many modern adolescent units may incorporate purpose-built intensive care suites, longer-term intensive care is best provided in purpose-built units where security can be more easily maintained, and where there is access to adequate resources including sports facilities. Patients admitted to such units must be under the Mental Health Act 1983 (amended 2007) or other statutory provisions. Severely disturbed adolescents or those who have committed offences in the context of mental illness may be referred to adolescent forensic inpatient services.

Children and adolescents with mild to moderate learning disabilities can usually be catered for in general inpatient units with consultation from learning disability services and by employing dually trained staff. Those with severe learning disabilities require separate provision because of the specialized needs and communication difficulties. Other specialist units include services for children and adolescents with autism.

Parental and family involvement

The involvement of parents is important, and for children parental involvement is obviously essential. For adolescents, the situation is not so straightforward: while younger adolescents require consent from parents for treatment, older adolescents can, if competent, make their own decisions, which cannot be overridden by parents. Psychoeducation for the patient and family is almost always necessary, and for some, such as the family-based treatment for eating disorders, family therapy is one of the major treatment agents. For all, communication and clarification of the aims and requirements of treatment are required. This can be summed up as *family work*, which does not necessarily imply any family psychopathology; however, this approach is particularly helpful with chaotic families. More formal therapy is useful where there are clear communication, hierarchy, and alliance problems, over- or under-involvement, and high or low expressed emotion.

The involvement of parents is complex. An appropriate level of engagement is essential, but hard to achieve, and it varies during the course of the admission. At the outset, anxieties and tensions are naturally at their height. Unit staff need to recognize this, explaining things clearly and often repeatedly. Attending to simple details can help build up a feeling of trust. After all, the parents are placing their 'ill' child in the unit's care as a judgement call, but often against deeply felt emotional wishes. The latter are heightened in the case of separation anxieties. These anxieties can be reduced by a calm, authoritative stance, that acknowledges the adolescent's and parents' worries and gives information on visiting times, possible length of stay, weekend leave when possible, and the date of planning or review meetings. At this time it is also useful to make arrangements to link with the referring agent and/or family physician. This gives the sense that admission is not the end, or final phase of treatment, but part of the ongoing process, and is time limited.

Modalities of treatment

Therapeutic function

Inpatient care encompasses a multitude of functions, including the provision of a broad range of evidence-based therapies such as pharmacotherapy, cognitive behavioural therapy, family therapy, supportive individual counselling, and possibly art and music therapy. There is no evidence that these treatments per se are more effective delivered in an inpatient setting, however, there is a belief that with more intensity and consistency these treatments can be more effective.

Inpatient treatment is not just 'residential' care with the provision of on-site therapies. A unit will have its own 'milieu or ethos' with some specifically designed, such as behavioural units or those adopting family therapy or indeed psychodynamic approaches. Core elements for 'milieu therapy' are consistency, boundaries, limit setting, role modelling led by staff, as well as open group forms for exploration and discussion of day-to-day emotional and psychological issues as they arise. A crucial component of inpatient care is physical and psychological containment (20). Patients will often be admitted following the breakdown of social relationships and appear in a distressed, unsettled, and fragmentary psychological state. The act of physical containment, alongside psychological support with boundaries seems essential to help settle the disorganized, and sometimes suicidal, patient.

Specific disorders and problems

Patients who self-harm

Commonly, patients admitted following a suicide attempt have previously engaged in repeated episodes of self-harm, of differing types. Some adolescent inpatients who self-harm meet criteria for emotionally dysregulated personality disorders, and show a reduced 'attraction to life' disposition, and significant depressive symptoms (21). Increasing age, female gender, a history of trauma, living with a step-parent, and a diagnosis of depression are risk factors for self-harm in psychiatric inpatients (22). Adolescents with emerging personality disorders are more likely to be admitted to hospital, be admitted as an emergency, and spend longer in hospital than those without personality disturbance (23). Sharp et al. (24) found that of those admitted for self-harm, 19% met criteria for borderline personality disorder and 39% for major depressive disorder.

Adolescent inpatients with borderline personality disorder can be notoriously difficult to help with the emergence of dependent, sometimes hostile dependent relationships. Hospital admissions can make the psychopathology associated with borderline personality disorder worse as result of disturbed transference relationships with caring staff; these relationships are often based upon distorted, sometimes oscillating types of attachment with a profound fear of abandonment (25). Also, 'contagion' of self-harm is seen in inpatient units. Dialectic behavioural therapy can significantly reduce behavioural incidents during admission when compared to inpatient treatment as usual (26). Both dialectic behavioural therapy and routine inpatient treatment demonstrate highly significant reductions in suicidal behaviour, depressive symptoms, and suicidal ideation

at 1 year (26). Likewise, mentalization therapy shows considerable promise in reducing self-harm in adolescent inpatients (27). Overall, it appears that adolescent inpatients with self-harm benefit more from a structured therapeutic approach.

Suicidal patients

The prevention of suicide and serious self-harm is one of the main functions of an adolescent psychiatric unit. However, the prevention of suicide and serious self-harm is by no means an easy task for a number of reasons. For adolescents admitted following suicide attempts, established risk factors (e.g. a history of suicide attempts) may not predict suicidality sufficiently well (28), rather, adolescents who remain depressed or hopeless, or who express a low value for life, or an abnormally high connection with the universe, are at higher risk for suicidality.

The risk of suicide varies and is raised at the time of admission, at discharge, and within the first of year post discharge. While suicidal behaviour is one of the most common reasons for admission, estimation of intent behind each act, and in a unit there may be several each day, is a constantly demanding task. One of the major techniques used to reduce serious self-harm and suicide within units is close nursing observation. This is a practised and standardized technique. Indeed, a standard protocol for the level of observations is essential so that communication between nurses and other members of the multidisciplinary team is clear. Without this, a highly suicidal patient could exploit any 'chinks in the amour' with potentially a serious, if not fatal outcome.

It is not immediately obvious that continuous observations themselves are therapeutic, however, experience shows they are a vital element in the care package. It is not that close nursing observation just 'buys' time, allowing other therapeutic interventions such as antidepressant medication to take effect; rather, the experience of close, supportive human contact can overcome the deep sense of isolation and despair that is associated with suicide and serious self-harm. Research has shown that suicides are often characterized by an increasing sense of isolation (29).

The worrying patient is the one who has planned his/her suicide and who quietly attempts this, having noted the routines within the unit, and chosen a potential 'down' time in the unit. This is everyone's nightmare, but the risks can be minimized: regular auditing of serious incidents of self-harm and suicide attempts can reveal patterns of timings, for instance, during early evenings when the rate of such incidents can peak, staffing levels can be adjusted accordingly. Building design can help reduce blind spots and potential ligature points. This can be combined with regular building inspections. At the individual patient level, it can be too easy to be lulled into a false sense of security, and as the admission progresses and a sense of familiarity and possible complacency develops. To overcome this, regular reviews of progress, and importantly the history with details of previous attempts, may help keep the focus on the potential risks. The latter review should include members of the multidisciplinary team at all levels, especially nursing assistants and those working directly with the patient and family. Communication is the key which involves listening to all those concerned. This especially applies to family members who may have a 'sense' something is wrong. The parents may have noticed a lowering of mood, odd fatalistic comments, or increasing hopelessness, possibly after a period of seeming improvement. Alternatively, the patient may be uncharacteristically cheerful, having, as described in the psychiatric literature, finally decided on suicide, and, therefore, feeling relaxed and free from previous worries. The unit must be able to respond to these concerns, which is not always easy, as these may not be openly expressed, or expressed at the last moment before leave, or arise amidst a number of similarly expressed worries. It is also helpful within an experienced team to be able to trust a staff member's intuition—a gut feeling that something is not right, even though formal risk assessments have indicated otherwise. It is hopefully the case that a well-functioning team is able to deal with conscious and unconscious communications.

There have been improvements in care: a prospective study (30) of all patients admitted to NHS inpatient psychiatric care in England between 1997 and 2008 showed a significant drop ($p <0.001$) in inpatient suicides from 0.4 to 0.1 per 100,000 population in the 15–24 years age range (N. Kapur, personal communication). For all ages, rates also fell for the most common suicide methods, particularly suicide by hanging (a 59% reduction). On a unit level, the design of the unit with the removal of ligature points is essential, and implementing procedures such as follow-up appointments within 7 days of discharge may contribute to better outcomes.

Psychosis

Recently, there has been a reduction in the proportion of those with psychosis admitted to adolescent units (31), partly as a result of the introduction of community early intervention psychosis services. This is to be welcomed, as research from the US Early Psychosis Intervention Center (EPICENTER) has found, over a 6-month follow-up period, a reduction in costs and improved outcome (32), the former being attributable to reduced inpatient care. This clearly implies, however, that those admitted, although fewer, are likely to be more severely affected. Indeed, those with early-onset psychosis are often more severely affected than those with adult-onset forms (33), and require intensive support, including the appropriate use of clozapine for treatment-resistant psychosis. The treatment of psychosis requires a multimodal approach with not only medication, but also psychological treatments such as behavioural family therapy, psychoeducation, or cognitive behavioural therapy.

One of the recently changing demographics within adolescent inpatient care is the increasing recognition of the association of childhood sexual abuse and psychosis (34). This risk of psychosis is thought to be mediated by elevated sensitivity and lack of resilience to socioenvironmental stress and enhanced threat anticipation.

Child abuse and post-traumatic stress disorder

Child maltreatment—physical and emotional ill-treatment, sexual abuse, neglect, and exploitation and 'polyvictimization', which also includes experiences of multiple forms of victimization, or abduction; witnessing of family and community violence; and cyberbullying—is unfortunately common, occurring in 10% of US children and adolescents aged 2–17 (35). Child maltreatment is associated with a range of psychopathology including PTSD, depression, and suicidality. Both sexes are affected, but girls are more frequently seen in hospital settings. The presentation of adolescents admitted to hospital following abuse can be very varied. Those admitted in the

acute phase, often in the midst of a disclosure, can be unsettled, confused, and angry, with evidence of self-harm and suicide attempts. PTSD is frequently seen, but unless specifically enquired about, and the question of abused raised, this diagnosis can be missed with the adolescent presenting with unexplained self-harm, which is often quite serious.

Inpatient care for these patients can sometimes be chaotic, with a distressed and depressed adolescent engaging in self-harming behaviours while indicating, but not fully disclosing, what is troubling him or her. The art of caring in this situation is to be patient and supportive, while providing a physically and psychologically safe environment. This may not be easy, especially in cases of intrafamilial abuse where the abuser may still, unbeknown to the medical staff, be having contact. A pattern of self-harm after visits, or after family arguments, may be clues. It is important in this situation not to direct an impressionable, distressed adolescent into making a disclosure by using tactics such as leading questions. Involvement of child protection agencies is essential. As part of the process it may be necessary to override patient confidentiality when abuse is suspected. While child protection measures are essential, the inpatient team needs to focus on the treatment needs, which can be difficult in the face of sometimes horrific and distressing accounts of maltreatment. An experienced team should be able to remain focused, with members of the team not so involved to be able to distance themselves from the powerful emotions and countertransference issues, and guide those working more directly with the adolescent and family.

The treatment of PTSD, depression, and psychosis in cases of child maltreatment usually requires a combination of psychological therapy—trauma-based cognitive behavioural therapy, medication, and a systemic approach involving the family and child protection agencies. Most adolescents are able to return home, particularly in cases of extrafamilial abuse, but some require foster care or alternative accommodation.

Autism and autistic spectrum disorders

There has been an increasing recognition of children and adolescents with autism and autistic spectrum disorders (ASD) (36, 37). In comparison with other children and adolescents, those with ASD are more likely to require hospital and emergency care (38). Hospital admission is not recommended for the treatment of the core symptoms of autism; however, treatment of comorbid conditions such as psychosis, depression, self-harm, and eating disorders quite frequently does necessitate admission. Children and adolescents with ASD in single-parent homes, those diagnosed at a later age, those engaging in self-injurious behaviour, aggressive behaviour, and those diagnosed with depression or obsessive–compulsive disorder are all more likely to be admitted to hospital (39). Inpatient care in these circumstances can be difficult (40) due to particular patient characteristics especially rigidity, sensory sensitivities, poor socialization, as well as high levels of irritability and hyperactivity, sometimes as comorbid attention deficit hyperactivity disorder. Intellectual disability can naturally add to the patient's difficulty in adapting to a busy ward environment. There is some evidence, however, from the US, that specialized inpatient services can reduce the length of hospital admission and improve outcomes (40). However, the provision of suitable aftercare remains a significant problem even with specialized ASD inpatient services (41).

Intellectual disability

Service for those with intellectual disability is probably one of the most neglected areas in medicine. Funding, resources, and academic support for this area of practice is poor, and the result, at least in England, is a dearth of available units, although those available are specialized and of a high standard. Young people with intellectual disability and mental disorders significantly improve clinically when admitted to hospital and do as well as non-disabled peers. However, patients with intellectual disability are more likely to be male, and have longer hospital stays (42)

The essential element of practice is the use of specialized behavioural programmes, overseen by psychologists. With attention to detail, clear ABC (antecedent, behaviour, and consequence) formulations, and workers skilled in behavioural techniques, crucially as a *whole team* approach, remarkable outcomes are achievable. This work can then be taught and supported with parents and/or carers. Indeed, this approach is essential; otherwise the few units that are available become 'log jammed' with patients unable to move back home or to residential units.

One of the most common problems is impulsive violence, which can be severe. Behavioural techniques provide the basis of treatment, with careful and judicious psychopharmacology. There is a danger of the use of multiple and large doses of medication if not regularly reviewed and audited. Of course, all psychiatric practice in inpatient unit should be reviewed and audited, and in this area in particular, external ethical review of behavioural programmes is advised.

This area demands expertise, and mental health nurses and psychiatrists in most countries require further specialist training to practice.

Structure and functioning of the unit

Unit management

Each unit can benefit from an external management group that can review policies and the operational running of the unit, to ensure against the unit becoming isolated and 'isolationist'. In the latter case, there is a real danger of therapeutic 'drift', and the unit adopting idiosyncratic practices, which at their worst become heavily rule bound and protectionist for staff, and ultimately of little benefit for patients. Fortunately, this situation has become less common with greater patient and parent involvement, and the setting up of national guidelines and standards.

An important management task is to set up the pathways for admission and discharge, integrating the inpatient service with day patient, outreach, and CAMHS. Modern practice is for a more horizontal service with equal allocation of resources between services, allowing more rapid and appropriate transfer of patients between levels of care (Figure 33.1).

Modern structure: horizontal more equal distribution of resources with shorter admissions.

Community services ←——→ Inpatient services

Older hierarchical structure with unequal distribution of resources and longer admissions (size of arrows refers to referral pressures).

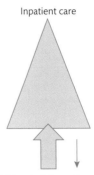

Inpatient care

Community child and adolescent psychiatric services

Figure 33.1 Differing arrangements of inpatient care.

Behavioural management

Complex behavioural regimes can be implemented within an inpatient service to underpin a psychological treatment programme for a variety of disorders such as obsessive–compulsive disorders. However, one of the main indications for the use of a behavioural regime is to treat aggression.

Physical aggression during admission is common, occurring in one study in up to 23% of inpatients (43). Factors that predict persistent physical aggression include a history of aggression and use of medication at presentation. Persistent aggression is also associated with an increased length of stay, but not necessarily a worse outcome. Broad-based behavioural management programmes lead to a reduction in aggression (44), emphasizing the importance of an organizational approach to behavioural management. Amongst inpatient staff, exposure to aggression is common—occurring in over 84% in one study (44). The impact on staff is considerable with difficulty attending work and other emotional and professional sequelae, highlighting the need for a cohesive staff group, and regular training to deal with violence.

Seclusion

Seclusion is defined as the placement of a patient in a specifically designed room in order to de-escalate behaviours, assure physical safety, and achieve behavioural control. Restraint refers to a physical intervention, either through therapeutic holding by a caregiver/staff member, or as in certain countries such mechanical restraining tools. Reasons for seclusion and restraint include threats (73%), agitation (63%), and physical aggression (63%) (45). A recent review showed that the use of both seclusion and restraint are reduced after behavioural interventions, or the more systematic use of restraint (46), and use of the correct legislation. In some countries such as the UK, mechanical restraints are very rarely used, while a Finnish study found mechanical restraint was used in 6.9% of adolescent inpatients (47).

Restraint in particular can have severe consequences including trauma for the individual, a reactivation of prior traumatic experiences, and serious physical side effects, such as asphyxia, aspiration, blunt trauma to the chest, thrombosis, and even death. One US study (48) reported 45 fatalities between 1993 and 2003 in child and adolescent psychiatric facilities related to restraints.

In certain cases, aggression or disturbed behaviour may be managed using medication. Rapid tranquillization techniques involve the administration of short-acting benzodiazepines, or antipsychotics intramuscularly or via rapidly absorbed oral preparations. Such procedures are safe provided there is a clear protocol, and regular physical monitoring by trained staff.

Risk management

The management and reduction of risk is a crucial function of an inpatient unit. Vital to this process is the detection and quantification of risk. A thorough and detailed history with corroborative evidence is essential. Finely tuned clinical skills can be enhanced in an inpatient setting with a multidisciplinary perspective, which adds an extra dimension—for example, by having both male and female viewpoints. Furthermore, it is possible to assess risk over time, and dynamically, via the interaction with observable stressors within the unit. A major advantage of residential psychiatric care is the possibility of modifying the milieu by various means—varying the level of nursing observations, excluding stressors and gradually reintroducing them.

Clinical skills based upon detailed observation are, therefore, at the heart of a risk assessment. Routine questionnaires can supplement the risk assessment for self-harm, but do not replace them. The limited research available indicates that violence towards others, unlike self-directed violence, can be successfully predicted using clinical judgement (49). Semi-structured assessments of violence such as the SAVRY (Structured Assessment of Violence Risk in Youth) have good predictive validity (50) and can be recommended. However, there is evidence that questionnaires do not help predict suicide (51), and therefore in this area reliance is based more upon informed, clinical judgement.

Building

The structure of the building of the unit is almost an entirely neglected consideration in textbooks of child and adolescent psychiatry; nevertheless, this is an important, if not crucial consideration for patient safety, welfare, and treatment, besides being an important consideration for staff comfort at work. An essential element in reducing inpatient suicides and serious suicide attempts by hanging is the design of the building so as to eliminate, as far as possible, any ligature points. This requires punctilious scrutiny at the design stage of any building. Improvements in general building design can help.

Besides safety, the ambience of the ward, the size of bedrooms and corridors, provision of good line of sight for nursing observations, lighting, and colour scheme all can contribute towards a more pleasant and safer working environment. A decision has to be made on the balance between how 'homely' or 'like a hospital'

an atmosphere the ward needs to be. This can be sensibly answered if one considers functionality, and the need to have some more intimate patient and family areas, alongside being able to deal safely and efficiently with any violent episodes, maintain good infection control, fire safety, etc.

Length of stay

There has been a marked change in the pattern of inpatient care with a trend for shorter admissions but with more complex presentations (52). While there may be concerns about this trend, shorter admissions have been shown not only to be feasible, but effective. In one study (53), the mean length of admission was 23.7 days for mood disorders, 18.9 days for anxiety disorders, and 46.9 days for the major psychosis diagnostic groups. Most improvements occurred during the first 3 weeks of admission. Importantly, readmission rates were not elevated. However, longer stays, positive therapeutic alliance, and better premorbid family functioning have been found independently to predict better outcome (54).

Readmission

Readmission occurs in just under half of cases—43% (55). Rehospitalization is highest during the first 30 days following discharge, and remains elevated for 3 months. Medication non-adherence and a history of childhood sexual abuse are associated with readmission (56). A real concern comes from the findings of a Danish 10-year follow-up study that 25% of those readmitted became 'long-term' psychiatric inpatients, particularly those with schizophrenia and affective psychoses (57).

Outcome studies

As treatment is understandably one of the major aims of any unit, it is surprising that more research has not been done in this area. Indeed, treatment processes are difficult to quantify: what treatments are offered, in what order, delivered by whom, to the patient and/or family, or conjointly. In order to meet the requirement for as short length of admission as possible, and to reduce the patient's suffering, often many interventions are started at the same time, and as a consequence it is often difficult to disentangle exactly what has been the important treatment agent.

The available global data from a meta-analysis of ten studies highlighted clear clinical improvements for inpatient care (58), while poor long-term prognosis has been noted for some early-onset disorders such as psychosis (59). A prospective study (54) found significant and clinically meaningful clinical improvements across all diagnoses, maintained at 1-year follow-up, following an average 16-week admission. The mean cost of admission was £24,100 (UK costs in 2007). Curiously, despite the clinical improvements, which enabled the patients to be subsequently treated within community mental health services (CAMHS), pre-admission and post-discharge support costs were similar. This finding for inpatient care contrasts with that from a community study of 56 severely disturbed adolescents in the UK (60) whose costs including placement in various residential units amounted to £56,000 per child/adolescent per year—over double that of psychiatric inpatient care with no appreciable change in the level of symptoms or functioning. Direct comparisons may not be possible, and while there is evidence pointing clearly to improvements for inpatient psychiatric care, it is evident, nonetheless, that residential care for severely disturbed children and adolescents is expensive.

The therapeutic factors that make a difference to outcome are difficult to discern, but appear from patient feedback, at least, to be the relationships that the adolescent makes during the admission. Adolescents particularly value the relationships they make with peers. This may be understandable when one understands that the adolescent often feels isolated, with depressive, paranoid thoughts, and unable to make sense of his/her mental state. Once the adolescent is able to overcome the initial fear and trepidation associated with admission, and experiences a warm, concerned approach from other adolescents, some of whom have similar experiences, they recognize that he/she is not alone, and may be able to see how others deal with these experiences and, hopefully, recover. Staff relationships are, of course, also important, but are not highlighted so much by the adolescent group.

Discharge and aftercare

There is some preliminary evidence from adults that the introduction of planned care coordination ('Care Programme Approach') results in better care with less community crisis team input, lower rates of readmission, and greater satisfaction for both patients and relatives following discharge (61). Curiously, a US and Canadian study found that while only 50% of discharged adolescents received aftercare, those that did were more likely to be readmitted (62). Disappointingly, follow-up research shows that only a proportion of inpatients receive the recommended services upon discharge (54). Even in services with variable, but high, engagement with outpatient treatment, rates of readmissions of up to 28% within a year are found (63).

Transition points into and out of an inpatient service and the transition of the older adolescent to adult mental health services are vital points in any care pathway because of the increased risk of disruption in continuity of care, disengagement from services, and possibly poorer clinical outcomes, including the risk of suicide. Some young people, such as those with neurodevelopmental disorders and complex needs, are at a greater risk of falling through the care gap during transition to adult services (64). This has led some to argue for the development of youth community services with an upper age range of 25 years.

Post discharge is recognized as a risk period. The death rate within 1 year of discharge from an adolescent inpatient service is six times higher than in the general population of the same age, although the total number of deaths following discharge from NHS child adolescent psychiatric units in England was low at 120 over a 6-year period (1998–2004) (5). The suicide rate is highest in the year after inpatient admission, with a Korean study showing that the standardized mortality ratio among former adolescent inpatients was 7.8 (95% confidence interval 4.7–12.3) for unnatural causes, and for suicide it was 14.2 (95% confidence interval 7.7–23.7) (65). Among the different diagnostic groups, patients with personality disorders, schizophrenia, or affective disorders had the highest risk for suicide.

REFERENCES

1. Rockett IR, Lilly CL, Jia H, et al. Self-injury mortality in the United States in the early 21st century: a comparison with proximally ranked diseases. *JAMA Psychiatry* 2016;73:1072–1081.
2. Collishaw S, Maughan B, Natarajan L, Pickles A. Trends in adolescent emotional problems in England: a comparison of two national cohorts twenty years apart. *J Child Psychol Psychiatry* 2010;51:885–894.
3. Holland J, Hall N, Yeates DG, Goldacre M. Trends in hospital admission rates for anorexia nervosa in Oxford (1968-2011) and England (1990-2011): database studies. *J R Soc Med* 2016;109:59–66.
4. Isaksen J, Diseth TH, Schjolberg S, Skjeldal OH. Autism spectrum disorders – are they really epidemic? *Eur J Paediatr Neurol* 2013;17:327–333.
5. James A, Clacey J, Seagroatt V, Goldacre M. Adolescent inpatient psychiatric admission rates and subsequent one-year mortality in England: 1998-2004. *J Child Psychol Psychiatry* 2010;51:1395–1404.
6. Blader JC. Acute inpatient care for psychiatric disorders in the United States, 1996 through 2007. *Arch Gen Psychiatry* 2011;68:1276–1283.
7. Ellila HT, Sourander A, Valimaki M, Warne T, Kaivosoja M. The involuntary treatment of adolescent psychiatric inpatients – a nation-wide survey from Finland. *J Adolesc* 2008;31:407–419.
8. Kaltiala-Heino R. Involuntary commitment and detainment in adolescent psychiatric inpatient care. *Soc Psychiatry Psychiatr Epidemiol* 2010;45:785–793.
9. Rytila-Manninen M, Lindberg N, Haravuori H, et al. Adverse childhood experiences as risk factors for serious mental disorders and inpatient hospitalization among adolescents. *Child Abuse Negl* 2014;38:2021–2032.
10. Kylmanen P, Hakko H, Rasanen P, Riala K. Is family size related to adolescence mental hospitalization? *Psychiatry Res* 2010;177:188–191.
11. Laukkanen M, Hakko H, Rasanen P, Riala K. Does the use of health care and special school services, prior to admission for psychiatric inpatient treatment, differ between adolescents housed by child welfare services and those living with their biological parent(s)? *Community Ment Health J* 2013;49:528–539.
12. McCann JB, James A, Wilson S, Dunn G. Prevalence of psychiatric disorders in young people in the care system. *BMJ* 1996;313:1529–1530.
13. Tonge BJ, Hughes GC, Pullen JM, Beaufoy J, Gold S. Comprehensive description of adolescents admitted to a public psychiatric inpatient unit and their families. *Aust N Z J Psychiatry* 2008;42:627–635.
14. Havens JF, Gudino OG, Biggs EA, Diamond UN, Weis JR, Cloitre M. Identification of trauma exposure and PTSD in adolescent psychiatric inpatients: an exploratory study. *J Trauma Stress* 2012;25:171–178.
15. Kaufman J, Birmaher B, Brent D, et al. Schedule for Affective Disorders and Schizophrenia for School-Age Children-Present and Lifetime Version (K-SADS-PL): initial reliability and validity data. *J Am Acad Child Adolesc Psychiatry* 1997;36:980–988.
16. James A, Hoang U, Seagroatt V, Clacey J, Goldacre M, Leibenluft E. A comparison of American and English hospital discharge rates for pediatric bipolar disorder, 2000 to 2010. *J Am Acad Child Adolesc Psychiatry* 2014;53:614–624.

17. Rice BJ, Woolston J, Stewart E, Kerker BD, Horwitz SM. Differences in younger, middle, and older children admitted to child psychiatric inpatient services. *Child Psychiatry Hum Dev* 2002;32:241–261.

18. O'Herlihy A, Worrall A, Lelliott P, Jaffa T, Hill P, Banerjee S. Distribution and characteristics of in-patient child and adolescent mental health services in England and Wales. *Br J Psychiatry* 2003;183:547–551.

19. Gowers SG, Clark AF, Roberts C, et al. A randomised controlled multicentre trial of treatments for adolescent anorexia nervosa including assessment of cost-effectiveness and patient acceptability—the TOuCAN trial. *Health Technol Assess* 2010;14:1–98.

20. Bion W. *Learning from Experience*. London: Heinemann; 1962.

21. Ferrara M, Terrinoni A, Williams R. Non-suicidal self-injury (NSSI) in adolescent inpatients: assessing personality features and attitude toward death. *Child Adolesc Psychiatry Ment Health* 2012;6:12.

22. de Kloet L, Starling J, Hainsworth C, Berntsen E, Chapman L, Hancock K. Risk factors for self-harm in children and adolescents admitted to a mental health inpatient unit. *Aust N Z J Psychiatry* 2011;45:749–755.

23. Magallon-Neri EM, Canalda G, De la Fuente JE, et al. The influence of personality disorders on the use of mental health services in adolescents with psychiatric disorders. *Compr Psychiatry* 2012;53:509–515.

24. Sharp C, Ha C, Michonski J, Venta A, Carbone C. Borderline personality disorder in adolescents: evidence in support of the Childhood Interview for DSM-IV Borderline Personality Disorder in a sample of adolescent inpatients. *Compr Psychiatry* 2012;53;765–774.

25. James A, Berelowitz M, Vereker M. Borderline personality disorder: study in adolescence. *Eur Child Adolesc Psychiatry* 1996;5:11–17.

26. Katz LY, Cox BJ, Gunasekara S, Miller AL. Feasibility of dialectical behavior therapy for suicidal adolescent inpatients. *J Am Acad Child Adolesc Psychiatry* 2004;43:276–282.

27. Sharp C, Ha C, Carbone C, et al. Hypermentalizing in adolescent inpatients: treatment effects and association with borderline traits. *J Pers Disord* 2013;27:3–18.

28. Consoli A, Cohen D, Bodeau N, et al. Risk and protective factors for suicidality at 6-month follow-up in adolescent inpatients who attempted suicide: an exploratory model. *Can J Psychiatry* 2015;60(2 Suppl 1):S27–36.

29. Miranda R, De Jaegere E, Restifo K, Shaffer D. Longitudinal follow-up study of adolescents who report a suicide attempt: aspects of suicidal behavior that increase risk of a future attempt. *Depress Anxiety* 2014;31:19–26.

30. Kapur N, Hunt IM, Windfuhr K, et al. Psychiatric in-patient care and suicide in England, 1997 to 2008: a longitudinal study. *Psychol Med* 2013;43:61–71.

31. Kronstrom K, Ellila H, Kuosmanen L, Kaljonen A, Sourander A. Changes in the clinical features of child and adolescent psychiatric inpatients: a nationwide time-trend study from Finland. *Nord J Psychiatry* 2016;7:436–441.

32. Breitborde NJ, Bell EK, Dawley D, et al. The Early Psychosis Intervention Center (EPICENTER): development and six-month outcomes of an American first-episode psychosis clinical service. *BMC Psychiatry* 2015;15:266.

33. Vyas NS, Gogtay N. Treatment of early onset schizophrenia: recent trends, challenges and future considerations. *Front Psychiatry* 2012;3:29.

34. Reininghaus U, Gayer-Anderson C, Valmaggia L, et al. Psychological processes underlying the association between childhood trauma and psychosis in daily life: an experience sampling study. *Psychol Med* 2016:1–15.

35. Finkelhor D, Ormrod RK, Turner HA. Poly-victimization: a neglected component in child victimization. *Child Abuse Negl* 2007;31:7–26.

36. Anon. Are rates of autism spectrum disorders increasing? Expanded diagnostic criteria and greater public awareness may explain why. *Harv Ment Health Lett* 2010;26:6.

37. Fombonne E. Epidemiology of autistic disorder and other pervasive developmental disorders. *J Clin Psychiatry* 2005;66(Suppl 10):3–8.

38. Schlenz AM, Carpenter LA, Bradley C, Charles J, Boan A. Age differences in emergency department visits and inpatient hospitalizations in preadolescent and adolescent youth with autism spectrum disorders. *J Autism Dev Disord* 2015;45:2382–2391.

39. Mandell DS. Psychiatric hospitalization among children with autism spectrum disorders. *J Autism Dev Disord* 2008;38:1059–1065.

40. Gabriels RL, Agnew JA, Beresford C, Morrow MA, Mesibov G, Wamboldt M. Improving psychiatric hospital care for pediatric patients with autism spectrum disorders and intellectual disabilities. *Autism Res Treat* 2012;2012:685053.

41. Siegel M, Doyle K, Chemelski B, et al. Specialized inpatient psychiatry units for children with autism and developmental disorders: a United States survey. *J Autism Dev Disord* 2012;42:1863–1869.

42. Chaplin R, Roach S, Johnson H, Thompson P. Inpatient children and adolescent mental health services (CAMHS): outcomes of young people with and without intellectual disability. *J Intellect Disabil Res* 2015;59:995–998.

43. Dean AJ, Duke SG, Scott J, Bor W, George M, McDermott BM. Physical aggression during admission to a child and adolescent inpatient unit: predictors and impact on clinical outcomes. *Aust N Z J Psychiatry* 2008;42:536–543.

44. Dean AJ, Gibbon P, McDermott BM, Davidson T, Scott J. Exposure to aggression and the impact on staff in a child and adolescent inpatient unit. *Arch Psychiatry Nurs* 2010;24:15–26.

45. Delaney KR, Fogg L. Patient characteristics and setting variables related to use of restraint on four inpatient psychiatric units for youths. *Psychiatr Serv* 2005;56:186–192.

46. De Hert M, Dirix N, Demunter H, Correll CU. Prevalence and correlates of seclusion and restraint use in children and adolescents: a systematic review. *Eur Child Adolesc Psychiatry* 2011;20:221–230.

47. Hottinen A, Valimaki M, Sailas E, et al. Mechanical restraint in adolescent psychiatry: a Finnish Register study. *Nord J Psychiatry* 2013;67:132–139.

48. Nunno MA, Holden MJ, Tollar A. Learning from tragedy: a survey of child and adolescent restraint fatalities. *Child Abuse Negl* 2006;30:1333–1342.

49. Phillips NL, Stargatt R, Brown A. Risk assessment of self- and other-directed aggression in adolescent psychiatric inpatient units. *Aust N Z J Psychiatry* 2012;46:40–46.

50. Singh JP, Grann M, Fazel S. A comparative study of violence risk assessment tools: a systematic review and metaregression analysis of 68 studies involving 25,980 participants. *Clin Psychol Rev* 2011;31:499–513.

51. Mulder R, Newton-Howes G, Coid JW. The futility of risk prediction in psychiatry. *Br J Psychiatry* 2016;209:271–272.

52. Olfson M, Gameroff MJ, Marcus SC, Greenberg T, Shaffer D. National trends in hospitalization of youth with intentional self-inflicted injuries. *Am J Psychiatry* 2005;162:1328–1335.

53. Swadi H, Bobier C. Hospital admission in adolescents with acute psychiatric disorder: how long should it be? *Australas Psychiatry* 2005;13:165–168.

54. Green J, Jacobs B, Beecham J, Dunn G, Kroll L, Tobias C, et al. Inpatient treatment in child and adolescent psychiatry – a prospective study of health gain and costs. *J Child Psychol Psychiatry* 2007;48:1259–1267.

55. James S, Charlemagne SJ, Gilman AB, et al. Post-discharge services and psychiatric rehospitalization among children and youth. *Adm Policy Ment Health* 2010;37:433–445.

56. Bobier C, Warwick M. Factors associated with readmission to adolescent psychiatric care. *Aust N Z J Psychiatry* 2005;39:600–606.

57. Pedersen J, Aarkrog T. A 10-year follow-up study of an adolescent psychiatric clientele and early predictors of readmission. *Nord J Psychiatry* 2001;55:11–16.

58. Pfeiffer SI, Strzelecki SC. Inpatient psychiatric treatment of children and adolescents: a review of outcome studies. *J Am Acad Child Adolesc Psychiatry* 1990;29:847–853.

59. Healy E, Fitzgerald M. A 16-year follow-up of a child inpatient population. *Eur Child Adolesc Psychiatry* 2000;9:46–53.

60. Clark F, O'Malley A, Woodham A, Barratt B, Byford S. Children with complex problems: needs, costs and predictors over 1 year. *Child Adolesc Ment Health* 2005;10:170–178.

61. Stewart MW, Wilson M, Bergquist K, Thorburn J. Care coordinators: a controlled evaluation of an inpatient mental health service innovation. *Int J Ment Health Nurs* 2012;21:82–91.

62. Carlisle CE, Mamdani M, Schachar R, To T. Aftercare, emergency department visits, and readmission in adolescents. *J Am Acad Child Adolesc Psychiatry* 2012;51:283–293.

63. Yen S, Fuller AK, Solomon J, Spirito A. Follow-up treatment utilization by hospitalized suicidal adolescents. *J Psychiatr Pract* 2014;20:353–362.

64. Singh SP. Transition of care from child to adult mental health services: the great divide. *Curr Opin Psychiatry* 2009;22:386–390.

65. Park S, Kim CY, Hong JP. Unnatural causes of death and suicide among former adolescent psychiatric patients. *J Adolesc Health* 2013;52:207–211.

34

Acute inpatient care in older adults

Brian Murray

Introduction

In the UK, specialist older adult mental health community teams provide care for the full range of mental health conditions affecting older adults, not just the 6.5% of the population over the age of 65 with dementia (1). Major depression, for instance, affects 8.5% of older adults (2) and depressive symptoms can affect up to 37% of the older adult population in acute care settings (3). Older adult inpatient units have been developed to help community services manage the particular needs of older adults, whose mental health problems play out against a psychosocial backdrop of retirement, loss of role, family relationships, and end of life concerns. In addition, the physiology of ageing requires a different approach to prescribing and a familiarity with the physical health problems that can affect older adults.

There is also a political element in that several reports point to historic underfunding and poor care for older adults with mental health problems (4), which the development of specialist services was designed to address. In fact, Hilton points out that the creation of the subspecialty was in no small measure an inpatient phenomenon; a reaction to the practice in the 1950s of consigning older adults with mental health problems to 'back wards' where active therapy was rarely a goal (5).

Despite international approval for the specialist community model for older adult mental health (6), and some evidence that it provides better care for older adults than generic mental health services (7), the preferred model for inpatient older adult mental health is less clear. Internationally, provision of inpatient services for older adults is a mixture of specialist older adult mental health wards, general mental health wards, community residential placements, and consultation-liaison services within 'general' acute hospitals. Each has its advantages and disadvantages. The 2004 World Health Organization report found that specialist older adult mental health units had better outcomes for older adults than general adult mental health services, joint wards, and liaison into acute medical/older adult wards. However, the report issues an important caveat that evidence is poor and head-to-head studies are lacking (6). Since then, integrated units have become popular: mental health wards in public hospitals in the US tend to have much greater emphasis on physical care with a range of wards designed to provide care depending on the balance of mental health needs versus physical

care needs (8). In the UK, similar integrated units are often hailed as centres of excellence, although it is unclear if the earlier discharge these units promise sufficiently compensates for the increased running costs (9, 10).

The Royal College of Psychiatrists' Faculty of the Psychiatry of Old Age comes down firmly in favour of specialist older adult mental health wards (11) and, given that this is still the predominant model in the UK, this chapter will focus on this model unless stated otherwise.

Who is an older adult?

In older adults' mental health services in the UK, people have traditionally transitioned from general adults of working age to older adult mental health services at the age of 65, according to need. However, across Europe, people are living longer and healthier lives, so retirement ages, and with them our traditional concept of the beginning of old age, are increasing.

Therefore, in many health care settings, a transition based largely or entirely on age is being abandoned and may be considered illegal if it can be proved that by enforcing transition the patient is being denied services. Although a minority of mental health trusts have adopted an 'ageless' model (12), the Royal College of Psychiatrists remains in favour of an (increased) age of transition, taking needs such as cognitive impairment and frailty into account (13).

National provision and resourcing for acute wards for older adult mental health

The Royal College's Faculty of the Psychiatry of Old Age report presents advice to commissioners and providers of inpatient mental health services for older adults (11). The authors argue that mixing older and younger patients on wards is a retrograde step and that wards dedicated to older adults are important to provide specialist expertise. The report advises close liaison with relevant community teams, although points out that specialist admission avoidance teams ('crisis teams') tend to be run by and for adults of working age with limited access for older adults in some areas. This may be no bad thing, as there is mixed evidence for the effectiveness of such

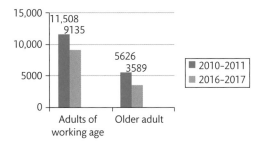

Figure 34.1 Average number of beds per mental health specialty: older adult beds have reduced by 36.2% versus 20.6% for adults of working age.
Source data from: Department of Health form KH03 24 May 2012 and 18 August 2016.

teams (14, 15), added to which the plethora of specialist teams for adults of working age risks patients being passed around or denied services at the whim of service boundaries rather than patient need. It is arguably to the advantage of older adult psychiatry that its main resource comprises relatively small, cohesive, multidisciplinary, and multifunctional teams with clear access pathways for primary care physicians and patients.

Overall bed numbers for mental health have reduced since the 1950s in the UK and in most countries. Although initially this was from a laudable desire to close asylums, in recent years this has become a cost-saving exercise (14). Unfortunately there is evidence that cost-saving has disproportionately affected services for older adults. Figure 34.1 shows that while both age groups have suffered large reductions in bed availability, older adults have suffered the most in recent years, meaning some of society's most vulnerable adults having to travel to distant locations, far from family support. Some of the reduction can be explained by loss of respite and continuing health care beds which have in recent years moved from the National Health Service into the private sector, but the impact of these changes is not negligible as it robs older adult services of flexibility when coping with demand for beds. This can add to the length of stay for patients with complex needs. Given the projected increase in the older adult population, the disproportionate reduction in older adult beds is hard to justify.

There is no objective guide to how many beds per population there should be and usage can be affected as much by availability of resources as background demand (16). Traditionally, adult mental health bed provision is calculated taking social deprivation into account whereas older mental health is not, but the rationale and evidence for this discrepancy is poor (17).

There is evidence that ward closure is offset to some extent by a corresponding increase in community support (14, 18). If done properly it can be highly appropriate to keep older adults at home for intensive or 'step-up' care. Background data collection for the Crisp report on acute adult psychiatric care also concluded that, given large variations in bed usage, better use of beds may still be possible (19), although the report cautions that the numbers of patients who may be inappropriately occupying inpatient beds may be offset by those inappropriately kept in the community by the current strictures.

In the UK, there is national guidance to maintain separate wards for patients of each sex in order to maintain patient dignity. Although this is aimed at all ages, it can be particularly important to patients from older generations. Where this is not practical, separate living space should be provided (e.g. separate corridors within a ward).

The Royal College report (11) also recommends separate functional and dementia wards for older adults but recognizes restricted resources mean this may not always be possible. When this occurs, the report recommends that within one ward there should be separate provision for the two diagnostic groups.

These requirements, to keep patients separate according to sex and diagnosis, would require each commissioning area to fund a minimum of four wards for older adults; however, we have already seen that, if anything, older adults have borne the brunt of bed closures in recent years. This creates a tension in ward planning and inventive use of ward space is required.

To illustrate the range of admissions a typical older adult mental health ward may have, Figure 34.2 shows the 103 admissions in the financial year from 2015–2016 on the author's mixed diagnosis 20-bed unit, broken down according to diagnosis (figures exclude occasional patients boarding from other services). Only the primary diagnosis is given, so the graph does not give a flavour of the frequent

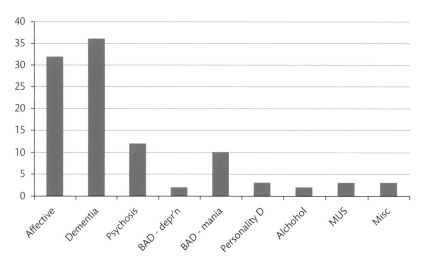

Figure 34.2 Numbers of inpatients for each primary diagnosis from April 2015 to the end of March 2016. MUS = medically unexplained symptoms.

overlap of diagnoses. Although dementia is the most frequent single diagnosis, it by no means predominates.

This is a small local audit but the distribution of diagnoses is in keeping with Tucker et al. (15). Further analysis (not shown here) showed a preponderance of male patients in the dementia category and a preponderance of female patients in the affective disorder category, which may be relevant in planning single-sex accommodation for older adults. Female admissions were more common, in keeping with previous studies of an older people's mental health inpatient population (15, 20).

Staffing

The Royal College of Psychiatrists runs accreditation schemes for mental health services, with specific standards for older adult inpatient services (Accreditation for Inpatient Mental Health Services for Older People (AIMS-OP), now renamed the Quality Network for Older Adult Mental Health Services (QNOAMHS)). Data provided by AIMS-OP shows older adult wards ranging in bed numbers from 9 to 30. For comparison, the Royal College recommends 18 beds for general psychiatric wards (21). AIMS-OP data shows an average of 1.04 whole-time equivalent consultant psychiatrists to each ward (Figure 34.3).

Consultant

Good consultant input is needed to provide clinical leadership, to handle the increasing bureaucracy of mental health legislation and clinical governance inspections, as well as to promote appropriate early discharge of patients. In order to achieve this, many wards now have a single 'ward consultant' post rather than multiple consultant ward rounds.

Any trainee can learn much on an older adult ward besides the management of specific conditions, namely communication skills, mental capacity assessment, and the management of long-term conditions. To support trainees the consultant needs space in his or her timetable to provide regular weekly supervision. Even a whole-time consultant cannot manage all this on his or her own: the assistance

of a good specialty doctor is recommended to support and provide cover for any consultant absence.

Nurses

Despite high rates of physical comorbidity on their wards, the basic training of older adult inpatient nurses is the same as other psychiatric nurses. The knowledge gap has to be filled with local training or by employing registered general nurses. In addition, Chaplin et al. found that nurses on older adult wards experience some of the highest staff assault rates in psychiatry (22). In this research, nurses on both mixed-diagnosis and dementia wards reported higher levels of aggression compared with their colleagues on general adult psychiatric wards. Patients reported less aggression, suggesting that the aggression was occurring when nurses were administering personal care, a role that is much less prevalent on wards for adults of working age. Employers need to work hard to make inpatient older adult nursing posts attractive given that there is already some evidence nurses find community posts more appealing (18).

Psychology

Traditionally, psychology input has been reserved for patients in the community as inpatients were assumed to be too unwell to engage with psychological therapy. However, this assumption is being challenged: the Royal College of Psychiatrists' AIMS scheme and the National Institute for Health and Care Excellence (NICE) (23) recommend psychology input to inpatient units.

On an older adult ward, specialist older adult psychology input is important: access to a neuropsychology opinion can be helpful in clarifying a diagnosis of an organic disorder; psychologists can also provide advice on the day-to-day management of someone presenting with behaviours that challenge (usually, but not exclusively, in the context of a diagnosis of dementia); finally, psychologists can provide systemic or other family-oriented psychological interventions for family and carers. This is only the direct patient-facing work: an important function of any inpatient psychologist is to support, supervise, and train all staff to be more psychologically aware. Kerfoot and colleagues, in a service evaluation from a generic psychiatric ward, showed that psychology input can reduce length of stay and reduce readmission rates (24).

Occupational therapy

Input from the occupational therapist (OT) is also important in providing crucial therapeutic activity on any ward. In addition, the OT has a specific role with older adults, for whom memory problems, physical comorbidity, and frailty may make activities of daily living difficult. Older adults' self-care can decline in a ward setting, compounded by longer lengths of stay. It is therefore important to have good OT input with a good assessment space (e.g. an OT kitchen) to assess the patient's ability to manage at home. The results of these assessments, plus OT advice on physical adaptations, can be crucial in discharge planning. In ward rounds, OTs provide invaluable feedback on patients' progress by interacting, rather than simply observing, them.

Other members of the multidisciplinary team

Although there is unlikely to be a need for a full-time ward-based physiotherapist, speech and language therapist, pharmacist, or

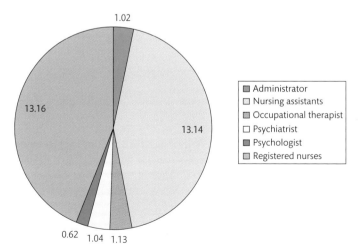

Figure 34.3 Mean whole-time equivalent staffing levels across 17 older people's mental health wards.
Reproduced with permission of the Royal College of Psychiatrists, AIMS-OP. © 2016

dietician, an older adult mental health ward should have ready access to their expertise. As with psychology input, it is preferable to provide specialist input from staff experienced with older adults.

Many older adults can spend days or even weeks in bed as a result of their mental illness. Although there is a lack of research specific to older adult mental health, extrapolating from the wealth of data supporting early mobilization in general medical settings, physiotherapy could assist discharge planning. Physiotherapy in this age group requires expertise, time, and patience: visiting a patient with cognitive impairment and leaving a set of instructions for exercises will have little impact on the patient's progress. The risk of falls (see 'Frailty, falls, and physical healthcare') can require a joint approach from physiotherapist and OT.

Access to speech and language therapy (SALT) is vital. Comorbidity can present with swallowing problems in the elderly: diseases such as Parkinson's disease as well as increased rates of oesophageal disease can cause problems with swallowing which can affect diet and predispose to aspiration pneumonias.

Pharmacokinetic changes with age mean that prescribing has to be undertaken with caution. Junior doctors may not be aware of the need to adjust dosing for older adults, or the increased risks of falls, sedation, or confusion. The rule when prescribing for older adults should be 'start low, go slow'. All prescribing on the ward should be kept under regular supervision from a trained pharmacist.

A social worker can be important on the ward to expedite discharge and to liaise with families and carers on aspects of social care. The social worker may be in a community mental health team and inreach to the ward or be on the ward and outreach to the community mental health team. Each model has its advantages but a good ward social worker familiar with the needs of the patient and the benefits of early discharge tends to be more effective from the ward's point of view.

Weight loss on an older adult mental health ward can be a significant issue. Nutrition therefore should be everyone's concern. 'Build-up' drinks are one solution but can be expensive and there is a strong case for routinely fortifying food on the ward: for the majority of older adults, there is no such thing as a bad calorie. For other patients with conditions such as diabetes, refeeding and other absorption syndromes, and swallowing difficulties, specialist advice is necessary.

Access to older adult medicine

Even in those wards which are not integrated with physical healthcare, the presence of physical comorbidity necessitates good access to care of the elderly medicine (geriatrics). At present, in the UK, large amounts of money are spent on psychiatric liaison services for acute hospitals, but the relatively small number of older adult mental health beds means that little thought goes into commissioning services in the other direction. The best scenario is usually when an older people's mental health ward happens to be located within an acute hospital, where custom and practice, rather than commissioning, result in an exchange of expertise between older adult specialties. Even where services are not on the same site, it is helpful to keep good relations with colleagues in older adult medicine. The ideal situation would be a commissioned arrangement in which one or two sessions a week of specialist geriatric time is brought in to help manage the physical comorbidity on the wards.

Ward environment and design

Design is important on any ward. Older adult wards and younger adult wards have the same challenge of striking a balance between providing a therapeutic environment and minimizing risk. Some of these tensions are shared, such as preventing inappropriate access or egress, however, while on younger adult wards design focuses on reducing ligature points, infection control, and violence, on an older adult ward other factors such as falls and physical frailty have to be taken into account as well.

It is hard to achieve randomized controlled trial levels of evidence in ward design as creating a proper 'control' would be formidably expensive, yet there has been much good work on design in dementia, the principles of which are summarized as follows:

1. The environment promotes meaningful interaction between patients, their families and staff.
2. The environment promotes well-being.
3. The environment encourages eating and drinking.
4. The environment promotes mobility.
5. The environment promotes continence and personal hygiene.
6. The environment promotes orientation.
7. The environment promotes calm, safety, and security.

The headings in the list have been taken from the 'Enhance the Healing Environment' audit tools provided by The King's Fund (25).

In order to achieve these goals, the ward should have a clear layout, including a reception area, areas for socializing, communal eating, and outdoor space. There should be cues for those with cognitive impairment, including age-appropriate signage, visible calendars, and easy-to-read (ideally analogue) clocks. There should be natural (or failing this, biodynamic) lighting, designed to reduce glare. Intrusive noise should be avoided. Continence should be promoted though personal toilets, easy-to-use appliances, and sanitary ware that is familiar to this population. Towels may be preferred to hand dryers. Good nutrition is aided by communal eating areas with plenty of space, constant access to fluids, access to snacks and finger food, and crockery designed with contrasting colours. All access (external and internal) needs to take poor mobility and other disability into account. Mobility can be further promoted by having the ward on a single level with high chairs and rails.

Although these design recommendations have been made with dementia in mind, they are invariably applicable to any older adult ward and would do no harm in even a younger adult setting (whereas the reverse is rarely true).

Common traps or misconceptions to avoid in designing older adult wards include the following:

1. *Not balancing all risks.* Ward design focusing on ligature control can result in door handles that are difficult to open for patients with arthritis, or sanitary appliances that older adults may struggle to use. Infection control can mean no carpets but this can be dangerous for patients at risk of falls. Fortunately flooring solutions are available.
2. *Avoiding the familiar.* Using a picture of, for example, a toilet on the toilet door may seem like a good idea, but in fact, people with memory problems will be more familiar with stick men and

women. Well-known but abstract signs may be better recognized than pictures of the object in question.

3. *Assumptions about the age range of the patient group.* Many patients on an older adult ward nowadays would have grown up in the years of the 1950s and 1960s, yet art and decorations in care homes and wards often reflect the taste of generations from the 1920s, 1930s, and 1940s.

4. *Colour scheme clichés.* While contrasting colours are often recommended, there is no one colour proven to work best for people with cognitive impairment or visual impairment. A myth has arisen that patients with dementia 'need' red toilet seats! This is not true, but it is worth experimenting with contrasting colours.

Some thought may need to go into what you may *not* want to draw attention to on the ward. It is recommended that staff areas are made less obtrusive by use of, for example, colour-neutral paint to avoid confusing patients. Although research evidence is mixed, there is a strong suggestion that doors with windows opening straight outside can act as a magnet for the disorientated patient.

Frailty, falls, and physical healthcare

A ward dedicated to the care of any group of older adults must provide appropriate care for their physical health needs. This includes a clinic room, used only for physical healthcare, with appropriate equipment for making observations (both electronic and manual), phlebotomy, and taking electrocardiogram readings. These tasks can fall to junior doctors, but it is preferable that there are staff such as physicians' assistants dedicated to the physical care of inpatients, or that the tasks are shared with nursing staff so that all staff groups manage a balance of providing physical and mental health care.

Frailty

Frailty is a complex condition which predicts susceptibility to minor illness, poor recovery from disease, and increases the individual's mortality. It is associated with age but can vary over time in an individual. In short, it does not fit into a traditional 'categorical diagnosis' view of illness. Frailty is conceptualized in at least two competing models. In the '*phenotype*' model, frailty is defined as a clinical syndrome based on the presence of specific physiological anomalies. Fried and colleagues define frailty as a condition in which three or more of the following criteria were present: unintentional weight loss, self-reported exhaustion, weakness (as measured by grip strength), slow walking speed, and low physical activity (26). Rockwood's alternative '*deficit*' model sees frailty as an accumulation of deficits (27).

Not all older adults are 'frail': frailty is a specific condition which only affects a proportion of older adults, although the lack of a universal model for frailty results in large variations in estimates of its prevalence, from 4.9% to 27.3% in the general population. Even when acute and chronic disease is excluded, frailty affects an average of 7% of the population over the age of 65 years (28).

There are a number of assessment tools that can be used to detect frailty (29). Scales that follow the phenotype model tend to be simpler (it has even been argued that a single measure such as grip strength could be used as a proxy for frailty), whereas the deficit model tends to lead to more complex evaluation. Of note to the psychiatrist, depression, cognitive impairment, and social support are all recognized as independent markers of frailty and usually included in both types of scale.

As frailty is on a dynamic spectrum, none of these scales is 'diagnostic', nor is there a silver bullet to manage frailty. The gold standard for managing frailty is the Comprehensive Geriatric Assessment, defined as 'a multidimensional, interdisciplinary diagnostic process to determine the medical, psychological and functional capabilities of a frail elderly person in order to develop a coordinated and integrated plan for treatment and long-term follow-up' and has been shown to improve outcomes for patients when conducted by a multidisciplinary team in a specialist older adult medical care unit (30). However the initial assessment alone can take at least 1.5 hours (29). This may limit its applicability to older adult mental health wards but, at its simplest, managing frailty can mean paying attention to issues long known to be associated with the ageing population: sensory deficit, functional ability, polypharmacy, mobility, and nutrition. All of these are common problems for patients on an older adult mental health ward and all map onto the ideal multidisciplinary team described earlier in this chapter under 'Staffing'. An awareness of frailty can also assist care planning, liaison with physical medical colleagues, and support the planning of staffing and ward design.

Falls

According to the National Patient Safety Agency (NPSA), older adult mental health inpatient units have the dubious distinction of being the clinical areas with the highest numbers of falls, with falls per 1000 bed days of 13.1–25 quoted from the international literature compared with the NPSA's calculated average of 2.8 per 1000 bed days across psychiatry generally (31). However, by its own admission, some of the data quoted by the NPSA have to be treated with some caution. An American study quoted showed 45 falls on a 28-bed unit in 6 months, which approximates to 8.8 falls per 1000 bed days (32).

Whatever the precise figures, there seems little doubt that patients with old age, depression, or dementia are at increased risk of falls and furthermore, are at increased risk of injury following fall, possibly as a result of poor reflexes (31).

NICE found that the following were most predictive of falls in an extended care setting: previous history of falls, gait deficit, balance deficit, visual impairment, and cognitive impairment. NICE recommends a multifactorial risk assessment tool while acknowledging that the evidence for these tools in an inpatient setting is of poor quality (33).

NICE found insufficient evidence to support the prevention of falls using low-intensity or group exercise, vitamin D replacement, cognitive behavioural therapy, or correction of sensory impairment. Furthermore, the evidence that hip protectors prevent injury after a fall is weak (and they are frequently unpopular with patients). A Cochrane review found little evidence that low-height beds and bed exit alarms made a difference in reducing falls in (generic) inpatient settings (34). However, NICE recommends medication review, exercise, psychoeducation, and correction of sensory impairment as part of a multifactorial care package.

A systematic review found no research of interventions for falls reduction among older adult mental health inpatients but did find some (albeit inconsistent) evidence that interventions in a group of cognitively impaired older adults could be effective (35). Again the evidence pointed towards multifactorial rather than single approaches.

There is often a focus on psychotropic medication as a cause of an increased risk of falls but risks have to be balanced: in depression and dementia, the underlying condition itself has a higher than average risk of falls (consider the risks posed to the patient—and others—by agitation or wandering at night), making it difficult to separate out the cause. Although the risk of falls is by no means confined to psychotropic medication, it is a major modifiable risk factor and psychiatrists are encouraged to constantly review patient medication using resources such as the Fallsafe project (36), or the AntiCholinergic Burden scale (37). Others, such as STOPP/START (38) merit geriatrician input.

The ideal admission

To ensure an admission is appropriate, it should be vetted by a senior clinical lead, ideally a consultant psychiatrist, in the community before admission is agreed with senior nurses or medical staff on the ward. Good communication is key: as a minimum, the ward needs to be clear on what the clinical issues are, who is asking for/authorizing the admission, and what clinical question the admission is designed to answer. An early meeting with the family or carers can also clarify the latter question and can avoid any misunderstandings and delays when the ward looks to discharge. It is often necessary to explain to families that the patient is on an acute ward and that this is not a long-term placement. It is also important to establish if there are any lasting powers of attorney, advance directives, or do-not-resuscitate orders.

Perhaps 20 years ago an older adult with dementia may have been admitted to an older adult unit for 'assessment' before moving to a care home. Patients gained nothing from these admissions other than the disruption of an unnecessary move. Nowadays, patients with dementia are kept at home for as long as possible and if necessary moved directly to care homes wherever possible. Respite (also known as replacement care) to reduce carer burden is now also usually provided in care homes although other settings exist.

Ideally, there should be a 72-hour period of assessment with minimal change in medication but this may not always be possible. A good physical health screen should be conducted at the first opportunity and certainly within 24 hours. Detecting delirium is not just important in dementia: a hypoactive delirium may mimic depression.

Many older adults stop eating and drinking when depressed, which, given an often lower body mass index and the physiology of ageing, puts them at risk. The combination of risk and treatment-resistant depression common in older adults (39) can mean a greater use of electroconvulsive therapy: the Royal College of Psychiatrists electroconvulsive therapy accreditation scheme found the mean average of use of electroconvulsive therapy was 61 years, and 65 for maintenance treatment (40).

Nurses should be encouraged to document an ABC chart (Antecedents—Behaviours–Consequences) to give clues to causes or precipitants of behavioural disturbance. This is an area where good psychology input can be helpful. OT can advise on activity management. It is important to screen patients for cognitive symptoms before they return home as depression and psychosis may be precursors for more significant memory disorders (39).

Good care planning necessitates a discharge planning meeting with family and the community team. While patients with functional mental illness may 'build up' leave in order to improve function before returning home, it can add to confusion for patients with dementia who may do better with a clear discharge date coordinated with local social services, community teams, and family. A short length of stay is desirable (20) and does not necessarily lead to higher rates of readmission (41).

As bed acuity has reduced, a greater proportion of patients are admitted under mental health legislation; even if they settle on the ward, patients with cognitive impairment may not be able to give meaningful consent and therefore legislation based on mental capacity may have to be used (Deprivation of Liberty Safeguarding authorization or DOLS). One advantage is that care homes are familiar with DOLS legislation and should be happy to accept patients requiring DOLS authorization.

REFERENCES

1. Matthews F, Arthur A, Barnes L, et al. A two decade comparison of prevalence of dementia in individuals aged 65 years and older from three geographical areas of England: results of the Cognitive Function and Ageing Study I and II. *Lancet* 2013;382:1405–1412.
2. McDougall F, Kvaal K, Matthews F, et al. Prevalence of depression in older people in England and Wales: the MRC CFA Study. *Psychol Med* 2007;37:1787–1795.
3. Taylor W. Depression in the elderly. *N Engl J Med* 2014;371:1228–1236.
4. Saad K, Bangash K. Ageless mental health services and the future of old age psychiatry in the UK. *J Geriatr Care Res* 2016;3:21–23.
5. Hilton C. Age inclusive services or separate old age and working age services? A historical analysis from the formative years of old age psychiatry c.1940—1989. *Br J Psychiatry Bull* 2015;39:90–95
6. Draper B, Low L. *What is the Effectiveness of Old-Age Mental Health Services?* Health Evidence Network Report. Copenhagen: WHO Regional Office for Europe; 2004. http://www.euro.who.int/document/E83685.pdf
7. Abdul-Hamid W, Lewis-Cole K, Holloway F, Silverman A. Comparison of how old age psychiatry and general adult psychiatry services meet the needs of elderly people with functional mental illness: cross-sectional survey. *Br J Psychiatry* 2015;207:440–443.
8. Lapid M, Rummans T. The medical psychiatry in patient unit. In: Abou-Saleh M, Katona C, Kumar A (eds), *Principles and Practice of Geriatric Psychiatry*, 3rd edition, pp. 785–789. Chichester: Wiley; 2011.
9. McCormack H. Integration of care and its impact on older people's mental health. Faculty report FR/OA/05. Faculty of the Psychiatry of Old Age of the Royal College of Psychiatrists; 2016. https://www.rcpsych.ac.uk/pdf/FR%20OA%2005_final.pdf
10. George J, Adamson J, Woodford H. Joint geriatric and psychiatric wards: a review of the literature. *Age Ageing* 2011;40:543–548.
11. Pinner G, Hillam J, Branton T, Ramakrishnan A. In-patient care for older people within mental health services. Faculty report FR/OA/1. Faculty of the Psychiatry of Old Age of the Royal College of Psychiatrists; 2011. https://www.rcpsych.ac.uk/pdf/FR_OA_1_forweb.pdf

12. Warner J, Old age psychiatry in the modern age. *Br J Psychiatry* 2015;207;375–376.

13. Faculty of the Psychiatry of Old Age of the Royal College of Psychiatrists. Criteria for old age psychiatry services in the UK. Faculty report FR/OA/4. 2015. https://www.rcpsych.ac.uk/pdf/FR%20OA%2004%20final.pdf

14. Crisp N. Improving acute inpatient psychiatric care for adults in England: interim report. The commission to review the provision of acute inpatient psychiatric care for adults. 2015. https://www.rcpsych.ac.uk/pdf/0e662e_a93c62b2ba4449f48695ed36b3cb24ab.pdf

15. Tucker S, Brand C, Wilberforce M, Abendstern M, Challis D. Identifying alternatives to old age psychiatry inpatient admission: an application of the balance of care approach to health and social care planning. *BMC Health Serv Res* 2015;15:267.

16. Imison C, Poteliakhoff E, Thompson J. *Older People and Emergency Bed Use: Exploring Variation*. London: The King's Fund; 2012.

17. Lund C, Stansfield S, De Silva M. Social determinants of mental health. In: Patel V, Minas H, Cohen A, Prince M (eds), *Global Mental Health: Principles and Practice*, pp. 116–136. New York; Oxford University Press; 2014.

18. Centre for Workforce Intelligence. In-depth review of the psychiatrist workforce. 2014. https://assets.publishing.service.gov.uk/government/uploads/system/uploads/attachment_data/file/507557/CfWI_Psychiatrist_in-depth_review.pdf

19. The Commission on Acute Adult Psychiatric Care. The Commission to Review the Provision of Acute Inpatient Psychiatric Care for Adults in England, Wales and Northern Ireland. Background briefing paper. 2015. http://media.wix.com/ugd/0e662e_5870bdbe49e4414cbf489252649eb10b.pdf

20. Bradshaw S, Purandare N. Inpatient services for older people with mental illness. *Ment Health Rev J* 2001;2:18–21.

21. Royal College of Psychiatrists. *Do the Right Thing: How to Judge a Good Ward; Ten Standards for Adult In-Patient Mental Healthcare*. Occasional Paper 79. London: Royal College of Psychiatrists; 2011.

22. Chaplin R, McGeorge M, Hinchcliffe G, Shinkwin L. Aggression on psychiatric inpatient units for older adults and adults of working age. *Int J Geriatr Psychiatry* 2008;23:874–876.

23. National Institute for Health and Care Excellence. Psychosis and schizophrenia in adults: prevention and management. Clinical guideline [CG 178]. 2014. https://www.nice.org.uk/guidance/cg178

24. Kerfoot G, Bamford Z, Jones S. Evaluation of psychological provision into an acute inpatient unit. *Ment Health Rev J* 2012;17:26–38.

25. The King's Fund. Enhance the Healing Environment: developing supportive design for people with dementia. http://www.kingsfund.org.uk/projects/enhancing-healing-environment/ehe-design-dementia

26. Fried L, Tangen C, Walston J, et al. Frailty in older adults: evidence for a phenotype. *J Gerontol* 2001;56A:146–156.

27. Rockwood K, Mitnitski A. How might deficit accumulation give rise to frailty? *J Frailty Aging* 2012;1:8–12.

28. Cha H. IAGG mission for frailty of older persons. In: Vellas B (ed), *The White Book on Frailty*, p. 3. New York: International Association of Gerontology and Geriatrics; 2016.

29. British Geriatrics Society. *Fit for Frailty: Consensus Best Practice Guidance for the Care of Older People Living with Frailty in Community and Outpatient Settings*. London: British Geriatrics Society; 2014

30. Ellis G, Whitehead M, O'Neill D, Langhorne P, Robinson D. Comprehensive geriatric assessment for older adults admitted to hospital. *Cochrane Database Syst Rev* 2011;7:CD006211.

31. National Patient Safety Association. *Slips, Trips and Falls in Hospital: The Third Report from the Patient Safety Observatory*. London: National Patient Safety Association; 2007.

32. Blair E, Gruman C. Falls in an inpatient geriatric psychiatric population. *J Am Psychiatr Nurses Assoc* 2006;11:351–354.

33. National Institute for Health and Care Excellence. Assessment and prevention of falls in older people. Clinical guideline [CG161]. 2013. https://www.nice.org.uk/guidance/cg161

34. Anderson O, Boshier PR, Hanna GB. Interventions designed to prevent healthcare bed-related injuries in patients. *Cochrane Database Syst Rev* 2012;1:CD008931.

35. Bunn F, Dickinson A, Simpson C, et al. Preventing falls among older people with mental health problems: a systematic review. *BMC Nurs* 2014;13:4.

36. Darowski A, Dwight J, Reynolds J. Medicines and falls in hospital: guidance sheet. Royal College of Physicians; 2011. https://www.rcplondon.ac.uk/guidelines-policy/fallsafe-resources-original

37. Fox C, Richardson K, Maidment I, et al. Anticholinergic medication use and cognitive impairment in the older population: the medical research council cognitive function and ageing study. *J Am Geriatr Soc* 2011;59:1477–1483.

38. O'Mahoney D, O'Sullivan, Byrne S, O'Connor M, Ryan C, Gallagher P. STOPP/START criteria for potentially in appropriate prescribing in older people: version 2. *Age Ageing* 2015;44:213–218.

39. Rodda J, Walker Z, Carter J. Depression in older adults. *BMJ* 2011;343:d5219.

40. Royal College of Physicians. ECTAS 5th National Report October 2011–October 2013. London: Royal College of Physicians; 2014. http://www.rcpsych.ac.uk/pdf/ECTAS%205th%20National%20Report.pdf

41. Babalola O, Gormez V, Alwan NA, Johnstone P, Sampson S. Length of hospitalisation for people with severe mental illness. *Cochrane Database Syst Rev* 2014;1:CD000384.

35

Psychiatric intensive care

Ashley Rule

Introduction

Sometimes a patient's presentation is such that they cannot be safely managed on an acute ward. This is usually because they are highly agitated and aggressive towards others. In order to manage such patients, the specialty of psychiatric intensive care was developed, and along with it, specialized psychiatric intensive care units (PICUs) were built. Psychiatric intensive care has been defined as a specialty within mental health inpatient services which specifically addresses acute need, for patients experiencing an acute mental disorder who require more rapid assessment and stabilization through active engagement and treatment (1).

PICUs are usually set up as small units, with more staff than acute (or 'open') wards and fewer patients (typically 14 or fewer (2)), and hence a correspondingly greater staff/patient ratio. They are usually designed to provide a safer physical environment than acute wards, with less access to potentially dangerous items (both in terms of the items that a patient may have in their possession and with regard to the physical environment), and with enhanced physical security (e.g. higher fences and air lock systems at entry points).

Patients are also occasionally admitted to a PICU to manage challenging behaviours other than violence to others, such as severe self-harming that requires intensive physical intervention by staff over a prolonged period, or in order to reduce the risk of absconding.

PICU staff will be trained in the management of challenging behaviour, particularly the management of violence and aggression, and may be more highly skilled and experienced in the use of interventions such as physical restraint, or the use of rapid tranquilization.

The ideal of PICU care is to provide a safe, 'low-stimulus' environment in which patients can be given intensive treatment for a short period of time until the harmful behaviours associated with their illness have lessened, and they can be cared for on an acute ward once again.

There is a significant overlap in terms of practice and physical environment between PICUs and the low and medium secure wards that are part of forensics services, but unlike on those wards, patients admitted to a PICU should expect to be there for a relatively brief period of time (a few days or weeks). In most cases, patients on a PICU will not have committed offences or be involved with the criminal justice system.

History of the psychiatric intensive care unit in the UK

Mentally unwell patients have been cared for in purpose-built establishments in the UK for several centuries (3)—the origins of the Bethlem hospital for the disturbed mentally ill go back at least 750 years. However, it was only in the twentieth century that patients were able to be admitted to such institutions on a voluntary basis. Indeed, it is only since the 1960s that most psychiatric wards have no longer been 'locked'.

In the 1970s, there was a trend towards establishing psychiatric wards within district general hospitals, but it soon became apparent that some patients with particularly disturbed behaviour were unable to be safely cared for in such settings. At the time, there was little option for such patients other than to be moved to establishments designed for the management of mentally disordered offenders, such as the 'special hospitals' (Broadmoor, Rampton, and Ashworth in England, and Carstairs in Scotland), or to be cared for in prisons. Even the establishment of Regional Secure Units (RSUs) in the 1970s after the publication of the Butler Report (4) in 1975 did not significantly improve the situation for these patients. The RSUs were built to provide secure wards for mentally disordered offenders who did not require the high security of the special hospitals, and even though they could in theory accept any patient who was sufficiently disturbed in behaviour, their focus was on offenders, and they were not linked with local mental health services in terms of their geographical location or funding.

As a result, the concept of the PICU emerged. The first psychiatric 'intensive care unit' (5) was described in New York in 1973, and it was designed to be a locked ward for the management of patients who could not be adequately managed in an open ward. Many of the patients who were treated there required a more secure environment in order to manage their risk of absconding, but within a few years, similar units were in operation across the world, including in the UK, and they were admitting patients whose main reason for being unmanageable in an open ward environment was violence.

Over the following two decades in the UK, psychiatric units specifically designed for the management of acutely unwell patients with challenging behaviours became more prevalent. Initially there were no universally accepted standards or practices for such units, and they often functioned in isolation from the main psychiatric wards and from other similar wards. As a result, the National Association of Psychiatric Intensive Care and Low Secure Units (NAPICU) was formed in 1996 with the aims of providing an identity for the developing field of PICU psychiatry in its own right, and of promoting evidence-based best practice with a multidisciplinary perspective.

The psychiatric intensive care unit model

According to the recently published 'Guidance for Commissioners of Psychiatric Intensive Care Units' (1), the primary function of a PICU is the rapid assessment and intensive management of acute mental disorder and behavioural disturbance. Patients admitted to a PICU will display a level of risk to themselves or others that cannot be safely managed in a non-PICU setting, and the treatment provided in a PICU will have a direct impact on reducing short- and medium-term clinical risk.

PICUs should be available for newly admitted patients and patients already being treated within inpatient services, who require rapid assessment, intensive treatment, and stabilization. The length of stay should be kept to a minimum, not normally exceeding 6–8 weeks.

In summary, PICUs should provide rapid, intensive interventions for acutely disturbed patients in a safe environment for a relatively short period of time, such that the patient can then complete their treatment on an open ward once the temporary stage of increased risk associated with the most acute period of their illness resolves.

In order to ensure that a PICU can fulfil this role effectively, there must be mechanisms in place to allow the unit to focus on treating the most acutely unwell patients who are likely to respond to a relatively brief intervention. Otherwise, a PICU with a small number of beds could very quickly be clogged up with its beds filled by patients who are no longer in the acute phase of their illness but who are unable to progress back to an open ward. This leaves the PICU unable to respond appropriately to the needs of the wider psychiatric population when future patients become unmanageable in a non-PICU setting.

For this reason, most units have inclusion and exclusion criteria with regard to patient suitability. Reasons for being admitted to a PICU would typically include externally directed aggression, or internally directed aggression with a corresponding high risk of suicide or serious injury, or high risk of absconding. There should be an agreement with the referring service that appropriate treatment cannot be provided safely in a less restrictive environment, and also a clear rationale for PICU assessment and treatment, including agreement on the expected benefits to be gained from a time-limited intervention.

Most patients admitted to a PICU will have been compulsorily detained under appropriate legislation, as the patient's liberty will have been deprived significantly by being on a PICU, and they may require treatment interventions to prevent harm to themselves or others to which they will be unwilling or unable to give informed consent.

Exclusion criteria for a PICU may include a primary diagnosis of substance misuse, intoxication, or dependence; or behaviour that is a direct consequence of substance misuse; patients with a primary diagnosis of brain injury, dementia, or learning disability; patients with borderline personality disorder without a concurrent psychosis or major mood disorder; or patients with significant physical frailty. It is self-evident that such presentations would not be suitable for PICU intervention as they are either not suitable for compulsory inpatient treatment at all (as is usually the case for the treatment of problems related to substance misuse) or they are not likely to be remediable with a brief intervention, as would be the case for brain injury, dementia, or learning disability.

PICUs should also have a well-defined upper threshold for the level of risk that they can safely manage. Some patients, for example, those with a history of significant violence or harm to others by the use of weapons, may pose too high a risk to the other patients and staff on a PICU and may require management in a forensic setting.

PICUs should be appropriately designed and staffed for particular age groups, and it would not be appropriate for children, adults of working age, and older adults to be managed on the same unit, given their differing physical, emotional, and psychological resiliencies and requirements.

There is a limited evidence base for the effectiveness of PICUs and direct comparisons of PICU care and care on an 'open' ward (e.g. by way of a randomized controlled trial) would be difficult to conduct due to the need to maintain safety. However, there is evidence that, despite significantly higher rates of violence towards staff and other patients on PICUs (6), the quality of care provided on PICUs is similar to that of open wards (7).

National minimum standards for psychiatric intensive care units in England

In 2014, the NAPICU, in collaboration with the Royal College of Psychiatrists, the Royal College of Nursing, the College of Mental Health Pharmacy, and the College of Occupational Therapists, published a set of national minimum standards for PICUs in general adult services (2). This document was an updated version of a set of minimum standards first published in 2002.

The document sets out a list of several hundred measurable standards of good practice, organized into 20 broad categories such as referral criteria, physical environment, risk assessment, interventions offered, staffing levels, management structure, user and carer involvement, record-keeping, and staff training needs (Box 35.1).

Individual PICUs that can demonstrate that they are meeting these standards can apply for accreditation from the Royal College of Psychiatrists as part of the Accreditation for Inpatient Mental Health Services (AIMS) initiative.

Management of the acutely disturbed patient

As previously discussed, the purpose of a PICU in general adult services is primarily concerned with the management of acutely disturbed behaviour. By and large, this is achieved by ensuring a safe environment; providing caring and compassionate support from ward staff; and promptly providing appropriate treatment and therapy, be it of a pharmacological, physical (e.g. electroconvulsive therapy), or psychological nature. This should be provided in a setting that is comfortable, that allows patients to maintain their dignity (e.g.

> **Box 35.1** Summary of the national minimum standards for PICUs in England
>
> - Admission criteria.
> - Core interventions.
> - Multidisciplinary team service structure and personnel.
> - Operations and clinical leadership.
> - PICU care pathway.
> - Physical environment.
> - Patient involvement.
> - Carer involvement.
> - Documentation.
> - Ethnicity, culture, and gender.
> - Supervision.
> - Liaison with other agencies.
> - Policies and procedures.
> - Clinical audit and monitoring.
> - Staff training.
> - Continuing professional development.
> - Security and risk assessment.
> - PICU support infrastructure.
> - Other types of psychiatric intensive care.
> - Staffing levels.

by providing individual, en-suite bedrooms), that offers appropriate recreational and occupational activities, and is supported by policies and protocols that can be sufficiently flexible to allow for care to be centred around the individual needs and preferences of the patient. In many of these ways, the care provided on a PICU will be similar to that which should be provided in any psychiatric inpatients setting.

However, there may be management strategies used in a PICU setting that will be far less commonly used elsewhere, particularly with regard to managing acutely disturbed behaviour. These can broadly be grouped into the following areas: enhanced security; the use of *pro re nata* (PRN, 'as required') medication; the use of restrictive interventions including patient segregation, restraint, and rapid tranquilization.

Security

At first glance, the word security may conjure up ideas of keeping patients locked away where they can't do any harm, but security is really about providing a safe environment for patients, as well as staff and the general public. The Department of Health published a document in 2010 entitled 'See Think Act' (8) which was specifically concerned with security in mental health settings.

Security can be thought of as three interrelated aspects: physical security, procedural security, and relational security. The first two aspects are concerned with such things as fences, locks, alarms, and the policies and protocols of the ward. However, the less easily defined 'relational security' is key to the successful functioning of a PICU.

Relational security is defined in 'See Think Act' as 'the knowledge and understanding staff have of a patient and of the environment, and the translation of that information into appropriate responses and care' (8). Successful relational security will involve staff and patients having clear understandings of how a patient's mental state

and behaviour are influenced by factors such as the layout of the ward, the other patients on the ward, the daily timetable of the ward, the impact of visits from family or friends, specific features of the patient's illness, or the patient's underlying personality. It also involves the overt defining of boundaries of expected behaviour from both the patient and the staff.

In many cases, acutely disturbed behaviour can be managed with little more than working collaboratively with the patient to understand their specific problems, formulating a shared understanding of these, and devising an individualized care plan with the patient that identifies stressors and flashpoints, aims to avoid them where possible, and suggests feasible strategies that the patient can employ in the escalation phase of anger before it becomes aggression. It may seem obvious that different patients will benefit from different distractions and coping strategies, and yet many wards fall foul of policy-driven, 'one-size-fits-all' approaches to the management of acute behavioural disturbance that may cause more harm than good. A well-thought through, patient-centred care plan, based on the ideas that are encompassed in relational security, may be all that is required to successfully prevent disturbed behaviour[9].

Use of 'as required' medication

Alongside a patient's regular medication, patients will often be prescribed medication that can be used on an as required (PRN) basis (10). On a PICU, such PRN medication might include anxiolytic medication such as the short- to medium-acting benzodiazepines lorazepam, clonazepam, or diazepam; sedative antihistamines such as promethazine; or sedative antipsychotic drugs such as olanzapine, haloperidol, or zuclopenthixol. Such medication can be useful for patients who recognize that they are feeling anxious or agitated, as they can request these tablets themselves. This can be a very effective way of preventing escalation of aggressive behaviour, or managing difficult emotional states. The use of PRN medication can also be empowering for the patient, as it allows the patient to have some control over their use of medication, as part of a mutually agreed care plan.

Restrictive interventions

In a PICU setting, it is inevitable that there will be occasions when aggressive behaviour cannot be prevented solely by the use of high-quality relational security or PRN medication, and the management of such aggression during the acute phase of a mental illness is arguably the primary purpose of a PICU. In circumstances such as these, PICU staff will need to make use of interventions that are intended to reduce the impact and duration of the disturbed behaviour, and to ensure the safety of the patient, as well as the other patients and staff on the ward. The Mental Health Act 'Code of Practice' (11) defines such strategies as 'restrictive interventions', as they will inevitably restrict someone's movement or freedom in order to take control of a dangerous situation, and to reduce danger to the person concerned or to others.

Restrictive interventions that may be employed to manage disturbed behaviour on a PICU include enhanced nursing observations, the use of de-escalation and seclusion rooms, manual restraint, and chemical restraint. Enhanced nursing observations (i.e. having a member of staff check on a patient frequently or be with them constantly) are a form of restrictive intervention that may be standard practice on most psychiatric wards and not specific to a PICU. The other forms of restrictive intervention, however, are much less commonly used in other settings.

Historically, mechanical restraint (i.e. the use of straps, belts, or other equipment to restrict movement) was used extensively, but this has become much less common since the introduction of safe and effective sedative medication, and it is now widely considered to be a strategy of last resort (12). In the UK, its use is largely confined to forensic settings, and would not be considered routine practice on a PICU.

Enhanced nursing observations

This area of clinical practice is discussed in Chapter 22.

De-escalation and seclusion rooms

It can be very helpful when a patient is angry or highly agitated to encourage them to spend some time in a quieter and safer area of the ward. The advantages of this are several.

Firstly, it removes the patient form the situation that is making them agitated, for example, it may be due to conflict with another patient or a particular member of staff.

Secondly, it allows the patient to be angry in a safe environment where there are fewer possibilities for causing harm to themselves or others, or to damage property. It takes time for anger or agitation to subside, and a safe 'de-escalation room' can allow the patient the time and physical space that they need to calm down, using whatever strategies are most helpful for them. These may include being allowed to shout, or to take out their physical aggression in a safe manner, for example, by hitting a foam mattress.

Thirdly, escorting a patient to a such an area of the ward allows staff to spend time talking with the patient in a quiet and private space away from other patients and staff, in order to explore their current thoughts and feelings, and to offer empathy, support, and practical solutions to help resolve their concerns.

There are occasions, however, when the patient may be so physically hostile during periods of acute agitation that it is not safe even for staff to be with them. In such circumstances, many PICUs will make use of seclusion (10) rooms. These rooms are safe, contained areas, where a patient can be isolated behind a locked door such that they cannot harm anybody. Seclusion rooms should be constructed such that they are comfortable and calming, but they should not contain objects or fittings that can be used as weapons or as a means of self-harm. The patient can then safely remain in the room until they have calmed sufficiently to be able to return to less restrictive areas of the ward. Seclusion rooms must be constructed such that the patient can be observed at all times, and able to interact with the staff observing them. As a minimum they should have a mattress, blankets, and bathroom facilities.

Spending time in seclusion can be very frightening and difficult for a patient, and so it is essential that patients are observed constantly by a member of staff with whom they can interact, and also that they are reviewed frequently in order to ensure that they can be safely moved to a less restrictive setting at the earliest opportunity. Typically this would mean a review of the seclusion at least every 1–2 hours. Patients should be monitored regularly for physical health problems, especially if they have been manually restrained or given medication by whatever route in order to help them to calm down.

Restraint

In a PICU setting, there will often be occasions when staff must intervene physically in order to manage a dangerous situation, prevent harm from being caused by a patient to themselves or to others, or in order to enforce treatment on an unwilling patient. Any type of physical intervention in which staff place hands on a patient is by definition restrictive, and although there may be a legal justification for its use, it should be considered to be an assault. It must, therefore, only be used when necessary. This would generally mean when other forms of non-restrictive intervention (such as the use of de-escalation techniques or PRN medication) or less restrictive intervention (such as enhanced nursing observations) have not been successful in managing the situation. Any intervention that leads to 'hands being laid' on a patient can be considered to be restraint (13–15).

Restraint may take many forms, and the guidelines for which techniques are safe and appropriate are frequently updated in light of the evidence base. There is a high risk of injures being caused to the patient or to staff during a restraint, and there may be a risk of death if the patient is restrained inappropriately for too long, or if they have underlying physical health problems. Restraining a patient in the prone (or face-down) position is particularly dangerous, as it can compromise their ability to breathe, and so should be avoided wherever possible. Special consideration must also be given to frail (e.g. elderly) or pregnant patients in need of restraint. It is essential that all staff who could be involved in restraint undertake appropriate training and that their skills are refreshed and assessed regularly.

In England, there are various pieces of legislation that can provide a legal basis for the use of restraint in a hospital setting, depending on the circumstances when it is used. These include common law (which can be used as a justification for using restraint to prevent harm to others or the commission of a crime), the Mental Capacity Act 2005 (which can used to justify forcibly administering treatment to a patient when it is believed to be in the best interests of the patient and they lack capacity to agree to or refuse such treatment), or the Mental Health Act 1983, amended 2007 (which provides a legal authority to provide treatment to patients who are detained under the Act when it is required to treat their mental disorder).

Rapid tranquilization

If a patient is highly agitated and engaging in behaviours that pose a high risk to self or others, there will be occasions when it is not possible to make successful use of the de-escalation strategies outlined in the previous section in order to manage the patient's risks. In these circumstances it may be necessary to give the patient medication against their will in order to help them to calm down as quickly as possible. Such interventions are known as rapid tranquilization. Typically, rapid tranquilization would entail the patient being given sedative medication via the intramuscular (IM) route.

It is not always clear when an intervention is rapid tranquilization, as many agitated patients will willingly take PRN medication orally, or even take oral medication reluctantly when they recognize that the alternative is to be given an injection. However, the National Institute for Health and Care Excellence (NICE) guidelines on the short-term management of violence and aggression in mental health, health, and community settings (10) define rapid tranquilization as the administration of sedative medication by injection. Although not always the case, it may be inferred that rapid tranquilization will probably also involve manual restraint of the patient, as a fully compliant patient would be likely to agree to take oral medication.

The NICE guidelines stress that there is a lack of evidence suggesting the superiority of any agent over another, and it therefore stresses the importance of patient choice and evidence of previous efficacy of a particular treatment, as well as consideration being given to comorbid physical health problems, potential interactions with other medication, and any history of adverse reactions to a medication. NICE suggests that, for most patients, the use of IM lorazepam would be a good first choice, and that the use of one medication at a time is good practice, particularly for the neuroleptic naïve patient.

NICE published an algorithm for rapid tranquilization in partnership with the Royal College of Psychiatrists in 2005 (16), and most mental health trusts have similar, more up-to-date guidelines as part of their own policies on rapid tranquilization. The widely available *Maudsley Prescribing Guidelines* (17) also include an algorithm for rapid tranquilization.

Although these various guidelines may have minor differences, and they are frequently updated, most advise initially offering oral lorazepam, and if this is not accepted by the patient, administering IM lorazepam. If this is not wholly effective, and the behavioural disturbance is in the context of a psychosis, then an IM antipsychotic such as haloperidol should be considered. IM olanzapine is an alternative, but must not be used within 1 hour of the use of IM lorazepam, due to the increased risk of cardiorespiratory depression when used together. Other sedative medications that may be used in rare situations include sedative antihistamines such as promethazine, intravenous diazepam, or IM paraldehyde.

After rapid tranquilization is used and the patient has settled, it is important that the patient is placed under constant nursing observations, and that vital signs are monitored frequently (e.g. every 15 minutes initially, reducing in frequency thereafter), at least until the patient is fully alert once again. Observing staff should be particularly wary of rare but severe adverse reactions such as respiratory depression, cardiac arrhythmias, anaphylaxis, or neuroleptic malignant syndrome, as well as more common adverse reactions such as extrapyramidal side effects including dystonias.

Due to the frequent revisions of national and local guidelines and algorithms for rapid tranquilization, in light of the evolution of the evidence base, prescribers with responsibility for rapid tranquilization are advised to consult the latest NICE guidelines or local policies for detailed advice.

Post-incident actions

Whenever an incident of violence or aggression has occurred in a hospital setting, particularly when this has necessitated the use of restrictive interventions as discussed previously, it is important that certain actions are taken after the incident. These will include reviewing the incident with the patient or patients involved, and debriefing staff or other service users who were involved in, or witnessed, the incident. This allows everybody involved an opportunity to try to understand what happened, to be reassured that the incident is over and that people are safe, to consider ways to avoid similar incidents in the future, and to express their own experiences and feelings in relation to what may have been a frightening and traumatizing event.

Injuries to patients or staff need to be assessed and dealt with accordingly. Any damage to the ward environment should be repaired or made safe as soon as possible, in order to maintain a safe environment. Police involvement may be required if it is felt that a crime has been committed, for example, assault or criminal damage.

It is also important that the incident is fully documented in the patient's clinical record, that incident reports are completed as per local policies, and that any safeguarding issues are managed. It may be appropriate for an independent serious incident investigation and root cause analysis to be conducted, in order to understand how the incident happened, and to identify learning points such that similar incidents can be made less likely to occur in the future.

The Oxford model

There are many ways to set up and run a PICU, and not every PICU will use the same model of care or utilize the same interventions as those described earlier.

In Oxford, the PICU operates to a model whereby all admissions must be referred and considered before being accepted. Less restrictive interventions that may enable the patient to be supported elsewhere are suggested wherever possible. Patients who are admitted are reviewed by a doctor upon admission, and an immediate risk assessment and management plan are formulated by the multidisciplinary team. This in turn leads to the formulation of an appropriate multidisciplinary care plan, wherever possible with the collaboration of the patient. Patients are assigned a named nurse and associate nurse, and where possible their family are contacted.

All patients are seen at least weekly for a senior medical review, and members of the community mental health team and family/carers are encouraged to attend.

The ward accepts male and female patients, and is laid out along two sex-specific corridors from a central quad area. Neither corridor can be entered by patients of the opposite sex, and both corridors have a sex-specific TV lounge area. All bedrooms have their own en-suite toilet and shower room. The ward also has a communal TV lounge, bathroom, dining room, treatment room, and occupational therapy activity room, as well as a communal enclosed garden, and a separate female-only garden. There are separate de-escalation and seclusion rooms along a third corridor, along with an appended Section 136 'Place of Safety' suite.

The ward has a total of 11 beds (eight male and three female), and the standard staffing levels are eight nursing staff (qualified and non-qualified) covering the two day shifts, and six nursing staff at night. The ward also has a full-time occupational therapist, two activity support workers, a ward clerk, dedicated input from a pharmacist and pharmacy technician, and dedicated psychology input. Senior nursing support is provided by a ward manager and modern matron, and medical support is provided by a consultant psychiatrist, a specialty doctor, and a foundation doctor.

Restrictive interventions are used as little as possible, and when they are used, this is for as short a time as necessary. Secluded patients are reviewed at least every 2 hours and seclusion can be terminated at any point by the nursing or multidisciplinary team, once it is felt that the patient no longer poses an immediate risk of harm to others.

The intermediate-acting IM antipsychotic zuclopenthixol acetate (Clopixol Acuphase) is used on the PICU more frequently than on any other ward, and often with good effect. Its use in Oxford is in line with local and national guidelines (including NICE), and it has proved to be a very effective treatment for patients who have had a positive response to it during previous episodes of illness, or for patients who have required repeated IM injections with shorter-acting antipsychotic agents and who are likely to continue to require repeated IM treatment in the short term. When it is used, zuclopenthixol acetate (Clopixol Acuphase) is used at a low dose initially, other antipsychotic medication is discontinued, and the patient is regularly monitored for extrapyramidal side effects and other adverse reactions. Its effects last for up to 72 hours, and it may be given up to four times over the course of several days.

As patients recover they are 'stepped down' to their local acute wards as soon as possible. However, they are able to access leave from the PICU, usually escorted by a member of staff, once the multidisciplinary team feel that this is safe.

Problems and pitfalls

The purpose, physical environment, treatment methods, and patient characteristics of a PICU set it apart from most other psychiatric wards. The PICU is a resource that helps the wider psychiatric service function safely and effectively. However, attempting to run a perfect PICU may be a worthy ideal, but it is unlikely to be achievable. Like any ward, a PICU will from time to time have to deal with problems such as staff shortages and serious untoward incidents. These difficulties are compounded by the fact that the very purpose of a PICU is to care safely for the most unwell patients, and so it is inevitable that there will often be patients who pose particular and unforeseen challenges with respect to their management. This in turn can lead to problems with staff morale, and then to difficulties recruiting and retaining staff.

In order to mitigate against these difficulties, careful thought must be given to how the ward is managed such that these challenges are addressed. This will involve consideration of the numbers of patients on the ward, whether the ward should be single or mixed sex, what the appropriate staffing levels should be, what the ward leadership structure should be, and what activities and therapies should be offered.

NAPICU guidelines state that children under the age of 16, and children under the age of 18 in full-time education, should never be cared for on an adult PICU (1). However, it may be necessary on occasion for adolescents to be cared for on an adult PICU. When this happens, it should be for the minimum amount of time until a more age-appropriate placement can be found, and care should be led by medical and nursing staff with specialist child and adolescent psychiatric training while the adolescent is on the adult PICU. As well as differences in the presentation of illness and behaviour between children/adolescents and adults, there are also important differences in the doses and licensed indications of pharmacological treatments, and methods of restrictive interventions such as restraint. All adolescents on an adult PICU will almost certainly require a specialist child and adolescent mental health services nurse with them at all times.

Consideration should be given as to whether the ward could and should have different policies and operating procedures compared with other wards. Whatever policies are in place, it is important that all staff are familiar with these and any other rules of the ward, and that they are applied consistently across all the patients. This requires good communication within the team, which in turn depends upon effective handovers and good staff supervision, and requires being honest and unambiguous in discussions with patients.

Flashpoints and triggers for anger and aggression are often caused by a small number of issues such as patients wanting to smoke, the availability of leave from the ward, promises being made by staff that are not kept, or emotionally difficult family visits. It is important, therefore, to anticipate these situations, and to explain the ward's rules and policies to new patients as soon as possible in an empathic and consistent manner.

Sometimes a patient's challenging behaviour is such that they cannot be safely managed even on a PICU, and so it is important to remember that a PICU has an upper threshold, as well as a lower threshold, for admission. It would be unreasonable for a PICU in adult services to be expected to care for a patient with a history or high risk of serious assaultive behaviour (e.g. with the use of weapons), and such patients would be more appropriately admitted to medium secure forensic settings.

Psychiatric practice, like all medical practice, takes place within an ever-changing healthcare environment, constrained by finite and often decreasing financial resources, and with regular turnover of staff. The pressures that can be placed on any one part of a psychiatric service by the needs of the wider service can have a significant impact on a ward like a PICU. This could lead to situations such as the PICU being used to admit patients who do not require PICU management because there is not a more suitable bed available elsewhere; patients being unable to step down from the PICU because of a lack of beds on the open wards; patients being discharged directly home from the PICU without any step down at all; or patients becoming 'informal' (i.e. not being subject to detention under the Mental Health Act or similar legislation) because their original Section has expired or has been discharged by a tribunal, and there is no bed on an open ward that the patient can be transferred to.

It may not always be possible to avoid situations such as these, and a well-run PICU must be flexible enough to deal with these occasions such that all patients are cared for with the least possible restrictions, while ensuring that the overall safety and integrity of the ward is not compromised.

Conclusion

A PICU represents the frontline of acute psychiatric services, and the purpose of a PICU is to provide safe and effective care to the most challenging patients in the acute psychiatric population. It is not possible to anticipate and plan for every possible situation that may occur on a PICU. However, a PICU that can attain the standards defined by AIMS; that provides individualized patient-centred care; that is mindful of the Mental Health Act Code of Practice and other relevant guidance; that has clear policies and protocols that are understood by all staff and explained clearly to all patients; that is fair and consistent in applying these policies; that has expertise and experience in applying restrictive practices; and that is inclusive to patients and their families and carers, and is supportive of its staff, will be a well-run PICU.

REFERENCES

1. National Association of Psychiatric Intensive Care and Low Secure Units. Guidance for commissioners of psychiatric intensive care units (PICUs). 2016. http://napicu.org.uk/wp-content/uploads/2016/04/Commissioning_Guidance_Apr16.pdf
2. National Association of Psychiatric Intensive Care and Low Secure Units. National minimum standards for psychiatric intensive care in general adult services. 2014. http://napicu.org.uk/wp-content/uploads/2014/12/NMS-2014-final.pdf
3. Beer MD, Pereira S, Paton C. Psychiatric intensive care: development and definition. In: Beer MD, Pereira S, Paton C (eds), *Psychiatric Intensive Care*, 2nd edition, pp. 3–11. Cambridge: Cambridge University Press; 2008.
4. Butler Report. *Committee on Mentally Abnormal Offenders.* London: HMSO; 1975.
5. Rachlin S. On the need for a closed ward in an open hospital: the psychiatric intensive care unit. *Hosp Community Psychiat* 1973;24: 829–833.
6. Loubser I, Chaplin R, Quirk A. Violence, alcohol and drugs: the views of nurses and patients on psychiatric intensive care units, acute adult wards and forensic wards. *J Psychiatr Intens Care* 2009;5:33–39.
7. Lemmey SJ, Glover N, Chaplin R. Comparison of the quality of care in psychiatric intensive care units and acute psychiatric wards. *J Psychiatr Intens Care* 2012;9:12–18.
8. Department of Health. Your guide to relational security: see think act. 2010. http://www.rcpsych.ac.uk/pdf/STA_hndbk_2ndEd_Web_2.pdf
9. Department of Health. Positive and proactive care: reducing the need for restrictive interventions. 2014. https://www.gov.uk/government/uploads/system/uploads/attachment_data/file/300291/JRA_DoH_Guidance_on_RH_Summary_web_accessible.pdf
10. National Institute for Health and Care Excellence. Violence and aggression: short-term management in mental health, health and community settings. NICE guideline [NG10]. 2015. https://www.nice.org.uk/guidance/ng10
11. Department of Health. Mental Health Act 1983: code of practice. 2015. https://www.gov.uk/government/uploads/system/uploads/attachment_data/file/435512/MHA_Code_of_Practice.PDF
12. Stewart D, Bowers L, Simpson A, Ryan C, Tziggili M. Mechanical restraint of adult psychiatric inpatients: a literature review. *J Psychiatr Ment Health Nurs* 2009;16:749–757.
13. Royal College of Nursing. Let's talk about restraint: rights, risks and responsibility. 2008. https://www.rcn.org.uk/professional-development/publications/pub-003208
14. Mind. Restraint in mental health services: what the guidance says. 2015. http://www.mind.org.uk/media/3352178/restraintguidanceweb.pdf
15. Care Quality Commission. Brief guide: restraint (physical and mechanical). 2015. https://www.cqc.org.uk/sites/default/files/20170126_briefguide-Restraint_physical_mechanical.pdf
16. National Institute for Health and Care Excellence. Quick reference guide: violence. 2005. http://www.nm.stir.ac.uk/documents/nice-quick-guide.pdf
17. Taylor D, Paton C, Kapur S. *Maudsley Prescribing Guidelines*, 12th edition. Chichester: Wiley Blackwell; 2015.

36

Eating disorders

Agnes Ayton

Introduction

There is increasing demand for inpatient treatment of severe eating disorders (1, 2), both in the UK and internationally. However, hospital treatment of severe eating disorders remains controversial, mainly because of poor long-term outcomes (3, 4). It is generally agreed that inpatient treatment should be available for those who do not respond to outpatient treatment, but the threshold for admission, and the length and model of treatment, varies a great deal, depending on local historical arrangements and the funding of health care.

There are also significant variations in the international guidelines. For example, the American Psychiatric Association (APA) guidance (5) cautions against delaying admission until the patient is medically unstable, and recommends consideration of hospitalization if there is:

> rapid or persistent decline in oral intake, a decline in weight despite maximally intensive outpatient or partial hospitalization interventions, the presence of additional stressors that may interfere with the patient's ability to eat, knowledge of the weight at which instability previously occurred in the patient, co-occurring psychiatric problems that merit hospitalization, and the degree of the patient's denial and resistance to participate in his or her own care in less intensively supervised settings.

It states that: 'generally, adult patients who weigh less than approximately 85% (body mass index (BMI) of 17.5) of their individually estimated healthy weights have considerable difficulty gaining weight outside of a highly structured programme'.

In the UK, by contrast, admission tends to be the last resort. Patients are usually only admitted when they are severely or extremely malnourished (a BMI of <15—often as low as a BMI of 10–12). While there is no set BMI limit for admission in the National Institute for Health and Care Excellence (NICE) guidelines (6), the Management of Really Sick Patients with Anorexia Nervosa (MARSIPAN) guidelines (7) recommend admission if there is medical instability and the patient's BMI is less than 13 (or for young people, <70% median BMI for age). The Australian guidelines advise psychiatric admission if the patient's BMI is less than 14, and medical admission if it is less than 12 (8). Hospital treatment tends to be more successful and shorter in duration if the patient is admitted relatively early—for example, once there is a clear indication that outpatient treatment is not going to achieve sufficient change—rather than when the patient is extremely ill. Most cohort studies show that admission and discharge weight predict long-term outcomes (9, 10). This is consistent with the US guidelines. Unfortunately, due to the shortage of specialist beds in the UK, many patients wait for admission until they are gravely ill, which is counterproductive.

Not surprisingly, the length of stay is also markedly different in different countries: on average it is much shorter in the US (50–60 days) (11) than in the UK (approximately 120 days with wide variations) (12, 13). Such variations in practice are partly explained by reference to the different healthcare systems and funding arrangements (11, 14), and partly by the difficulties involved in evaluating the effectiveness of complex interventions, such as hospital treatment.

Hospital treatment is definitely helpful to improve patients' physical health, at least in the short term. Cohort studies consistently show that while most patients gain weight in a hospital setting (13, 15), the core eating disorder psychopathology often remains unresolved, with relapse rates high after discharge (16). However, this can be viewed as a 'chicken and egg' dilemma. If only the most severely ill patients are admitted to hospital, it should not be surprising that recovery rates are lower than for those responding to outpatient treatment alone. Extreme malnutrition has been repeatedly shown to be a poor prognostic factor (9, 10).

Large, well-designed trials are badly needed. However, evaluating the long-term benefits of complex interventions, such as hospital treatment for high-risk patients, is challenging in randomized controlled trials (RCTs), due to number of difficulties, such as those concerning recruitment, consent, high drop-out rates, and the achievement of true double blinding. Furthermore, severe eating disorders, such as anorexia nervosa, pose additional ethical problems for clinical trials. Because the risk of mortality is significant, not all patients can be included in randomized trials, hence the sickest patients, who need inpatient treatment most, are often excluded. As a consequence, research evidence is available only for moderately/mildly ill patients. Furthermore, certain interventions can never be randomized. For example, researchers cannot randomly allocate patients into voluntary and involuntary treatment. This means that there will never be randomized controlled evidence about the pros and cons of admission against the will of the patient. Consequently, when making decisions about compulsory treatment, clinicians rely on a few observational studies (17, 18) and their clinical judgement of risk.

Treatment models

The majority of specialist eating disorder units offer a range of eclectic interventions, with varying emphasis on physical or psychological treatment. One notable exception is the pioneering new model of inpatient cognitive behavioural therapy for eating disorders (CBT-E) (19). The purpose of hospital treatment depends on the length of stay. Brief admissions are usually labelled as 'medical stabilization', while longer ones tend to aim for recovery.

'Medical stabilization'—or crisis admission

Medical stabilization is often used to describe brief admissions, but at present, there is a wide variation of interpretation as to what 'medical stabilization' actually means in this context. For example, patients presenting to accident and emergency departments with life-threatening electrolyte imbalances may be temporarily 'stabilized' by intravenous replacement, but unless the eating disorder is addressed, the crisis will rapidly recur. In many UK units, patients with severe and enduring anorexia are admitted for a time-limited 'medical stabilization admission' of a few weeks (e.g. to improve the BMI from 12 to 14, and with no individual psychological treatment). The effectiveness of these practices has never been formally evaluated. While they can help to keep the patient alive and reduce the cost of prolonged hospitalization, whether this approach contributes to the maintenance of the illness is uncertain: it could give the impression to the sufferer that prolonged extreme malnutrition can be 'stable'. The reality is that very few patients are able to maintain an abnormally low weight. The majority lose weight and rapidly deteriorate (20, 21), but even those who maintain a very low BMI, do this at the cost of their deteriorating physical and mental health and of social isolation.

In the author's opinion, it would be much clearer if we used the term 'crisis management' for these admissions: it would be less misleading for both patients and carers. If a patient is discharged when still extremely malnourished, she or he may be over an immediate crisis, but is not stable. Recovery from severe eating disorders takes a long time. Short admissions tend to be more effective if the admission is part of an integrated care programme. This would mirror crisis admissions for other long-term conditions, such as diabetes: correcting blood sugar level in hospital can be lifesaving, but it would be ineffective in the long term without appropriate aftercare. Short-term hospitalization combined with family-based treatment (22), or day hospital (23), for adolescents has been evaluated in RCTs recently.

Madden's group in Sydney, Australia, compared short 'medical stabilization' admission, followed by 20 sessions of family-based treatment over a year after discharge, with admission for weight restoration in a sample of 82 adolescents. Surprisingly, there was no significant difference between the length of stay during the index admission (22 versus 27 days). However, although the participants were 'medically unstable' on admission, they were not extremely underweight (77–80% median BMI for age), and the 'medical stabilization' group was discharged at 84.4% BMI. This was mild malnutrition, so the term was being used very differently from how it is used in the UK—referring to patients discharged when still extremely malnourished (BMI <15). The conclusion from this study is that admission for 3–4 weeks may achieve similar outcomes if the patient is moderately underweight and if there is appropriate aftercare using evidence-based treatment. However, readmission rates were 35%, and remission rates 30%, within the first 12 months, which is poor for adolescents.

A larger German study compared 3 weeks' admission followed by day treatment or inpatient treatment in a sample of 172 adolescents (23). The length of day treatment was 16 weeks in the day-treatment arm, and 14 weeks in the inpatient arm. All patients were followed by outpatient treatment for a minimum of a year. The authors concluded that the short admission followed by day treatment was not inferior in moderately ill patients. The readmission rate was 20% in the sample.

Very few eating disorder services in the UK have such an integrated approach. Furthermore, the majority of patients are admitted when they are severely or extremely malnourished, and moderately ill patients are usually managed in the community. Consequently, the generalizability of these studies to the UK is poor. There are no similar studies in adult patient populations; only a few cohort studies reporting short-term outcomes, which do not provide information about overall patient outcomes (15, 24).

Recovery models

The majority of specialist eating disorder units in the UK offer admission with the aim of working towards recovery. This is particularly the case in child and adolescent mental health services (CAMHS), but most adult units in the UK also offer this option to the 'motivated' patient. Such treatment usually aims to achieve full weight restoration to a BMI of 19–20, supported by multidisciplinary interventions addressing malnutrition, abnormal eating behaviours, and psychological and family factors. Most units offer an eclectic combination of approaches. These include weight restoration with dietetic advice and medical monitoring, support, and supervision by the nursing team at mealtimes and after meals to prevent compensatory behaviours. In addition, most units offer various psychological and occupational therapy group programmes, as well as individual and family therapy, and education for young people.

While it is recognized that lengthy hospital admissions can be counterproductive, normalization of weight may be very difficult for the extremely malnourished patient outside of a hospital setting, because of the temptation to restrict their diet or use unhelpful compensatory behaviours to prevent weight gain. As malnutrition and dietary restriction are important maintaining factors, they need to be addressed in treatment. If the patient needs to gain 10–20 kg in weight to reach a minimum healthy BMI, that will take a long time.

The weakness of the eclectic programmes is that there is often a risk of conflicting messages given to the patient, as the various interventions were never designed to complement each other. For example, if the medical and nursing team focus on weight restoration, while the psychologist delivers non-directive psychodynamic therapy at the same time, this would cause direct conflict between different therapeutic models. Indeed, there is a real risk of professional rivalries, due to different training backgrounds in opposing theoretical frameworks. This is unhelpful in a patient population with a high level of ambivalence towards treatment and recovery. Not surprisingly, disengagement and self-discharge is common—as much as 60% in some studies (25, 26).

One solution is to stagger the interventions. The APA guidelines recommend psychodynamic therapy after weight restoration. The Australian guidelines state that research has not yet unearthed a cure; but, in the main, they recommend supportive counselling or cognitive behavioural therapy as a second step after nutritional rehabilitation. In the UK, psychological input to inpatient services tends to be limited, so supportive therapy is usually provided by the nursing team, and group work by occupational therapists.

Inpatient cognitive behavioural therapy for eating disorders

To address the common inconsistencies, Dalle Grave's team in Garda, Italy, have developed a new, revolutionary inpatient programme that builds on CBT-E (19). The novelty of this programme is the clear theoretical underpinning of treatment, which is in contrast with the traditional eclectic models. The treatment focuses on helping patients to become their own expert of their illness and address the maintaining factors.

There are many strengths of this inpatient model. There is a strong emphasis on patient autonomy, even when the patient is severely unwell, which helps with engaging the patient. All team members are trained in CBT-E and all interventions are designed with the same principles in mind. Furthermore, there is much less restriction and supervision than in traditional inpatient units: the focus of the team is to help the patient address their eating disorder rather than force them to do something they do not want to do. For example, treatment intensity is chosen with the patient and depends on need (outpatient, intensive day treatment, or hospital treatment). Psychological treatment starts before admission and continues after discharge (40 sessions in total), providing continuity, consistency, and a stepped care.

Dalle Grave has published a manual (19) and several papers to describe the method and evaluate outcomes, and what these publications demonstrate are impressive outcomes and completion rates compared to traditional eclectic models. Furthermore, the approach seems to benefit a wide range of patient groups, from adolescents to chronic and enduring anorexia nervosa (27–29). There have been a number of attempts to implement this treatment approach internationally: in Norway, the US, and the Netherlands. Replication studies are on the way (30). As the length of inpatient admission is 13 weeks, implementation of the inpatient CBT-E in the National Health Service (NHS) would offer both cost saving, better outcomes, and improved patient satisfaction. Our team in Oxford has been working on adopting the model for the NHS.

Quality Network for Eating Disorders in the UK

Patients can be admitted to either general psychiatric wards or specialist eating disorder units. There is a significant difference between adult and CAMHS inpatient units in this respect: most adult patients with eating disorders tend to be admitted to specialist units in the UK, while the majority of children and young people are treated within general CAMHS units in the NHS (31). General adult psychiatric wards rarely have sufficient expertise to manage a patient with a severe eating disorder. This is mainly due to insufficient training of staff working on these units. Inpatient services offering treatment

for severe eating disorders need to have the training and facilities to manage both the physical and psychological aspects of eating disorders.

Given the wide variation in services, the Royal College of Psychiatrists' Centre for Quality Improvement has developed national quality standards for specialist eating disorder inpatient units and general units offering eating disorder treatment. These were built on existing quality networks, such as the Quality Network for Inpatient CAMHS (32) for children and adolescents and Adult Inpatient Mental Health Services for adults.

The standards are divided into five main sections:

1. Staffing, training, and policies.
2. Timely and purposeful admission.
3. Safety.
4. Environment and facilities (including quality of food).
5. Therapies and activities (including refeeding).

The current standards are freely available on the Royal College of Psychiatrists' website (33).

The first national Quality Network for Eating Disorders (QED) report of adult services was published in 2016 (34). Twenty-five services out of 32 in the UK were accredited. The data showed 'significant diversity in clinical ethos and approach', as well as in 'size of units and length of treatment'. Occupancy levels were nationally high, leaving limited time to prepare patients and carers for admission. Patients commented that this would be helpful. This is in line with Dalle Grave's work, which shows that preparation for admission is fundamentally important for improving motivation and treatment outcomes. The mean length of stay was 116 days with wide variations.

Problems with staffing levels and use of agency staff were found in many units in the UK, resulting in cancellation of planned activities. Recruitment and retention of staff, particularly nursing, is a challenge for most inpatient services in the UK. Working with patients with severe eating disorders is emotionally demanding, so training, supervision, and a supportive team culture are essential. Compassionate and cohesive leadership is essential to create a positive therapeutic milieu, which is important for the well-being of both the patient and staff. It is important that nursing levels allow for taking breaks, time for handovers, training, supervision, reflection, and team discussions. In addition to these, our unit also uses patient and carer feedback to refine the treatment programme. This approach has helped reduce incidents and improved the therapeutic milieu.

QED standards have been helpful in improving the environment and facilities on inpatient units. However, the requirement to separate male and female patients has caused practical difficulties: as the male-to-female ratio tends to be 1:10 in eating disorder units, having separate facilities for men is difficult to provide if space is limited. This has led to closing male beds in some hospitals.

The multidisciplinary team is led by a consultant psychiatrist, and consists of junior doctors, nursing staff, psychologists, dieticians, occupational therapists, and social workers. CAMHS units also have teachers providing education while young people are in hospital. In Oxford, we allocate a psychologist to each patient to ensure that there is continuity of psychological treatment before, during, and after admission. Patients highly value this. Clarity of roles is essential for good multidisciplinary team working. The psychiatrists offer assessment and advise on investigations and medical treatment depending on individual comorbidity. The nursing staff take the lead on monitoring the patients' nutritional and psychological progress, help with assisted eating, and provide emotional support. The dietician works closely with the medical and nursing team to ensure safe weight restoration and normalization of eating behaviours. The occupational therapists take the lead on the group programme and in helping the patient regain confidence in their relevant skills such as cooking and shopping. The social worker can help with benefits, and the physiotherapist helps with exercise and any mobility issues.

Components of treatment

Given the diversity of practices and poor evidence base, what treatments should eating disorder inpatient services provide? Specialist teams should have the expertise in managing a severely unwell patient in an emergency, as well as in providing a meaningful and comprehensive psychosocial intervention. It is also important to be mindful that inpatient treatment is always a time-limited intervention in an illness that lasts for several years, and therefore admission and discharge planning are both fundamentally important. An integrated, evidence-based psychological approach would help to improve treatment adherence and long-term outcomes.

Preparation for admission

Preparation for admission is fundamental for the success of inpatient CBT-E, even for the physically compromised patient (19). This is because a high level of ambivalence towards treatment and recovery is inherent in the illness. Furthermore, the control of diet and weight and shape is central to the psychopathology, and unless the patient is fully signed up to the treatment, premature discharge is a high risk. Ideally, patients should start psychological treatment before admission, or if this is not available, have a care coordinator who can provide continuity between inpatient and outpatient treatment. The patient and the carers should have an opportunity to visit the unit and familiarize themselves with the treatment available. This is essential in managing anxiety and to start therapeutic engagement. The preparation for admission may take more than one visit, but it is time well spent.

Managing the physically compromised patient: MARSIPAN guidelines

A significant proportion of patients with eating disorders are admitted in an extremely malnourished state, often as an emergency. It is therefore essential that the team has sufficient expertise to manage the physically compromised patient safely and well.

The Royal College of Psychiatrists has developed the MARSIPAN guidelines to improve patient safety in this area (7, 35). It is important to note that the guidance was built on limited evidence. However, the working group included experts from all relevant professional groups and involved various other organizations. The guidelines help with assessing and managing risks in patients who are extremely malnourished: they provide advice regarding treatment setting and service organizations, as well as for using compulsory treatment. As a general rule, the MARSIPAN guidelines recommend that even patients who are severely ill should be managed in specialized eating disorder units, unless there are complications which need acute hospital equipment, such as intravenous replacement of electrolytes, or advanced life support. In such cases, joint working between the acute hospital and the specialist eating disorder service is essential to engage the patient and prevent any compensatory behaviours that may sabotage refeeding.

The most important lifesaving intervention for an extremely malnourished patient is safe refeeding. The MARSIPAN guidelines emphasize that underfeeding is equally, if not more dangerous than fast refeeding. This is absolutely true: refeeding complications, such as low phosphate and potassium levels, can be safely managed by an experienced team (36, 37). However, there is no treatment of underfeeding other than feeding itself. It is surprising that despite this, the guidelines recommend starting refeeding with 5–10 kcal/kg/day, albeit increasing this quickly. There is considerable debate whether this is an overcautious approach, as patients with anorexia do not have an underlying physical illness, so they can usually tolerate refeeding better. Recent RCTs have shown that patients tolerate well a refeeding diet starting with 1200–1500 kcal/day (38, 39). Using parenteral vitamin replacements can be helpful to prevent severe vitamin deficiencies, such as pellagra and beri-beri.

The other contentious recommendation in the MARSIPAN guidelines is bed rest. Historically, it was usual practice to keep severely underweight patients on bed rest in hospital, even though the patient would be fully mobile before admission. This was often part of a behavioural programme, when patients were expected to 'earn privileges' by weight gain. Such behavioural programmes are counterproductive psychologically as they will alienate the patient, and they are no longer recommended. However, bed rest has remained an intervention often used in a hospital setting. While it is important to ensure that the patient does not exercise excessively, it is important to be mindful that bed rest carries significant physical risks. These include worsening muscular atrophy (both skeletal and cardiac muscle), bone turnover (40, 41), deep vein thrombosis, and the risk of pressure sores and infections. Allowing the patient to move around gently on the ward is a cheap and effective intervention. A special mattress to prevent pressure sores and deep vein thrombosis prophylaxis may also be necessary. On balance, it is always better to increase the diet than restrict the patient's movement. Skilled nursing observation and support can help to ensure that the movements are not excessive, and that the patient has sufficient rest during the day.

Assessing and monitoring risks

A thorough physical examination is essential on admission. This should include a neurological examination and an electrocardiogram. In terms of baseline blood tests, the MARSIPAN guidelines recommend the following:

- Full blood count.
- Urea, creatinine, electrolytes (sodium, potassium, chloride, and bicarbonate); phosphate, calcium, magnesium, albumin; C-reactive protein; liver functions tests; amylase.
- Glucose.
- Thyroid function.
- Iron, ferritin.
- Vitamin B12, folate, and vitamin D.

- Urine biochemistry—sodium, potassium, chloride, osmolality, creatinine—may be useful in hypokalaemia, hyponatraemia, or altered hydration status.
- Optional micronutrients: zinc, copper, selenium, vitamin A/E, carotene.

The frequency of monitoring of blood tests is best decided depending on the patient's risk. It is important to be aware that patients who are severely malnourished often have normal blood test results. This is because the body regulates blood levels of various essential electrolytes, proteins, and lipids very carefully. It will try to maintain, for example, a normal blood calcium level, even at the cost of using it up from the bones and other tissues. This explains why patients, who seem stable, can decompensate very rapidly in the final stages of their illness: there are no further reserves to draw on. In patients who purge, the most commonly found abnormality in blood tests is a low potassium level. This can be corrected by potassium supplements, but stopping vomiting is the only effective long-term solution.

Hypoglycaemia is not uncommon and can be asymptomatic. It usually occurs when people are so severely emaciated that there are insufficient carbohydrate reserves in the body. Patients with anorexia who have type 1 diabetes are at high risk of medical consequences, as they tend to disregard medical advice about healthy eating patterns, resulting in poor blood sugar control and the risk of hypoglycaemia and sudden death.

The most common refeeding complications are hypophosphataemia and thiamine deficiency. Both of these can easily be managed by supplementation. The MARSIPAN guidance recommends prophylactic administration of Pabrinex®, which can be given intramuscularly rather than intravenously, with good effects (patients need to be monitored for rare anaphylactic reaction). If needed, patients usually tolerate oral phosphate supplementation as well. Refeeding oedema can occur, and it can be particularly severe if the patient uses high doses of laxatives. It tends to resolve spontaneously, but occasionally diuretics are needed.

The initial assessment also should carefully assess psychological risks. A patient who is extremely ill is often unaware of the risk to their life, and may refuse treatment, or they may be extremely anxious about the prospect of weight gain and may use various covert strategies to undermine treatment, such as excessive exercise, purging, or secreting food. Furthermore, comorbid psychiatric disorders are common, particularly depression, and the risk of suicide needs to be carefully assessed. The nursing staff have an important role in monitoring risks during the initial stages of refeeding. The level of monitoring needs to be decided based on the patient's individual risk, and will take account of the degree of malnutrition, any physical comorbidity, compensatory behaviours, and engagement with treatment.

Weight restoration

The rate of expected weight gain according to the NICE guidelines is approximately 1 kg/week in a hospital setting. Slower weight restoration would prolong the hospital stay, and is often associated with poor outcomes. Faster weight restoration (approximately 1.5 kg/week) is entirely safe from a biological point of view and has, indeed, been recommended by Dalle Grave (19).

The diet is usually discussed with the dietician and the patient, with medical input if there are any specific concerns. On our unit, in the first week we usually start with a diet of about 500 kcal per day more than the diet the patient has been on before starting treatment. For example, if the patient has been allowing themselves only about 500–600 kcal per day, weight restoration in the first week starts with about 1000–1200 kcal/day. This can be recommended for only a few days, as having a diet at this level would be dangerously low. During the second week, the diet could be increased to 1500–1800 kcal/day, and later (depending on the rate of weight restoration) the diet could be increased further. After a few weeks, most people require a minimum of 2500–3000 kcal/day for weight restoration, depending on their gender and activity levels. Men require more energy than women. About 500 kcal extra calories a day are needed for weight gain of 0.5 kg per week. This is almost impossible to achieve without the introduction of higher-energy density foods. Some experts suggest the temporary use of high-energy drinks, such as Fortisip®, Ensure®, and so on. This is best negotiated with the patient depending on their individual preference in the short term, but bearing in mind that it is important to widen their food choices to achieve the best long-term outcomes. Often it is helpful to address 'fear foods' in a gradual way, in a similar fashion to addressing other anxieties.

Artificial feeding

There are a lot of myths about nasogastric (NG) feeding, with some people regarding it as 'horrific' and 'inhumane'. There is nothing inhumane about saving a person's life by whatever means necessary. On the contrary, doctors and nurses would be negligent if they left a person to die of starvation, when feeding would help. The overwhelming majority of patients understand that not being able to eat is dangerous, and therefore accept NG feeding as a helpful medical intervention, just as they would accept other interventions, such as a drip or blood tests. NG feeding is similar to having a drip, but much safer. There are various methods of using tube feeding. Most paediatric units tend to use overnight feeding with a pump, while most eating disorder services prefer to use several smaller portions of feed during the day, usually following mealtimes (42). This latter method allows the body to get used to regular mealtimes. If the team works well with the patient, it is very rare for NG feeding to be administered against the patient's will. Most patients understand that this is an intervention to keep them alive, and when severely ill they may find artificial feeding easier than coping with their anxiety and guilt regarding eating. Using NG feeding is always a short-term intervention, and it is important to encourage the patient to start eating normally as soon as possible. The NICE guidelines state that NG feeding against the patient's will should only be administered by a highly skilled team, and under the relevant legal framework.

In extreme situations, a percutaneous endoscopic gastrostomy (PEG) tube may be necessary (43). This is usually used if a person has problems swallowing, or if a patient with anorexia is unable to eat for a long time. Fortunately, this is very rarely necessary. The PEG allows the person to be discharged from hospital, as long as she or he accepts the feed through the PEG voluntarily.

Weighing the patient

Weighing is an essential part of risk management and progress monitoring, but it can be highly anxiety provoking for the patient. All evidence-based psychological treatments (CBT-E and family-based treatment for adolescents) emphasize the importance of collaborative weighing. It is important that the patient understands the reasons for weight monitoring and the need for weight restoration: malnutrition is one of the main maintaining factors of severe eating disorders. While it may take time, most patients recognize that this is necessary and will cooperate with treatment. It may, however, be challenging if the patient is treated against their will. Under these circumstances it is important for nursing staff to be vigilant, watching out for the manipulation of weight by water loading or the use of weights.

Most units weigh patients first thing in the morning, after voiding, and either in underwear, or in minimal clothing. Patients accept the rationale for this if it is done sensitively (44). It is useful to chart weight restoration regularly, with clear expectation of a consistent weight gain week by week. The inpatient CBT-E treatment includes asking the patient to draw a weight gain chart showing the effect of both 1 kg/week and 1.5 kg/week gains. This can help the patient consider the pros and cons of faster weight restoration. Although most people with anorexia nervosa are anxious about any weight gain and would prefer a slower rate, the longer the weight restoration takes, the longer the time to achieve recovery. So, there is a trade-off: quicker weight restoration may be more anxiety provoking in the short term, but it also shortens the time to recovery. Keeping a weight chart can also help to challenge the associated fears, such as that which associates rapid weight gain with the eating of certain foods (chocolate, etc.). It is also helpful to agree on how to monitor weight restoration. Most specialist units use one or two weighing days per week, depending on progress.

Helping the patient normalize eating behaviours

Dietary restriction is another maintaining factor of eating disorders. So, introducing regular meals is essential for helping the patient, not just from a physical point of view, but also to address their psychopathology. It is beneficial to introduce meals every few hours, because this helps to provide a regular energy supply for the body, and for a starving person it is easier to digest smaller, but frequent meals. This is particularly important after severe weight loss, as by this time the body's reserves are exhausted. Most units provide three main meals and three snacks (including one before bedtime) as the best way of managing this. Smaller, frequent meals also help to prevent bingeing and break the vicious circle of bingeing and vomiting. Regular eating is one of the most important interventions in CBT-E and, more generally, inpatient units can help to reinstate regular eating, encouraging the patient to learn about the right amount and range of foods.

In the UK, most specialist units offer intensive nursing support and supervision at mealtimes. This is one of the most difficult tasks for the staff, as patients can be highly distressed at mealtimes, and frequently show abnormal behaviours. People with anorexia are often afraid of certain foods and exclude them from their diet, but this avoidance makes their fears of normal foods worse. For this reason it is also necessary to exclude 'diet foods' from the very beginning. Many of these are nutritionally quite poor. Fat-free foods, for example, are usually high in sugars. Usually, as the patient progresses in treatment, they gradually take over responsibility for cooking and managing their meals. In preparation for discharge, it is important to include a variety of foods that fit family traditions and lifestyle, and to practise meals away from the hospital environment.

The inpatient CBT-E introduces patient autonomy much earlier. While the dieticians help to devise meals, and replace any food that was not consumed, patients are expected to use self-monitoring and distraction strategies during mealtimes.

Psychological interventions

The NICE guidelines recommend CBT-E (45), supportive clinical management, and the Maudsley Model of Anorexia Nervosa Treatment for Adults (MANTRA) (46) for the psychological treatment of anorexia nervosa in adults, and family-based treatment for children and young people. Although therapeutic groups are encouraged on inpatient units, there is limited evidence to support their effectiveness.

Individual therapies

Individual psychological treatment usually starts after some weight restoration (such as a BMI of 15) on most units. This is consistent with the APA guidelines recommending individual psychotherapy after weight restoration. The main rationale for this is that starvation has a negative effect on the brain. People who are severely starved tend to have real difficulty thinking rationally and reflecting on their problems. However, in our experience, most patients would prefer starting psychological therapy immediately, and recent evidence suggests that they can benefit even if they are extremely underweight (27).

Supportive clinical management

This is a commonly used, non-specific approach that is offered in parallel with weight restoration. Therapists draw upon a variety of insights and techniques from differing psychotherapeutic traditions that are relevant to an individual's strengths and difficulties. Manuals for supportive clinical management exist.

Psychoeducation

All guidelines include psychoeducation as part of the treatment, and it is an integral part of CBT-E. While this is clearly essential, many patients initially find it difficult to take on board the information, or believe that it does not apply to them. This is partly the result of denial and partly the consequence of impaired thinking caused by starvation. Because of this, it is important to revisit the information from time to time. Books can be helpful, as they can be picked up again and again. On our unit we use *Anorexia Nervosa: Hope for Recovery* (47) and *Overcoming Binge Eating* (48). Similarly, carers are in a much better position to help if they are fully aware of the complex issues relating to anorexia. Apart from reading materials, psychoeducation is often delivered in groups for patients and for carers.

Cognitive behavioural therapy

During the past 30 years, there has been significant research focusing on CBT-E, based on its success in bulimia nervosa. CBT-E is concerned with the factors that maintain the condition once it has become established. By focusing on the link between thoughts, feelings, and behaviours, it aims to challenge thoughts and behaviours in order to achieve a positive change in feelings, and therefore break the maintenance cycle. Enhanced CBT-E also offers modules addressing perfectionism, mood intolerance, and low self-esteem, tailored to the patient's needs. The benefits of using CBT-E in an inpatient setting have been shown by the Villa Garda group (49).

They have also successfully challenged the dogma that extremely malnourished patients are unable to start psychological treatment. In fact, they recommend starting CBT-E before admission, and continue during and after inpatient treatment. In our initial experience of implementation of the model, patients highly value this approach.

Family-based treatment

All guidelines recommend family therapy for children and young people. In contrast with individual and group therapies, family interventions oriented towards eating disorders have been found, in several RCTs, to be helpful for young people with anorexia nervosa (50, 51). The emphasis is on assisting parents to find ways to help their child, both with weight restoration and to address underlying emotional difficulties. Treasure's new approach seeks to use these principles for carers of adults too. Her team emphasizes the benefits of helping carers to develop new skills to support a loved one with an eating disorder (52). There is emerging evidence that family therapy integrated with inpatient treatment can significantly reduce the length of stay and improve outcomes (22, 53).

Group therapies

The underlying rationale for group work is that sharing problems with other people with similar conditions can help to relieve the experience of shame and isolation. In addition, they also help structure the time in hospital. Our unit, like most others, offers a range of groups focusing on psychoeducation, nutrition, self-esteem, assertiveness, and various skills, such as cooking and social eating. Patients also participate in other activities, such as arts and crafts, literature, music, or exercise, such as gentle stretching or yoga. The group programme is regularly reviewed with the patients. We also offer groups supporting carers.

Medication

Psychotropics

Medication is not recommended as a sole treatment for anorexia nervosa, because the evidence for its effectiveness is poor (54, 55). However, comorbidity in anorexia, such as underlying depression or obsessive–compulsive disorder is common. These problems may need to be treated by medication, particularly if there is no response to psychological treatment.

Despite the high rate of comorbid depression, the jury is still out on whether the use of antidepressants is beneficial when people are malnourished. There is some evidence that it is ineffective in starved patients, but further trials are needed. Furthermore, concerns have been raised that there is an increased risk of self-harm while on these medicines, particularly in adolescents. As with any other treatment, the potential side effects and benefits need to be balanced very carefully before treatment decisions are made.

Anxiolytics are often used in hospitals as a temporary measure to manage the high levels of anxiety associated with initial weight restoration. They have never been tested for anorexia in formal clinical trials, but at the same time there is no evidence of harm in the literature, so if they are used cautiously, they can be helpful in managing severe anxiety and distress in the short term.

Olanzapine and other atypical antipsychotics are sometimes used if patients are very highly distressed and agitated, or if anorexic beliefs are of an almost delusional intensity and resistant to any rational discussion. Apart from reducing the delusional level of preoccupation, they can also help to reduce intense anxiety and mood swings. There is some evidence to show that olanzapine can be beneficial in these difficult-to-treat cases of anorexia, as part of a comprehensive treatment (55–57). The main side effects of olanzapine are drowsiness and low blood pressure in underweight patients. Interestingly, olanzapine can cause increased appetite and associated weight gain in other patient groups, such as those suffering from psychosis or bipolar disorder, but this almost never happens in anorexia. The reason for this is unknown, but this fact should be reassuring for anorexia patients. The optimal length of treatment in anorexia is unknown, but it is likely to be several months. Reduced anxiety can also help patients to use psychotherapies more effectively. Patients need to be carefully monitored for metabolic side effects. Some advocate using aripiprazole as an alternative. The author has seen a number of patients rapidly lose weight while on aripiprazole, so this may be a significant risk for some patients.

Other medications

Oestrogens or bisphosphonates are sometimes used to prevent deterioration of osteoporosis. The evidence for this is mixed. The best prevention of osteoporosis is full weight restoration with a nutritionally balanced diet. Some experts recommend the use of vitamin D and calcium supplements. As long as these are not used instead of a balanced diet, they may be helpful.

Vitamins and omega-3 supplements can be useful at the beginning of refeeding. They may be helpful in restoring reserves of essential nutrients in the body, but it is important to recognize that they cannot replace a normal mixed diet. Vitamin D and thiamine deficiencies are common, and need to be replaced.

During weight restoration, abdominal complaints are common. These include reflux, constipation, and abdominal bloating. It is important to keep gastroenterological medication limited: the problems usually resolve with time. On our unit, we have been using Fox's Glacier Mints to reduce abdominal discomfort with good effect. This also normalizes eating behaviours, as mints are often served after meals in restaurants. In terms of laxatives, macrogols should be the first line of treatment. If the patient has irritable bowel syndrome, probiotics can be helpful.

Educational in hospitals

In UK law, hospitals need to provide education for all young people. This is particularly important in the case of hospital treatment of anorexia because the length of stay tends to be several months. Even on adult units it is helpful to support patients to continue their studies and to take exams—as long as this is not undermining their treatment.

Compulsory treatment

Most countries have a legal framework that allows for the compulsory treatment of people with mental disorders. However, there is often confusion about anorexia, as it is sometimes regarded as a personal choice rather than an illness. In England and Wales, the Care Quality Commission issued a 'Guidance Note on the Treatment of Anorexia Nervosa' with the Mental Health Act 1983 to help clinicians with treatment decisions when the patient refuses treatment. This guidance emphasized that in general, 'compulsory measures are unnecessary in the treatment of anorexia nervosa because it may be counterproductive to patient autonomy in the long term'. However, they recognized that in 'rare cases, when the patients' physical health or survival is seriously threatened by food or fluid refusal, compulsory treatment may be necessary'.

It is striking that in this guidance, anorexia nervosa is viewed differently from other mental disorders. The physical risk to the patient is emphasized rather than the general conditions for compulsory treatment such as risk to health, safety of self, or safety of others. It may be questioned whether there is any theoretical reason to assume that patient autonomy is more important in anorexia nervosa than, for example, in depression or psychosis. The risk of mortality is higher in anorexia nervosa than in other mental disorders, and a significant proportion of sufferers commit suicide rather than die of the consequences of starvation. Therefore, the different approach cannot be justified on the basis of the risk to the patient. Furthermore, there is no evidence that the patient's engagement or long-term outcome is irrevocably harmed by compulsory treatment (18, 58, 59).

In English law, parents can consent to treatment on behalf of a non-consenting child under the age of 16 years. The NICE guidelines emphasize the importance of a collaborative approach in the treatment of young people with eating disorders, just as with adults. NICE state that 'when feeding against the patient's will becomes necessary, it is recommended that this should only be done in the context of the Mental Health Act (MHA) or the Children's Act'. The NICE guidelines stress that although parental consent can be used to override the young person's refusal of treatment, relying 'indefinitely' on parental consent to treatment should be avoided. The NICE guidelines add that if both the patient with anorexia nervosa and those with parental responsibility refuse treatment, legal advice should be sought in order to consider proceedings under the Children's Act.

Waiting too long for compulsory treatment (with all the best intentions to honour the patient's wishes) can have tragic consequences, so clinicians need to be mindful that compulsory treatment is not the worst thing that can happen to a patient. This is also emphasized in the MARSIPAN Guidelines.

Criteria for discharge

Inpatient units vary as to whether discharge occurs after stabilization of a healthy weight, or prior to reaching a healthy weight, for continued work in the community. If the patient is to be discharged prior to achieving a healthy weight, it is essential that there is an intensive package of care in the community, as relapse following inpatient admission is high. The APA guidelines strongly recommend full weight restoration and stabilization for relapse prevention before discharge from hospital.

In usual clinical practice, the decision about discharge is always negotiated with the person and the family, based on the likely response to further outpatient treatment. If the patient is able to complete his or her weight restoration at home, that is fine, but if there is a high level of anxiety or reluctance to do so, it is better to complete weight restoration in hospital where intensive support is available. Otherwise, the risk of relapse would be almost 100%.

REFERENCES

1. Holland J, Hall N, Yeates DG, Goldacre M. Trends in hospital admission rates for anorexia nervosa in Oxford (1968-2011) and England (1990-2011): database studies. *J R Soc Med* 2016;109:59–66.
2. Gammelmark C, Jensen SO, Plessen KJ, Skadhede S, Larsen JT, Munk-Jorgensen P. Incidence of eating disorders in Danish psychiatric secondary healthcare 1970-2008. *Aust N Z J Psychiatry* 2015;49:724–730.
3. Madden S, Hay P, Touyz S. Systematic review of evidence for different treatment settings in anorexia nervosa. *World J* 2015;5:147–153.
4. Ben-Tovim DI, Walker K, Gilchrist P, Freeman R, Kalucy R, Esterman A. Outcome in patients with eating disorders: a 5-year study. *Lancet* 2001;357:1254–1257.
5. American Psychiatric Association. Practice guideline for the treatment of patients with eating disorders, third edition. *Am J Psychiatry* 2006;163:1–128.
6. National Institute for Health and Care Excellence. Eating disorders: recognition and treatment. NICE guideline [NG69]. 2017. https://www.nice.org.uk/guidance/ng69
7. Royal College of Psychiatrists. *MARSIPAN: Management of Really Sick Patients with Anorexia Nervosa.* CR189. London: Royal College of Psychiatrists; 2014.
8. Hay P, Chinn D, Forbes D, et al. Royal Australian and New Zealand College of Psychiatrists clinical practice guidelines for the treatment of eating disorders. *Aust N Z J Psychiatry* 2014;48:977–1008.
9. Sly R, Bamford B. Why are we waiting? The relationship between low admission weight and end of treatment weight outcomes. *Eur Eat Disord Rev* 2011;19:407–410.
10. Wales J, Brewin N, Cashmore R, et al. Predictors of positive treatment outcome in people with anorexia nervosa treated in a specialized inpatient unit: the role of early response to treatment. *Eur Eat Disord Rev* 2016;24:417–424.
11. Kalisvaart JL, Hergenroeder AC. Hospitalization of patients with eating disorders on adolescent medical units is threatened by current reimbursement systems. *Int J Adolesc Med Health* 2007;19:155–165.
12. Morris J, Simpson AV, Voy SJ. Length of stay of inpatients with eating disorders. *Clin Psychol Psychother* 2015;22:45–53.
13. Goddard E, Hibbs R, Raenker S, et al. A multi-centre cohort study of short term outcomes of hospital treatment for anorexia nervosa in the UK. *BMC Psychiatry* 2013;13:287.
14. Guarda AS, Schreyer CC, Fischer LK, et al. Intensive treatment for adults with anorexia nervosa: the cost of weight restoration. *Int J Eat Disord* 2017;50:302–306.
15. Gaudiani JL, Brinton JT, Sabel AL, Rylander M, Catanach B, Mehler PS. Medical outcomes for adults hospitalized with severe anorexia nervosa: an analysis by age group. *Int J Eat Disord* 2016;49:378–385.
16. Fennig S, Brunstein Klomek A, Shahar B, Sarel-Michnik Z, Hadas A. Inpatient treatment has no impact on the core thoughts and perceptions in adolescents with anorexia nervosa. *Early Interv Psychiatry* 2017;11:200–207.
17. Ward A, Ramsay R, Russell G, Treasure J. Follow-up mortality study of compulsorily treated patients with anorexia nervosa. [Erratum appears in *Int J Eat Disord* 2016;49:435]. *Int J Eat Disord* 2015;48:860–865.

18. Ayton A, Keen C, Lask B. Pros and cons of using the Mental Health Act for severe eating disorders in adolescents. *Eur Eat Disord Rev* 2009;17:14–23.

19. Dalle Grave R. *Intensive Cognitive Behavior Therapy for Eating Disorders: Eating Disorders in the 21st Century*. New York: Nova Science Pub Inc; 2012.

20. Baran SA, Weltzin TE, Kaye WH. Low discharge weight and outcome in anorexia nervosa. *Am J Psychiatry* 1995;152:1070–1072.

21. Willer MG, Thuras P, Crow SJ. Implications of the changing use of hospitalization to treat anorexia nervosa. *Am J Psychiatry* 2005;162:2374–2376.

22. Madden S, Miskovic-Wheatley J, Wallis A, et al. A randomized controlled trial of in-patient treatment for anorexia nervosa in medically unstable adolescents. *Psychol Med* 2015;45:415–427.

23. Herpertz-Dahlmann B, Schwarte R, Krei M, et al. Day-patient treatment after short inpatient care versus continued inpatient treatment in adolescents with anorexia nervosa (ANDI): a multicentre, randomised, open-label, non-inferiority trial. *Lancet* 2014;383:1222–1229.

24. Gaudiani JL, Sabel AL, Mascolo M, Mehler PS. Severe anorexia nervosa: outcomes from a medical stabilization unit. *Int J Eat Disord* 2012;45:85–92.

25. Sly R, Morgan JF, Mountford VA, Lacey JH. Predicting premature termination of hospitalised treatment for anorexia nervosa: the roles of therapeutic alliance, motivation, and behaviour change. *Eat Behav* 2013;14:119–123.

26. Gentile MG, Manna GM, Ciceri R, Rodeschini E. Efficacy of in-patient treatment in severely malnourished anorexia nervosa patients. *Eat Weight Disord* 2008;13:191–197.

27. Calugi S, El Ghoch M, Dalle Grave R. Intensive enhanced cognitive behavioural therapy for severe and enduring anorexia nervosa: a longitudinal outcome study. *Behav Res Ther* 2017;89:41–48.

28. Dalle Grave R, Calugi S, El Ghoch M, Conti M, Fairburn CG. Inpatient cognitive behavior therapy for adolescents with anorexia nervosa: immediate and longer-term effects. *Front Psychiatr* 2014;5:14.

29. Dalle Grave R, Calugi S, Conti M, Doll H, Fairburn CG. Inpatient cognitive behaviour therapy for anorexia nervosa: a randomized controlled trial. *Psychother Psychosom* 2013;82:390–398.

30. Danielsen YS, Ardal Rekkedal G, Frostad S, Kessler U. Effectiveness of enhanced cognitive behavioral therapy (CBT-E) in the treatment of anorexia nervosa: a prospective multidisciplinary study. *BMC Psychiatry* 2016;16:342.

31. Tulloch S, Lelliott P, Bannister D, et al. The Costs, Outcomes and Satisfaction for Inpatient Child and Adolescent Psychiatric Services (COSI-CAPS) study. Report for the National Coordinating Centre for NHS Service Delivery and Organisation R&D (NCCSDO). 2008. http://www.netscc.ac.uk/hsdr/files/project/SDO_FR_08-1304-062_V01.pdf

32. Thompson P, Clarke H. Quality Network for Inpatient CAMHS: service standards. Royal College of Psychiatrists; 2016. https://www.rcpsych.ac.uk/pdf/QNIC_Standards_2016_AW.pdf

33. Clarke H, Gardner M. Standards for adult inpatient eating disorder services, 2nd edition. Royal College of Psychiatrists; 2017. https://www.rcpsych.ac.uk/pdf/QED%202nd%20Edition%20Standards.pdf

34. Azmoodeh K, Beavon M, Clarke H. Quality Network for Eating Disorders (QED): 1st national report. Royal College of Psychiatrists; 2016. https://www.rcpsych.ac.uk/pdf/QED%201st%20National%20Report%20-%20July%202016.pdf

35. Marikar D, Reynolds S, Moghraby OS. Junior MARSIPAN (Management of Really Sick Patients with Anorexia Nervosa). *Arch Dis Child Educ Pract Ed* 2016;101:140–143.

36. Leitner M, Burstein B, Agostino H. Prophylactic phosphate supplementation for the inpatient treatment of restrictive eating disorders. *J Adolesc Health* 2016;58:616–620.

37. Redgrave GW, Coughlin JW, Schreyer CC, et al. Refeeding and weight restoration outcomes in anorexia nervosa: challenging current guidelines. *Int J Eat Disord* 2015;48:866–873.

38. O'Connor G, Nicholls D, Hudson L, Singhal A. Refeeding low weight hospitalized adolescents with anorexia nervosa: a multicenter randomized controlled trial. *Nutr Clin Pract* 2016;31:681–689.

39. Garber AK, Sawyer SM, Golden NH, et al. A systematic review of approaches to refeeding in patients with anorexia nervosa. *Int J Eat Disord* 2016;49:293–310.

40. DiVasta AD, Feldman HA, Quach AE, Balestrino M, Gordon CM. The effect of bed rest on bone turnover in young women hospitalized for anorexia nervosa: a pilot study. *J Clin Endocrinol Metab* 2009;94:1650–1655.

41. Caiani EG, Massabuau P, Weinert L, Vaida P, Lang RM. Effects of 5 days of head-down bed rest, with and without short-arm centrifugation as countermeasure, on cardiac function in males (BR-AG1 study). *J Appl Physiol (1985)* 2014;117:624–632.

42. Hart S, Franklin RC, Russell J, Abraham S. A review of feeding methods used in the treatment of anorexia nervosa. *J Eat Disord* 2013;1:36.

43. Born C, de la Fontaine L, Winter B, et al. First results of a refeeding program in a psychiatric intensive care unit for patients with extreme anorexia nervosa. *BMC Psychiatry* 2015;15:57.

44. Jaffa T, Davies S, Sardesai A. What patients with anorexia nervosa should wear when they are being weighed: report of two pilot surveys. *Eur Eat Disord Rev* 2011;19:368–370.

45. Fairburn CG, Cooper Z, Doll HA, O'Connor ME, Palmer RL, Dalle Grave R. Enhanced cognitive behaviour therapy for adults with anorexia nervosa: a UK-Italy study. *Behav Res Ther*. 2013;51(1):R2–8.

46. Schmidt U, Ryan EG, Bartholdy S, et al. Two-year follow-up of the MOSAIC trial: a multicenter randomized controlled trial comparing two psychological treatments in adult outpatients with broadly defined anorexia nervosa. *Int J Eat Disord* 2016;49:793–800.

47. Ayton A. *Anorexia Nervosa: Hope for Recovery*. London: Hammersmith Press Limited; 2011.

48. Fairburn CG. *Overcoming Binge Eating*. New York: Guilford Press; 2013.

49. Dalle Grave R, El Ghoch M, Sartirana M, Calugi S. Cognitive behavioral therapy for anorexia nervosa: an update. *Curr Psychiatry Rep* 2016;18:2.

50. Madden S, Miskovic-Wheatley J, Wallis A, Kohn M, Hay P, Touyz S. Early weight gain in family-based treatment predicts greater weight gain and remission at the end of treatment and remission at 12-month follow-up in adolescent anorexia nervosa. *Int J Eat Disord* 2015;48:919–922.

51. Godart N, Berthoz S, Curt F, et al. A randomized controlled trial of adjunctive family therapy and treatment as usual following inpatient treatment for anorexia nervosa adolescents. *PLoS One* 2012;7:e28249.

52. Magill N, Rhind C, Hibbs R, et al. Two-year follow-up of a pragmatic randomised controlled trial examining the effect of adding a carer's skill training intervention in inpatients with anorexia nervosa. *Eur Eat Disord Rev* 2016;24:122–130.

53. Lock J, Agras WS, Bryson SW, et al. Does family-based treatment reduce the need for hospitalization in adolescent anorexia nervosa? *Int J Eat Disord* 2016;49:891–894.

54. Suarez-Pinilla P, Pena-Perez C, Arbaizar-Barrenechea B, et al. Inpatient treatment for anorexia nervosa: a systematic review of randomized controlled trials. *J Psychiatr Pract* 2015;21:49–59.

55. Bissada H, Tasca GA, Barber AM, Bradwejn J. Olanzapine in the treatment of low body weight and obsessive thinking in women with anorexia nervosa: a randomized, double-blind, placebo-controlled trial. *Am J Psychiatry* 2008;165:1281–1288.

56. Dold M, Aigner M, Klabunde M, Treasure J, Kasper S. Second-generation antipsychotic drugs in anorexia nervosa: a meta-analysis of randomized controlled trials. *Psychother Psychosom* 2015;84:110–116.

57. Attia E, Kaplan AS, Walsh BT, et al. Olanzapine versus placebo for out-patients with anorexia nervosa. *Psychol Med* 2011; 41:2177–2182.

58. Elzakkers IF, Danner UN, Hoek HW, Schmidt U, van Elburg AA. Compulsory treatment in anorexia nervosa: a review. *Int J Eat Disord* 2014;47:845–852.

59. Tan JO, Stewart A, Fitzpatrick R, Hope T. Attitudes of patients with anorexia nervosa to compulsory treatment and coercion. *Int J Law Psychiatry* 2010;33:13–19.

Index